SPORTS IN SOCIETY

SPORTS IN SOCIETY

Issues and Controversies

TWELFTH EDITION

Jay Coakley, Ph.D.
University of Colorado
Colorado Springs

Mc Graw Hill Education

SPORTS IN SOCIETY: ISSUES AND CONTROVERSIES, TWELFTH EDITION

Published by McGraw-Hill Education, 2 Penn Plaza, New York, NY 10121. Copyright © 2017 by McGraw-Hill Education. All rights reserved. Printed in the United States of America. Previous editions © 2015, 2009, and 2007. No part of this publication may be reproduced or distributed in any form or by any means, or stored in a database or retrieval system, without the prior written consent of McGraw-Hill Education, including, but not limited to, in any network or other electronic storage or transmission, or broadcast for distance learning.

Some ancillaries, including electronic and print components, may not be available to customers outside the United States.

This book is printed on acid-free paper.

1 2 3 4 5 6 7 8 9 DOC 21 20 19 18 17 16

ISBN 978-0-07-352354-5
MHID 0-07-352354-2

Senior Vice President, Products & Markets: *G. Scott Virkler*
Vice President, General Manager, Products & Markets: *Michael Ryan*
Managing Director: *Gina Boedecker*
Brand Manager: *Penina Braffman*
Director, Product Development: *Meghan Campbell*
Product Developer: *Anthony McHugh*
Marketing Manager: *Meredith Leo*
Director, Content Design & Delivery: *Terri Schiesl*
Program Manager: *Jennifer Shekleton*
Content Project Managers: *Jessica Portz, George Theofanopoulos, Sandra Schnee*
Buyer: *Laura M. Fuller*
Design: *Studio Montage, St. Louis, MO*
Content Licensing Specialist (Text): *Shannon Manderscheid*
Cover Image: *Copyright © Ernie Barnes "His Effort"*
Compositor: *SPi Global*
Printer: *R.R. Donnelley*

All credits appearing on page or at the end of the book are considered to be an extension of the copyright page.

Library of Congress Cataloging-in-Publication Data

Names: Coakley, Jay J. author.
Title: Sports in society : issues and controversies / Jay Coakley, Ph.D.,
   University of Colorado, Colorado Springs.
Description: Tweleth edition. | New York, NY : McGraw-Hill Education, [2017]
Identifiers: LCCN 2016017236 | ISBN 9780073523545 (acid-free paper)
Subjects: LCSH: Sports—Social aspects. | Sports—Psychological aspects.
Classification: LCC GV706.5 .C63 2017 | DDC 306.4/83—dc23 LC record available at https://lccn.loc.gov/2016017236

The Internet addresses listed in the text were accurate at the time of publication. The inclusion of a website does not indicate an endorsement by the authors or McGraw-Hill Education, and McGraw-Hill Education does not guarantee the accuracy of the information presented at these sites.

mheducation.com/highered

To the memory of Ernie Barnes—a uniquely perceptive artist whose drawings and paintings capture the movement and spirit of athletic bodies in ways that inspire people worldwide.

ABOUT THE AUTHOR

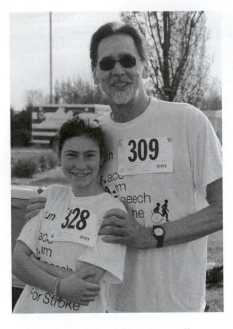

Jay Coakley and granddaughter, Ally, are running buddies in local Colorado races. (*Source:* © Jay Coakley)

Jay Coakley is Professor Emeritus of Sociology at the University of Colorado in Colorado Springs. He received a Ph.D. in sociology at the University of Notre Dame and has since taught and done research on play, games, and sports, among other topics in sociology. Dr. Coakley has received many teaching, service, and professional awards, and is an internationally respected scholar, author, and journal editor. In 2007 the Institute for International Sport selected him as one of the 100 Most Influential Sports Educators, and the University of Chichester in West Sussex, England awarded him an Honorary Fellowship in recognition of his outstanding leadership in the sociology of sport; in 2009, the National Association for Sport and Physical Education inducted Coakley into its Hall of Fame; and in 2015 he was named an Honorary Member of the International Sociology of Sport Association.

A former intercollegiate athlete, Coakley continues to use concepts, research, and theories in sociology to critically examine social phenomena and promote changes that make social worlds more democratic and humane. He currently lives in Fort Collins, Colorado with his wife, Nancy.

ABOUT THE COVER ARTIST

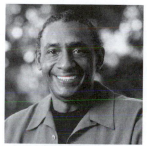

© Peter Read Miller

The cover image, *His Effort,* is a painting by the late Ernie Barnes (1938–2009), an internationally known artist, a former professional football player, and an unforgettable friend.

Barnes was born during Jim Crow in Durham, North Carolina. As a child, he was shy, introverted and bullied. In junior high school, he learned about weightlifting and training. By his senior year of high school, he was captain of the football team and state shot put champion. On an athletic scholarship, he majored in art at North Carolina College at Durham (now NCCU).

In 1959 he was drafted by the Baltimore Colts and later played offensive guard for the San Diego Chargers (1960–62) and Denver Broncos (1963–64). In his final season, a football team owner paid him "to just paint." A year later, Barnes had his first solo exhibition and retired from football at age 28 to devote himself to art. His autobiography, *From Pads to Palette,* chronicles this transition.

Barnes' ability to uniquely capture the athlete's experience earned him "America's Best Painter of Sports" by the American Sports Museum. In 1984 he was appointed the Sports Artist of the 1984 Olympic Games in Los Angeles. Recently his beloved football painting *The Bench* was presented to the Pro Football Hall of Fame for their permanent collection.

His artwork first became known in pop culture when it was used during the 1970s television show *Good Times.* The iconic dance scene, *The Sugar Shack* by Ernie Barnes, on a Marvin Gaye album is one of the most recognizable works of art.

A remarkable feature of Barnes' work is his use of elongation and distortion to represent energy, power, grace, intensity, and fluidity in his art. His sports background provided a distinct vantage point for observing bodies in movement, and he used his unique understanding of the human anatomy to portray not only athletes but everyday mannerisms in delayed motion. As a result, his images communicate an intimate sense of human physicality.

For many people, Ernie Barnes captures the spirit and determination of athletes as they express themselves through movement. His images present to us the kinesthetic soul of sports.

This is the seventh consecutive cover of *Sports in Society* that presents the art of Ernie Barnes. He spoke to students regularly, bringing his work to show that art, sport, and academic learning could come together in their lives. This particular cover image was chosen to represent Barnes's legacy based on *his effort* to represent the wonder and endurance of the human spirit.

For more information, please visit his official website: www.ErnieBarnes.com. My thanks go to Ernie's longtime friend and assistant, Luz Rodriguez and his family for sharing *His Effort* for the eleventh and twelfth editions of *Sports in Society.*

CONTENTS

PREFACE

PURPOSE OF THIS TEXT

The twelfth edition of *Sports in Society: Issues and Controversies* provides a detailed introduction to the sociology of sport. It uses sociological concepts, theories, and research to raise critical questions about sports and explore the dynamic relationship between sports, culture, and society. The chapters are organized around controversial and curiosity-arousing issues that have been systematically studied in sociology and related fields. Research on these issues is summarized so that readers can critically examine them.

Chapter content is guided by sociological research and theory and based on the assumption that a full understanding of sports must take into account the social and cultural contexts in which sports are created, played, given meaning, and integrated into people's lives. At a time when we too often think that a "website search" provides everything we need to know, I intend this text as a thoughtful scholarly work that integrates research on sports as social phenomena, makes sense of the expanding body of work in the sociology of sport, and inspires critical thinking.

FOR WHOM IS IT WRITTEN?

Sports in Society is written for everyone taking a first critical look at the relationships between sports, culture, and society. Readers don't need a background in sociology to understand and benefit from discussions in each chapter; nor do they need detailed knowledge of sport jargon and statistics. My goal is to help readers identify and explore issues related to sports in their personal experiences, families, schools, communities, and societies.

The emphasis on issues and controversies makes each chapter useful for people concerned with sport-related policies and programs. I've always tried to use knowledge to make sports more democratic, accessible, inclusive, and humane, and I hope to provide readers with the information and desire to do the same.

WRITING THIS REVISION

As soon as the extensively revised eleventh edition of *Sports in Society* went to press I began research for this edition. This involves reading six newspapers each day, including *USA Today, The New York Times, The Wall Street Journal,* and *The Financial Times.* I also read two sports magazines—*Sports Illustrated* and *ESPN The Magazine*—and other magazines that often publish articles about the social dimensions of sports. But most of my research involves reading abstracts for articles published in the major journals dealing with sports as social phenomena. I regularly survey the tables of contents of a few dozen journals in sociology and related fields to find articles on sport-related topics. Although I do not read every article or every book in the field, I read many and take notes as I do.

Finally, I track photos that I might buy for the edition, and I take thousands of photos myself, always hoping to have ten to twenty new ones for each new edition. I regularly ask friends to take photos if they are in unique sport settings. In the final photo selection I usually review 250 photos for every one I choose to include in the book.

In all, this amounts to thousands of hours of research, writing, and discussing issues with people from many walks of life in the United States and other parts of the world I've had opportunities to visit.

CHANGES TO THIS TWELFTH EDITION

This edition builds on and updates the fully revised eleventh edition. New chapter-opening quotes, photos, and examples maintain the timeliness of content.

New research and theoretical developments are integrated into each chapter. There are over 2000 references to assist those writing papers and doing research. Most new references identify materials published after 2009.

The sociology of sport has expanded so much in recent years that *Sports in Society* is now an introduction to the field more than a comprehensive overview.

Revision Themes and New Materials

This edition updates all time sensitive materials and continues to provide readers with a brief Chapter Outline, and Learning Objectives. At the end of each chapter are lists of Supplemental Readings that are accessible through the Instructor Resources section in Connect, along with selected sport management discussion issues related to the chapter content.

Chapter 1 introduces "the great sport myth"— the widespread belief that all sports are essentially pure and good, and that their purity and goodness are transferred to those who participate in or watch sports. This concept helps readers understand how and why sports are perceived in such positive terms worldwide and why it is difficult to promote critical thinking about sports in society. References to the great sport myth appear in most of the chapters. Chapter 1 also has a new explanation of ideology to give readers a clearer idea of how sports are cultural practices linked with the perspectives we use to make sense of our everyday lives.

Chapter 2 contains information and diagrams that explain the knowledge production process and the primary data collection methods used in sociology of sport research. There is an explanation of gender as meaning, performance, and organization in social worlds, and discussion of the differences between quantitative and qualitative research.

Chapter 3 focuses on socialization. It contains a section on "Family Culture and the Sport Participation of Children," which examines families as the immediate contexts in which socialization into sports is initiated and nurtured. There are discussions of sports participation and socialization experiences, the transition out of competitive sports careers, and current approaches to sports and socialization as a community process.

Chapter 4, on youth sports, presents a discussion of how the culture of childhood play has nearly disappeared in most segments of post-industrial society. There's also an expanded discussion of the possibility that in the United States some upper-middle-class parents use youth sports as a way to create mobility opportunities and reproduce privilege for their children. Finally, there is a discussion of how and why youth sport programs in the United States are fragmented and exist independently of any theory-based approach to teaching age-appropriate physical skills and promoting lifelong involvement in sports and physical activities.

Chapter 5, on deviance, contains a discussion of the relationship between deviant overconformity and injuries, concussions, and repetitive head trauma in sports. There's also an explanation of how widespread acceptance of the great sports myth leads people to deny or ignore certain forms of deviance in sports and use punitive social control methods that focus on individuals rather than the systemic problems that exist in various forms of sport. This is followed by a discussion of new surveillance technologies being used to police and control athletes, especially in connection with the use of performance-enhancing substances.

Chapter 6, on violence in sports, discusses why violent sports have become commercially successful in certain cultures. The issue of concussions and repetitive head trauma is also discussed in connection with the culture of violence that is widely accepted in heavy-contact sports. Finally, there is an expanded discussion of how the threat of terrorism is perceived and how it influences the dynamics of social control at sport events.

Chapter 7, on gender and sports, introduces the concept of *orthodox gender ideology* to help readers understand the cultural origins of gender inequality and why sports are one of the last spheres of social life in which the two-sex approach is accepted in a way that normalizes gender segregation. This chapter also contains a section on "Progress Toward Gender Equity," which identifies girls' and women's increased participation as the single most dramatic change in sports over the past two generations. There is an updated *Reflect on Sports* box that examines Title IX compliance and "what counts as equity in sports." A new table presents data on female and male athletes at recent Paralympic Games, and a section, "The Global Women's Rights Movement," discusses the belief that girls and women are enhanced as human beings when they develop their intellectual *and* physical abilities. Discussions of the media coverage of women in sports and the impact of budget cuts and the privatization of sports are presented to show that programs for women and girls remain vulnerable to cuts because they lack a strong market presence and have not been profit producing.

Chapter 8, on race and ethnicity, presents a revised discussion of how racial ideology influences sports participation. A *Reflect on Sports* box deals with "Vénus Noire: A legacy of Racism After 200 years," and a discussion of the isolation often experienced by women of color participating in or coaching college sports. Research is presented to show the ways that some Japanese parents use youth sports leagues to establish relationships with other Japanese families and connect their children with Asian American peers. Finally, there is a section on race, ethnicity, and sports in a global perspective in which efforts to control the expression of racism at sport events is discussed.

Chapter 9, on social class, has expanded discussions of whether building a new stadium triggers new jobs for the surrounding community and how the economic downturn has impacted sports participation in the United States. There is a discussion of research on whether local boxing gyms help participants bond with one another and acquire forms of social capital that alter their structural position in society, as well as a discussion of data on the impact of income and wealth on sport participation patterns.

Chapter 10, written with Elizabeth Pike, my colleague from the University of Chichester in England, focuses on issues and controversies related to age and ability in sports. The framework of this chapter is built on research showing how social definitions of age and ability impact the provision of sport participation opportunities and the decisions made by people to become and stay involved in sports. The sections on masters events, the Paralympics, the Special Olympics, and related forms of sport provision illustrate the complexity of sports when they are viewed in a general social and cultural context in which age and ability influence how people are perceived and how they include physical activities in their lives.

Chapter 11 deals with the commercialization of sports. It explains how the great sport myth is used to appropriate public money to build sport venues and subsidize sport teams. Labor relations in sports are discussed in more depth, with explanations of collective bargaining agreements, lockouts, and the role of players' associations.

Chapter 12, on sports and the media, now contains much material on the changing media landscape and how it is related to sports. There is a discussion of fantasy sports as an arena in which participation is influenced by gender and the quest to sustain white male privilege. There's material on how social media are used by established sport organizations and by athletes practicing emerging sport activities around the world. Changes in media coverage are discussed, with attention given to how masculinity and sexuality are presented in sports media. Finally, there is a new discussion of how entertainment journalism has replaced investigative journalism in sports media.

Chapter 13, on politics, government, and global processes, is updated in its coverage of sport and national identity in global relations, and how the Olympics and men's World Cup have become tools for generating profits for the International Olympic Committee and FIFA at the same time that the countries hosting these games incur increasing debt for debatable returns. Research on recent sport mega-events is used to discuss the challenges and the pros and cons of hosting such events. There is an updated discussion of the new political realities of sports—where team owner-ship and event sponsorship have become global in scope, where athletes seek opportunities world-wide, where global media make it easy to follow the sporting events of teams from all over the world, and where fans' loyalties are no longer lim-ited to teams from their own regions or countries. Research is presented to show that these realities are linked with corporate expansion, the global flow of capital, the business strategy of global media companies, and processes of *glocalization* through which global sports are integrated into people's everyday lives on a local level.

Chapter 14, on high school and college sports, includes new research findings related to issues such as the rising costs of sport programs, who benefits from the revenues generated by certain sports, the dramatic increase of inequality among programs at both the high school and college lev-els, and young people's perceptions of athletic and academic achievement in schools with high-profile sport programs. There are updated sections on budget issues, the uncertainty that faces school sports today, and the issues currently faced by the NCAA as it tries to control a college sport system that is increasingly unmanageable and inconsistent with the goals of higher education.

Chapter 15, on religion and sports, presents information on world religions and how they influ-ence conceptions of the body, evaluations of phys-ical movement, and sport participation. There also is updated information about the ways in which individuals and organizations combine sport with religious beliefs, and how this has spread beyond the United States in recent years.

Chapter 16 has been shortened and now focuses primarily on the process of making change in sports rather than describing what the future of sports might be. This is because there is a need for us to acknowledge the power of corporations in shaping sports to fit their interests and to develop strategies for creating sport forms that directly serve the needs of individuals and communities.

Supplemental Readings and New Website Resources

Each chapter is followed by a list of Supplemen-tal Readings that provide useful information about topics in the chapters. The Supplemental Read-ings for each chapter can be accessed through the Instructor Resources within Connect.

New Visual Materials

There are 118 photos, 20 figures, and 30 cartoons in this edition. These images are combined with updated tables to illustrate important substantive points, visually enhance the text, and make reading more interesting.

connect

The twelfth edition of *Sports in Society,* is now available online with Connect, McGraw-Hill Edu-cation's integrated assignment and assessment platform. Connect also offers SmartBook for the new edition, which is the first adaptive reading experience proven to improve grades and help stu-dents study more effectively. All of the title's web-site and ancillary content is also available through Connect, including:

- A full Test Bank of multiple choice questions that test students on central concepts and ideas in each chapter
- An Instructor's Manual for each chapter with full chapter outlines, sample test questions, and discussion topics
- Supplemental Readings that add depth and background to current chapter topics
- Group projects
- Previous chapters on coaches, competition, history (from the tenth edition), and social theories (from the ninth edition)
- True/false self-tests for each chapter
- A cumulative 275-page bibliography that lists all references from this and the last six editions of *Sports in Society*
- A complete glossary of key terms integrated into the index

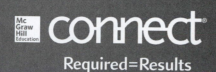 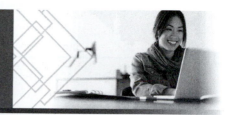

Required=Results

McGraw-Hill Connect®
Learn Without Limits

Connect is a teaching and learning platform that is proven to deliver better results for students and instructors.

Connect empowers students by continually adapting to deliver precisely what they need, when they need it and how they need it, so your class time is more engaging and effective.

Course outcomes improve with Connect.

Exam Scores — 80.4% / 74.7%
Pass Rates — 83.7% / 72.9%
Attendance Rates — 92.5% / 74.5%
Retention Rates — 87.5% / 71.1%

With Connect / Without Connect

Using **Connect** improves passing rates by **10.8%** and retention by **16.4%**.

88% of instructors who use **Connect** require it; instructor satisfaction **increases** by 38% when **Connect** is required.

Analytics

Connect Insight®

Connect Insight is Connect's new one-of-a-kind visual analytics dashboard—now available for both instructors and students—that provides at-a-glance information regarding student performance, which is immediately actionable. By presenting assignment, assessment, and topical performance results together with a time metric that is easily visible for aggregate or individual results, Connect Insight gives the user the ability to take a just-in-time approach to teaching and learning, which was never before available. Connect Insight presents data that empowers students and helps instructors improve class performance in a way that is efficient and effective.

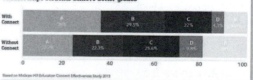

Connect helps students achieve better grades

Based on McGraw-Hill Education Connect Effectiveness Study 2013

Students can view their results for any **Connect** course.

Mobile

Connect's new, intuitive mobile interface gives students and instructors flexible and convenient, anytime–anywhere access to all components of the Connect platform.

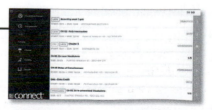

Adaptive

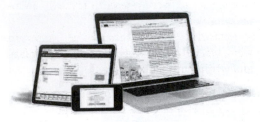

THE FIRST AND ONLY **ADAPTIVE READING EXPERIENCE** DESIGNED TO TRANSFORM THE WAY STUDENTS READ

More students earn **A's** and **B's** when they use McGraw-Hill Education **Adaptive** products.

SmartBook®

Proven to help students improve grades and study more efficiently, SmartBook contains the same content within the print book, but actively tailors that content to the needs of the individual. SmartBook's adaptive technology provides precise, personalized instruction on what the student should do next, guiding the student to master and remember key concepts, targeting gaps in knowledge and offering customized feedback, driving the student toward comprehension and retention of the subject matter. Available on smartphones and tablets, SmartBook puts learning at the student's fingertips—anywhere, anytime.

Over **4 billion questions** have been answered making McGraw-Hill Education products more intelligent, reliable & precise.

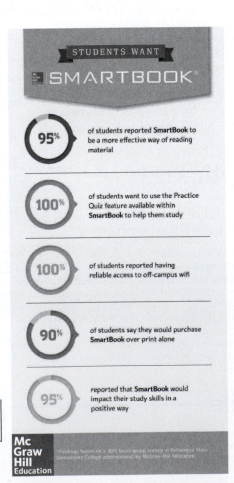

STUDENTS WANT

SMARTBOOK®

95% of students reported **SmartBook** to be a more effective way of reading material

100% of students want to use the Practice Quiz feature available within **SmartBook** to help them study

100% of students reported having reliable access to off-campus wifi

90% of students say they would purchase **SmartBook** over print alone

95% reported that **SmartBook** would impact their study skills in a positive way

Mc Graw Hill Education

*Findings based on a 2015 focus group survey at Hattiesburg State Community College administered by McGraw-Hill Education.

ACKNOWLEDGMENTS

This book draws on ideas from many sources. Thanks go to students, colleagues, and friends who have provided constructive criticisms over the years. Students regularly open my eyes to new ways of viewing and analyzing sports as social phenomena.

Special thanks go to friends and colleagues who influence my thinking, provide valuable source materials, and willingly discuss ideas and information with me. Elizabeth Pike, Chris Hallinan, and Cora Burnett influenced my thinking as I worked with them on versions of *Sports in Society* for the United Kingdom, Australia/New Zealand, and Southern Africa, respectively. Peter Donnelly, co-author of past Canadian versions, has provided special support for this edition and influenced my thinking about many important issues. Laurel Davis-Delano deserves special thanks for her constructive critiques of recent past editions. Thanks also go to photographers and colleagues, Lara Killick, Barbara Schausteck de Almeida, Elizabeth Pike, Bobek Ha'Eri, Becky Beal, Kevin Young, Jay Johnson Michael Boyd, Tim Russo, Basia Borzecka and my daughter, Danielle Hicks, for permission to use their photos. Rachel Spielberg, a recent Smith College grad, coach, and artist contributed cartoons to this edition; thanks to her for working with me. Thanks also to artist Fred Eyer, whose cartoons have been used in this and previous editions.

Thanks also to my Development Editors, Ashwin Amalraj and Erin Guendelsberger, and the entire McGraw-Hill team for their help during the course of this revision.

Finally, thanks go to Nancy Coakley, who has lived through twelve editions of *Sports in Society* and assisted with each one in more ways than I can list here. She keeps me in touch with popular culture sources related to sports, and tells me when my ideas should be revised or kept to myself—a frequent occurrence.

My appreciation also goes to the following reviewers, whose suggestions were crucial in planning and writing this edition:

Amanda K. Curtis, Lake Erie College
Susan Dargan, Framingham State College
Bruce Haller, Dowling College
Ken Muir, Appalachian State University
Tracy W. Olrich, Central Michigan University
Gary Sailes, Indiana University
Stephen Shapiro, Old Dominion University
Angela Smith-Nix, University of
    Arkansas–Fayetteville
Jessica Sparks Howell, Mississippi State
    University
Ashley VandeVeen, Mayville State University

Finally, thanks to the many students and colleagues who have e-mailed comments about previous editions and ideas for future editions. I take them seriously and appreciate their thoughtfulness—keep the responses coming.

Jay Coakley
Fort Collins, CO

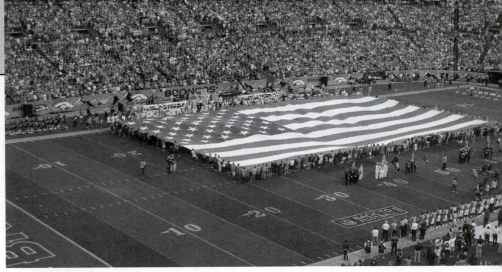

chapter

1

(*Source:* © Jay Coakley)

THE SOCIOLOGY OF SPORT

What Is It and Why Study It?

Our sports belong to us. They came up from the people. They were invented for reasons having nothing to do with money or ego. Our sports weren't created by wealthy sports and entertainment barons like the ones running sports today.

> —**Ken Reed, Sport Policy Director,**
> **League of Fans (2011).**

Why should we play sport? Why not just have everyone exercise? [. . . Because sport] takes you to the edge of a cliff, and it's at that edge of the cliff where you understand your creative soul.

> —**Brian Hainline, chief medical officer,**
> **NCAA (in Wolverton, 2014)**

New York joins 34 other states and the District of Columbia in recognizing competitive cheerleading as a sport. Section VI and the state will make a distinction between traditional, sideline cheerleading and competitive cheerleading, he said. Schools will decide for themselves which type of team they want.

> —**Barbara O'Brien, staff reporter,**
> **Buffalo News (2014).**

Sports is real. . . . Sports is Oprah for guys. . . . Sports is woven deeper into American life than you know. You may change religion or politics, but not sport teams.

> —**Rick Reilly (2009)**

Chapter Outline

Learning Objectives

- Explain what sociologists study about sports and why sociology of sport knowledge is different from information in sports media and everyday conversations.

- Understand issues related to defining sports and why a sociological definition differs from official definitions used by high schools, universities, and other organizations.

- Explain what it means to say that sports are social constructions and contested activities.

- Explain why sociology of sport knowledge may be controversial among people associated with sports.

- Understand the meaning of "ideology" and how ideologies related to gender, race, social class, and ability are connected with sports.

ABOUT THIS BOOK

If you're reading this book, you have an interest in sports or know people who play or watch them. Unlike most books about sports, this one is written to take you beyond scores, statistics, and sports personalities. The goal is to focus on the "deeper game" associated with sports, the game through which sports become part of the social and cultural worlds in which we live.

Fortunately, we can draw on our experiences as we consider this deeper game. Take high school sports in the United States as an example. When students play on a high school basketball team, we know that it can affect their status in the school and the treatment they receive from teachers and peers. We know it has potential implications for their prestige in the community, self-images and self-esteem, future relationships, opportunities in education and the job market, and their overall enjoyment of life.

Building on this knowledge enables us to move further into the deeper game associated with high school sports. For example, why do so many Americans place such importance on sports and accord such high status to elite athletes? Are there connections between high school sports and widespread beliefs about masculinity and femininity, achievement and competition, pleasure and pain, winning and fair play, and other important aspects of U.S. culture?

Underlying these questions is the assumption that sports are more than games, meets, and matches. They're important aspects of social life that have meanings going far beyond scores and performance statistics. Sports are integral parts of the social and cultural contexts in which we live, and they provide stories and images that many of us use to evaluate our experiences and the world around us.

Those of us who study sports in society are concerned with these deeper meanings and stories associated with sports. We do research to increase our understanding of (1) the cultures and societies in which sports exist; (2) the social worlds created around sports; and (3) the experiences of individuals and groups associated with sports.

ABOUT THIS CHAPTER

This chapter is organized to answer four questions:

1. What is sociology, and how is it used to study sports in society?
2. What are sports, and how can we identify them in ways that increase our understanding of their place and value in society?
3. What is the sociology of sport?
4. Who studies sports in society, and for what purposes?

The answers to these questions will be our guides for understanding the material in the rest of the book.

USING SOCIOLOGY TO STUDY SPORTS

Sociology provides useful tools for investigating sports as social phenomena. This is because **sociology** *is the study of the social worlds that people create, maintain, and change through their relationships with each other.*[1] The concept of **social world** refers to *an identifiable sphere of everyday actions and relationships* (Unruh, 1980). Social worlds are created by people, but they involve much more than individuals doing their own things for their own reasons. Our actions, relationships, and collective activities form patterns that could not be predicted only with information about each of us as individuals. These patterns constitute identifiable ways of life and social

---

[1]Important concepts used in each chapter are identified in **boldface.** Unless they are accompanied by a footnote that contains a definition, the definition will be given in the text itself. This puts the definition in context rather than separating it in a glossary. Definitions are also provided in the Subject Glindex.

arrangements that are maintained or changed over time as people interact with one other.

Social worlds can be as large and impersonal as an entire nation, such as the United States or Brazil, or as personal and intimate as your own family. But regardless of size, they encompass all aspects of social life: (a) the values and beliefs that we use to make sense of our lives; (b) our everyday actions and relationships; and (c) the groups, organizations, communities, and societies that we form as we make choices, develop relationships, and participate in social life.

Sociologists often refer to **society,** *which is a relatively self-sufficient collection of people who maintain a way of life in a particular territory.* In most cases, a society and a nation are one and the same, such as Brazil and Brazilian society. But there are cases where a society is not a nation, such as Amish Mennonite society as it exists in Ohio, Pennsylvania, and other parts of the United States.

The goal of sociology is to describe and explain social worlds, including societies—how they are created, re-created, and changed; how they are organized; and how they influence our lives and our relationships with each other. In the process of doing sociology we learn to see our lives and the lives of others "in context"—that is, in the social worlds in which we live. This enables us to identify the social conditions that set limits or create possibilities in people's lives. On a personal level, knowing about these influential conditions also helps us anticipate and sometimes work around the constraints we face at the same time that we look for and take advantage of the possibilities. Ideally, it helps us gain more control over our lives as well as an understanding of other people and the conditions that influence their lives.

Key Sociology Concepts

Sociologists use the concepts of culture, social interaction, and social structure to help them understand sports as social activities.

Culture consists of *the shared ways of life and shared understandings that people develop as they live together.* Once a culture exists, it influences relationships and social interaction.

Social interaction consists of *people taking each other into account and, in the process, influencing each other's feelings, thoughts, and actions.* Through interaction, we learn to anticipate the thoughts and actions of others and predict how others may respond to what we think and do.

Social structure consists of *the established patterns of relationships and social arrangements that take shape as people live, work, and play with each other.* This is the basis for order and organization in all social worlds.

These three concepts—culture, social interaction, and social structure—represent the central interconnected aspects of all social worlds. For example, a high school soccer team is a social world formed by players, coaches, team parents, and regular supporters. Over time every team creates and maintains a particular *culture* or a way of life consisting of values, beliefs, norms, and everyday social routines. Everyone involved with the team engages in *social interaction* as they take each other into account during their everyday activities on and off the playing field. Additionally, the recurring actions, relationships, and social arrangements that emerge as these people interact with each other make up the *social structure* of the team. This combination of culture, social interaction, and social structure comprises the team as a social world, and it is connected with the larger social world in which it exists.

Peer groups, cliques, and athletic teams are social worlds in which participants are known to one another. Communities, societies, concert crowds, and online chat rooms are social worlds in which participants are generally unknown to each other. This means that the boundaries of social worlds may be clear, fuzzy, or overlapping, but we generally know when we enter or leave a social world because each has identifying features related to culture, social interaction, and social structure.

We move back and forth between familiar social worlds without thinking. We make nearly automatic shifts in how we talk and act as we accommodate changing cultural, interactional, and structural features in each social world. However, when we enter or participate in a new or unfamiliar social world, we usually pay special attention to what is happening. We watch what people are doing, how they interact with each other, and we develop a sense of the recurring patterns that exist in their actions and relationships. If you've done this, then you're ready to use sociology to study sports in society.

Sociological Knowledge Is Based on Research and Theory

My goal in writing this book is to accurately represent research in the sociology of sport and discuss issues of interest to students. At a time when online searches provide us with infinite facts, figures, and opinions about sports, I am primarily interested in the knowledge produced through systematic research. I use newspaper articles and other media as sources for examples, but I depend on research results when making substantive points and drawing conclusions. This means that my statements about sports and sport experiences are based, as much as possible, on studies that use surveys, questionnaires, interviews, observations, content analyses, and other accepted methods of research in sociology.

The material in this book is different than material in blogs, talk radio, television news shows, game and event commentaries, and most of our everyday conversations about sports. It is organized to help you critically examine sports as they exist in people's lives. I use research findings to describe and explain as accurately as possible the important connections between sports, society, and culture. I try to be fair when using research to make sense of the social aspects of sports and sport experiences. This is why over 1700 sources are cited as references for the information and analysis in this book.

Of course, I want to hold your attention as you read, but I don't exaggerate, purposely withhold, or present information out of context to impress you and boost my "ratings." In the process, I hope you will extend your critical thinking abilities so you can assess what people believe and say about sports in society. This will enable you to make informed decisions about sports in your life and the social worlds in which you live.

DEFINING SPORTS

Most of us know enough about the meaning of sports to talk about them with others. However, when we study sports, it helps to precisely define our topic. For example, is it a sport when young people choose teams and play a baseball game in the street or when thirty people of various ages spend an afternoon learning and performing tricks at a skateboard park? These activities are sociologically different from what occurs at major league baseball games and X Games skateboard competitions. These differences become significant when parents ask if playing sports builds the character of their children, when community leaders ask if they should use tax money to fund sports, and when school principals ask if sports are valid educational activities.

When I say that I study sports, people ask if that includes jogging, double-dutch, weight lifting, hunting, scuba diving, darts, auto racing, chess, poker, ultimate fighting, paintball, piano competitions, ballroom dancing, skateboarding, Quidditch, and so on. To respond is not easy, because there is no single definition that precisely identifies sports in all cultures at all times (Lagaert & Roose, 2014).

According to definitions used widely in North America and much of Europe, **sports** *are physical activities that involve challenges or competitive contests.* They are usually organized so that participants can assess their performances and compare them to the performances of others or to their own performances from one situation to

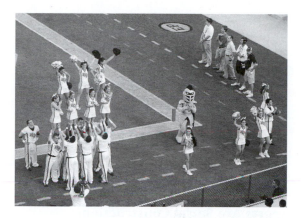

Is "Competitive Cheer" and sideline cheerleading a sport? The answer to this question is important because it impacts the budgets, participation rates, and gender equity decisions in U.S. high school and college sport programs. Sociologists study why certain activities are considered to be sports, who has the power to make such decisions, and how those decisions affect people's lives (Lamb & Priyadharshini, 2015). (*Source:* © Jay Coakley)

another. However, the organization, meaning, and purpose of sports often vary from one cultural context to another.

Some sports are organized to emphasize free-flowing, playful action and exist primarily for the pleasure of the participants. Examples include 5K fun runs, spontaneous games of Ultimate in open areas, and skateboarding in the streets or local skate parks. In contrast, other sports are organized to include scheduled and regulated action with participants displaying their skills for the pleasure of spectators. These include professional and other elite sports that people follow through media and pay to see in person. NFL games, matches in professional soccer leagues, and major golf tournaments are examples.

Most sports, however, are organized in ways that fall somewhere between these two extremes. They are formally organized and, even though people may watch them, they exist mostly for participants, who enjoy them, value the skills needed to play

them, and receive external rewards, such as peer or family approval, social status, or formal awards for playing them. Softball leagues, scheduled volleyball tournaments, and most organized youth sports are examples.

Scholars who study sports as social phenomena generally use a flexible and inclusive definition of sport. Although past research in the sociology of sport has focused mainly on what you and I would describe as "organized sports," current research often focuses on **physical culture,** *which includes all forms of movement and physical activities that people in particular social worlds create, sustain, and regularly include in their collective lives.* This could be tai chi done in a Beijing park, capoeira in a Sao Paulo plaza, parkour in a Paris neighborhood, or break-dancing in New York City's Central Park.

Of course, organized sports are a central and often dominant component of physical culture in many societies today, but it has not always been this way and there continue to be societies in which traditional folk games and expressive forms of movement are more important than formally organized, competitive sports. Research on physical culture is important because it helps us understand how people think and feel about their bodies and how they define movement and integrate it into their lives. Additionally, it provides a foundation for critically examining the deeper game associated with sports in society.

Official Definitions of Sports

Defining *sport* in official terms and choosing specific activities that qualify as sports is an important process in organizations, communities, and societies. Being classified as an official sport gives special status to an activity and is likely to increase participation, funding, community support, and general visibility. For example, in Switzerland and the Scandinavian countries, walking, bicycling, and certain forms of general exercise are considered to be "sports." Therefore, those who participate regularly in these activities often see themselves as "sportspersons" and are treated that way by their peers. Additionally, public policies are likely to provide common spaces for these activities and financial support for events that include them.

The official definitions of sport used by organizations and officials in the United States are more exclusive in that they give priority to formally organized, competitive activities. Therefore, even though walking is encouraged for general health purposes, most people in the United States would not consider walking a sport, nor would they ever describe walkers as sportspersons. This is important because it also may mean that walking trails and walking events will receive much less financial and political support than stadiums and arenas in which elite and professional sports are played and watched—because these are seen as the "real" or official sports.

According to most people in the United States, Canada, and a growing number of other societies, sports involve rules, competition, scoring, winners and losers, schedules and seasons, records, coaches, referees, and governing bodies that set rules and sponsor championships. Additionally, organizations such as local park and recreation departments, state high school athletic federations, the National Collegiate Athletic Association (NCAA), and the United States Olympic Committee use their own criteria for defining *sport* and selecting activities for official recognition as sports for purposes of funding and support.

Official definitions of sport have important implications. When a definition emphasizes rules, competition, and high performance, many people will be excluded from participation, and decide that they are not fit to play, or avoid other physical activities that are defined as "second class." For example, when a twelve-year-old is cut from an exclusive club soccer team, she may not want to play in the local league sponsored by the park and recreation department because she sees it as "recreational activity" rather than a real sport. This can create a situation in which most people

are physically inactive at the same time that a small number of people perform at relatively high levels for large numbers of spectators—a situation that negatively impacts health and increases health-care costs in a society or community. When sport is defined to include a wide range of physical activities that are played for pleasure and integrated into local expressions of social life, physical activity rates will be high and overall health benefits are likely.

Sports Are Social Constructions

Understanding the sociology of sport is easier if you learn to think of sports as **social constructions**—that is, as *parts of the social world that are created by people as they interact with one another under particular social, political, and economic conditions*. This means that the kinds of sports that exist and gain popularity often tell us much about the values and orientations of those who play, watch, or sponsor them. They also tell us about who has power in a social world.

Just as defining and identifying *official* sports is part of a political process, with outcomes that benefit some people more than others, so is the process of creating and sustaining sports in a social world. This becomes apparent when we examine the struggles that often occur over whose ideas will be used when making decisions about the following sport-related issues:

1. What is the meaning and primary purpose of sports, and how should sports be organized to fit that meaning and purpose?
2. Who will play sports with whom, and under what conditions will they play?
3. What agencies or organizations will sponsor and control sports?

Heated debates occur when people have different answers to these questions. History shows that some of these debates have caused conflicts and led to lawsuits, government intervention, and the passage of laws. For example, people often disagree about the meaning, purpose, and organization of cheerleading in U.S. high schools. School officials have traditionally said that cheerleading is not a sport because its primary purpose is to support high school teams. But as competitive cheer teams have been organized to train and compete against other teams at least 34 state high school activities associations now define "cheer" as an official sport. This is important because the stakes are high: being designated an official sport brings funding and other support that changes its status and meaning in schools, communities, and society.

Disagreements and struggles over the purpose, meaning, and organization of sports occur most often when they involve the funding priorities of government agencies. For example, if the primary purpose of sport is to improve health and fitness for everyone, then funding should go to sports with widespread participation resulting in net positive effects on physical well-being. But if people see sports as "wars without weapons" with the purpose being to push the limits of human ability, then funding should go to sports organized to produce high-performance athletes who can achieve competitive victories. This issue is regularly contested at the national and local levels of government, in universities and public school districts, and even in families, as people decide how to use resources to support physical activities.

These examples show that sports are **contested activities**—that is, *activities for which there are no timeless and universal agreements about what they mean, why they exist, or how they should be organized.* This is also illustrated by historical disagreements over who is allowed to play sports and the conditions under which certain people can play. Cases involving extended struggles are listed in the box, "Who Plays and Who Doesn't" (p. 10).

The third issue that makes sports contested activities focuses on who should provide the resources needed to play them and who should control them. When people see sports contributing to the common good, it is likely that sport facilities and programs will be supported by government agencies and tax money. When people see sports as primarily contributing to individual development, it is likely that sport facilities and programs will be supported by individuals, families, and private-corporate sponsors. However, in both cases there will be struggles over the extent to which sponsors control sports and the extent to which sports are organized to be consistent with community values.

Struggles over these three issues show that using a single definition of sports may lead us to overlook important factors in a particular social world, such as who has power and resources and how meanings are given to particular activities at different times in a community or society. Being aware of these factors enables us to *put sports into context* and understand them in the terms used by those who create, play, and support them. It also helps us see that the definition of sports in any context usually represents the ideas and interests of some people more than others. In the sociology of sport, this leads to questions and research on whose ideas and interests count the most when it comes to determining (1) the meaning, purpose, and organization of sports; (2) who plays under what conditions; and (3) how sports will be sponsored and controlled. Material in each of the following chapters summarizes the findings of this research.

WHAT IS THE SOCIOLOGY OF SPORT?

The **sociology of sport** *is primarily a subdiscipline of sociology and physical education that studies sports as social phenomena.* Most research and writing in the field focuses on "organized, competitive sports," although people increasingly study other forms of physical activities that are health and fitness oriented and informally organized. These include recreational, extreme, adventure,

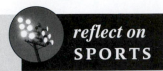

reflect on **SPORTS**

Who Plays and Who Doesn't
Contesting a Place in Sports

Being cut from a youth sport team is a disappointing personal experience. But being in a category of people that is wholly excluded from all or some sports is more than disappointing—it is unfair and occasionally illegal. Most cases of categorical exclusion are related to gender and sexuality, skin color and ethnicity, ability and disability, age and weight, nationality and citizenship, and other "eligibility" criteria. Struggles occur in connection with questions such as these:

- Will females be allowed to play sports and, if they are, will they play the same sports at the same time and on the same teams that males play, and will the rewards for achievement be the same for females and males?
- Will sports be open to people regardless of social class and wealth? Will wealthy and poor people play and watch sports together or separately?
- Will people from different racial and ethnic backgrounds play together or in segregated settings? Will the meanings given to skin color or ethnicity influence participation patterns or opportunities to play sports?
- Will age influence eligibility to play sports, and should sports be age integrated or segregated?

Will people of different ages have the same access to participation opportunities?
- Will able-bodied people and people with a disability have the same opportunities to play sports, and will they play together or separately? What meanings will be given to the accomplishments of athletes with a disability compared to the accomplishments of athletes defined as able-bodied?
- Will lesbians, gay men, bisexuals, and transsexuals play alongside heterosexuals and, if they do, will they be treated fairly?
- Will athletes control the conditions under which they play sports and have the power to change those conditions to meet their needs and interests?
- Will athletes be rewarded for playing, what form will the rewards take, and how will they be determined?

Federal and local laws may mandate particular answers to these questions. However, traditions, local customs, and personal beliefs often support various forms of exclusion. The resulting struggles illustrate that sports can be hotly contested activities.

Think about sports in your school, community, and society: how have these questions been answered?

and virtual sports as well as fitness and exercise activities.

Research in the sociology of sport generally seeks to answer the following questions:

1. Why are some activities, and not others, selected and designated as sports in particular groups and societies?
2. Why are sports created and organized in different ways at different times and in different places?
3. How do people include sports and sport participation in their lives, and does participation affect individual development and social relationships?
4. How do sports and sport participation affect our ideas about bodies, human movement work, fun, social class, masculinity and femininity, race and ethnicity, ability and disability, achievement and competition, pleasure and pain, deviance and conformity, and aggression and violence?
5. How do various sports compare with other physical activities in producing positive health and fitness outcomes?

6. How do sports contribute to overall community and societal development, and why do so many people assume that they do?
7. How is the meaning, purpose, and organization of sports related to the culture, social structure, and resources of a society?
8. How are sports related to important spheres of social life such as family, education, politics, the economy, media, and religion?
9. How do people use their sport experiences and knowledge about sports as they interact with others and explain what occurs in their lives and the world around them?
10. How can people use sociological knowledge about sports to understand and participate more actively and effectively in society, especially as agents of progressive change?

For those of us doing research to answer these and other questions, sport provides windows into the societies and cultures in which they exist. This means that the sociology of sport tells us about more than sports in society; in reality, it tells us about the organization and dynamics of relationships in society, and about how people see themselves and others in relation to the world at large.

The *Great Sport Myth* and Resistance to the Sociology of Sport

As organized sports have spread around the world, so has the myth that sport is essentially pure and good, and that its purity and goodness is transferred to all who participate in it. This myth supports related beliefs that sport builds character, and that anyone who plays sport will be a better person for doing so. The great sport myth is outlined in Figure 1.1.

Evidence clearly shows that the essential purity and goodness of sport is a myth and that merely participating in or consuming sports does not guarantee any particular outcomes related to character development or increased purity and goodness. In fact, we hear every day about cases that contradict the great sport myth. But that doesn't seem to weaken its uncritical acceptance by many people.

Sport is essentially pure and good, and its purity and goodness are transferred to anyone who plays, consumes, or sponsors sports.

THEREFORE

There is no need to study and evaluate sports for the purpose of transforming or making them better, because they are already what they should be.

FIGURE 1.1 The great sport myth.

In fact, when the actions of athletes, coaches, spectators, and others associated with sports are inconsistent with the perceived inherent purity and goodness of sport, those who accept the myth dismiss them as exceptions—as the actions of people so morally flawed that they resist the lessons that are inherent in sports.

The great sport myth implies that there is no need to study sports or seek ways to make them better. The sociology of sport is unnecessary, say the myth-believers, because sport is inherently positive. The source of problems, they say, is the morally flawed individuals who must be purged from sports so that goodness and purity will prevail. Sport, according to myth believers, is already as it should be—a source of inspiration and pure excitement that is not available in any other activity or sphere of life.

Throughout this book, we will see how the great sport myth influences many important decisions—from creating and funding organized sport programs for "at-risk" youth to making multibillion-dollar bids to host the Olympic Games, the FIFA World Cup (for men), and other sport mega-events. The myth supports a strong belief in the power of sports to bring purity and goodness to individuals in the form of positive character traits and to cities and nations in the form of revitalized civic spirit and desired development.

Using the Sociology of Sport

Knowledge produced by research in the sociology of sport can be useful to athletes, coaches, parents, and people in sport management, recreation, physical education, public health, and community planning and development. For example, it can inform parents and coaches about the conditions under which youth sport participation is most likely to produce positive developmental effects (NASPE, 2013). It explains why some sports have higher rates of violence than others and how to effectively control sports violence (Young, 2012).

Like knowledge produced in other fields, sociology of sport knowledge can be used for negative and selfish purposes unless it is combined with concerns for fairness and social justice. For example, it can inform football coaches that they can effectively control young men in U.S. culture by threatening their masculinity and making them dependent on the coaching staff for approval of their worth as men. And it also shows that this strategy can be used to increase the willingness of young men to sacrifice their bodies "for the good of the team"—an orientation that some football coaches favor and promote.

This example shows that the sociology of sport, like other scientific disciplines, can be used for many purposes. Like others who produce and distribute knowledge, those of us who study sports in society must consider why we ask certain research questions and how our research findings might affect people's lives. We can't escape the fact that social life is complex and characterized by inequalities, power differences, and conflicts of interests between different categories of people. Therefore, using knowledge in the sociology of sport is not a simple process that automatically brings about equal and positive benefits for everyone. In fact, it must also involve critical thinking about the potential consequences of what we know about sports in society. Hopefully, after reading this book you will be prepared and willing to do the following:

1. Think critically about sports so you can identify and understand the issues and controversies associated with them.
2. Look beyond performance statistics and win–loss records to see sports as social constructions that can have both positive and negative effects on people's lives.
3. Learn things about sports that enable you to make informed choices about your sport participation and the place of sports in your family, community, and society.
4. See sports as social constructions and strive to change them when they systematically and unfairly disadvantage some categories of people as they privilege others.

> **Sociology has always attempted to defatalize and denaturalize the present, demonstrating that the world could be otherwise.** —Editor, *Global Dialogue* (2011)

Controversies Created by the Sociology of Sport

Research in the sociology of sport can be controversial when it provides evidence that changes are needed in the ways that sports and social worlds are organized. Such evidence threatens some people, especially those who control sport organizations, benefit from the current organization of sports, or think that the current organization of sports is "right and natural."

People in positions of power know that social and cultural changes can jeopardize their control over others and the privileges that come with it. Therefore, they prefer approaches to sports that blame problems on the weaknesses and failures of individuals. When individuals are identified as the problem, solutions emphasize the need to control individuals more effectively and teach them how to adjust to social worlds as they are currently organized.

The potential for controversy created by a sociological analysis of sports is illustrated by reviewing research findings on sport participation among women around the world. Research shows that women, especially women in poor and working-class households, have lower rates of sport participation than do other categories of people (Donnelly and Harvey, 2007; Elling and Janssens, 2009; Tomlinson, 2007; Van Tuyckom et al., 2010). Research also shows that there are many reasons for this, including the following (Taniguchi and Shupe, 2012):

1. Women are less likely than men to have the time, freedom, "cultural permission," and money needed to play sports regularly.
2. Women have little or no control of the facilities where sports are played or the programs in those facilities.
3. Women have less access to transportation and less overall freedom to move around at will and without fear.
4. Women often are expected to take full-time responsibility for the social and emotional needs of family members—a job that seldom allows them time to play sports.
5. Most sport programs around the world are organized around the values, interests, and experiences of men.

These reasons all contribute to the fact that many women worldwide don't see sports as appropriate activities for them to take seriously.

It is easy to see the potential for controversy associated with these findings. They suggest that opportunities and resources to play sports should be increased for women, that women and men should share control of sports, and that new sports organized around the values, interests, and resources of women should be developed. They also suggest that there should be changes in ideas about masculinity and femininity, gender relations, family structures, the allocation of child-care responsibilities, the organization of work, and the distribution of resources in society.

People who benefit from sports and social life as they are currently organized are likely to oppose and reject the need for these changes. They might

even argue that the sociology of sport is too critical and idealistic and that the "natural" order would be turned upside down if sociological knowledge were used to organize social worlds. However, good research always inspires critical approaches to the social conditions that affect our lives. This is why studying sports with a critical eye usually occurs when researchers have informed visions of what sports and society could and should be in the future. Without these visions, often born of idealism, what would motivate and guide us as we participate in our communities, societies, and world? People who make a difference and change the world for the better have always been idealistic and unafraid of promoting structural changes in societies.

Regardless of controversies, research and popular interest in the sociology of sport has increased significantly in recent years. This growth will continue as long as scholars in the field do research and produce knowledge that people find useful as they try to understand social life and participate effectively as citizens in their communities and societies (Burawoy, 2005; Donnelly et al., 2011).

WHY STUDY SPORTS IN SOCIETY?

We study sports because they are socially significant activities for many people, they reinforce important ideas and beliefs in many societies, and they've been integrated into major spheres of social life such as the family, religion, education, the economy, politics, and the media.

Sports Are Socially Significant Activities

As we look around us, we see that the Olympic Games, soccer's World Cup, American football's Super Bowl, the Rugby World Cup, the Tour de France, the tennis championships at Wimbledon, and other sport mega-events attract global attention and media coverage. The biggest of these events are watched by billions of people in over two hundred countries. The media coverage of sports provides vivid images and stories that entertain, inspire, and provide for people the words and ideas they often use to make sense of their experiences and the world around them. Even people with little or no interest in sports cannot ignore them when family and friends insist on taking them to games and talking about sports.

People worldwide talk about sports at work, at home, in bars, on campuses, at dinner tables, in school, with friends, and even with strangers at bus stops, airports, and other public places. Relationships often revolve around sports. People identify with teams and athletes so closely that the outcomes of games influence their moods, identities, and sense of well-being. In a general sense, sports create opportunities for conversations that enable people to form and nurture relationships and even enhance their personal status as they describe and critique athletes, games, teams, coaching decisions, and media commentaries. When people use sports this way, they often broaden their social networks related to work, politics, education, and other spheres of their lives. This increases their **social capital,** that is, *the social resources that link them positively to social worlds* (Harvey et al., 2007).

> In the space of a few decades, the world has come to take sport more seriously than ever before. —Simon Kuper, journalist, *The Financial Times* (2012)

When people play sports, their experiences are often remembered as special and important in their lives. The emotional intensity, group camaraderie, and sense of accomplishment that often occur in sports make sport participation more memorable than many other activities.

For all these reasons, sports are logical topics for the attention of sociologists and others concerned with social life today.

Sports Reaffirm Important Ideas and Beliefs

We also study sports because they often are organized to reaffirm ideas and beliefs that influence how people see and evaluate the world around them. In fact, a key research topic in the sociology of sport is the relationship between sports and cultural ideologies.

We are not born with ideologies. We learn them as we interact with others and accept ideas and beliefs that are generally taken for granted in our culture. An **ideology** is a *shared interpretive framework that people use to make sense of and evaluate themselves, others, and events in their social worlds.* We learn ideologies as people around us consistently give meaning to and make sense of social phenomena in certain ways. Even if we don't agree with a particular ideology it represents the principles, perspectives, and viewpoints that are widely shared in our culture.

Most ideologies serve the interests of a particular category of people and are presented as accurate and truthful representations of the world as it is or as influential people think it should be. In this way, ideologies serve a social function and in that they can be used to justify certain decisions and actions.

When we study sports in society, it is important to know about four ideologies that influence how sports are organized and who controls and participates in them. These ideologies are organized around ideas and beliefs about gender, race, social class, and ability. Each of these ideologies is explained in terms of how it is related to sports in our lives.

Gender Ideology

Gender ideology consists of *interrelated ideas and beliefs that are widely used to define masculinity and femininity, identify people as male or female, evaluate forms of sexual expression, and determine the appropriate roles of men and women in society.* The most widely shared or *dominant* gender ideology used in many societies is organized around three central ideas and beliefs:

1. Human beings are either female or male.

2. Heterosexuality is nature's foundation for human reproduction; other expressions of sexual feelings, thoughts, and actions are abnormal, deviant, or immoral.
3. Men are physically stronger and more rational than women; therefore, they are more naturally suited to possess power and assume leadership positions in the public spheres of society.

Debates about the truth of these ideas and beliefs have become common worldwide and they are part of (a) larger struggles over what it means to be a man or a woman; (b) what is defined as normal, natural, moral, legal, and socially acceptable when it comes to gender and expressing sexuality; and (c) who should have power in the major spheres of life such as the economy, politics, law, religion, family, education, health care, and sports. Today, many people have come to realize that dominant gender ideology privileges heterosexual males, gives them access to positions of power, and disadvantages women and those not socially or biologically classified as a heterosexual.

Fortunately, ideologies can be changed. But those whose interests are directly served by a dominant ideology usually possess the power and resources to resist changes and demonize those advocating alternative ideas and beliefs. For example, the girls and women who first challenged gender ideology by entering the male world of sports were generally defined as abnormal, immoral, and unnatural (see Chapter 7). The demonization of these "gender benders" was especially strong in the case of women who played sports involving power and strength and women who did not conform to norms of heterosexual femininity. Men with power and resources banned females from certain sports, refused to fund their participation, excluded them from sport facilities, labeled them as deviant, and publicly promoted ideas and beliefs that supported their discriminatory actions discrimination against females (Sartore et al., 2010; Travers, 2011; Vannini and Fornssler, 2011).

The struggles around gender ideology also influence the lives of men—most directly, those who don't conform to prevailing ideas and beliefs about heterosexual masculinity (Anderson, 2011b; Harrison et al., 2009). In this sense certain sports, such as American football, ice hockey, boxing, and mixed martial arts, are organized, played, and described in ways that reaffirm an ideology that privileges certain boys and men over others. But as women and gender nonconforming men increasingly demonstrate their physical skills, they raise questions about and discredit dominant gender ideology (McGrath and Chananie-Hill, 2009). This means that sports are *sites,* or *social places,* where ideas and beliefs about gender are reaffirmed at the same time that oppositional ideas and beliefs are expressed. In this way, sports are important in ideological struggles related to the meaning and implication of gender in society and our everyday lives.

Racial Ideology

Racial ideology consists of *interrelated ideas and beliefs that are widely used to classify human beings into categories assumed to be biological and related to attributes such as intelligence, temperament, and physical abilities.* These ideas and beliefs vary greatly from culture to culture, due to historical factors, but racial ideologies are usually divisive forces that privilege a particular category of people and disadvantage others.

Racial ideology in the United States has been and continues to be unique. Its roots date back to the seventeenth century, but it was not fully developed until slavery came to an end and white people faced a new reality in which former slaves could claim citizenship and the rights that came with it. Fear, guilt, ignorance, rumors, stereotypes, and a desire to retain power and control over blacks led whites to develop a complex set of ideas and beliefs promoting white superiority and black inferiority as facts of nature. The resulting ideology was organized around these three major ideas and beliefs:

1. Human beings can be classified into races on the basis of biologically inherited or genetically based characteristics.

2. Intellectual and physiological characteristics vary by race, with white people being intellectually and morally superior to black people and all people of color.
3. People classified as white have only white ancestors, and anyone with one or more black ancestors is classified as a black person.

The ideology based on these ideas and beliefs was used to justify segregation and discrimination based on skin color and deny that black people were real "Americans" in the full legal sense of the term.

The connections between racial ideology and sports are complex (see Chapter 8). Through much of the twentieth century whites in the United States used racial ideology to exclude African Americans and other dark-skinned people from many sports, especially those occurring in gender-mixed social settings, such as golf, tennis, and swimming.

For many years whites also believed that blacks had physical weaknesses that prevented them from excelling in certain sports. But, when blacks demonstrated physical skills that rivaled or surpassed those of whites, dominant racial ideology was revised to describe blacks as less evolved than whites and, therefore, dependent on their innate physicality for survival. At the same time, whites saw themselves at a more advanced stage of evolution and dependent on their innate intellectual abilities for survival—abilities they believed were not possessed by blacks.

This racial ideology has been challenged and factually discredited during struggles over civil rights. But its roots are so deep in U.S. culture that it still influences patterns of sport participation, beliefs about skin color and abilities, and the ways that people view sports and integrate them into their lives.

Social Class Ideology

Social class ideology consists of *interrelated ideas and beliefs that are widely shared and used by people to evaluate their material status; explain why economic success, failure, and inequalities exist; and what should be done about economic differences in a group or society*. The dominant class ideology in the United States is organized around three major ideas and beliefs:

1. All people have opportunities to achieve economic success.
2. The United States is a **meritocracy** *where deserving people become successful and where failure is the result of inability, poor choices, and a lack of motivation.*
3. Income and wealth inequality is normal and inevitable because some people work hard, develop their abilities, and make smart choices and others do not.

Although some people question the truth of these ideas and beliefs, the class ideology that they support is heavily promoted and remains in existence because it serves the interests of people with power and wealth.

Competitive sports in the United States have been organized and described to inspire stories and slogans that reaffirm this ideology and help sustain its popularity (see Chapter 9). Coaches, media commentators, and sport fans consistently proclaim that people can achieve anything through hard work and discipline, and that failure is the result of laziness and poor choices.

This way of thinking leads to the conclusion that wealth and power are earned by hardworking people of good character and that poverty befalls those who are careless, unwilling to work, and have weak character. As a result, there is little sympathy for the poor at the same time that winning athletes and coaches—and wealthy people generally—are widely seen as models of smart choice-making and strong character. To the extent that people accept this class ideology, socioeconomic inequality is justified and the wealth and privilege of economic elites is protected. Therefore, economic elites and the corporations they control are major sponsors of high profile, competitive sports that are organized and presented in ways that inspire widespread acceptance of this class ideology.

Ableist Ideology

Ableist ideology consists of *interrelated ideas and beliefs that are widely used to identify people as physically or intellectually disabled, to justify treating them as inferior, and to organize social worlds and physical spaces without taking them into account.* This ideology in many cultures today is organized around three major ideas and beliefs:

1. People can be classified as normal *or* disabled.
2. Disability exists when physical or mental impairments interfere with a person's ability to function normally in everyday life.
3. Disabled people are inferior to normal people.

Underlying these ideas and beliefs is the general perspective of **ableism,** that is, *attitudes, actions, and policies based on the belief that people perceived as lacking certain abilities are inferior and, therefore, incapable of full participation in mainstream activities.* Therefore, when people use ableist ideology, they tend to patronize, pathologize, or pity those whose abilities don't "measure up" to their standards. This ideology leads to forms of social organization in which people are sorted into the categories of *able-bodied* and *disabled.*

Ableist ideology denies that there is natural variation in the physical and intellectual abilities of human beings, that abilities are situation- and task-specific, and that the abilities of all human beings change over time.

Everyday experience shows us that there are many different abilities used for many different purposes, and each of us is more or less able, depending on the situation or task. Additionally, people often forget that being *able-bodied* is not a permanent condition, because abilities change due to accidents, disease, and the normal process of aging. This means that we cannot neatly categorize everyone as either able-bodied or disabled. We can rank people from low to high on a particular ability in a particular situation or when doing a specific task, but it is impossible to have one ability-based ranking system across all situations and tasks encountered in everyday life, or even in sports.

Variations across all physical and intellectual abilities are a normal part of human life. But ableist ideology and ableism obscure this fact and prevent us from realistically dealing with ability differences in society.

In summary, ideologies are important parts of culture. People are usually unaware of them because they are simply taken for granted in their lives. As ideologies are widely shared and used as a basis for establishing, organizing, and evaluating social relationships and all forms of social organization, they are woven over time into the fabric of a society. This makes them different from the ideas and beliefs of individuals or those shared only with family members and friends.

Ideologies also resist change. They are defended by those who use them to make sense of the world and those whose privilege depends on them. Sometimes they are connected with religious beliefs and given intrinsic moral value, which fosters intense resistance to change. Although we rarely acknowledge our ideologies, we frequently recognize the ideologies of people from other cultures because they challenge our taken-for-granted assumptions. When this occurs we often criticize "foreign" ideologies while we leave our own unexamined. However, in this book we will take a critical look at dominant gender, racial, class, and ableist ideologies in Chapters 7–10.

Sports Are Integrated into Major Spheres of Social Life

Another reason for using sociology to study sports is that they are clearly connected to major spheres of social life. This will become increasingly clear in the following chapters. For example, Chapters 4 and 5 deal with family relationships and how they influence sport participation and how sports influence family life today. Issues involving the economy are covered in most chapters, and Chapter 11 is dedicated to examining the commercialization of sports and the changes that come with it. The media are closely connected with contemporary sports, and new social media are now changing the ways in which fans engage athletes and consume sports. This is explained in Chapter 12.

Government and politics are no strangers to sports, although their influence has changed as sports have become increasingly global and less dependent on nation-states. This is the topic of Chapter 13. The connections between interscholastic sports, the lives of students, the academic mission of schools, and the organization of high schools and colleges is the focus of Chapter 14. Finally, Chapter 15 deals with the complex relationships between major world religions and sports. Overall, sports are not only visible and important activities in themselves, but they are linked to major spheres of life in today's societies.

summary

WHY STUDY THE SOCIOLOGY OF SPORT?

Sociology is the study of *the social worlds that people create, organize, maintain, and change through their relationships with each other.* Sociologists use concepts, research, and theories to describe and explain social worlds. In the process, they enable us to put the lives of individuals and groups into context. This makes us aware of the circumstances that set limits and create possibilities in people's lives. For most sociologists, the ultimate goal is to create and distribute knowledge that enables people to understand, control, and improve the conditions of their lives and the social worlds in which they live.

Sociologists use the concepts of culture, social interaction, and social structure as they investigate social worlds. Sociological knowledge about sports and other social worlds is based on data systematically collected in research. This makes it different from statements about sports that are based only on personal experience and opinions.

Defining sports presents a challenge. If we use a single definition that emphasizes organization and competition, it can lead us to ignore people who have neither the resources nor the desire to develop formally organized and competitive physical activities. For this reason, many of us in the sociology of sport prefer an alternative definitional approach based on the assumption that sports are social constructions and that conceptions of sports vary over time and from one social world to another.

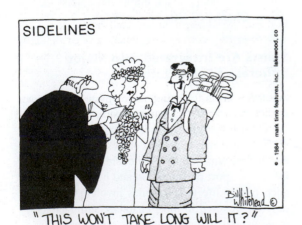

"THIS WON'T TAKE LONG WILL IT?"
(*Source:* By permission of William Whitehead)

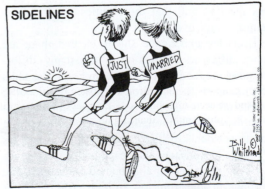

(*Source:* By permission of William Whitehead)

Families and family schedules often are shaped by sport involvement, sometimes interfering with family relationships (left) and sometimes creating enjoyable time together (right).

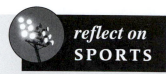

The Body Is More than Physical
Sports Influence Meanings Given to the Body

Until recently, most people viewed the body as a fixed fact of nature; it was biological only. But many scholars and scientists now recognize that a full understanding of the body requires that we view it in social and cultural terms (Adelman & Ruggi, 2015; Dworkin and Wachs, 2009; Eichberg, 2011; Hargreaves and Vertinsky, 2006; Wellard, 2012). For example, medical historians explain that the body and body parts have been identified and defined differently through history and from one culture to another. This is important because it affects medical practice, government policies, social theories, sport participation, and our everyday experiences.

The meanings given to the body and body parts in any culture are the foundation for people's ideas and beliefs about sex, gender, sex and gender differences, sexuality, beauty, self-image, body image, fashion, hygiene, health, nutrition, eating, fitness, ability and disability, age and aging, racial classification systems, disease, drugs and drug testing, violence and power, and other factors that affect our lives.

Cultural definitions of the body influence deep personal feelings such as pleasure, pain, sexual desires, and other sensations that we use to assess personal well-being, relationships, and quality of life. For example, people in Europe and North America during the nineteenth century identified insensitivity to physical pain as a sign that a person had serious character defects, and they saw a muscular body as an indicator of a criminal disposition, immorality, and lower-class status (Hoberman, 1992).

Cultural definitions of the body have changed so that today we see a person's ability to ignore pain, especially in sports, as an indicator of strong moral character, and we see a muscular body as proof of self-control and discipline rather than immorality and criminal tendencies. But in either case, our identities and experiences are inherently embodied, and our bodies are identified in connection with social and cultural definitions of age, sex, sexuality, race, ethnicity, and ability, among other factors.

Definitions of the body are strongly related to sports in many societies. For example, our conception of the

"ideal body," especially the ideal male body, is strongly influenced by the athletic body (van Amsterdam et al., 2012). In fact, the bodies of athletes are used as models of health and fitness, strength and power, control and discipline, and overall ability.

In today's competitive sports, the body is measured, monitored, classified, conditioned, trained, regulated, and assessed in terms of its performance under various conditions. Instead of being experienced as a source of pleasure and joy, the body is more often viewed as a machine used to achieve important goals. As a machine, its parts must be developed, coordinated, maintained, monitored, and repaired. Additionally, when the athletic body fails due to injuries, impairments, and age, it is reclassified in ways that alter a person's identity, relationships, and status.

Socially constructing the body in this way emphasizes control and rationality. It leads people to accept forms of body regulation such as weigh-ins, measuring body-fat percentage, testing for aerobic and anaerobic capacity, observing physiological responses to stressors, doing blood analysis, dieting, using drugs and other substances, drug testing, and on and on. For example, the members of the U.S. women's national soccer team must wear heart monitors on their chest and GPS devices in specially designed sport bras during practices so coaches and trainers can determine how hard they work, their fitness level, and their on-field strategy awareness (Reilly, 2012). Similar technology is now used by other coaches to monitor the energy and effort being exerted by athletes while on the field of play (Newcomb, 2012a, 2012b). All this helps coaches know how to "discipline" athletes' bodies and achieve performance goals.

Cultural conceptions of *body as machine* and *sport as performance* make it likely that athletes will use brain manipulations, hormonal regulation, body-part replacements, and genetic engineering as methods of disciplining, controlling, and managing their bodies. Measurable performance outcomes then become more important than subjective experiences of physical pleasure and joy. As a result, the ability to endure pain and stay in the game is an indicator of the "disciplined body;" and bodies that

Continued

The Body Is More than Physical (*continued*)

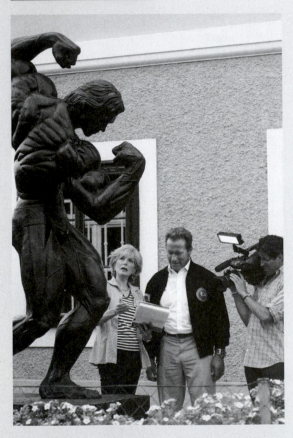

The ideal male body? Before he gained fame as "Conan the Destroyer" and "The Terminator" in films and became the governor of California (2003–2011), Austria-born Arnold Schwarzenegger was a legendary bodybuilder who won five Mr. Universe and seven Mr. Olympia titles. This statue outside the Schwarzenegger Museum in Austria captures one of his signature poses, which have had a worldwide impact on ideas about the male body and its representation of power and strength. However, ideas about the body change over time *and* are shaped by many social and cultural factors. (*Source*: © MARKUS LEODOLTER/epa/Corbis)

are starved to reduce body fat to unhealthy levels are ironically viewed as "fit" and "in shape."

When we realize that human life is embodied and that bodies are socially constructed in the context of culture, those who think critically ask the following questions:

1. What are the origins of prevailing ideas about natural, ideal, and deviant bodies in sports and in society?
2. What are the moral and social implications of the ways that the body is protected, probed, monitored, tested, trained, disciplined, evaluated, manipulated, and rehabilitated in sports?
3. How are bodies in sports marked and categorized by gender, skin color, ethnicity, (dis)ability, and age, and what are the social implications of such body marking and categorization?
4. How are athletic bodies represented in the media and popular culture, and how do those representations influence identities, relationships, and forms of social organization in society?
5. Who owns the body of an athlete, including the athletes' tattoos, and under what conditions can bodies or tattoos be used to promote products, services, beliefs, or ideas?
6. If moving the body were seen primarily as a source of pleasure rather than tool for achievement and weight control, would more people engage in physical activity?

These questions challenge taken-for-granted ideas about nature, beauty, health, and competitive sports. Ask yourself: *how have your ideas about bodies, including your own, been influenced by sports and the culture in which you live?*

Therefore, we try to explain why certain activities, and not others, are identified as sports in a particular group or society, why some sports are more strongly supported and funded than others, and how various categories of people are affected by commonly used definitions of sports and related funding priorities.

This alternative approach to defining sports also emphasizes that they are contested activities, because people can disagree about their meaning, purpose, and organization. Furthermore, people often have different ideas about who should play sports and the conditions under which participation should occur. Debates over who plays and who is excluded can create heated exchanges and bitter feelings, because they are tied to notions of fairness and the allocation of resources in social worlds. Finally, people can also disagree over which sports will be sponsored, who will sponsor them, and how much control sponsors should have over sports.

Asking critical questions about sports in society is the starting point for doing the sociology of sport. This forces us to think about why sports take particular forms and who is advantaged and disadvantaged by the current organization of sports in a social world. The sociology of sport often struggles for acceptance in societies where many people accept the great sport myth—that is, the assumption that sports are pure and good and that all who play or consume them will share in this purity and goodness. This assumption leads to the conclusion that it is not necessary to study and critically evaluate sport because it is essentially good as it is.

When sociologists study sports in society, they often discover problems related to the structure and organization of sports or the social worlds in which sports exist. Although we might be well informed about social issues, we usually lack the political power or influence to bring about change. Additionally, our recommendations may threaten those who benefit by maintaining the status quo in sports. This leads some people to see the sociology of sport as controversial, but we continue to do research and produce knowledge that can be used to promote fairness and social justice.

People study sports in society because sports are socially significant activities for many people; they provide excitement, memorable experiences, and opportunities to initiate and extend social relationships. Sports also reaffirm and sometimes challenge important ideas and beliefs, especially those related to gender, race and ethnicity, social class, and ability.

Finally, sports are studied because they are closely tied to major spheres of social life such as family, economy, media, politics, education, and religion.

Overall, sports are such an integral part of everyday life that they cannot be ignored by anyone concerned with the organization and dynamics of social life today.

SUPPLEMENTAL READINGS:

Reading 1. Why should I take sociology of sport as a college course?
Reading 2. The sociology and psychology of sport: what's the difference?
Reading 3. Play, games, and sports: They're all related to each other
Reading 4. Professional associations in the sociology of sport
Reading 5. Where to find sociology of sport research
Reading 6. Basketball: An idea becomes a sport

SPORT MANAGEMENT ISSUES

- You work for a sport management consulting firm. A client wants to invent a new sport that will attract participants as well as eventual media coverage, and asks you to submit a proposal covering what must occur and how long it might take. Describe the outline you will use for your "create a sport" proposal.

- You have a teaching assistantship as you pursue your doctorate in sport management. Your advisor says that you must teach a sociology of sport course to the first-year undergraduate sport management students. Describe what you will say on the first day of class to convince your students that it is important for them to take the course seriously.

- One of the major challenges faced in sport management is to deal with the influence of the great sport myth in contemporary cultures. Explain this challenge and how people in sport management might cope with it as they do their jobs.

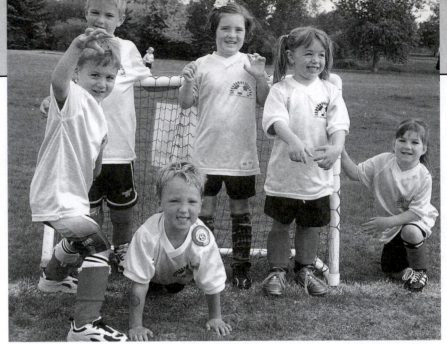

(*Source:* © Jay Coakley)

PRODUCING KNOWLEDGE ABOUT SPORTS IN SOCIETY

How Is Knowledge Produced In the Sociology of Sport?

"The first lesson of modern sociology is that the individual cannot understand his own experience or gauge his own fate without locating himself within the trends of his epoch and the life-chances of all the individuals of his social layer"

> —C. Wright Mills,
> social theorist and activist (1951)

. . . there is a difference between an open mind and an empty head. To analyse data, we need to use accumulated knowledge, not dispense with it.

> —Ian Dey, Social policy expert,
> University of Edinburgh, Scotland (1993)

The idea of real utopia is rooted in . . . the foundational claim of all forms of critical sociology: we live in a world in which many forms of human suffering and many deficits in human flourishing are the result of the way our social structures and institutions are organized.

> —Erik Wright, past president,
> American Sociological Association (2011)

We all work with concepts. . . . We have no choice. . . . Without concepts, you don't know where to look, what to look for, or how to recognize what you were looking for when you find it.

> —Howard Becker, sociologist (1998)

Chapter Outline

Learning Objectives

- Understand how and why our personal theories about social life differ from theories used in the sociology of sport.
- Identify the five steps involved in the production of knowledge.
- Explain the differences between cultural, interactionist, and structural theories.
- Understand what it means to say that gender exists as meaning, performance, and organization.
- Know the differences between a quantitative approach and qualitative approach and when it would be best to use one over the other when doing social research.
- Identify and describe the three major research methods used in the sociology of sport.
- Describe what it means to say that sports are more than reflections of society.
- Know the key features of a critical approach to producing knowledge in the sociology of sport.

The sociology of sport focuses on the deeper game associated with sports in society. We learn about that deeper game by using research and theories to understand the following:

1. The social and cultural contexts in which sports exist
2. The connections between those contexts and sports
3. The social worlds that people create as they participate in sports
4. The experiences of individuals and groups associated with those social worlds

Our research is motivated by combinations of curiosity, interest in sports, and a desire to expand what we know about social worlds. Most of us also want to use what we know about sports in society to promote social justice, expose and challenge the exploitive use of power, and empower people so they can effectively participate in political processes and change the social conditions that have a negative impact on their lives and their sport participation.

As we study sports, we use research and theories to produce knowledge. **Social research** consists of *investigations in which we seek answers to questions about social worlds by systematically gathering and analyzing data.* Research is the primary tool that we use to expand what we know and to develop, revise, and refine theories about sports in society.

Social theories are *logically interrelated explanations of the actions and relationships of human beings and the organization and dynamics of social worlds.* Theories provide frameworks for asking research questions, interpreting information, and applying the knowledge we produce about sports.

Research and theories go hand in hand because we use research to create and test the validity of theories, and we use theories to help us ask good research questions and make sense of the data we collect in our studies.

The goal of doing sociology is to describe and explain social worlds logically and in ways that are consistent with evidence that is systematically collected and analyzed. When sociologists achieve this goal, their research and theories add to our knowledge about social worlds. This makes knowledge in the sociology of sport a more valid and reliable source of information than what we read or hear in the media and online, where much of the content is based on a desire to entertain and attract audience.

In practical terms, the knowledge produced in the sociology of sport helps us understand more fully the actions of individuals, the dynamics of social relationships, and the organization of social worlds. This, in turn, enables us to be more informed citizens as we participate in our schools, communities, and society.

The goal of this chapter is to answer these questions:

1. How is knowledge produced in the sociology of sport?
2. What are the primary research methods used by scholars who study sports in society?
3. Why do scholars often use a critical approach when doing research and developing theories in the sociology of sport?

PRODUCING KNOWLEDGE IN THE SOCIOLOGY OF SPORT

Most people manage their lives and navigate social worlds by using personal, practical knowledge. They acquire this knowledge by keeping their eyes and ears open and developing explanations of everyday experiences and events. For example, consider how you manage your life at home, school, work, and with friends. What strategies do you use to understand what occurs around you, and how do you make decisions about what to do in connection with the people and events in your life?

If you're like most people, you learn to navigate social worlds and manage your life by observing how others act and what occurs in various situations. Then you use this information to develop experience-based explanations or "personal theories" about your own actions, the actions of others, and the social worlds you encounter. These **personal theories** *are summaries of your ideas and explanations of social life and the contexts in which it occurs.* All of us use them as guides when we make decisions and interact with others throughout the day.

Think about your family life as an example. You collect information and develop explanations to make sense of your family and your involvement in it. You may even consider how your family is related to the larger community and society in which you live. In the process, you develop "educated hunches" for why your family is more or less loving, strict, organized, wealthy, or supportive than other families. You may also try to explain the impact of external factors on your family, such as (a) the closing of your local high school that forced you to be bused 20 miles to another school, (b) a nationwide economic recession during which your father lost his job, and (c) the local decision to build a major highway that cut your neighborhood off from a previously accessible recreation center where you played sports.

The goal of our personal, experience-based data collection and theorizing is to make sense and gain control of our lives and the social worlds in which we live. Personal theories are forms of practical knowledge that we use to anticipate events, the actions of others, and the consequences of our own actions in various situations. Without them, we would be passive responders in our social worlds—victims of culture and society. But with theories, we become potentially active agents with the ability to participate intentionally and strategically in social worlds, reproducing or changing them as we take action alone and with others.

When Pierre Bourdieu, a famous French sociologist, discussed the practical knowledge that people develop through their personal experiences, he referred to it as "cultural capital" (Bourdieu, 1986). He explained that each of us can acquire and accumulate cultural capital as we expand our social and cultural experiences and make sense of them in ways that increase our understanding of ourselves, our relationships, and the ways that social worlds operate. Although each of us has different opportunities and experiences, we can convert our personal theories into cultural capital. Like money, cultural capital has value as we use it to navigate, manage, and control our lives. But unlike money, cultural capital can be used over and over again without running up our bills.

As you consider these points, you may wonder how your personal observations and theories compare with research and theories in the sociology of sport. In what ways are they different? Can research and theories in the sociology of sport be used in combination with personal research and theories? Can they take their place? Are they more accurate and reliable? These questions will be answered in the rest of the chapter and throughout this book.

Our personal observations and theories are useful in our everyday lives, but they differ from research and theories in the sociology of sport. Personal research focuses on our immediate social worlds. We gather and analyze information, but we don't use carefully developed methods and follow systematic and rigorous guidelines as we do so. Similarly, we develop personal theories for our own use. We don't systematically test them, compare them with related theories, and make them public so that others can examine them and determine their overall validity in different social worlds.

Research in the sociology of sport, unlike personal research, is designed to answer questions that go beyond the experiences and the social situations encountered by one person. In sociological

> . . . theories are like maps: the test of a map lies not in arbitrarily checking random points but in whether people find it useful to get somewhere. —Kevin Clarke and David Primo, political science professors, University of Rochester, 2012

research, we collect data from people or in situations that are chosen because they can provide information to answer particular questions. We then analyze the data by using methods that have been developed and refined by other sociologists. If the analysis leads to clear conclusions, we try to connect them with the conclusions and theories of other sociologists in the hope of expanding knowledge about the dynamics and organization of social life. Finally, we are expected to publish our studies so that others can critically examine them to see if they have flaws that would invalidate our findings.

People in the sociology of sport may study particular topics because they have a personal interest in them, but the process of doing research involves using methods that minimize the influence of our personal values and experiences on the findings and conclusions. Basic research methods used in sociology of sport research are

described later in the chapter (pp. 33–37), but first we'll examine a case study that illustrates how social research is done and how theory is used in the process of producing knowledge in the sociology of sport.

DOING RESEARCH AND USING THEORY IN THE SOCIOLOGY OF SPORT: A CASE STUDY

Micheal Messner is a well-known and respected sociologist at the University of Southern California. One of his books, *Taking the Field: Women, Men, and Sports* (2002), was named best book of the year by his colleagues in the sociology of sport. In the first chapter of Messner's book, he described a situation that, in part, inspired him to do in-depth sociological research on the connections between sport and gender in the United States. The situation

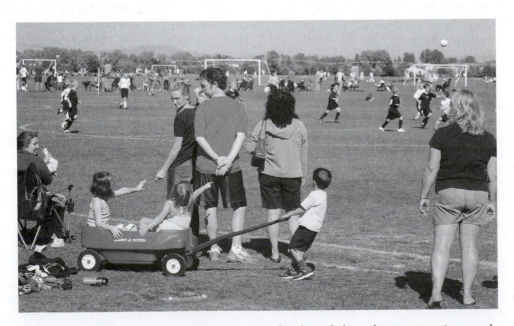

The social worlds created around sports are so complex that it helps to have systematic research methods and logical theories to study and understand them. I attend youth sports events for personal reasons, but I also use knowledge produced by Micheal Messner and others in the sociology of sport to help me make sense of what occurs at the events. (*Source*: © Jay Coakley)

occurred as he accompanied his son to the opening ceremony of a youth soccer season. Here are his words:

> The Sea Monsters is a team of four- and five-year old boys. Later this day, they will play their first ever soccer game. . . . Like other teams, they were assigned team colors—in this case, green and blue—and asked to choose their team name at their first team meeting. . . . A grandmother of one of the boys created the spiffy team banner, which was awarded a prize this morning. While they wait for the ceremony to begin, the boys inspect and then proudly pose for pictures in front of their new award-winning team banner. The parents stand a few feet away, some taking pictures, some just watching. . . .
>
> Queued up one group away from the Sea Monsters is a team of four- and five-year-old girls in green and white uniforms. . . . They have chosen the name Barbie Girls and they too have a new team banner. But the girls are pretty much ignoring their banner, for they have created another, more powerful symbol around which to rally. In fact, they are the only team among the 156 marching today with a team float—a red Radio Flyer wagon base, on which sits a Sony boom box playing music, and a three-foot-plus tall Barbie doll on a rotating pedestal. Barbie is dressed in the team colors; indeed, she sports a custom-made green and white cheerleader-style outfit, with the Barbie Girls' names written on the skirt. Her normally all-blond hair has been streaked with Barbie Girl green and features a green bow with polka dots. Several of the girls on the team have supplemented their uniforms with green bows in their hair as well.
>
> The volume on the boom box nudges up, and four or five girls begin to sing a Barbie song. Barbie is now slowly rotating on her pedestal, and as the girls sing more gleefully and more loudly, some of them begin to hold hands and walk around the float, in synch with Barbie's rotation. Other same-aged girls from other teams are drawn to the celebration and, eventually, perhaps a dozen girls are singing the Barbie song. . . .
>
> While the Sea Monsters mill around their banner, some of them begin to notice and then begin to watch and listen when the Barbie Girls rally around their float. At first, the boys are watching as individuals, seemingly unaware of each other's shared

> interest. . . . I notice slight smiles on a couple of their faces, as though they are drawn to the Barbie Girls' celebratory fun. Then, with side glances, some of the boys begin to notice each other's attention on the Barbie Girls. Their faces begin to show signs of distaste. One of them yells out, "NO BARBIE!" Suddenly, they all begin to move, jumping up and down, nudging, and bumping one another, and join in a group chant; "NO BARBIE! NO BARBIE! NO BARBIE!" They now appear to be every bit as gleeful as the girls as they laugh, yell, and chant against the Barbie Girls.
>
> The parents watch the whole scene with rapt attention. . . . "They are SO different!" exclaims one smiling mother approvingly. A male coach offers a more in-depth analysis: "When I was in college," he says, "I took these classes from professors who showed us research that showed that boys and girls are the same. I believed it, until I had my own kids and saw how different they are." "Yeah," another dad responds. "Just look at them! They are so different!"
>
> The girls meanwhile, show no evidence that they hear, see, or are even aware of the presence of the boys, who are now so loudly proclaiming their opposition to the Barbie Girls' songs and totem. The girls continue to sing, dance, laugh, and rally around the Barbie for few more minutes, before they are called to reassemble in their groups for the beginning of the parade.
>
> After the parade, the teams reassemble on the infield of the track, but now in a less organized manner. The Sea Monsters once again find themselves in the general vicinity of the Barbie Girls and take up the "NO BARBIE!" chant. Perhaps put out by the lack of response to their chant, they begin to dash, in twos and threes, invading the girls' space and yelling menacingly. With this, the Barbie Girls have little choice but to recognize the presence of the boys; some look puzzled and shrink back, some engage the boys and chase them off. The chasing seems only to incite more excitement among the boys. Finally, parents intervene and defuse the situation, leading their children off to their cars, homes, and eventually to their soccer games (from Messner, 2002, pp. 3–6).

As Messner observed these things, it caused him to think critically about youth sports. As a father, he was concerned about the way his son would make sense of these experiences as a five-year-old boy in twenty-first-century America. He even thought about what he would say to help his son define them in ways that would impact his development positively. But as a sociologist, Messner's thoughts went beyond his immediate experiences and his role as a father. He wondered why parents at the soccer ceremony accepted without questioning the idea that boys and girls are naturally different, even though many of the boys were initially interested in the playful actions of the girls and their use of the Barbie icon. Taking this thought a step further, he wondered if people who use "nature" to explain the actions of their children tend to overlook similarities between boys and girls and feel no need to discuss strategies to help their children understand that boys don't "naturally" try to intimidate girls.

Even though the boys' "playful actions" at the soccer ceremony did not physically hurt anyone, Messner wondered if certain sports are organized to reaffirm ideas about masculinity and femininity so that they make it seem normal for boys and men to express aggression and intimidate others. This also made him think about the decision of the American Youth Soccer Organization (AYSO) officials to segregate soccer teams by sex, thereby eliminating opportunities for boys and girls to play together and discover that they often share interests and other characteristics. Without such opportunities, are boys and girls more likely to grow up thinking that males and females are naturally "opposites," even though they share many attributes? And if this is so, what implications does it have for how we identify ourselves, form relationships, and organize our social worlds? As Messner asked these critical questions about sports and gender, he decided that he should do a study to expand sociological knowledge about this topic.

At this point, Messner was at the beginning of a five-step process for producing knowledge in the sociology of sport and in science generally. These steps are listed in Figure 2.1, and we can use them as a guide as we discuss this case study.

Step 1: Develop Research Questions

Producing knowledge always begins with observations of the world followed by questions about what is and is not observed. In this case, Messner observed a particular event and combined what he witnessed with his previous observations and knowledge of sports.

As he thought more deeply about his observations, he asked a series of critical questions about culture, social interaction, and social structure—the three concepts around which much sociological knowledge is organized. In connection with culture, he asked these questions:

- What gender-related words, meanings, and symbols do American children learn to use as they identify themselves and others?
- How do children learn and use cultural ideas and beliefs to separate human beings into two distinct, nonoverlapping, and "opposite" sex categories, even though males and females share many social, psychological, and physiological attributes and are not biological "opposites"?

In connection with social interaction, he asked:

- How do children perform gender in their everyday lives, and how do they learn to successfully present themselves to others as boys or girls?
- What happens in their relationships when they don't perform gender as others expect them to?

In connection with social structure, he asked:

- How is gender a part of the overall organization of the AYSO (American Youth Soccer Organization) and other sport programs?
- How does the organization of sports at all levels create constraints and possibilities that influence the lives of boys and men in different ways than they influence the lives of girls and women?

To see if other researchers had already answered these questions or developed theories to guide his

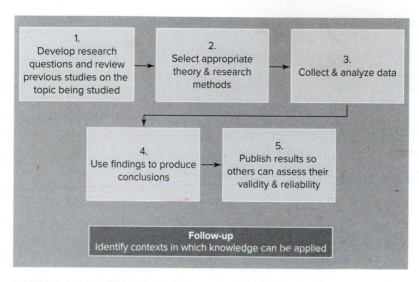

FIGURE 2.1 Producing knowledge in the sociology of sport.

study, Messner reviewed many of the 326 sources he listed as references in his book. This "review of the literature," as it is called by researchers, indicated that there was a need to know more about the relationship between sports and how people learn and incorporate ideas about gender into their identities, relationships, and the organization of social worlds.

Step 2: Select Appropriate Theory and Research Methods

This is a crucial step in the knowledge production process. When you have selected a theory, or a combination of theories, you then have a guide for thinking about your research questions and connecting them to what is already known about the organization and dynamics of social worlds. Additionally, there are different research methods that can be used to collect and analyze the information that will help you answer your research questions. Because Messner was asking so many questions in his project, he decided to use a combination of theories and methods.

Selecting Theories   As he designed his research project, Messner knew that human beings, social

relationships, and social worlds are complex and must be viewed from different angles and vantage points to describe and explain them accurately. Therefore, he used a combination of cultural, interactionist, and structural theories as guides for conceptualizing his project. Each of these theories focuses on different aspects of social life. Table 2.1 summarizes the central features of these theories, showing that each one explains different aspects of social worlds, has a different focus of analysis, uses different concepts, and addresses different issues.

Messner used **cultural theories** because they *explain what we know about the ways that people think and express their values, ideas, and beliefs as they live together and create social worlds.* Research based on cultural theories focuses on the processes through which people create, maintain, and change ideas and beliefs about their lives and the social worlds in which they live.

Cultural theories emphasize that people create symbols and give meaning to aspects of their worlds that are important to them; in turn, those symbols and meanings influence their feelings, thoughts, and actions.

Cultural theories utilize concepts such as values, norms, ideas, beliefs, ideology, symbols, and

Table 2.1   Central features of major types of theories used in the sociology of sport

Type of Theory	Help to Explain	Major Focus of Analysis	Major Concepts Used	Examples of Research*
Cultural Theories	Processes through which people create, maintain, and change values, norms, ideas, and beliefs as they play and watch sports	The ways people define and make sense of their bodies, experiences, and relationships as sport participants and consumers	Values, norms, ideas, beliefs, ideology, symbols, and narratives associated with sports	- imagery and narratives in media coverage of men's and women's sports - impact of racial ideology on the sport participation choices of individuals
Interactionist Theories	Social interaction and relationships in the social worlds created in connection with sports	Social development; the relationships through which people give meaning to sport experiences and integrate them into their lives	Interaction, socialization, role models, significant others, self-concept, identity, labeling, deviance, and stereotyping	- process of normalizing pain and injury when playing sports - process of developing and maintaining athletic identities
Structural Theories	The social organization and patterns of relationships that influence opportunities, decisions, and actions in sports	Impact of social organization on access to power, authority, status, resources, and economic opportunities in sports and society	Status, roles, groups, authority, power relations, social control, social inequality, social institutions, organizations, and societies	- gender equity in school sport programs - who benefits when public money builds stadiums for pro sport teams

*See Messner (2002) Chapters 2, 3, and 4 for examples of these and other studies. Chapter 4, "Center of Attention: The Gender of Sports Media," summarizes studies guided by cultural theories. Chapter 2, "Playing Center: The Triad of Violence in Men's Sports," summarizes studies guided by interactionist theories. Chapter 3, "Center of the Diamond: The Institutional Core of Sport," summarizes studies guided by structural theories.

language because they are the tools and reference points that people use to make sense of and give meaning to themselves, their experiences, and the world around them. In most cases, people who use cultural theories assume that culture is messy—its boundaries are fuzzy and difficult to identify, it contains inconsistencies and contradictions, and it is dynamic, meaning that culture is always changing as people develop new ideas, beliefs, values, and norms (McCarthy et al., 2005).

Cultural theories alerted Messner to the importance of symbols, such as the names, colors, uniforms, banners, songs, and chants that were used

to represent teams in the AYSO. Further, they directed his attention to specific **narratives,** which are *the explanations that people use—or the stories they tell—to explain and make sense of their choices and actions.* Therefore, Messner focused on the ways that ideas and beliefs about masculinity and femininity were included in the narratives that were used in the context of youth sports.

Messner also used **interactionist theories** because they *explain what we know about the origins, dynamics, and consequences of social interaction among people in particular social worlds.* These theories focus on processes of social learning and development. They deal with how people come to know and give meaning to themselves, others, and the things and events in their lives.

Interactionist theories use concepts such as social interaction, socialization, role models, significant others, self-concept, identity, labeling, deviance, and stereotyping to study social development during childhood, adolescence, and adulthood. This alerted Messner to the ways that youth sports are **sites,** or *identifiable social places or contexts,* where people learn what it means to be a man or woman, how to perform masculinity or femininity as they interact with others, and the ways that ideas and beliefs about gender are integrated into the organization of social worlds.

Finally, Messner used **structural theories** because they *explain what we know about different forms of social organization and how they influence actions and relationships.* These theories focus on the ways that relationships are organized and how they influence people's access to power, authority, material resources, economic opportunities, and other resources.

Structural theories help us identify and understand the social impact of recurring social relationships and patterns of social organization that exist in different spheres of everyday life, such as the family, religion, education, the economy, politics, and the media. They emphasize concepts such as status, roles, authority, power, social class, and social inequality to explain that the constraints and opportunities that exist in social worlds affect people differently, depending on their social positions and relationships with others. Therefore, these theories alerted Messner to the ways that sport organizations are "gendered" in terms of the jobs done by women and men, and who has authority and power on AYSO teams, in the AYSO administration, and in sports generally.

Selecting Research Methods   After selecting the theories he would use to guide his research, Messner selected a combination of research methods for collecting and analyzing data. Depending on the topic being studied, most researchers use either quantitative or qualitative methods, but Messner was asking such a variety of questions that he decided to use both.

Quantitative methods *involve collecting information (data) about people and social worlds, converting the information into numbers, and analyzing the numbers by using statistical procedures and tests.* Data may be collected by using a written questionnaire administered to a randomly selected sample of people that represents a larger population, or by quantifying particular facts in a sample or series of official records, reports, documents, or media content. The facts or data are usually presented in graphs and tables to represent statistical profiles and the quantifiable aspects of people, relationships, events, and social worlds (Aubel and Lefevre, 2013; Borgers et al., 2013).

Quantitative methods are used when social realities can be explained and understood by creating an overall view—a "big statistical picture"—of a population, media content, event, or social world. For example, they would be used to study general patterns and relationships, such as the differences between the grade point averages of U.S. high school students who play sports compared to those who don't play on school teams, or the patterns of keywords used in newspaper articles about different sports.

Qualitative methods *involve collecting information about specific people, media content, events, or social worlds; identifying patterns and unique features; and analyzing information by using interpretive procedures and tests.* Data are usually collected by doing in-depth interviews with a carefully selected sample of respondents, by observing particular events and social worlds, or by collecting a sample of documents or media content for analysis. These data are analyzed to provide detailed descriptions of what people say and do, and what occurs in social events and social worlds.

Qualitative methods are used when researchers want to discover the meanings and ideologies that underlie what people say and do, or when they want to understand the precise details of what occurs in relationships, groups, and social worlds.

For example, qualitative methods might be used to discover and understand why young people drop out of sports, the meanings people give to their sport experiences, or athletes' decisions to play when injured.

When sociologists study sports in society, they generally use surveys and interviews, observations, and text analysis to collect data (see Figure 2.2). Examples of these methods and how they are used in actual research are provided in the following sections.

SURVEYS AND INTERVIEWS: ASKING PEOPLE QUESTIONS
Social scientists often collect data by using surveys, which involve asking people questions through written questionnaires or person-to-person interviews. Questions must be clearly worded so that respondents understand them, and formulated so they do not influence or bias the answers given by study participants.

Each of us has responded to survey questionnaires in which we are asked about our attitudes, opinions, preferences, backgrounds, or current circumstances. Additionally, we're usually asked to provide demographic data such as our age, gender, education, occupation, income, race and ethnicity, and place of residence. The goal of many surveys is to construct statistical profiles of the characteristics, attitudes, beliefs, and actions of respondents who represent or statistically match a larger collection of people. Researchers then compare and analyze those profiles to describe and even predict the patterns of how people will think and act in particular situations.

Survey questionnaires are also used to identify recurring patterns and relationships in social life and to see if they support or contradict predictions based on a particular theory. As more people have access to computers and online connections, written questionnaires are more often being sent and replied to online.

In Messner's research project on gender and sports, he used data collected in a national survey of 800 boys and 400 girls, ten- to seventeen-years-old, equally distributed across four ethnic backgrounds: White, African American, Latino, and Asian American. The data were collected through written questionnaires, and they indicated that boys

SURVEYS	OBSERVATIONS	TEXT ANALYSIS
• **Written questionnaries** that participants complete by checking response boxes or providing brief written responses	• **Nonparticipant observation** in which the researcher is an outside observer who notes what is seen and heard	•**Scan** a large quantity of text, audio, or video content to extract keywords, identify patterns and priorities, or condense the text
• **Interviews** in which participants are asked brief or in-depth questions that are answered by telephone or face-to-face	• **Participant observation** in which the researcher is a full participant in a social world and notes what is seen and heard	• **Deconstruct*** texts to identify the logic, values, ideological assumptions, and contradictions that are built into them

* Text deconstruction is a special method of analyzing documents, literary materials, webpages, ads, billboards, graffiti, paintings, photographs, and all forms of media content. It uses defined strategies to uncover the logic, values, and assumptions underlying the narratives and/or images that constitute *the text*. This method also identifies the ideology that informs the text and the contradictions that are contained in it.

FIGURE 2.2 Data collection methods for studying sports in society.

were five times more likely than girls to regularly watch sports on television. Thirty percent of boys across the four ethnic groups watched sports every day, whereas only 6 percent of girls did so.

When it isn't practical to use written questionnaires, or when the goal is to do an in-depth investigation of people's feelings, thoughts, and actions, data may be collected through interviews. When questions are brief and straightforward, it has been customary to do person-to-person telephone interviews that can be completed in 5 minutes or less. But this method is used less frequently now that cell phones are replacing land lines, and area codes no longer identify the general location of the people being called.

In-depth interviews are used instead of written questionnaires when researchers seek open-ended information about the details and underlying meanings of what people say and do. Conducting in-depth interviews is a time-consuming method of collecting data. Usually, they are done with people who have been chosen because of their experiences, positions in an organization or community, or vantage point for viewing one or more social worlds. Interviewers attempt to develop trust and rapport to maximize the truthfulness of responses. Interview questions are presented in a clear, understandable manner, and the interviewer listens carefully to what *is* and *is not* said. Usually interviews are recorded for later transcription and analysis, but in the case of interviews done in the field, notes may be taken by hand rather than using a recording.

Messner used data from in-depth interviews that he conducted with thirty men who were former elite athletes (Messner, 1992). He learned that these men began playing sports with already-gendered identities, that is, with certain ideas about how to be a man in U.S. culture. As their athletic careers progressed, the men had experiences and formed attitudes consistent with dominant ideas about manhood. They believed that gender was grounded in nature and biological destiny, and this belief influenced the ways they performed masculinity in public, defined and interacted with women, and

evaluated their position and relative privilege in the overall organization of social worlds.

In summary, when data are collected by using questionnaires or interviews, researchers seek knowledge about general patterns and relationships in social worlds or knowledge about the details of everyday experiences and the meanings that people give to them.

OBSERVATIONS: SEEING AND HEARING WHAT PEOPLE DO AND SAY   Researchers in the sociology of sport often collect data by observing people in everyday life situations. They do this as (1) "nonparticipants" or outside observers, who are detached from the people and situations being studied, or as (2) "participant observers" who are or become personally involved in the social worlds being studied. For example, Noel Dyke studied youth sports by collecting data as an outside observer who attended practices and games and interviewed players and adults (Dyke, 2012); the late Janet Chafetz studied youth sports as participant observer/"team helper" for her son's baseball team (Chafetz and Kotarba, 1999).

Collecting data through observational methods is time intensive. Relationships must be established so there is trust and rapport developed with the people being studied. Actions, relationships, and social patterns and dynamics must be studied over time and from different vantage points so the data accurately depict the people and social worlds being studied. The goal of some sociologists who do observational research is to extend or challenge our knowledge of familiar groups and social worlds or introduce us to marginalized groups and unique social worlds about which we have little or no knowledge (Anderson, 2005b, 2011d; Atencio and Beal, 2011; Atencio and Wright, 2008; Brittain, 2004b; Huang and Brittain, 2006; Ravel and Rail, 2006, 2007; Shipway et al., 2013).

Observational methods generally involve **fieldwork,** that is, *"on-site" data collection.* An **ethnography** *is fieldwork that involves both observations and interviews;* in fact, ethnography literally means writing about people and how they live with each other (Adler and Adler, 2003; Hammersley, 2007). Ethnographies may take years to complete. They provide detailed descriptions and analyses of particular people and social worlds, such as sport teams, organizations, and communities.

Sociologist Reuben May (2008) did an ethnography in which he studied young men on a basketball team in a high school located in a poor neighborhood of a midsize southern U.S. city. As the assistant coach of the team, he was a participant observer. May's observations and interviews occurred over seven years because he wanted to accurately represent the experiences and lives of the young men he coached—all African Americans. He organized his study to allow the young men to speak for themselves and describe their view of the world in which they lived. As he presented their stories, May put them into a social and cultural context so that he and his readers could make sense of them and extend our knowledge of sports in the lives of young African American men growing up in resource deprived, urban neighborhoods today. In the process, he described the complexity and contradictions associated with sports in such a social world and identified the serious dilemmas faced by coaches as they try to help these young men make the transition from high school to the rest of their lives.

Ethnographies are limited because they focus on particular social worlds, and it is difficult to know whether the knowledge they produce can be used to understand other social worlds. However, they provide detailed information about the organization and dynamics of the social worlds studied. This enables us to understand how actions and relationships create, sustain, and change those worlds; how they become unique; and how the meanings created in them influence the decisions and actions of the people who inhabit them. For example, recent ethnographies about flat track roller derby enable us to understand how particular women have created a form of sport that fits their interests and life circumstances (Beaver, 2012; Donnelly, 2013; Gieseler, 2014; Pavlidis and Fullagar, 2013, 2015).

TEXT ANALYSIS: STUDYING DOCUMENTS AND MEDIA
Research in the sociology of sport often involves some form of text analysis in which data are collected from any source in which there are narratives and images that represent ideas, people, objects, and events associated with sports. **Narratives** are *the stories that people tell about themselves and their social worlds.* They are an integral part of conversations, social interaction, and the media. They represent factual or fictional realities and they're often combined with **images**—that is, *visual representations of ideas, people, and things.*

These narratives and images are pervasive in connection with sports in society today. For example, sociology of sport scholars have analyzed data collected from sport team media brochures, newspaper articles, media commentaries during the Olympics and other sport events, the ads in sports magazines, the commercials aired during televised sport events, and sport books and films—and many of these studies are discussed in Chapter 12 on media and sport. For documents and media content that are digitized, special software programs can be used to identify patterns and themes in a large quantity of text. In other cases, researchers focus on a smaller number of documents or selected media content and carefully deconstruct it to identify underlying meanings and assumptions contained in the narratives and images in the texts.

In a series of studies, Messner and his colleagues analyzed the content of network sports news from 1989 through 2009 (Table 2.2), and they also analyzed at regular intervals during 2009 the content of ESPN's one-hour evening *Sports Center* program and sports coverage by two network stations (Table 2.3). The data indicated that stories about men's sports dominated television coverage between 1989 and 2009, despite dramatic increases in women's sport participation during that period. For example, during ESPN's prime time *Sports Center* program, only 1.3 percent of total airtime was given to women's sports (Cooky et al., 2013). Messner and his colleagues concluded that this type of mainstream television news coverage

Table 2.2   Gender focus of network sports news stories, 1989–2009 (in percentages)

Stories	1989	1993	1999	2009
About men	92.0	93.8	88.2	96.3
About women	5.0	5.1	8.7	1.6
Neutral/About both	3.0	1.1	3.1	2.1

Source: Cooky, Messner, and Hextrum, 2013.

Table 2.3   Percentage of 2009 sports coverage, by sex, on ESPN *Sports Center* and KCBS and KNBC (Southern California)

	ESPN	KCBS and KNBC
Men's Sports	96.4	95.9
Women's Sports	2.7	3.2
Both/Neutral	1.0	1.0

Source: Cooky, Messner, and Hextrum, 2013.

perpetuates the notion that elite sports is a masculine activity in U.S. culture.

Messner and his colleagues also did a more in-depth analysis in which they *deconstructed* narratives and images to identify the logic, values, assumptions, and underlying ideologies used by those who produce media content about sports (Messner et al., 2000). This method of analyzing data enabled them to identify a master narrative that media people used to describe masculinity. This narrative emphasized the following: sports are a man's world, sports are wars and athletes are warriors, boys will be boys, boys are basically violent, aggressive guys win and nice guys lose, women are sexy props, men sacrifice their bodies for their teams, and the measure of a man is his "guts." Messner and his colleagues concluded that these assumptions formed a "Televised Sports Manhood Formula" that was consistently presented in sports programming.

These quantitative and qualitative methods of investigating the content of documents and media

help us understand the complex connections between sports and other spheres of our lives. Scanning, analyzing, and deconstructing narratives and images associated with sports enables researchers to identify widely accepted ideas and beliefs about competition, authority structures, teamwork, dedication achievement, and success.

Step 3: Collect and Analyze Data

Using cultural theories as a guide, Messner also collected information on the team names that players and coaches selected for the 156 AYSO teams that season. Names, along with colors, uniforms, banners, and songs or chants, are symbols that people often use to represent sport teams in U.S. culture. **Symbols** are important to sociologists because they *are concrete representations of the values, beliefs, and moral principles around which people organize their ways of life.*

When Messner analyzed the 156 team names, he found that 15 percent of the girls' teams and 1 percent of the boys' teams chose sweet, cutesy names such as the Pink Flamingos, Blue Butterflies, Sunflowers, and Barbie Girls.[1] "Neutral" or paradoxical names such as Team Flubber, Galaxy, Blue and Green Lizards, and Blue Ice were selected by 32 percent of the girls' teams and 13 percent of the boys' teams; and power names such as Shooting Stars, Raptor Attack, Sea Monsters, Sharks, and Killer Whales were selected by 52 percent of the girls' teams and 82 percent of the boys' teams.

Overall, boys were much more likely to avoid sweet, cutesy names in favor of power names. This is consistent with past research showing that people represent themselves and their groups with symbols and names that reaffirm their favored identity. In this case, the boys and girls selected names that fit their gendered sense of who they were and how they wished to be perceived in the social world of AYSO youth soccer.

When Messner used interactionist theory as a guide, he observed the actions of people at AYSO

---

[1]*Smurfs* was the only "sweet" name chosen by a boys' team.

events to see how they performed gender as they interacted with others. His observations of the children indicated that their performances clarified *and* blurred traditional gender distinctions. But the most noticeable gender performances occurred when the boys vocally objected to the girls' celebration of their Barbie icon and attempted to physically disrupt the girls' celebration. At the same time, the girls were surprised by the boys' actions and either withdrew due to fear or stood their ground to challenge the boys. The parents reaffirmed the normalcy of these performances by attributing them to natural differences between boys and girls; they did not consider that the children's actions could be due to cultural norms, the interactional dynamics of the opening AYSO ceremony, or the overall social organization of the soccer league and most sports in the United States.

Using structural theory as a guide, Messner also collected data on the adult divisions of labor and who held power positions in the AYSO and on each of the 156 teams. He found that there were gender-based limits for the actions and relationships of some children and adults, and gender-based possibilities for others. For example, the commissioner and assistant commissioners were men, as were twenty-one of thirty board members. Over 80 percent of the head and assistant coaches were men, whereas 86 percent of the team managers, or "team moms," as most people referred to them, were women. The coaches had formal authority at the league and team levels, and the "team moms" performed support roles that were labor intensive, time consuming, and behind the scenes.

Even when the soccer experiences of women surpassed those of men, they were less likely to volunteer as coaches. Men volunteered because they believed it was appropriate for them to play such a role, whereas the women felt less so—and men didn't see themselves as "team moms" or even as "team dads" doing what team moms did.

As Messner collected and analyzed data on the organization of the AYSO, he also found that patterns of authority were *informally* gendered by the adults, whereas gender was *formally* and officially

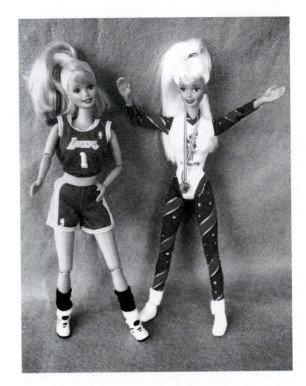

What does it mean when five-year-old girls choose Barbie as a representation of their team? Barbie represents traditional feminine values and ideals in U.S. culture, but the girls in Messner's study connected Barbie to their sport participation. Is this a sign that traditional feminine values are changing, that the girls are creating a new form of femininity, or that the girls value traditional femininity more than playing sports? The sociologists most likely to ask these questions are guided primarily by cultural theories. (*Source:* © Jay Coakley)

used to segregate boys and girls into separate leagues. According to AYSO leaders, the teams at all age levels were segregated by sex "to promote team unity." For the leaders, this made gender "appear to disappear" in the organization and in the decision-making processes of the leagues. By using sex to segregate the leagues and teams, gender was erased from the day-to-day consciousness of coaches, officials, parents, players, and administrators, even though it was the primary organizing principle for the entire AYSO and the experiences of nearly 2000 young people.

Messner pointed out that this type of social structure creates highly gendered experiences while they give everyone the impression that gender is irrelevant. For example, as the children played on sex-segregated teams, they had no opportunities to observe similarities in the skills, personalities, interests, and emotions of boys and girls or to be teammates and friends with differently gendered peers. Coaches treated boys as they felt boys should be treated and girls as they felt girls should be treated without realizing that ideas and beliefs about gender influenced the entire social context in which they coached. Gender was erased from their awareness at the same time that it organized and structured the experiences of everyone associated with the AYSO.

Collecting and analyzing data about the AYSO was a very small part of Messner's overall research project. He had already done many studies of sports and gender in different contexts, and he and his colleagues had studied gender in media coverage of sports, commentaries during sport events, ads during sport events and in sport publications, and patterns of corporate sponsorships for sports. In other words, his systematic collection and analysis of data went far beyond the opening ceremony, the Sea Monsters and Barbie Girls, and the AYSO.

Step 4: Use Findings to Produce Conclusions

Messner's analysis of all the data he collected enabled him to present detailed explanations of the connections between gender and sports in the United States. He used cultural, interactionist, and structural theories to make sense of these connections and make knowledge statements about gender in social worlds. Messner's overall conclusion was that **gender** is much more than a social category or trait that identifies a person; instead, it *consists of interrelated meanings, performances, and organization that become important aspects of social worlds.*

Figure 2.3 depicts Messner's description of gender as a multidimensional concept. *Gender as meaning* refers to the fact that in a particular culture people often learn to identify certain colors, names, and objects as "masculine" or "feminine." Gestures, actions, and elements of physical appearance may also be identified in this way. These socially agreed-upon cultural meanings are part of a larger cultural process of constructing the gender categories that people use to identify themselves and make sense of what occurs in their relationships and experiences. For example, boys or men in the United States don't select pink as a team color because they have learned that it is associated with femininity. The five-year-old boys observed by Messner had already learned *gender as meaning* to the extent that they did not name themselves the "Barbie Boys" or "Pink Monsters." This example may seem trivial, but gender as meaning influences people's choices and interpretations of the world around them. Significant here is the fact that sports serve as an important site at which this meaning is learned, reaffirmed, and sometimes even challenged and changed.

Gender as performance (Figure 2.3) refers to the fact that people "do" gender as they interact with others. In the process they reproduce existing meanings and organization, or they offer alternatives. The five-year-olds observed by Messner had clearly learned to perform gender in certain ways and evaluate each other in terms of what it meant for them to "act like a boy" or "act like a girl" in their social worlds. In this sense, *gender is performance*. For example, a coach might refer to boys on his team as "girls" when they don't perform well. Similarly, a player on a girls' team who spits regularly on the field may be told by her coach to "act like a lady"—meaning that she is not performing gender as expected in U.S. culture.

Gender as organization (Figure 2.3) refers to the ways that positions, roles, and responsibilities are structured around gender. For example, in most sports the coaches are more likely to be men than women, because it is widely believed that masculinity is more compatible with the demands of

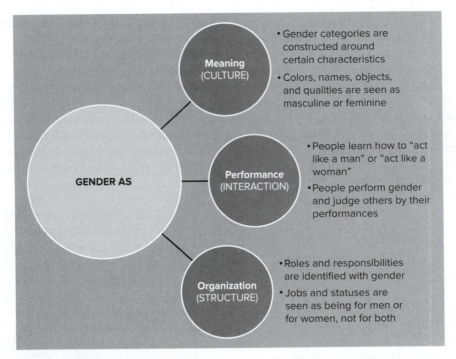

FIGURE 2.3 Gender as meaning, performance, and organization in social worlds.

coaching than femininity is. This is why men coach nearly all men's teams and most women's teams, whereas women coach a minority of women's teams and almost no men's teams.

The pattern of men in positions of control and women in support positions was clear in the AYSO, where the commissioner and assistant commissioners were men, as were twenty-one of the thirty members of the board of directors, and 85 percent of the 156 head coaches. In this sense, organization is clearly gendered.

Part of Messner's contribution to what we know about gender and sport is showing us how gender constitutes a combination of meaning, performance, and organization in social worlds, especially those constructed around sports. This is important because it explains why it is so difficult to "ungender" sport. As long as we uncritically accept current meanings, performances, and organization, sport will remain gendered in ways that preclude equal treatment for men and women. However, once we see gender in these terms, it's possible to develop strategies to create equity.

Step 5: **Publish Results**

After completing his project, Messner wrote research papers that explained what he had done and what he had discovered about gender and sports in the United States. At least three of these papers were written as articles and submitted for possible publication in academic journals, and a long manuscript was written as a possible book and submitted to the University of Minnesota Press. The journal and book editors each asked scholars who were experts on the topic of gender and sports to critically review Messner's manuscripts and recommend whether they should be published. These reviewers assessed the overall quality and accuracy of Messner's work: Did he ask good questions, collect useful data from appropriate sources, analyze the data with care and accuracy, come to logical conclusions based on the data, and make thoughtful knowledge statements about sport and gender?

After receiving favorable reviews calling only for minor revisions, each of Messner's manuscripts was accepted for publication. One of his articles was published in the journal, *Gender & Society* (Messner, 2000), and his book manuscript was published by the University of Minnesota Press (Messner, 2002).[2] In both cases, the editors and reviewers concluded that Messner's research produced worthwhile knowledge about sports and the ways that gender becomes a key part of social worlds.

Even though Messner was an established scholar and had tenure at the University of Southern California, he, like most researchers, was expected to publish his work so that his contributions to sociology knowledge could be verified by a community of scholars who study gender, sports, and related topics. This is because knowledge production in science is never a one-person job; it always depends on the critical review of a community of scholars. Messner understood this and published his research so that others could evaluate it. Although his manuscripts were published, most manuscripts submitted for publication are rejected because reviewers find them lacking in quality or not contributing to knowledge production in a particular field.

Messner's claim that gender was more than a social category and should be viewed as a combination of meaning, performance, and organization was an important addition to sociological knowledge, and very useful for people who study gender. In his own research, Messner used this knowledge to theorize about sports as sites where ideas and

beliefs about gender are created, maintained, and sometimes challenged and changed.

This knowledge is important because many people describe sports simply as a reflection of society—sites where aspects of culture and society are revealed to those who take a close look. But Messner's research findings challenged this view and provided evidence that sports are more than reflections of society; in fact, they are sites where ideas and beliefs about gender and other important

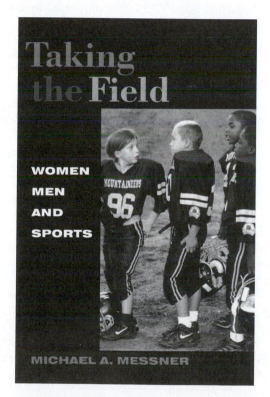

Reviewers determined that Messner's research was valid, that is, it measured what Messner claimed it measured and his conclusions were supported by the data. When research lacks validity in the eyes of reviewers, it is not published. Messner's book, pictured here, was also named the Outstanding Book of the Year by his colleagues in the North American Society for the Sociology of Sport. (*Source*: Used with permission from University of Minnesota Press)

---

[2]Other publications based on this research are Cooky, Messner, and Hextrum, 2013; Messner, 2007, 2009, 2011; Messner, Dunbar, and Hunt, 2000; Messner, Duncan, and Cooky, 2003; Messner, Hunt, and Dunbar, 1999; and Messner and Stevens, 2002.

aspects of our lives are created, reproduced, and changed. Therefore, sports constitute a significant social world to study, and the people associated with sports are most accurately viewed as agents actively involved in shaping social worlds rather than passive subjects determined by culture and society. This issue is discussed further in the box, "Sports Are More Than Reflections of Society."

Messner's research made an important contribution to knowledge. His article in *Gender & Society*, "Barbie Girls vs. Sea Monsters: Children Constructing Gender," is frequently used by others as they develop ideas and do their own research on gender, sports, childhood, and other topics. His book, *Taking the Field*, received positive reviews and in 2004 was named the Outstanding Book of the Year by his colleagues in the North American Society for the Sociology of Sport. In 2007 and 2009, Messner published two additional books, *Out of Play: Critical Essays on Gender and Sport* and *It's All for the Kids: Gender, Family, and Youth Sports*, which built on and extended the work he began a decade earlier. In 2012, he became the first man to be given a special award from the American Sociological Association for expanding sociological knowledge about gender in society.

THE IMPACT OF SOCIOLOGY OF SPORT KNOWLEDGE

After reading about *how* to do research in the sociology of sport, it is reasonable to ask *why* we do this research—in other words, for what purpose do we produce knowledge about sports in society?

Those of us who do research on the social aspects of sports hope that the knowledge we produce does not just sit on the pages of journals and books. When considering the application of this knowledge, it is important to be aware of the following:

1. Social science research does not produce "ultimate truth" in the form of knowledge that eliminates all doubt and uncertainty in everyday life.

2. Research, theories, and knowledge in the sociology of sport will never lead to the creation of a single strategy to prevent social problems and forever guarantee fairness and justice in sports and sport organizations.

3. Knowledge about social worlds is never complete, and using knowledge to solve current problems does not mean that the solutions will be free of challenges and problems.

This does not mean that social research and theories should be ignored in our personal decisions about sports or in planning, making, and funding policies and programs related to sports, but it reminds us of our limitations as social scientists.

With that said, sociology of sport knowledge can help us detect bias and validity problems in our personal theories and enable us to make more fully informed choices about sports in our lives. For example, the research of Micheal Messner and others (see Chapters 4 and 5) is clearly useful when we select sport programs for our children, become coaches in schools or youth programs, create policies to increase healthy sport participation in our communities, develop sport programs for employees at our workplaces, or vote on ballot issues regarding the use of public money to build local recreational centers or new stadiums for men's professional teams. Overall, knowledge produced in the sociology of sport enables us to view sports from multiple perspectives that go beyond our personal experiences and vantage points in social worlds.

It is difficult to know whether and how sociology of sport knowledge is used. Although many of us work with sport programs and serve as sources of information for people who make decisions about the provision and organization of sports, we don't control how that knowledge is used in all circumstances. We may produce science-based knowledge, but we seldom have official power in sport organizations, so we generally depend on others to apply sociology of sport knowledge in real-world situations.

There is resistance to the application of research-based knowledge when it raises questions about the

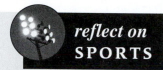

Sports Are More Than Reflections of Society

When people study the social aspects of sports, they often say that sports are reflections of society. This is true, but sports are much more than reflections. In fact, they are social practices that actively influence what people do and how social worlds are organized. For example, many sports in the United States are organized in ways that perpetuate very limited ideas and beliefs about race, skin color, and race relations. This encourages people to accept these ideas and beliefs and avoid the following: (1) asking critical questions about race in social worlds; (2) considering the meaning of race and the racial categories that people use to classify themselves and others; (3) identifying the ways that ideas about race influence people's actions, their choices of what sports to play, and their expectations of how they might excel at certain sports; or (4) becoming aware of how race is woven into the organization of sports and social worlds generally.

At the same time, sports are also **sites,** that is, *identifiable social contexts,* where people can challenge and even change ideas and beliefs about race and skin color—as Jackie Robinson did when he became the first African American to play in modern Major League

Baseball in 1947, or when Tony Dungy became the first black head coach to win a Super Bowl in 2007.

This way of thinking about sports in society recognizes that people organize, perform, and give meaning to sports in many different ways, and that sports are sites at which ideas, beliefs, and approaches to social relationships are created, maintained, and changed. Therefore, instead of merely reflecting society, sports comprise the "social stuff" from which society and culture are forever being created and reproduced. This makes them sociologically important.

When we understand the dynamic nature of social life, we realize that each of us is an agent that is involved in creating, maintaining, and changing the social and cultural worlds in which we live. Therefore, we are not destined to think about or do sports as they are portrayed in the narratives and images presented by media companies, Coca-Cola, Nike, Red Bull, Budweiser, or other sponsors of sports today. This opens our minds and makes it possible for us to think critically about sports and to work with others to make them what we want them to be in our lives. *If you could change one thing about sports in your school or community, what would it be?*

status quo. Such knowledge—usually produced by researchers who ask critical questions—is often seen as threatening or even subversive by those who benefit from the current organization of sports. This is why it is important for access to knowledge to be widespread so that decisions about putting knowledge to use can be part of a democratic political process rather than part of a strategy to enhance the control exercised by powerful people. In this sense, research and knowledge production are a starting point rather than an end point for many of us in the sociology of sport. We want to see knowledge used for the common good and to make sports more humane, democratic, and inclusive.

What inspired Micheal Messner to do his research were his initial observations of the youth soccer program in which his son wanted to participate. These observations led to questions about what his son might learn as he played soccer, why the leagues and teams were sex-segregated, why parents and coaches supported this segregation, how gender was performed by the children and adults, how gender was integrated into the organization of the leagues and teams, and how gender is related to more general forms of social organization in society.

Messner knew that widely held ideas and beliefs about femininity, masculinity, and male-female relationships created constraints for males and females and supported a system of social organization that often privileged men and disadvantaged women, especially in terms of their access to positions of power in most spheres of social life, including sports. Therefore, he was inclined to use a critical approach as he designed his research project. He wanted to understand and explain why the meanings that people give to sports, the actions of females and males in sports, and the organization of sports are gendered and how this might affect other parts of society. Using a critical approach, Messner's goal was to produce knowledge that could be used to find solutions to social problems, identify and eliminate injustices, and shrink the "the gap between what is and what could be" in social worlds (Burawoy, 2004). Therefore, he wanted that knowledge to empower people as they participate in a process of creating sustainable, just, and equitable ways of life.

USING A CRITICAL APPROACH TO PRODUCE KNOWLEDGE

When using a critical approach to study sports in society, our research is guided by one or more of the following questions:

- What values, ideas, and beliefs are promoted through sports, and who is advantaged or disadvantaged by them?
- What are the meanings currently given to sports and sport participation, and who is advantaged or disadvantaged by those meanings?
- How are sports organized, and who is advantaged or disadvantaged by existing forms of organization in sports?
- Who has power in sports, to what ends is power used, and how are various categories of people affected by power relations associated with sports?
- Who accepts and who resists the organization of mainstream sports, and what happens to those who resist?

- What strategies effectively foster progressive changes in sports and the social worlds around them?

These questions show that a critical approach is organized around an awareness that people are positioned differently in social worlds, and they are affected differently by the meaning, purpose, and organization of mainstream sports. In other words, everyone does not benefit from sports in the same ways, and some people may be disadvantaged by how they are organized and played in a particular social world. For example, an emphasis on high-performance or elite sports in a society may exclude or discourage participation among many people who could benefit from sports organized for recreational purposes.

Additionally, a critical approach heightens one's awareness that knowledge about social worlds can be applied in many ways. For example, Messner understood that knowledge about the relationship between masculinity and the cultures that exist in certain sports could be used to transform those cultures, thereby reducing male-on-male violence and the serious injuries that boys and men often learn to accept as "part of the game." Therefore he organized the last chapter of his book to answer the question: "Just do *what?*" The chapter presents thirty pages of recommendations for critically informed actions to make sports more humane, equitable, and democratic.

Referring to the Nike marketing slogan "*Just do it!*," Messner emphasizes that without critically assessing what "it" is, we reproduce sports as they are rather than actively changing and developing them to be fair and equitable as they provide people with excitement, physical challenges, and joy. For example, he called for more activities that give boys and young men opportunities to make healthy, respectful connections with others (2002, p. 166). Similarly, he urged that we must reorganize certain sports so that boys and men do not have their "need for closeness, intimacy, and respect thwarted [and] converted into a narrow form of group-oriented bonding based on competitive one-upmanship,

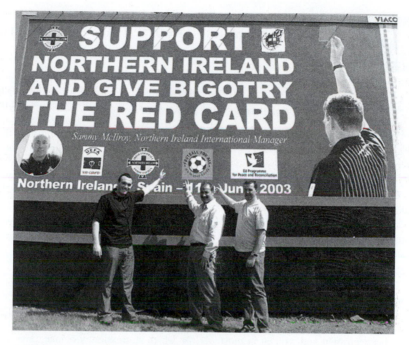

A critical approach to knowledge production in Northern Ireland focuses on the role of sport in eliminating sectarian (Protestant versus Catholic) violence. Administrators in the Irish Football Association have consulted with scholars in the sociology of sport as they develop strategies to make soccer more inclusive, just, and supportive of the well-being of athletes and spectators. (*Source:* © Michael Boyd, Irish Football Association)

self-destructive behaviors, silent conformity to group norms, and sexually aggressive denigration of others" (2002, p. 166).

Along with Messner and many of my colleagues in the sociology of sport, I also use a critical approach to guide my thinking and research on sports in society. Our sense is that if we only did research that reflected and reaffirmed sports as they are, there would be no point to our professional existence. Unless our work is based on a critical approach, raises questions about sport, and causes people to think about the place of sports in our lives, we contribute nothing of value to the world around us. This is why you will notice that the following chapters often focus on issues and controversies that deal with fairness, access to sport

participation, and equity. Underlying these critical discussions is my desire to make available to more people the excitement, physical challenges, and joy that can be part of sport participation.

summary

HOW IS KNOWLEDGE PRODUCED IN THE SOCIOLOGY OF SPORT?

Sociology of sport knowledge is produced through research and theories. Research provides data and systematic analyses to answer questions and validate or revise existing theories about sports in society. Theories provide logical explanations of

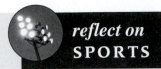

reflect on SPORTS

Critical Feminist Theory Today
From the Margins to Mainstream

Prior to the 1970s, science was much like sport—it was a man's world, created by and for men and based on their interests and experiences. Men dominated all fields of study and produced knowledge based on their questions, observations, analyses, and theorizing about the world. This did not make science wrong, but it certainly made it incomplete, and occasionally it was so biased that it misrepresented physical and social realities.

When women entered science and pointed this out, most men became defensive and used their power to question the ability of female scientists and the quality of their work. This led to conflicts between men and women in most scientific disciplines, from biology to sociology. These conflicts are less common today because many male scientists now realize that women scholars using a feminist approach raised valid points and did research that made important contributions to their fields. In fact, many male scholars today use feminist theories to inform their own work. In the sociology of sport, feminist theories have become mainstream with few questions about their legitimacy or usefulness when trying to understand sports in society.

During the 1970s and 1980s, feminist research and theory in sociology focused on making apparent the patriarchal organization of nearly all societies and explaining how the values, experiences, and interests of men, especially men with power, had shaped social relationships and social life generally. They showed that the privileges accorded to men were directly linked to systemic disadvantages experienced by women. In other words, more important than sexist attitudes and feelings was the fact that relationships and society were organized around particular meanings given to gender.

There are several different forms of feminist theory, but most scholars in the sociology of sport favor critical feminist theory because it focuses on issues of ideology,

Despite stereotypes that paint feminists as forever negative—doing feminist work requires boundless optimism. It means believing that people have the ability to be better, that culture can change, and maybe even that people who hate can learn to love. It's exhausting. —Jessica Valenti, journalist, 2013

power, and the need to ask critical questions about the meaning, purpose, and organization of sports in society.

Like feminist theories generally, critical feminist theory is based on the assumption that knowledge about social life requires an understanding of how gender and gender relations operate in our lives. It takes seriously the insights and research done by women as part of the knowledge production process.

In the sociology of sport, critical feminist theory explains that sports are gendered activities—their meaning, purpose, and organization lead to a celebration of a form of masculinity in which aggression, violence, physical domination, and conquest are highly valued. Relatedly, it explains how and why the bodies, abilities, orientations, and relationships of girls and women are systematically devalued in sports. Finally, it explains why gender equity and the transformation of the culture and structure of sports are in the best interests of both females and males.

Research based on critical feminist theory generally focuses on one or more of the following questions:

1. How have girls and women been excluded or discouraged from participating in sports, and why do some men continue to resist gender equity in sports?
2. How are sports involved in producing and maintaining ideas about what it means to be a man in society and why tough and aggressive men are valued more than men with other traits?
3. How are sports and sport participation involved in the production of gendered ideas about physicality, sexuality, and the body?
4. Why do many people assume that men who play sports are heterosexual, and why have men's locker rooms served for so long as sites for the expression of homophobia, gay-bashing jokes, and comments that demean women?

5. Why have gay men been so hesitant to come out in high-profile sports, and why do some women continue to fear being called lesbians if they become strong and powerful athletes?

6. How are media sports produced to give differential coverage to women's and men's sports, and how do media representations of male and female athletes influence gender ideology in society?

7. Why are sports promoted as healthy developmental activities when the injury rates in certain sports are so high?

8. What strategies are effective in transforming the male-centered gender ideology that is promoted and reproduced through most competitive sports?

These questions, inspired by critical feminist theory, deal with issues that affect our lives every day. In fact, unless we have thoughtful answers to them, we really don't know much about sports or society.

Like all theories, critical feminist theory is revised as its weaknesses and oversights are identified. For example, today it focuses more directly on understanding gender in terms of how it is connected with other categories of experience, including age, sexuality, race and ethnicity, social class, ability, religion, and nationality—in order to gain a full understanding of its importance in everyday life. Additionally, critical feminist theory today is no longer just about women (Adams, 2011; Allain, 2008; Anderson, 2008a, 2008b, 2011a, 2011b; Baker and Hotek, 2011; Chimot and Louveau, 2010; Crocket, 2012; Fogel, 2011; Martin, 2012; Messner, 2011; Thorpe, 2009a; Yochim, 2010). Much of the focus is now on social justice, equality of opportunities, and analyzing ideologies that undermine fairness and social inclusion related to gender and other identity categories (Bose, 2012; Flintoff, 2008; Hardin and Whiteside, 2009; Dorothy Smith, 2009; Travers, 2008, 2011, 2013a, 2013b; Travers and Deri, 2011). For this reason, critical feminist research now looks at how gender intersects with other socially significant factors to influence people's lives.

Younger scholars today often use critical feminist theory, but they are less likely than their older peers to describe themselves as feminists. They accept feminist principles, but want to move beyond the weaknesses and oversights of past feminist approaches that often focused too much on the lives of upper-middle-class, able-bodied, white, heterosexual women and were not as inclusive as they should have been. They know that the meaning and real-life implications of gender vary in the lives of women and men who face different social circumstances depending on their access to resources, jobs, medical care, and community support. Therefore, feminism may be less visible today than in the 1980s and 1990s because so many people now take it for granted, but feminism and critical feminist theory remain as viable as ever.

We have not yet entered what some describe as a postfeminist world. Gender and gender relations remain contentious issues in many spheres, and they continue to be central concerns for those of us who study sports in society. Since the beginning of this century feminist theories have been increasingly integrated into sociology and the sociology of sport and combined with other theories to the point that feminism is no longer considered a separate project seeking legitimacy and challenging the way social research is done. In this sense, the emerging legacy of feminism influences our lives and makes us aware of the problems associated with systematically excluding particular categories of people as we try to understand sports in society.

Finally, from a practical standpoint, as organizations, communities, and societies seek to revive physical activity and sport participation in everyday life, the concepts and research inspired by critical feminist theory are invaluable tools. Without awareness of the challenges faced when seeking inclusion and participation, people who manage or work in sport programs often find that they serve a select few and reproduce existing patterns of inactivity. Young people hoping to work in sport programs are much less likely to find jobs if participation rates do not increase in all demographic sectors. *How might familiarity with research guided by critical feminist theory help bring about increased participation in sports?*

people's actions and relationships and the organization and dynamics of social worlds. Additionally, theories guide research and the interpretation of research findings. This makes knowledge in the sociology of sport more valid and reliable than most of what we read, see, or hear in the media and discuss in our everyday conversations about sports.

Personal experience is a useful starting point for understanding the role of research and theory in knowledge production. This is because each of us gathers information about the people and things around us and uses it to develop experience-based explanations or "personal theories" about people, relationships, events, and social worlds.

We use personal theories to anticipate events, the actions of others, and the consequences of our actions in various situations. But these theories are limited because they focus on our individual circumstances and immediate social worlds. On the other hand, research and theories in the sociology of sport take us beyond the limitations of our own experiences and worlds.

Social research follows systematic and rigorous guidelines for collecting and analyzing data, and social theories are systematically tested, compared with related theories, and presented for others to examine. The goal of social research and theory in the sociology of sport is to develop logical and verifiable explanations of the social worlds created in association with sports and the actions and relationships of people in those social worlds.

The case study of Michael Messner's research illustrates that scholars in the sociology of sport use systematic and carefully planned methods as they study and develop explanations of sports. The five-stage process of producing knowledge consists of (1) developing research questions; (2) selecting appropriate theory and research methods; (3) collecting and analyzing data; (4) using research findings to produce conclusions; and (5) publishing results so that others may assess their validity and reliability.

Three types of theories guide most sociology of sport research. *Cultural theories* help us study and understand the meanings that people give to sports, sport experiences, and relationships formed in and through sports. *Interactionist theories* help us study and understand the origins, dynamics, and consequences of social relationships connected with sports. And *structural theories* help us study and understand the ways that various forms of social organization influence actions and relationships in sports and the social worlds associated with sports in society.

Depending on the research topic and the goals of the project, researchers use either a quantitative or a qualitative approach when collecting and analyzing data, or a combination of the two. Data in sociology of sport studies are usually collected through surveys, interviews, observations, or text analysis.

Many people in the sociology of sport use a critical approach as they do research and develop theory. This means that they are committed to producing knowledge that can be used to promote fairness and equity in sports and society, expose and challenge exploitation, and empower those who are disadvantaged by the current organization of sports in society. Overall, critical scholars are dedicated to the idea that sociological knowledge should be used to create and sustain social worlds in which basic human needs can be satisfied fairly and equitably.

Research and theories in the sociology of sport help us understand that sports are more than mere reflections of society. Instead, sports are sites where meanings, relationships, and forms of social organization are created, maintained, and changed. Learning about the knowledge production process in the sociology of sport is part of the process of thinking critically about the issues and controversies discussed in the following chapters. When we use research and theories critically, we become aware of the deeper game associated with sports in society and this makes us more informed participants in our families, schools, communities, and societies. How we use this knowledge depends on how we are engaged as citizens of our schools, communities, and society.

SUPPLEMENTAL READINGS:

Reading 1. Sociologists use more than one theoretical approach

Reading 2. The meaning of pain: Interactionist
theory as a research guide

Reading 3. Specific theories used in the sociology
of sport

Reading 4. Feminist theories in the sociology of
sport

Reading 5. Sociology of sport research today is
based on a critical approach

Reading 6. A European approach: Figurational
theory

SPORT MANAGEMENT ISSUES

• You are hired to study why athletes are
willing to play while they are in pain or
injured. Explain which theory (cultural, interactionist, structural) you would use to guide
your research. What research questions would
you ask, what would be the focus of your
analysis, and what concepts would you use in
your study?

• You are hired to study the pros and cons of
intercollegiate sports on your campus. Today
you report on the steps in your research project.
Identify the steps and briefly explain each as
you will do them.

• As a sport management consultant you are
hired by the Women's Center at a major university to study gender and sports on their campus.
You use some of Messner's work as a model
for your project. Explain the data collection
methods you will use.

• Research using a critical approach may produce
findings that challenge individuals in sport
management positions. Identify examples
of possible research findings that might be
rejected or ignored by executives for a professional sport team.

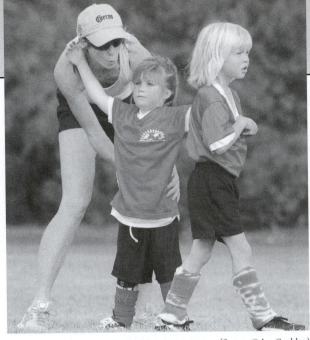

(*Source:* © Jay Coakley)

SPORTS AND SOCIALIZATION

Who Plays and What Happens to Them?

I know how to manage a football game. The problem with me is, sometimes, managing my life.

—Lawrence Taylor, NFL Hall of Fame player (Associated Press, 2012)

Why do we even pretend that sportspeople are models of propriety? Or rather why do we need them to be? . . . we continue to project an irrational desire for the physically perfect to be spiritually strong.

—Julia Baird, journalist (2004)

. . . so many kids don't even know what they could be good at because they're only playing one sport since they were eight years old. So, I look back and I'm grateful that I had the opportunity to play those other sports.

—Jennie Finch, Gold medalist softball pitcher (Jacobson, 2010)

If I have a shot at the championship and there's two races to go and my head is hurting and I just came through a wreck . . . I'm not going to say anything.

—Jeff Gordon, NASCAR driver (Moore, 2012)

Chapter Outline

Learning Objectives

- Describe what occurs during the socialization process, and explain why it is important to study socialization as an interactive learning process.
- Identify key factors involved in the process of becoming and staying involved in sports.
- Describe key factors involved in the process of changing or ending sport participation, and explain when the retirement process is most likely to be difficult for a former athlete.
- Understand why sport participation does not have the same socialization effects for everyone who plays sports.
- Differentiate pleasure and participation sports from power and performance sports, and explain why it is important to

know these differences when discussing socialization in sports.

- Identify the conditions under which sport participation is most likely or least likely to have positive socialization effects on those who play sports.
- Explain why sport participation does not automatically lead to physical fitness and well-being and why it may not reduce obesity rates in a society.
- Identify examples of how sports are sites at which ideological messages are communicated to people in society.
- Explain what sociologists mean when they say that socialization is a community and cultural process.

Whenever we discuss why people play sports, why they stop playing, and what happens to them as they play, we deal with the process of social learning and development that sociologists call socialization.

For more than half a century, people in the sociology of sport have done research to learn about three topics that are central to discussions of sports and socialization:

1. The process of becoming involved and staying involved in sports
2. The process of changing or ending sport participation
3. The consequences, both positive and negative, of being involved in sports

This chapter is organized around these topics. As you read, you'll see that we've learned much about socialization and sports, but our understanding remains incomplete. Some of what we've learned is so complex that the discussions carry over to subsequent chapters.

The chapter closes with a discussion of socialization as a community and cultural process affecting many people at once.

WHAT IS SOCIALIZATION?

Socialization *is a process of learning and social development, which occurs as we interact with one another and become familiar with social worlds.* It involves forming ideas about who we are and what is important in our lives. We are *not* simply passive learners in this process. We actively participate in our own socialization as we form relationships and are influenced by others at the same time that we influence them. We actively interpret what we see and hear, and we accept, resist, and revise messages that we receive from others about who we are and how we are connected with social worlds. Therefore, socialization is not simply a one-way process of being molded and shaped by our social environment. Instead, it is an interactive process through which we make decisions about

our relationships, our interpretation of information that comes to us through interaction, and what we will say and do. It is through these decisions that we become who we are and influence the social worlds in which we participate.

Each of us experiences socialization as we learn about social worlds and use our knowledge to construct our own lives. In this sense, socialization, social development, and identity formation are interconnected processes. We make choices in this process, but our choices are influenced by the options available to us, the resources we have to assess them, and the context in which we make them (Van de Walle, 2011).

The *consequences* of these choices for our lives also depend on the contexts in which we make them. For example, one person might have opportunities to play many different sports and then be able to choose the one in which she or he has the best chances of succeeding, whereas another person might have an opportunity to play only one sport. Additionally, one person might play a sport in a context where there is excellent coaching, good support from others, and good mentors, whereas another person might play in a context where there is no one around to be a coach or mentor. Therefore, some of us are in better positions than others when it comes to using socialization experiences to our advantage and extending our knowledge, experience, and developmental opportunities.

This explanation of *socialization* is based on a *social interaction model* that is organized around a combination of cultural, interactionist, and structural theories. It leads researchers to assume that human beings learn values and norms and develop as individuals as they interact with others and participate in social worlds. For example, as children interact with their parents, other family members, teachers, and peers, they learn norms about safety and risk-taking and they learn to give meaning to the pain that comes with the bumps, bruises, and cuts that are a part of childhood. However, if they play organized sports, their interaction with coaches and teammates may lead them to define pain as a normal part of playing sports and to see sports injuries as symbols of their commitment to a team and their identity as an athlete. In this way sense, socialization can be is a powerful and influential process.

The social interaction model is widely used in the sociology of sport today, but some scholars continue to use a *personal internalization model* of socialization when they study sports. This model emphasizes that social learning occurs when people internalize the rules of society as they grow up in families, attend school, interact with peers, and receive messages through media. This approach has inspired many studies of socialization, but it mistakenly assumes that socialization is a one-way process in which learning occurs automatically.

Most studies based on the personal internalization model produce inconsistent and contradictory findings about why people play sports, why they stop, and what happens to them as they play. However, a few studies using this model of socialization have been carefully designed and provide detailed statistical analyses of the complex connections between sport participation and other aspects of people's lives (Berger et al., 2008; Guest and Schneider, 2003; Hershow et al., 2015; Hwang et al., 2013; Kraaykamp et al., 2012; Lee, 2013; Sabo et al., 2005; Shakib and Veliz, 2013). The findings in these studies identify three things: (1) general patterns in sport participation through the life course; (2) the barriers that prevent or discourage some people from playing sports; and (3) connections between sport participation and educational achievement, occupational success, sexual behavior and pregnancy rates, health and wellness, and general self-esteem. These findings are discussed throughout this chapter.

Most studies of sports and socialization today are based on a social interaction model and use qualitative rather than quantitative research methods. Instead of using written questionnaires or other quantitative methods that provide snapshots of people's lives, they use in-depth interviews and field observations to study smaller collections of people over time. This provides continuous videos rather than snapshots. Their goal is to obtain detailed descriptions of sport experiences as they occur in people's lives and then analyze the processes

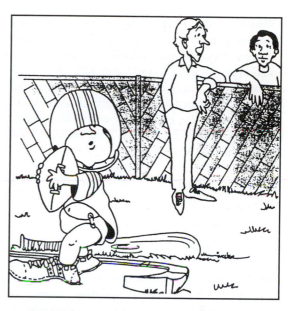

"I know this is starting early, but I can't let him get too far behind the other kids if he's going to succeed in life."

Research guided by structural theories focuses on who influences the sport participation patterns of children. Fathers and other family members are usually identified as *significant others* who influence when, how, and where children play sports.

through which people make decisions about sport participation and give meaning to sport experiences. Finally, they seek to connect those decisions and meanings with the cultural and structural contexts in which sports and sport participation exist. This approach captures the complexity of the processes through which people become and stay involved in sports, change or end sport participation, and incorporate sports into their lives. The rest of this chapter uses both research snapshots and videos to explain what we know about sports and socialization today.

BECOMING AND STAYING INVOLVED IN SPORTS

Who plays sports consistently over time, who plays and drops out, and who never plays? This three-part question is important today, as many societies deal with health problems that are partly related to a lack of regular physical exercise (Nike, Inc. 2012).

Carefully designed studies based on structural theories and a personal internalization model of socialization have found that sport participation is related to three factors: (1) a person's abilities, characteristics, and resources; (2) the influence of significant others, including parents, siblings, teachers, peers, and role models; and (3) the availability of opportunities to play sports in ways that are personally satisfying. These are the snapshot research findings that help us explain how and why people become involved and stay involved in sports. However, a more complete explanation is provided by detailed stories from people about their sport participation. When these stories are collected in research based on a social interaction model, they provide socialization videos rather than single snapshots.

Studies using in-depth interviews and participant observation indicate that sport participation is connected to multiple and diverse processes that make up people's lives, and it occurs as people interact with others and make decisions based on available opportunities and the meanings they give to sports in connection with what they want to happen in their lives. These decisions and meanings are not permanent and often change as social conditions and relationships change. Furthermore, as people stay involved in sports, their reasons for participating usually change over time. When there are no reasons, they discontinue or change their sport participation—until things change again and there are new reasons to become re-involved.

Current knowledge about the processes through which people become and stay involved in sports has been produced through multiple studies across various populations of people in different situations. The most effective way to learn what we know about socialization is to review a few studies that highlight key aspects of these processes. The following summaries provide three sociological

videos illustrating processes of becoming and staying involved in sports.

Example 1: Family Culture and the Sport Participation of Children

Sociologist Sharon Wheeler studies sport education and development in England. In one of her research projects she conducted semi-structured interviews with elementary school children identified as "sporty"—that is, playing sports was important in their lives—and their parents. She found that the parents in each family defined sport participation as important for young people and willingly dedicated considerable family time, money, and energy to support their children as they sampled different sport activities in various programs. Transporting them to practices and games and attending games were part of the family routine and overall lifestyle. Their support, however, had limits in that they did not coach or critique their children nor did they provide anything other than verbal encouragement as they participated (Wheeler, 2012, 2014).

Because these families lived in the United Kingdom, parents were not obsessed with pushing their children to excel so they might obtain athletic scholarships to college, as many parents do in the United States. These UK families also were relatively well off, meaning that they had the resources to sustain a lifestyle that included sport participation. This lifestyle was linked with a culture created and sustained by a network of families with similar beliefs and lifestyles. This culture of family sport participation then served as a context in which playing sports was seamlessly integrated into the lives of the children. Sports for these children were simply a taken-for-granted part of family life.

Of course, families with fewer resources and less access to sport programs would have different lifestyles in which such a culture would be more difficult to create and sustain. This would also be the case for single-parent families and families

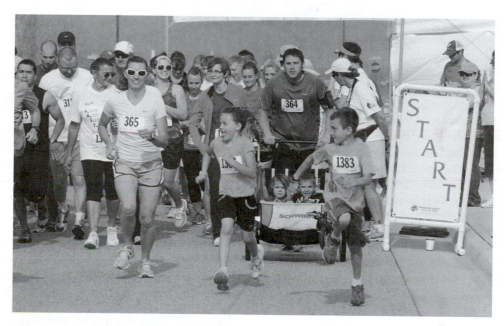

When physical activities and sport participation are incorporated into everyday family life, children are more likely to remain physically active through their lives. The four children in this family are learning that running is an enjoyable activity for men and women, young and old. The positive memories from "fun runs" such as this will be factors that encourage these children to be active in the future. (*Source:* © Jay Coakley)

in which sports were given a low priority for the expenditure of resources.

Wheeler notes that it is important to study families as the immediate contexts in which sport participation is initiated and nurtured. This is especially the case as publicly funded sport programs are eliminated and selectively replaced by private fee-based programs that require parental support and family resources for transportation, uniforms, equipment, and paid coaches.

Wheeler's findings are consistent with other research in which family culture has been found to provide a context in which children see sport involvement as a normal part of their everyday lives and continue playing sports as they become adolescents and young adults (Birchwood et al., 2008; Hennessy et al., 2010; Kraaykamp et al., 2012; Quarmby and Dagkas, 2010). Her findings also suggest that short-term interventions designed to increase sport participation among young people outside of this culture are likely to fail if they ignore the extent to which families now serve as the contexts in which participation decisions are made and supported. For example, young people cannot develop or sustain a commitment to sport participation if their families lack the resources to pay for their opportunities to sample different sports and select one or more programs that suit their interests. Additionally, if they don't become involved during childhood or early adolescence, they are less like to feel comfortable playing sports later in their lives.

Wheeler's research shows us that the process of becoming and staying involved in sports is closely tied to family dynamics and decisions, and these are influenced by structural and cultural factors.

Structural factors include the availability of sport facilities, equipment, financial support, coaching, and competition opportunities (Wheeler and Green, 2014). Cultural factors include the importance given to particular sports and to the ways that one's age, gender, race, ethnicity, sexuality, and ability influence the meaning of being an athlete. For example, data from a national sample of young people in the United States indicates that African American youth are more likely than their white, Latino, and Asian counterparts to receive encouragement for sport participation through all their relationships, including family, teachers, coaches, peers, and friends (Shakib and Veliz, 2013). This is partly because many people in the United States assume that there is a connection between sport and race and that African Americans are either better at or more interested in sports than others, and that sports provide them with mobility opportunities that are less accessible in other realms of life.

Example 2: To Participate or Not to Participate

When I worked at the University of Chichester in England, my colleague Anita White and I received a grant to study why most young people did not participate in a highly publicized, state-sponsored sport program. We designed a study in which we used in-depth interviews to explore how British adolescents in a working-class area east of London made decisions about what they did in their free time (Coakley and White, 1999).

Data from our interviews indicated that the young people took a combination of factors into account as they made decisions about sport participation. These factors included the following:

1. Their ideas about the connection between sport participation and other interests and goals in their lives
2. Their desires to develop and display competence so they could gain recognition and respect from others
3. Social support for participation plus access to the resources needed for participation (time, transportation, equipment, and money)

4. Memories of past experiences with physical activities and sports
5. Sport-related images and meanings that were part of their social worlds

Overall, the young people decided to play sports when it helped them extend control over their lives, achieve development and career goals, and present themselves to others as competent. We also found that young women were less likely than young men to imagine that they could accomplish those things by playing sports. Therefore, the young women took sports less seriously and chose to participate less often.

The young people in our study made their decisions by determining if sport participation would add something positive to their lives. They didn't passively respond to the world around them, and their decisions and sport participation patterns shifted over time, depending on access to opportunities, available resources, and changes in their identities. Therefore, socialization into sports was a *continuous, interactive process* grounded in the social and cultural contexts in which they lived.

Our study also found that people make decisions to participate in sports for different reasons at different points in their lives. This is consistent with theories stating that personal growth depends on accomplishing developmental tasks associated with various stages of childhood, adolescence, young adulthood, and adulthood. Therefore, the issues considered by seven-year-olds as they make decisions about sport participation differ from the issues considered by fourteen-year-olds, forty-year-olds, and sixty-year-olds. Furthermore, when seven-year-olds make decisions about sport participation today, they do so in different social and cultural contexts than the contexts in which seven-year-olds lived in 1980 or will live in 2030.

After analyzing our interview data, it was clear to Anita and me that sport participation decisions among these young people were tied to their perceptions of the cultural importance of sports and the links between playing sports, gaining social acceptance, and achieving personal goals.

Therefore, when we study why people become and stay involved in sports, we should take into account people's perceptions of how sport participation is related to their own growth and development, how sports are integrated into their social worlds, and the extent to which participation is supported by widely accepted ideologies in their culture.

I was reminded of these points when I read that some parents in Ethiopia now accept competitive running as a way for their daughters to achieve financial success. This change has allowed girls to take up running as a strategy to stay in school, avoid an arranged marriage (as a young teen), and seek a life that consists of more than washing laundry, preparing food, and obeying a husband who is likely to define her as a form of property. Running, for girls lucky enough to be identified as talented, opens up developmental opportunities, gives them more control over their lives, and enables them to claim their bodies as their own. This is why thirteen-year-old Ethiopian girls are more likely to define running as a desirable activity than thirteen-year-old girls living in air-conditioned homes in Beverly Hills, California—the context and consequences of their decisions are much different.

Example 3: The Process of Being Accepted as an Athlete

Peter Donnelly and Kevin Young (1999) are sociologists who have studied sports as social worlds in which people form relationships and unique ways of life organized around shared interests. One of their studies focused on the process through which people became accepted members of sport cultures.

Using data that Donnelly collected from expert rock climbers and Young collected from elite rugby players, they concluded that playing sports occurs in connection with processes of identity formation. They explained that becoming an athlete in a particular sport culture occurs through a four-phase process:

1. Acquiring knowledge about the sport
2. Interacting with people involved in the sport
3. Learning how participation occurs and what people in the sport expect from each other as athletes
4. Becoming recognized and fully accepted as an athlete in the sport culture

This finding shows that becoming an athlete in a particular sport depends on learning to "talk the talk and walk the walk" so that one is identified and accepted as an athlete *by other athletes*. This process of identification and acceptance is continuous; it doesn't happen once and for all time. When athletes can no longer talk the talk and walk the walk, interaction with other athletes declines, and support for their identity fades away. Membership in a sport culture is always temporary; it depends on what you do today, not what you did in the past.

To understand Donnelly and Young's findings, observe skateboarders, in-line skaters, snowboarders, beach volleyball players, basketball players, or members of any sport culture. Each culture has a unique vocabulary, its own way of referring to its members and what they do, unique ways of thinking about and doing their sports, and special understandings of what they expect from each other. New participants are tested and "pushed" by the "veterans" before being accepted as true skaters, riders, boarders, volleyball players, or ballers. Vocabularies may change over time, but the process of being accepted as an athlete exists in all sport cultures.

Donnelly and Young help us understand that becoming and staying involved in a sport often depends on establishing social connections, being accepted in a sport culture, and receiving social support for the formation of an athlete identity (see also, Light et al., 2013). This finding also helps explain why there are so few girls and women in alternative sport cultures. Boys and men have defined riding on a board, whether it is down a mountain, a wave, or a sidewalk curb as an activity that conveys a valued form of masculinity. In the process, they create cultures that make it very difficult for girls and women to be accepted as authentic "board athletes." In other words, becoming and staying involved in sports is a complex, *interactive* socialization and *identity formation* process.

In summary, these three studies provide complementary videos about the process of becoming and staying involved in sports. They show that people don't make decisions about sport participation once and for all time; they make them day after day as they consider how playing a sport is related to their lives. These decisions are made in particular social and cultural contexts and they are influenced by access to resources and the meanings attached to gender, class, skin color, ethnicity, age, and physical abilities.

CHANGING OR ENDING SPORT PARTICIPATION

Questions about becoming and staying involved in sports are usually accompanied by questions about changing or ending involvement. Research done during the latter half of the twentieth century helped us understand the following basic facts about changing and ending sport participation:

• When people drop out of a particular sport, they don't drop out of all sports forever, nor do they cut all ties with sports.

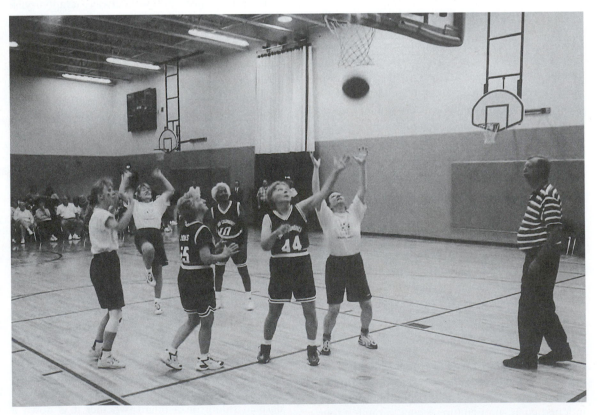

Although people may drop out of sports at one point in the life course, they may return at a later point. This team of women, all over seventy years old, is playing an exhibition game against a group of younger women. The team is raising funds to travel to the national finals in the Senior Games. Most of these older women had not played competitive basketball for thirty to fifty years. (*Source:* © Jay Coakley)

- Many people play different and less-competitive sports as they become older, or they move into other sport roles such as coach, administrator, or sports businessperson.
- Dropping out of sports is usually connected with developmental changes and transitions in the rest of a person's life—changing schools, graduating, getting a job, getting married, having children, and so on.
- Dropping out of sports is not always the result of negative experiences, although injuries, exploitation, poor coaching, and abuse from coaches influence some decisions to change or end participation.
- Problems may occur for those who end long careers in sports, especially those who have no identities apart from sports or lack social and material resources for making transitions into other careers and relationships.

More recent studies, especially those using qualitative research methods and a social interactionist model of socialization, have built on these findings and extended our understanding of the process of changing or ending sport participation. The following summaries of three studies are representative of this research.

Example 1: Burnout Among Young Athletes

My work with coaches and my interest in identity issues led me to study young people who decided to quit sport at a time when they were experiencing great success, often as age-group champions in their sports (Coakley, 1992, 2011a). People described these young people as "burned out," so I decided to interview former elite adolescent athletes who were identified as cases of burnout.

Data collected through in-depth interviews indicated that burnout during adolescence was grounded in the organization and authority structure of many high-performance sports for young people. It occurred when young athletes felt they

no longer had control over their lives and could not explore, develop, and nurture identities apart from sports. This led to increased stress and decreased fun as they did their sports. Burnout occurred when stress became high and fun declined to the point that they no longer felt that continued participation was worth their effort.

The data also indicated that stress increased and fun decreased when sport programs were organized so that successful young athletes felt that they could not accomplish important developmental tasks during adolescence. My conclusion was that burnout could be prevented only if sport programs were reorganized so that young athletes had more control over their lives. Stress management strategies might delay burnout, but they would not change the underlying organizational and development barriers that caused burnout. Overall, my study led me to conclude that young people sometimes end sport participation during late adolescence when they feel that their career in a sport prevents them from developing the autonomy and the multiple identities necessary to effectively claim adult status in U.S. culture.

Example 2: Getting out of Sports and Getting on with Life

Konstantinos Koukouris (1994, 2005) is a physical educator from Greece who wanted to know why seriously committed athletes ended or reduced their sport participation. After analyzing questionnaire data from 157 former national athletes, Koukouris identified thirty-four who had ceased or reduced sport participation between the ages of eighteen and twenty-four. In-depth interviews with these people enabled him to identify patterns in the disengagement process.

His data indicated that ending or reducing sport participation was a voluntary decision among these athletes. But this decision was often part of a process during which they stopped playing and then started again more than once. In other words, they hadn't gone "cold turkey" as they withdrew from sport. Their decisions were usually associated with two practical factors: (1) the need to obtain a job and support themselves and (2) realistic judgments about their sport skills and the chances of advancing to higher levels of competition. As they graduated from high school or college, the athletes faced the expectation that they should work and be responsible for their livelihoods. But jobs interfered with the time needed to train and play sports at an elite level. Furthermore, as they spent money to establish adult lifestyles, there was little left to pay for serious training. At the same time, their demanding training programs conflicted with new responsibilities in their adult lives.

When they ended serious training, many of these young adults sought other ways to be physically active or involved in sports. Some encountered problems, but most of them grew and developed in positive ways, much like their peers who had never played elite sports. Most of the former athletes perceived the end of their serious training and competition as an inevitable, necessary, and usually beneficial developmental change in their lives.

Koukouris (2005) also did in-depth interviews with nineteen elite gymnasts and found that their disengagement from sport often occurred prematurely due to a combination of mental and physical exhaustion, lack of support from coaches and administrators, and the politics of judging and Federation governance. Unlike the athletes in Koukouris's previous study, the gymnasts began their elite careers at a very young age and required more guidance and support to prevent them from becoming disillusioned and gradually disengaging from their sport.

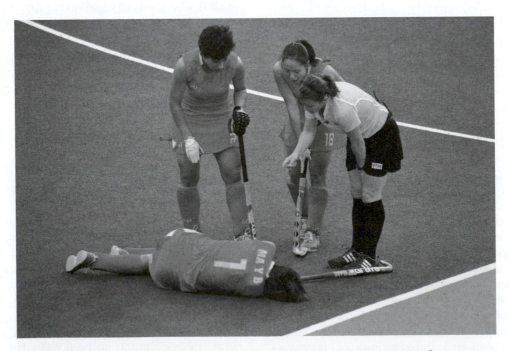

Many factors influence the decisions to drop out of sports or shift participation from one sport to another. Although identity changes, access to resources, and life course issues are involved, injuries often force people to make changes. In all these cases, as our circumstances change, so do our ideas about ourselves and about sports and sport participation. (*Source:* © Lara Killick)

Example 3: Changing Personal Investments in Sport Careers

Garry Wheeler at the University of Alberta, has been concerned with the careers of athletes with a disability and what happens when their playing careers end. Building on a previous study of Paralympic athletes, Wheeler and his fellow researchers interviewed forty athletes from the United Kingdom, Canada, Israel, and the United States (Wheeler et al., 1999). The data indicated that athletes in each of these countries became deeply involved in sports and often achieved a high level of success in a relatively short time. Through sports they developed a sense of personal competence and established identities as elite athletes.

Ending active sport participation and making the transition into other spheres of life often presented challenges for these athletes. Retirement generally came suddenly and forced them to reinvest time and energy into other activities and relationships. As they reconnected with family members and friends, returned to school, and resumed occupational careers, some of the former athletes experienced emotional problems. However, most stayed connected with sports and sport organizations as coaches, administrators, or recreational athletes. Those few who hoped to regain their elite athlete status usually experienced difficulties during the retirement transition, whereas those who accepted the end of their competitive careers had fewer adjustment problems.

In summary, research shows that ending or changing sport participation often involves the same interactive and decision-making processes that occur as a person becomes and stays involved in sports. Changes in participation are often the result of decisions associated with other life events, social relationships, and cultural expectations related to development. This means that theories explaining why people play sports and change their participation over time must take into account identity issues and developmental processes that are part of the social and cultural contexts in which people make decisions about sports in their lives (van Houten et al., 2015).

Furthermore, theories must take into account the personal, social, and material resources that former athletes possess as they make transitions to other relationships, activities, and careers. When problems occur during this transition, they are associated with an unwillingness to transition into identities unrelated to sports and a lack of the personal and material resources needed to negotiate the transitional challenges they face (Tinley, 2015).

Research suggests that changes and retirement transitions are less likely to involve problems if sport participation has *expanded* a person's identities, experiences, relationships, and resources. Difficulties are most likely when athletes have never had the desire or the chance to live outside the culture of elite sports and learn to negotiate their lives in nonsport social worlds. This is highlighted in Scott Tinley's fifteen year study of retired professional and elite athletes. In one of many interviews, a former NFL player disclosed this identity-related statement: "Without football, without my ability to express myself through football I am nobody. I will disappear. Football has been my life and I have so little else" (Tinley, 2015, p. 133).

BEING INVOLVED IN SPORTS: WHAT HAPPENS?

Beliefs about the consequences of sport participation vary from culture to culture, but many people in North America and Europe accept what was described in Chapter 1 (p. 11) as the *great sport myth*. In other words, they believe that playing sports builds character and improves health and well-being. These beliefs create encouragement for children to play sports, and they lead to support for funding sports programs in schools, building stadiums, promoting teams and leagues, and sponsoring international events such as the Olympic Games, the Paralympics, and world championships.

Do Sports Build Character?

For over a half century, researchers have tried to prove that "sport builds character." Their studies have compared the traits, attitudes, and behaviors of those who play organized sports with those who don't. These one time snapshot comparisons have produced inconsistent and confusing findings. This is because researchers have used inconsistent definitions of *character* and have designed their studies around two faulty assumptions (McCormack and Chalip, 1988). First, they've wrongly assumed that *all* athletes have the same or similar experiences in *all* organized competitive sports. Second, they've wrongly assumed that organized sports provide unique experiences that are not available in other activities. These assumptions have caused researchers to overlook the following important things when they study sports and socialization:

1. Sport experiences are diverse, because sport programs and teams are organized in vastly different ways. Therefore, we cannot make unqualified general statements about the consequences of sport participation. This point is explained further in Reflect on Sports, pp. 64–66.
2. People who choose or are selected to play sports often have different character traits than those who do not choose to play or are not selected by coaches. Therefore, sports may not *build* character as much as they are organized to *select* people who already possess certain character traits that are valued by coaches and compatible with highly organized, competitive, physical activities.
3. The meanings that people give to sport experiences vary from one person to another, even when they play in the same programs and on the same teams. Therefore, there are important variations in what athletes learn when they play sports and in how they apply what they learn to their lives.
4. As people change and grow older they often alter the meanings they give to their past sport experiences and integrate them into their lives in new ways as they develop new ideas and values.
5. Socialization occurs through the social interaction that accompanies sport participation. Therefore, the meaning and importance of playing sports depend on a person's social relationships and the social and cultural contexts in which participation occurs.
6. The socialization that occurs in sports may also occur in other activities. Therefore, people who do not play sports may have developmental experiences similar to the experiences of athletes.

Due to these oversights, studies that compare "athletes" with "nonathletes" have produced inconsistent and misleading research results about the impact of sport participation in people's lives. After evaluating these studies, I've concluded that sport participation is most likely to have positive socialization consequences when it provides athletes with the following things:

- Opportunities to explore and develop identities apart from playing sports
- Knowledge-building experiences that go beyond the locker room and playing field
- New relationships, especially with people who are not connected with sports and do not base their interaction on a person's status or identity as an athlete
- Explicit examples of how lessons learned in sports may be applied to specific situations apart from sports (skills transfer)
- Opportunities to develop and display competence in nonsport activities that are observed by other people who can serve as mentors and advocates outside sports

In other words, positive socialization outcomes *do not* occur automatically.

My review of past research also suggests that when playing sports *constricts* opportunities, experiences, relationships, and general competence apart from sports, it is likely to have negative

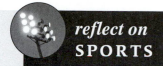

reflect on
SPORTS

Power and Performance *versus* Pleasure and Participation
Different Sports, Different Experiences, Different Consequences

Sport experiences are diverse. It's a mistake to assume that all sports are organized around the same goals and orientations, played in the same spirit, or defined in the same way. For example, there are highly organized competitive sports, informal sports, adventure sports, recreational sports, extreme sports, alternative sports, cooperative sports, folk sports, contact sports, artistic sports, team sports, individual sports, and so on. However, at this point in history, the most dominant sport form in wealthy postindustrial nations is organized around a **power and performance model.**

Power and performance sports are highly organized and competitive; they emphasize the following factors:

- Using strength, speed, and power to push human limits and achieve competitive success
- Proving excellence through competitive success and attributing success to dedication, hard work, and sacrifice
- Being willing to risk physical well-being and play with pain
- Exclusive processes through which participants are cut from teams if they do not meet elite performance standards

- A chain of command in which owners and administrators control coaches, and coaches control athletes
- Competing against opponents and defining them as enemies to be conquered

These points exaggerate the characteristics of power and performance sports to show that experiences in these sports are very different from experiences in other sport forms. Although, many people use the power and performance model as a standard for defining "real" sports, it is not the only model around which sports are organized. For example, people in many societies often play other forms of sport, including various revisions of, alternatives to, and reactions against dominant sports.

The sport forms most unlike power and performance sports today are organized around a **pleasure and participation model,** and they emphasize the following factors:

- Active participation revolves around connections between people, integration of mind and body, and harmony with the environment

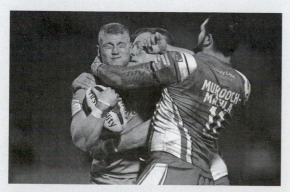

Power and performance sports involve the use of strength, speed, and power to dominate opponents in the quest for competitive victories. (*Source:* © Al Bello/ Getty Images)

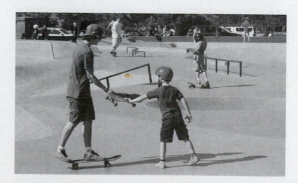

Pleasure and participation sports may involve competition, but the primary emphasis is on connections between people and personal expression through participation. This is often seen at skateboard parks where participants support and encourage each other. (*Source:* © Jay Coakley)

Continued

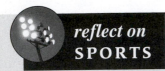

Power and Performance *versus* Pleasure and Participation (*continued*)

- A spirit of personal expression, enjoyment, growth, good health, and mutual concern among participants
- Personal empowerment created by gaining knowledge about and pleasure from the body
- Inclusive processes through which participation is encouraged by accommodating ability differences
- Democratic decision-making structures in which relationships are characterized by cooperation and sharing power
- An emphasis on participating and competing *with* others who are defined as partners in creating and meeting physical challenges

Again, these points exaggerate the characteristics of pleasure and participation sports, but they show that experiences in these sports are very different from experiences in power and participation sports.

These two sport forms do *not* represent all the ways that sports might be organized, played, and defined. There are sports that contain elements of both forms and reflect diverse ideas about what is important in physical activities. However, power and performance sports remain dominant today because they receive the most attention, support, and sponsorship. When people play or watch these sports, their socialization experiences are different from their socialization experiences in pleasure and participation sports.

WHY ARE POWER AND PERFORMANCE SPORTS SO DOMINANT TODAY?

Power and performance sports are dominant today because, they foster the interests of people and organizations with the resources to sponsor and stage large sport events. History shows that wealthy and influential people in societies around the world have used different strategies to maintain their privileged positions. Some have used coercive strategies such as employing the police and military to maintain their control over resources and people, but most have used cultural or "soft" strategies that foster the belief that they deserve their wealth and power and that society benefits from their resources.

In countries where wealth and power have been controlled by a monarchy, the privileged position of the royal family is based on the belief that it is their birthright to rule over others. Therefore, kings and queens maintain their privileged positions as long as their "subjects" believe that birthrights represent legitimate claims to wealth and power. This is why the church and state have usually been closely aligned in societies with monarchies—kings and queens use the clergy to promote the belief that their wealth and power are bestowed on them by a divine, supernatural source, such as a god.

In democratic countries, most people use *merit,* or "personal achievement," as a standard when judging whether the possession of wealth and power is legitimate. Therefore, it is only when most people believe that wealth and power are rightfully earned that those who possess them are seen in a positive way. When a democracy is characterized by widespread inequality, as in the United States today, people with wealth and power promote the idea that they have earned their privileged positions through hard work and intelligence and that society as a whole benefits from their control and influence. In recent history, this idea has been promoted by emphasizing that *competition* is a natural part of social life and the only fair basis for determining who gets what in society. When there is widespread acceptance of this idea, people generally idealize and defer to wealthy and powerful people and believe that they deserve what they have.

Power and performance sports are widely promoted and sponsored by people with wealth and power because these sports are based on an ideology that celebrates competitive winners and defines competition as the only fair and natural way to distribute rewards. This ideology also explains and justifies economic inequalities as part of the natural order of things. The executives of major corporations realize this and collectively allocate billions of dollars annually to sponsor power and performance sports worldwide. They personally believe that rewards should go to winners, that winners deserve wealth and power, and that the ranking of people on the basis of wealth and power is fair and natural. By sponsoring power and performance sports and making them a major source of enjoyment and excitement in people's lives, they promote these beliefs at the same time that they profit from selling the vehicles, fast food, soft drinks, and beer advertised during sports events.

The sport forms that challenge this ideology may be popular among some people, but they don't receive many sponsorship dollars from wealthy and powerful people. For example, alternative sports such as skateboarding and disk sport (Frisbee) were often banned and associated with deviance until they were organized around a power and performance model. Free-flowing, expressive alternative sports that don't produce winners and losers receive little attention from powerful sponsors. But when ESPN used a power and performance model to restructure these sports in the X Games, corporate sponsors began to support them. Today, many of these sports have lost their alternative character. Celebrity athletes now hawk corporate products and lifestyles of consumption. At the same time, participation comes to be tied with brands and the quest for the latest piece of equipment, clothing, or energy drink endorsed by the athletes. The masses watch and idolize the select few at the top. This raises questions about who benefits from the ways sports are currently organized and supported worldwide.

Are there ways to preserve and promote pleasure and participation sports under these circumstances? Is this important to do in today's societies? From a policy and management perspective these are important questions to answer.

· ·

consequences for a person's overall development. Therefore, we cannot make a general statement that sports build *or* undermine character development. Neither positive nor negative character is automatically developed by playing sports. Sport experiences are diverse, and they are given meaning and incorporated into people's lives in various ways, depending on the social and cultural contexts in which they live (Denise Anderson, 2009; Hartmann, 2008; Light, 2010; Robbins, 2012; Swanson, 2009; Taylor and Turek, 2010; Taylor et al., 2010a, 2010b; Van Ingen, 2011).

This conclusion does *not* mean that sports and sport participation are irrelevant in people's lives. We know that discourses, images, and experiences related to sports are vivid and powerful in many social worlds. Sports *do* affect our lives and the world around us. However, we cannot separate those affects from the meanings that we give to sports and how we integrate them into our lives. Therefore, if we want to know what happens in sports, we must study sport experiences in the contexts in which they occur. This type of research provides insights into the complex connections between sports and socialization and helps us understand the conditions under which positive or negative outcomes occur among those who play sports (Holt, 2016).

Do Sports Improve Health and Physical Well-Being?

An international organization called Sport for Development and Peace asked a team of scholars at the University of Toronto to answer this question (SDP/IWG, 2007). After a critical review of English language studies worldwide, the scholars came to this conclusion:

> The physiological effects of participation in sport and physical activity are widely known, and one of the best established findings in the research literature. It is important to note that the effects are not a result of sport, . . . but of physical activity more generally. . . . Given clean air, adequate nutrition, and a variety of moderate levels of exercise, *there is a well-established direct positive relationship between physical health and physical activity,* including feelings of well-being associated with increasing

physical fitness. In addition, research increasingly points to both the preventive and rehabilitative effects of physical activity with respect to some diseases. (SDP/IWG Secretariat, p. 4)

This is a carefully worded statement because the authors knew that it was important to distinguish between *exercise, physical activity,* and *sports* when talking about physical health and well-being. Similarly, a report by the US Department of Health and Human Services (2008), "competitive athletes who participate and train at high levels (e.g., elite, professional sports, National Teams, Olympic athletes) in sports requiring high joint impact (e.g., football, track and field, soccer) for many years have higher rates of incident knee or hip OA [osteoarthritis] than do non-athletes" (p. G5–20). These athletes also incur abnormally high rates of joint injuries that result in eventual surgeries over the life course.

The Sport–Health Connection   The relationship between sports, exercise, and health has been widely studied (Ng and Popkin, 2012; Nike, Inc., 2012; USDHHS, 2008). When sociologist Ivan Waddington (2000a, 2000b, 2007) reviewed research on this topic, he concluded that the healthiest of all physical activities were rhythmic, noncompetitive exercises in which individuals control and regulate their own body movements. The research also indicated that health benefits decline when there is a shift from self-controlled exercise to competitive sports. This is because the injury rates in competitive sports are high enough to increase health costs above what is considered "average" in most populations. This benefit–cost ratio becomes even less favorable when there is a shift from noncontact to contact sports and from recreational sports to elite sports in which participants train intensely for more than 15 hours per week, play while injured, and perceive their bodies as tools for achieving competitive success.

The connection between sport and health is being viewed more critically now that mainstream media have published numerous stories about concussions, brain trauma, sudden cardiac arrest, heat stroke, overuse injuries, ACL injuries, and others

sustained regularly by athletes (Abrams, 2013; Cook, 2012; Gregory, 2012; Le Batard, 2013; Longman, 2011b; Pennington, 2013; USDHHS, 2008; Wiedeman, 2013).

Dr. Edward Wojtys, director of sport medicine at the University of Michigan, notes that ACL injuries are so frequent, especially among female athletes, that they are becoming a public health problem (Longman, 2011b). Athletes tear or rupture ligaments in over 250,000 knees each year and sustain between two and four million concussions. Knee surgeries and rehabilitation are major health-care costs in the United States. Overuse injuries among child athletes are increasingly common—about 300,000 per year—and it costs about $1.8 billion to treat those injuries (Zernicke et al., 2009). Additionally, about 5000 former NFL players and their families sued the NFL in 2013 for withholding information about the consequences of head trauma and other injuries that are causing them chronic problems and leading to massive health care costs. College athletes have filed suit against the NCAA for similar reasons. Football, hockey, lacrosse, and other sports now publicize new efforts to make participation safer for athletes. Research on these issues is discussed in Chapter 6, but at this point people must clarify what they mean when they say that "sports improve health and physical well-being."

In practical terms, if you lack health insurance, it is best to stay fit by doing aerobics, walking, swimming, and jumping rope; and if you play football, rugby, hockey, or other competitive contact sports, you should have good health insurance because your medical bills are likely to be higher than average. If you play sports in which you sustain concussions, receive repetitive hits to the head, or collide violently with other players, you may also want to have long-term-care insurance in case you develop chronic traumatic encephalopathy (CTE) and are not able to function on your own in later life. Even if you play golf, softball, soccer, and other sports that require sudden and forceful twisting motions or sprinting from a dead stop, it is important to have health-care insurance.

The Sport–Obesity Connection Obesity is a highly publicized health issue today. Nearly, every discussion of this issue ends with the conclusion that eating right and exercising regularly is the best way to avoid unhealthy weight gains.

Some people think that as sports become increasingly popular in a society, obesity rates decline, but data in the United States indicate the exact opposite: Obesity rates among young people and adults have more than doubled between 1985 and 2012—a period when competitive sports grew significantly in popularity. This does not mean that sports cause obesity, but it does mean that the popularity of sports in a society does not automatically inspire people to exercise and change their eating habits in ways that reduce obesity.

Like the connection between sports and health, the connection between sports and weight is complex. Some competitive sports such as wrestling and gymnastics emphasize extreme forms of weight control; others emphasize weight gain for some or all participants. Many football players at the high school, college, and professional levels are encouraged to gain weight to the point that they would be classified as overweight or obese according to the body mass index (BMI). Although the BMI is not always a good measure for assessing the relationship between weight and health (Etchison, 2011), there is good reason to believe that playing football does not routinely promote healthy weight control.

Expectations in football today often encourage excessive eating, taking untested nutritional supplements, or using drugs to gain size. A consequence of these expectations is illustrated in Table 3.1. Unlike in 1920–1985, when no more than eight NFL players weighed over 300 pounds, in 2010 there were 394 players over 300 pounds, and they claim to have gained weight by overeating. This takes a toll on overall health (Briggs, 2002; Longman, 2007b, 2011a).

Research also shows that these patterns exist in college and high school football, which together have by far the most participants of all school-sponsored sports (Keller, 2007; Laurson and

Table 3.1 Number of 300-pound players in the NFL, 1970–2012

Year	Number of Players
1970	1
1980	3
1990	94
2000	301
2010	394
2012	361

Source: Stats LLC & NFL (2012).
Note: At the beginning of training camps in 2010, there were 532 NFL players who weighed more than 300 pounds (Longman, 2011a).

Eisenmann, 2007; Longman, 2007b). In fact, young men who play the line positions on high school football teams regularly have obesity rates that are twice as high as others of their age. As one 332-pound fifteen-year-old high school lineman said, "They're going to notice me because of my size. . . . Most linemen in the NFL are 290 or 300" (Longman, 2007b).

Football is unique, but like other sports, it exists in a social world where expectations focus on competitive success rather than healthy actions and overall fitness. If playing sports is to have a positive impact on the long-term physical well-being of people, regardless of age, it should be accompanied by information about nutrition and health combined with effective encouragement to use this information in connection with sport participation. As it is now, participation in certain elite sports leads to forms of training and competition that create both acute and chronic health problems for some athletes.

HOW DO SPORTS AFFECT OUR LIVES?

Sports and sport participation affect the lives of many people around the world. We're learning more about this impact through three types of studies based on a combination of cultural, interactionist, and structural theories:

1. Studies of sport experiences as presented through the voices of sport participants
2. Studies of the social worlds that are created and maintained in connection with particular sports
3. Studies of sports as sites, or "social locations," where dominant ideas and ideologies are expressed and sometimes challenged and changed

Most of these studies are grounded in a critical approach. Taken together, they help us rethink socialization issues and expand our understanding of how social learning occurs in social worlds.

Today most of us in the sociology of sport view sports as *sites* for socialization experiences, rather than the *causes* of specific socialization outcomes. This is an important distinction that highlights two things. First, sports are social locations rich in their potential for providing memorable and meaningful personal, social, and cultural experiences. Second, sports *by themselves* do not cause particular changes in the character traits, attitudes, and actions of athletes or spectators. Therefore, when positive or negative socialization outcomes occur in connection with sports, we don't simply say that sports caused them. Instead, we view sports as sites where people have potentially influential experiences and then we look for and try to understand the relationships and social processes through which particular forms of socialization occur.

The following summaries of selected studies illustrate how this approach to socialization enables us to understand more fully the social dimensions of sports and the connections between sports and the larger social and cultural contexts in which they are produced, reproduced, and changed.

Athletes' Voices: Giving Meaning to Sport Experiences

The following examples provide two socialization "videos." They present the perspectives of the participants themselves, and they help us understand how people give meaning to sport experiences and integrate them into their lives.

Example 1: Giving Meaning to Ice Hockey   Sociologist Nancy Theberge (1999, 2000b) spent two years studying an elite women's ice hockey team in Canada. As she observed and interviewed team members, she noted that their experiences and orientations were influenced by the fact that men controlled the team, the league, and the sport itself. Within this structure, the women developed a professional approach to participation. They focused on hockey and were serious about playing well and winning games. In the process, they developed close connections with each other. The team became a community with its own dynamics and internal organization. Within this constructed community, the athletes learned about hockey, their teammates, and themselves. The meanings that the players gave to their hockey experiences and the ways they integrated those experiences into their lives emerged as they interacted with each other both on the ice and off.

The locker room was a key place for interacting with teammates and giving meaning to their sport experiences. Its emotional climate, especially *after* a practice or a game, encouraged talk about their lives outside hockey. This talk gave shape and meaning to what they did on the ice. It also served as a means for expressing feelings and thoughts about men, sexuality, intimate partners, and families.

The women talked and joked about men but didn't degrade or reduce them to body parts in their comments. They made references to sex and sexuality in their conversations, but the substance of these references was neither hostile nor based on stereotypes. This was very different from what has reportedly occurred in some men's locker rooms, where women have been routinely derogated and objectified, and homosexuality has been scorned if it is discussed at all (Clayton and Humberstone, 2006; Gregory, 2015; Holden, 2013).

Theberge's study shows us that playing sports is both a physical and a social experience. Hockey

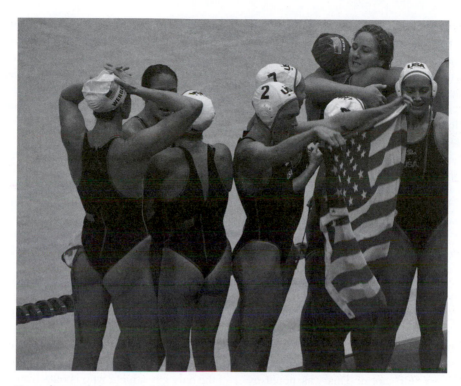

To understand the impact of sport experiences it is necessary to study them in connection with the meanings they are given and how those meaning are integrated into athletes' lives. (*Source*: © Lara Killick)

was a site for memorable experiences, but it was only *through social relationships* that those experiences were given meaning and incorporated into the women's lives. Theberge also gathered data on relationships between the athletes and others, including coaches, managers, trainers, friends, family members, sport reporters, and even fans. She realized that if she wanted to know what happens in sports, she had to understand the relationships and interaction through which socialization occurs among athletes.

Example 2: Coming Out Then and Now   The meanings given to sport experiences vary from one person to another because social relationships are influenced by social definitions given to age, gender, socioeconomic status, ethnicity, skin color, (dis)abilities, and sexuality. This point has been made by sociologist Eric Anderson in his two decades of research on sports and homosexuality (Anderson, 2008a, 2008b, 2009b, 2011a, 2011b, 2011c, 2011d; 2014; Anderson and Bullingham, 2015; Anderson and McGuire, 2010; Magrath et al., 2013).[1] Anderson's studies cover multiple topics related to the experiences of gay and lesbian athletes, and he has recently investigated how those experiences changed between 2000 and 2010. In 2010 he interviewed twenty-six openly

---

[1] Most of Anderson's research focuses on gay men. However, if we combine the work of Pat Griffin (1998) with recent studies by Anderson and his colleagues (Anderson and Billingham, 2013), the trends discussed in this section are similar for lesbian athletes. That is, openly lesbian athletes face less homohysteria today than even a decade ago.

gay U.S. high school and college athletes and compared what they said about their experiences with statements made by twenty-six openly gay athletes interviewed in 2000 (Anderson, 2002, 2011b). The athletes in both samples were predominantly white and middle class.

The athletes interviewed in 2000 generally feared that coming out, would result in their being marginalized, excluded, or physically threatened, but their counterparts in 2010 did not express the same fears. Typical of the 2002 athletes was Jason, a track and cross-country runner who said this about coming out: "One of the things that was holding me back . . . was . . . my own fear of locker room situations. . . . I didn't want to make other people uncomfortable around me in the locker room, and I didn't want them to make it an issue. . . . I'd heard some horror stories from some of my friends. . . . One of my friend's friend was beaten to a bloody pulp because they thought he was gay" (2002, p. 868).

Most of the athletes in 2000 faced an unstated "don't ask, don't tell" norm. This was noted by Ken, a champion college runner who said, "Even to this day, people know, but people just won't say it. . . . It's like they just can't talk about it. It makes me so uncomfortable knowing that some people know, but then they still ask me about girls . . . it's really frustrating. . . . Not one time on the team did anyone ask me, 'Ken, are you gay?'" (p. 870).

After analyzing the data collected in 2000, Anderson explained that the widely accepted homophobic, anti-gay discourse during that time assumed that being gay was an inferior form of masculinity. This pushed gay athletes to the margins of their teams and prevented them from merging their sexual and athlete identities and feeling fully comfortable as team members. Even though Anderson was encouraged by the gay athletes who had confronted homophobia by coming out and generally had positive experiences, he concluded that it would take years before heterosexual athletes would accept gay males as their equals.

Now fast-forward to 2010. When Anderson interviewed Neil, an openly gay soccer player attending a Catholic college in the rural Midwest, Neil described his teammates as very supportive of him after he came out. He went on to say, "I think it's good that we played together for a long time. So they got to know me before I came out. But they have been amazing. Absolutely nothing has changed since I came out. . . . I should have come out earlier" (2011d, p. 257).

Similarly, Tom, a high school runner, said that he was confident that coming out would not be a problem because there were "at least a dozen openly gay kids at my school." He explained that they had no problems, "so I knew I wouldn't either." He also added, "It just doesn't make sense to be homophobic today, everybody has gay friends" (2011d, p. 258).

Many of the athletes in the 2010 study also explained that they talked openly with teammates who acknowledged their identity and discussed it in ways that made them feel comfortable, In fact, Mark said, "I think it's fair to say that I'm known as 'the gay hockey player' at my high school. I'm the only gay athlete who is out, even though I suspect a few more. . . . It's funny, I'll be at a party, and meet someone new and they will be like, 'Hey, I heard of you. You're the gay hockey player, huh?'" (2011d, p. 260).

These responses did not surprise Anderson, because his many studies in 2000–2010 had found a trend of declining homophobia. In his analysis he explained that as homophobia declines, men would feel increasingly free to define masculinity in more varied, fluid, and flexible terms. In turn, this would reduce the compulsion to strictly police gender boundaries and would open up cultural space for different ways to be men and express manhood. In his conclusion, Anderson prophetically noted that as of 2011 we had reached a point where there was "acceptance of gay male athletes" (2011b). It took another two years for an athlete in one of the major men's sports in the United States to come out, but when NBA player Jason Collins announced that he was gay, he experienced widespread acceptance (Beck and Branch, 2013).

These findings do not mean that homophobia no longer exists in sports or society (Gregory, 2015). It continues to exist, but its social significance and meaning is changing in many sport cultures. This, in turn, changes relationships and socialization experiences for many athletes.

Social Worlds: Living in Sports

Sociologists also study socialization processes in connection with the social worlds in which they occur. In Chapter 1, a **social world** is defined as *an identifiable sphere of everyday actions and relationships*. These actions and relationships revolve around a focus and "worldview" that unites people in terms of a shared mind-set. For example, "the tennis world," "the football world," and "the motocross world" each can be viewed and studied as a unique social world.

Qualitative research methods are most often used to study social worlds. Researchers use participant observation and interviews to view sport participation in the overall context in which it occurs. Studies are based on the assumption that we can't understand who athletes are, what they do, and how sports influence their lives unless we also understand the social worlds in which they give meaning to sport experiences and integrate them into their lives. This is especially true when the lives of athletes revolve completely around a particular sport—that is, when the social world of their sport is their entire world.

Studies of the social worlds created around specific sports provide useful information about socialization processes and experiences. The following summaries of two ethnographic studies are representative of this type of research.

Example 1: Learning to Be a Hero   Sociologists Patti and Peter Adler spent nearly ten years studying the social world of a high-profile college basketball team. Much of their data, presented in the book *Backboards and Blackboards* (1991), focuses on how the self-conceptions of young men changed as they lived in the social world of big-time college basketball. The Adlers found that the young men, about 70 percent of whom were African Americans, usually became deeply engulfed in their roles as athletes. This influenced how they viewed themselves and allocated their time between basketball, social life, and academics. This "role engulfment" intensified as the young men became increasingly committed to their identities that were formed around relationships with teammates, coaches, and others associated with basketball. Everyone they met supported and reinforced their athlete identity. As a result, college basketball became the context in which the young men identified themselves, set their goals, and viewed the rest of the world.

The Adlers noted that the young men learned to set goals, focus their attention on specific tasks, and make sacrifices to succeed in basketball. However, there was no apparent evidence that the athletes applied these lessons to other aspects of their lives. The social world of basketball separated them so much from the rest of life that the lessons they learned in that world stayed there.

The Adlers' study raises an important point about socialization: When the social world in which athletes play their sport is so separate from other spheres of life and role engulfment confines athletes to that world, it is difficult to take the learning that occurs through sport participation and transfer it to nonsport worlds.

Example 2: Surviving in a Ghetto   Sociologist Loïc Wacquant (1992, 2004) spent three years studying the social world of boxers in a gym located in a black neighborhood in Chicago. His observations, interviews, and experiences as a boxer helped him uncover the ideas and meanings that constitute the life and craft of boxing. He explained that the social world of the boxing gym was very complex: It was created in connection with social forces in an ethnically segregated ghetto and its masculine street culture, but it also shelters black men from the full destructive impact of those forces.

To learn the "social art" of boxing, the men at the gym engaged in an intense regimen of body regulation focused on the physical, visual, and mental requirements of boxing. They had to "eat, drink, sleep, and live boxing," and in the process, they developed what Wacquant described as a *socialized lived body,* which was at the very core of their identities and actions.

The social world of the boxing gym was a workplace, a refuge, and a place where dreams were pursued by men dedicated to disciplining their bodies and souls (Wacquant, 2004). Immersing themselves in this world separated the men from their peers on the streets and kept them alive by helping them navigate their lives in dangerous neighborhoods devoid of hope or opportunity. For these men, boxing was a powerful socialization experience, but it can be understood only in connection with social and material conditions that constituted the social world of their everyday lives. In fact, the gym studied by Wacquant would never exist in an upper-middle-class white neighborhood; it would make no sense there.

In summary, these two studies of social worlds created around sports help us understand more fully the contexts in which athletes and others connected with sports form identities, make decisions, and give meaning to their experiences. Research that takes us into those worlds helps us make sense of actions that sometimes appear strange or even irrational from an outsider's perspective. This doesn't mean that we approve of everything that occurs in those worlds, but insightful research provides the information needed to make sports more humane and healthy activities.

Ideology: Sports as Sites for Presenting Ideas and Beliefs

Socialization research has focused mostly on what occurs in the lives of individuals within bounded social worlds. However, researchers now use a combination of cultural theories and text analysis to do studies of *socialization as a community and cultural process.* These studies go beyond investigating the experiences and characteristics of athletes and the organization of social worlds. Instead, they focus on sports as sites at which people collectively create and learn "stories," which they use to give meaning to and make sense of realities outside of sports. These stories are sociologically relevant because so many people use them as vehicles for presenting ideas and beliefs about everything from morality and work to capitalism and lifestyles of consumption. They often have their own vocabularies and images and the meanings in these stories shift, depending on who tells and hears them. Researchers in the sociology of sport conduct studies to identify these stories, explain how they fit into the culture, and show how people use them as a guide for what they think and do.

Researchers using cultural theories and a poststructuralist approach are primarily concerned with whose stories about sports become dominant in a culture and whose stories are ignored. The dominant or most widely told stories are important because they are based on ideological assumptions of what is natural, normal, and legitimate in social worlds; therefore, they promote ideas and beliefs that often privilege some people more than others. For example, sports stories often revolve around heroic figures—warriors who are big, strong, aggressive, record-setting competitors. As researchers have deconstructed these stories to examine the logic, values, and ideological assumptions on which they are based, they've found that many of them celebrate ideas and beliefs that serve the interests of unregulated capitalist expansion and traditional notions of masculinity based on the ability to dominate others through the use of physical strength, power, and speed (Burstyn, 1999).

Researchers using a poststructuralist approach also study more privately told stories representing voices that are silenced or "erased" from the widely circulated and accepted stories in the dominant culture. Additionally, they've analyzed sports media coverage to learn what *is* and what *is not* contained in commentaries, images, and other representations that spectators consume during mediated sport events. These studies are important because they give us a fuller understanding of the ways that sports influence how people think and what they do.

This type of research is difficult to do because it requires a deep knowledge of history and the conditions under which sports and sport stories become a part of people's lives. But it is important in the knowledge-building process because it deals with the ways that sports influence culture, society, and the lives of people even when they don't participate in or care about sports.

Socialization as a Community and Cultural Process   Critical research on socialization as a community and cultural process is partly inspired by the ideas of the Italian political theorist Antonio Gramsci. When the fascist government in Italy imprisoned Gramsci for speaking out against their oppressive policies, he used his time in prison (1928–1935) to think about why people in Italy and elsewhere had not revolted against exploitive forms of capitalism in Western societies. Gramsci concluded that revolutions had not occurred because popular notions of common sense and widely accepted ideas about organizing society were actually supportive of the powerful people who exploited and oppressed the general population.

After carefully studying historical evidence from around the world, Gramsci explained that leaders often maintained power by convincing the people that they governed of three things: (1) that life was as good as it could be under present conditions; (2) that any positive things that people experienced were due to the goodwill and power of current leaders; and (3) that changing the current structure of their society would threaten everything that people valued.

Although Gramsci never talked about sports, he used historical data to conclude that current leaders could most effectively maintain their power by providing people with exciting and pleasurable experiences that promoted particular ideas and beliefs in support of their positions. In other words, by sponsoring forms of popular entertainment that perpetuated ideological perspectives supportive of current economic and political structures, leaders could retain their power without using coercion and fear. If this was done successfully, there would

be little support for radical or structural changes because people would not want to undermine the primary sources of excitement and pleasure in their lives (Chappell, 2007).

Gramsci's analysis explains why large corporations spend billions of dollars every year to sponsor power and performance sports and present their commercial messages in connection with them. For example, Coca-Cola and McDonald's each spent close to $2.5 billion sponsoring and presenting advertising messages during the Olympic Games from 2000 through 2016. These expenditures were made to promote sales, but more important, they were made to use the Olympics as a site for delivering cultural messages that encouraged people to see these transnational corporations as benevolent sources of excitement and pleasure. If these messages were widely accepted, people would be less likely to criticize these corporations or support legislation that would curb their power and influence. Therefore, the corporate executives who made the decisions to sponsor the Olympics wanted people watching the events to agree that competition was the fair and natural way to allocate rewards. They realized that this belief and the free market ideology that it supported were the foundation of their personal status and wealth as well as the success of the corporations for which they worked. For them, Olympic sports provide a model of life that fits their interests.

The people who run Coca-Cola and McDonalds want to sell Coke and fast food, but they don't spend billions of sponsorship dollars only to boost sales figures. Their more important goal is to effectively promote lifestyles organized around consumption and the use of corporate brands and logos as status and identity symbols. They want to convince people that corporations are the source of their excitement and pleasure, and the sponsors of the athletes, teams, and sports they love so dearly. Coke and McDonalds executives want people to associate their good and memorable times with corporations and their products and to use consumption as the primary measure of progress and prosperity. To the extent that people in society accept this ideology, the power of corporations is nearly guaranteed. This is why the marketing departments of major corporations often use power and performance sports as sites to promote their interests.

TV viewers of the Super Bowl may not realize it, but the biggest stakes associated with that event have nothing to do with the score and everything to do with how viewers integrate into their lives the cultural messages that are deeply embedded in the narratives and images presented in everything from the pregame show through the game, commercials, and postgame shows.

Many sociologists refer to this process of forming consent around a particular ideology as the process of establishing hegemony (heh-ġem-ō-nee). In political science and sociology, **hegemony** is a *process of maintaining leadership and control by gaining the consent and approval of other groups, including those who are being led or controlled.* For example, American hegemony in the world exists when people worldwide accept U.S. power and influence as legitimate. Hegemony is never permanent, but it can be maintained as long as most people feel that their lives are as good as can be expected and there is no compelling reason to change things.

Similarly, corporate hegemony is maintained as long as most people accept a view of the world that discourages them from objecting to corporate policies, profits, and executive pay packages. Like Gramsci, corporate executives know that preserving corporate power depends on establishing "ideological outposts" in people's heads. Sports, because they are exciting and pleasurable activities for so many people, are important sites for constructing these mental outposts. Once established, they serve as relay terminals for delivering corporate messages directly into the popular psyche. To highlight Gramsci's conclusion about hegemony, it can be said that "it is difficult to fight an enemy that has outposts in your head."[2]

---

[2]This phrase was popularized by Sally Kempton, a feminist and spiritual teacher.

Research on Socialization as a Community and Cultural Process It is difficult to understand socialization as a community and cultural process unless we see it in action. The following examples of research highlight this approach to sports and socialization.

When anthropologist Doug Foley (1999a) did an ethnographic study of a small town in southern Texas, he focused part of his attention on the connection between sports and community socialization processes. High school football games were the most visible and popular events in the town, and the local team was important in the lives of many townspeople.

As Foley observed social dynamics in the town and interviewed people about local events, he discovered that the stories created around high school football reaffirmed established ways of thinking and doing things in the town. As a result, sports served as a site for maintaining forms of social inequality that made life good for a few and difficult for many residents. For example, even though a young Mexicana could become a cheerleader and a young Mexicano from a poor family could be a star on the football team, this did nothing to improve the political and economic status of women, citizens with Mexican heritage, and low-income people in the town.

The experiences and meanings associated with football reproduced ideologies that supported and justified inequalities of gender, ethnicity, and social class. Even though particular individuals benefited from sport participation, the vocabularies and images associated with sports perpetuated actions and forms of social organization that maintained existing patterns of power and privilege. Foley summarized the findings of his ethnography in this way:

> Local sports, especially football, socialize every new generation of youth into the local status hierarchy, both inside and outside the school. Each new generation of males learns to be individualistic, aggressive, and competitive within a group structure. . . . (1999a, p. 138)

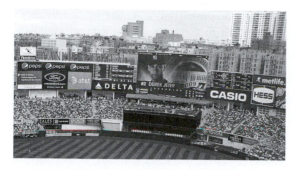

When corporations invest money to have their names, logos, and products associated with sports, they are looking for more than sales. In the long run, their executives hope that people will believe that their enjoyment of sports depends on corporations. This will make people more likely to support and less likely to interfere with corporate interests. (*Source*: © Jay Coakley)

Other studies have used a similar methodological approach and focused on the ways that popular images connected with sports become influential cultural symbols as they are represented in the media and everyday conversations. For example, physical cultural studies scholar David Andrews and his colleagues have studied Michael Jordan as an iconic figure that influenced the attitudes and experiences of people worldwide, especially a generation of young people in the United States (Andrews, 1996a, 1996b, 2001; Andrews and Jackson, 2001; and McDonald and Andrews, 2001). These researchers meticulously deconstructed the cultural stories that were created around Jordan, mostly between 1982 and 1995. This involved analyzing commercials, commentaries, and various forms of media coverage. One of their findings was that the "Jordan persona" was severed from African American experiences and culture so that white America, seeking evidence that it was color blind and open to all, could comfortably identify with it and approve of their children hanging Jordan posters on bedroom walls in their all-white neighborhoods. Race and skin color were strategically erased from Jordan's public

persona thereby allowing it to become a sign that could be attached to any corporate brand, including Nike, Wilson, Hanes underwear, Jordan brand apparel, Bijan (the Michael Jordan fragrance), Coca-Cola, Gatorade, McDonald's, Wheaties, Ball Park Franks, Quaker Oats, Sara Lee, CBS SportsLine, MJ's sports videos, MCI telephone long-distance service, General Motors, Chevrolet, Rayovac, and others (Andrews, 2001; McDonald and Andrews, 2001). This strategy continues to be successful today as Jordan makes more money annually on endorsement deals than any current or former athlete (Badenhausen, 2015).

In the United States, Jordan's persona was shaped in connection with capitalism and traditional family values, and he was represented as both a brand sign and a family man (Andrews, 2001; Andrews and Jackson, 2001). As the media transmitted the Jordan persona around the world, it was often associated with American capitalist expansion and the power of transnational corporations such as Nike. However, among Black Britons striving to transcend the legacy of being colonized by white people from England, the Jordan persona represented black empowerment and resistance to white supremacy. Among whites in New Zealand, it represented the NBA, American popular culture, and African American prowess in sports. In Poland, the Jordan persona represented the American Dream, freedom, independence, the self-made man, opportunity, wealth, and other American values that stood in opposition to the communism that Poles had recently rejected in their lives.

The research by Andrews and his colleagues shows that sports and celebrity athletes are given multiple and sometimes contradictory meanings by different people in different cultural contexts. Therefore, the significance of sports in the socialization that occurs at the community and cultural level can be understood only in connection with local history, ideologies, and power relations. In other words, the influence of sports on people's lives cannot be captured in a single statement about building character, bringing people together, creating responsible citizens, promoting conformity, or

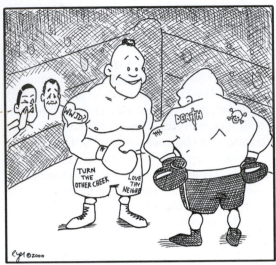

(*Source:* © Frederic A. Eyer)

*"I think these guys give different meanings
to their boxing experiences."*

**The meanings given to sports vary from one person
to another. However, many power and performance
sports are organized to encourage orientations that
emphasize domination over others. Those who do
not hold this orientation may not fit very well in
these sports.**

fostering warfare. The connection between sports
and socialization is much more complex than that
and can be explained only by studying sports in the
contexts in which people give them meaning and
make them a part of their lives.

summary

WHO PLAYS AND WHAT HAPPENS?

Socialization is a complex, interactive process
through which people learn about themselves and
the social worlds in which they participate. This
process occurs in connection with sports and other
activities in people's lives. Research indicates that
playing sports is a social experience as well as a
physical one.

Becoming involved and staying involved in
sports occur in connection with general socialization processes in people's lives. Decisions to play
sports are influenced by the availability of opportunities, the existence of social support, processes
of identity formation, and the cultural context in
which decisions are made.

Research also indicates that people do not make
decisions about sport participation once and for all
time. They make them day after day, as they set and
revise priorities throughout their lives. Research on
sport-related decisions indicates that significant
others influence those decisions and that reasons
for staying in sports change over time as people's
lives change. Therefore, to understand sport participation it is important to study the changing contexts in which decisions are made.

Changing or ending active sport participation
also occurs in connection with general socialization processes. These processes are interactive and
influenced by personal, social, and cultural factors.
Changes in sport participation are usually tied to
a combination of identity, developmental, and life
course issues. Ending sport participation involves
a transition process, during which a person dis-
engages from sport, redefines personal identity,
reconnects with friends and family members, and
uses available resources to become involved in
other activities and careers. Just as people are not
socialized into sports, they are not simply socialized out of sports. Research shows that changing
or ending a career as a competitive athlete occurs
over time and is often tied to events and life course
issues apart from sports. These connections are best
studied by using research methods that enable us to
identify and analyze long-term transition processes.

Socialization that occurs as people participate in
sports has been widely studied, especially by people wanting to know if and how sports build character and promote positive development. Much of
this research has produced inconsistent findings
because it has been based on oversimplified ideas
about sports, sport experiences, and socialization.

Reviews of this research indicate that the most
informative studies of sports and socialization take

into account variations in the ways that sports are organized, played, and integrated into people's lives. This is important because different sports involve different experiences that influence socialization outcomes. For example, the experience and meaning of playing power and performance sports is different from the experience and meaning of playing pleasure and participation sports. The continued visibility and popularity of power and performance sports are related to issues of wealth and power in society because they promote an ideology that supports the interests of existing leaders and wealthy people.

We know that sports have an impact on people's lives. The most informative research on what happens in sports deals with (1) the everyday experiences of people who play sports; (2) the social worlds created around sports; and (3) community and cultural processes through which ideologies are created, reproduced, and changed. As we listen to the voices of those who participate in sports, study their lives in sports, and identify the ideological messages associated with sports, we learn that there is a complex relationship between sports and socialization.

Most scholars who study sports in society now see sports as sites for socialization experiences, rather than the causes of specific socialization outcomes. This distinction recognizes that powerful and memorable experiences can occur in connection with sports, but the impact of those experiences depends on the relationships through which they are given meaning and the social and cultural factors that influence how those meanings are integrated into people's lives. Therefore, the most useful research in the sociology of sport focuses on the importance of social relationships and the contexts in which sport experiences occur.

SUPPLEMENTAL READINGS

Reading 1. Socialization and sports: A brief overview

Reading 2. Making decisions about sport participation during adolescence

Reading 3. Burnout among adolescent athletes: A sociological approach

Reading 4. Sport and character development among adolescents

Reading 5. Why do people believe that "sport builds character"?

Reading 6. Using Mead's theory of the self to organize youth sport programs

Reading 7. Saving the world with youth sports: Who is doing it and are they succeeding?

SPORT MANAGEMENT ISSUES

- You work in the parks and recreation department of a city with a high rate of obesity among people of all ages. Your job is to create programs that will increase the physical activity rate across the general population. Using research as support, outline your plan and specify how it will interface with sport programs in the city.

- You are the athletic director of a new private school with a student body of fewer than 600 students. The parents and teachers want to discuss with you whether the new sports program will emphasize power and performance sports or pleasure and participation sports. You plan to identify the pros and cons of each alternative from the perspective of the students' overall educational experience. Create a handout that does that.

- You are now working for an NFL team, and you want to thoughtfully consider the ideological impact of the team on its fans and the surrounding community. Identify at least three of the ideological messages that are highlighted in the media coverage of the NFL and discuss who is most likely to be advantaged or disadvantaged by each of them.

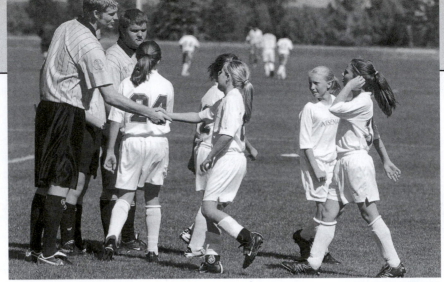

SPORTS FOR CHILDREN

Are Organized Programs Worth the Effort?

As in the focus of a magnifying glass, play contains all developmental tendencies in a condensed form and is itself a major source of development . . . A child's greatest achievements are possible in play, achievements that tomorrow will become her basic level of real action and morality.

> **—Lev Vygotsky, Psychologist (1980)**

The perception is you train early and only do a single sport and do as much as you can until you're better than everyone else. I think it's pretty clear from the injury and performance-data side that that's a terrible developmental model.

> **—Neeru Jayanthi, Medical Director, Primary Care Sports Medicine, Loyola University Health System (in Reddy, 2014).**

Despite all the elite teams and high-powered youth leagues across the U.S., . . . statistics show that many children are dropping out of sports early—in droves—often because they can't afford to play.

> **—Patti Neighmond, Reporter, National Public Radio (2015)**

[Today's youth sports] emphasize performance over participation well before kids' bodies, minds, and interests mature. And we tend to value the child who can help win games or whose families can afford the rising fees. The risks for that child are overuse injuries, concussion, and burnout.

> **—Project Play Report (2015, p. 7; http://youthreport. projectplay.us/the-problem)**

Chapter Outline

Origin and Development of Organized Youth Sports

Major Trends in Youth Sports Today

Informal, Player-Controlled Sports: A Case of the Generation Gap

Youth Sports Today: Assessing Our Efforts

The Challenge of Improving Youth Sports

Recommendations for Improving Youth Sports

Summary: Are Organized Programs Worth the Effort?

Learning Objectives

- Explain how social changes related to family and childhood have influenced the growth of organized youth sports in the United States since 1950.

- Identify the sponsors of organized youth sports today, and explain why children's sport experiences may vary depending on who sponsors their sport programs.

- Explain how the trend toward privatization in youth sports affects youth sport experiences.

- Define what is meant by the performance ethic, and explain why it has become especially important in private and elite youth sport training programs.

- Explain why parents today take youth sports so seriously.

- Explain why alternative sports have become increasingly popular with many young people today.

- Distinguish the differences between organized sports and informal games, and explain why informal games are played less today than in the past.

- Use the grades that experts have given to organized youth sports in the United States to identify the major problems in those programs.

- Identify recommendations that will increase the positive experiences of children in youth sports.

According to Census Bureau estimates, there were about 50 million six- to eighteen-year-olds living in the United States in 2016. Widely cited estimates of youth sport participation range from 15 million to 46 million six- to eighteen-year-olds, depending on who does the counting and what counts as sports. But best as I can tell, during a given year, about 23 million U.S. children and youth participate in organized sports, including high school teams.[1]

When, how, why, and to what end children play these sports are the questions that concern parents, community leaders, and child advocates worldwide.

When sociologists study youth sports, they focus on the experiences of participants and how those experiences vary depending on the social and cultural contexts in which they occur. Research by sociologists has influenced how some people think about and organize youth sports, and it continues to provide valuable information that parents, coaches, and program administrators can use when organizing and evaluating youth programs.

This chapter summarizes part of that research as we discuss five topics that are central to understanding youth sports today. These are

1. The origin and development of organized youth sports
2. Major trends in youth sports
3. Variations in the organization of youth sports and in the sport experiences of young people
4. Youth sports and issues related to access, psychosocial development, and family dynamics
5. Recommendations for improving youth sports

An underlying question that guides our discussion of these topics is this: Are organized youth sports worth the massive amount of time, money, and effort that people put into them? I continue to ask and help people answer this question as I talk with parents and work with coaches and others who are committed to organizing sports for young people.

ORIGIN AND DEVELOPMENT OF ORGANIZED YOUTH SPORTS

During the latter half of the nineteenth century, people in Europe and North America began to realize that child development was influenced by the social environment. This created a movement to organize children's social worlds with the goal of building their character and turning them into hard-working, productive, and patriotic adults in rapidly expanding capitalist economies (Chudacoff, 2007).

It wasn't long before organized sports for young boys were organized and sponsored by schools, communities, and church groups. The organizers hoped that sports, especially team sports, would teach boys from working-class families to obey rules and work together productively. They also hoped that sports would toughen middle- and upper-class boys and turn them into competitive men, despite the "feminized" values they learned from their stay-at-home mothers. At the same time, girls were provided activities that taught them to be good wives, mothers, and homemakers. The prevailing belief was that girls should learn domestic skills rather than sport skills when they went to schools and playgrounds. There were exceptions to these patterns, but after World War II, youth programs were organized this way in Western Europe and North America.

---

[1]The data on youth sport participation are confusing because some figures double and triple count children who play two or more sports; some figures include informal physical activities, such as riding a skateboard once during a year or wading in the water at a beach, as participating in a sport; and other figures are based only on official counts from national youth sport organizations, such as Little League, Inc., US Youth Soccer, the American Youth Soccer Organization, and others. For example, the Sports and Fitness Industry Association counts being in the water for a few minutes at a local pool as "participation in swimming," because it involves buying and wearing a bathing suit, which concerns members of this organization.

The Postwar Baby Boom and the Growth of Youth Sports

The baby-boom generation was born between 1946 and 1964. Young married couples during these years were optimistic about the future and eager to become parents. As the first wave of baby boomers moved through childhood during the 1950s and 1960s, organized youth sports grew dramatically, especially in the United States. Programs were sponsored by public, private, and commercial organizations. Parents also entered the scene, believing that their sons' characters would be built through organized competitive sports. Fathers became coaches, managers, and league administrators. Mothers did laundry and became chauffeurs and short-order cooks so their sons were ready for practices and games.

Most programs were for boys eight to fourteen-years-old, and they were organized with the belief that playing sports would prepare them to participate productively in a competitive economy. Until the 1970s, girls were largely ignored by these organizers and sat in the bleachers during their brothers' games and, in the United States, given the hope of becoming high school cheerleaders. Then came the women's movement, the fitness movement, and government legislation prohibiting sex discrimination in education, including school-sponsored sports. These changes stimulated the growth of sport programs for girls beginning in the mid-1970s. By the 1990s girls had nearly as many opportunities as boys.

Participation in organized youth sports is now a valued part of growing up in most wealthy nations. Parents and communities use their resources to sponsor, organize, and administer a variety of youth sports. However, some parents today question the benefits of programs in which winning is more important than overall child development; others seek out win-oriented programs, hoping their children will become the winners. A few parents

> For a century now, youth sport has been more proving ground than playground—an enterprise laced with purpose and emotion, even the hopes of a nation.
> —Tom Farrey, ESPN (in *Game On,* 2008, p. 99)

encourage their children to engage in unstructured, noncompetitive physical activities—an alternative that many young people prefer over organized, adult-controlled sports.

Social Change and the Growth of Organized Youth Sports

Since the 1950s, an increasing amount of children's after-school time and physical activity has occurred in adult-controlled organized programs. This growth is partly related to changing ideas about family life and childhood in **neoliberal societies,** that is, *societies where individualism and material success are highly valued and where publicly funded programs and services are being eliminated and selectively replaced by private programs.* The following six changes are especially relevant to the growth and current status of organized youth sports.

First, the number of families with both parents working outside the home has increased dramatically. This has created a demand for organized and adult supervised after-school and summer programs. Organized sports have grown because many parents believe they offer their children opportunities to have fun, learn adult values, become physically fit, and acquire positive status among their peers.

Second, since the early 1980s, there's been a major cultural shift in what it means to be a "good parent." Good parents today are those who can account for the whereabouts and actions of their children 24/7—an expectation that leads many parents to seek organized, adult-supervised programs in which their children are monitored and controlled. Organized sports are also favored by parents because they provide predictable schedules, adult leadership for children, and measurable indicators of a child's accomplishments. When children succeed, parents can claim that they are meeting cultural expectations. In fact, many

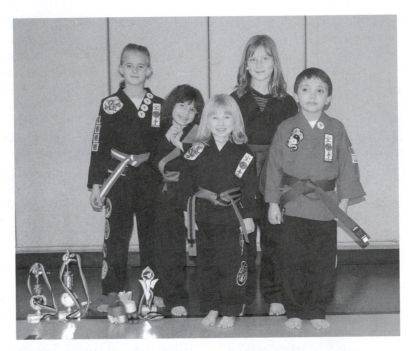

To meet cultural expectations for the "good parent," mothers and
fathers often are attracted to youth sport programs that use symbols of
progressive achievement and skill development. Karate, with achievement
levels signified by belt colors, is appealing to some because the visible and
quantifiable achievements of their children can be used as proof of their
parental moral worth. (*Source:* © Jay Coakley)

mothers and fathers feel that their moral worth as
parents is associated with the visible achievements
of their children—a factor that further intensifies
parental commitment to youth sports.

Third, many people today believe that informal, child-controlled activities inevitably lead to
trouble—much like what occurs in the novel, *Lord
of the Flies.* When young people are seen as threats
to social order, organized sports are seen as ideal
activities to keep them occupied, out of trouble,
and under the control of adults.

Fourth, many parents, responding to fear-
producing news stories about murders and child
abductions now see the world outside the home as
dangerous for their children. They regard organized
sports as safe alternatives to informal activities that
occur outside the home without adult supervision.

Even when organized sports have high injury rates
and uncertified coaches, parents still feel that organized programs are needed to protect their children.

Fifth, the visibility of high-performance and
professional sports has increased awareness of
organized competitive sports as a valued part of
culture. As children watch sports on television,
listen to parents and friends talk about sports, and
hear about the wealth and fame of popular athletes, they often see organized youth sports, especially those modeled after professional sports, as
attractive activities. And when children say they
want to be gymnasts or basketball players, parents
often try to nurture these dreams by seeking the
best-organized programs in those sports. Therefore, organized youth sports have become popular
partly because children see them as enjoyable and

culturally valued activities that will enhance their status among peers and adults.

Sixth, the culture of childhood play has nearly disappeared in most segments of post-industrial society, especially in the United States. Children today have few opportunities to engage in spontaneous play—activities that involve creativity, expressiveness, joy, and "ownership" possessed by the participants themselves (Christakis and Christakis, 2010). Structured, achievement-oriented activities now begin early in children's lives (Hyman, 2012). These activities, including organized sports for preschoolers, are controlled by adults and provide few opportunities for children to play, which often is seen as a "waste of time." Instead, the focus is on improvement and measurable development that will pay off for a child in the future. Parents seek developmental activities that they hope will help their children experience academic and future occupational success.

Time for play has become a low priority in most families (Glenn et al., 2013; Singh and Gupta, 2012). Parents also restrict the spaces for play by keeping children in the house and yard, unless they live on a cul-de-sac where there is no traffic and where children know they are being watched by one neighbor or another (Hochschild, 2013). Even the language of play has nearly disappeared as children learn to describe and evaluate their experiences in instrumental terms rather than by using a vocabulary of emotions and expression—so they talk about activities in terms of what they have learned and accomplished rather than how they felt while they participated.

Together, these six social changes have boosted the popularity of organized youth sports in recent decades. Knowing about them helps to explain why parents invest so many family resources into the organized sports participation of their children. The amount of money that parents spend on participation fees, equipment, travel, personal coaches, high-performance training sessions, and other items defined as necessary in many programs has skyrocketed in recent years (Farrey, 2008; Hyman, 2012). For example, the parents of elite youth hockey players who travel to regional and national tournaments often spend more than $10,000 per year to support their sons' hockey participation. They justify the costs by saying that being a hockey player benefits their sons in many ways. Other parents have gone even further—remortgaging houses and spending hundreds of thousands of dollars to nurture the sport dreams of a child (Hyman, 2012; Weir, 2006).

One of the troubling issues raised by these changes is that mothers and fathers in working-class and lower-income households are increasingly defined as irresponsible and "bad" parents because they lack the resources to fund sport participation for their children as wealthier parents do. Parents without resources may also be perceived as uninterested in nurturing the dreams of their children, even though this is far from true. In this way, organized sports for children become linked to political issues and debates about family values and the moral worth of parents in lower-income households.

> Children's play is so focused on lessons and leagues [that] kids aren't getting a chance to practice policing themselves. When they have that opportunity, . . . the results are clear: Self-regulation improves —Alix Spiegel, PBS, Morning Edition (2008)

MAJOR TRENDS IN YOUTH SPORTS TODAY

In addition to their growing popularity, youth sports are changing in five socially significant ways.

First, organized programs are becoming increasingly privatized. This means that more youth sports today are sponsored by private and commercial organizations, and fewer are sponsored by public, tax-supported organizations such as park and recreation departments.

Second, organized programs increasingly emphasize the "performance ethic." This means that participants in youth sports, even in recreational programs, are encouraged to evaluate experiences in terms of their progress in developing technical skills and moving to higher levels of competition.

Third, there's an increase in private, elite sport-training facilities dedicated to producing highly skilled and specialized athletes who can compete at the highest levels of youth sports. This means that parents often spend significant amounts of money to buy sport training for their children, and they see youth sport expenditures as financial investments in their children's future.

Fourth, parents are increasingly involved in and concerned about the participation and success of their children in organized youth sports. This means that youth sports are now serious activities for both adults and children, and adults are more likely to act in extreme ways as they advocate what they perceive to be the interests of their children.

Fifth, participation in alternative and action sports has increased. This means that many young people prefer unstructured, participant-controlled activities such as skateboarding, in-line skating, snowboarding, BMX biking, disc golf, Ultimate, slacklining, footbag (hacky sack), climbing, jumping rope, and other sports that have local or regional relevance.

These five trends have an impact on who plays and what happens in organized youth sports. This is discussed in the following sections and in the box "Sponsorship Matters: Variations in the Purpose of Organized Youth Sports."

The Privatization of Organized Programs

Privatization is a prevalent trend in youth sports today. Although organized sports are widely popular

> **If a family doesn't think their huge investment in expensive sport is going to turn their child into an Olympian or professional athlete, they are often walking away from sport completely.** —Barry Shepley, Hall of Fame Triathlon Coach, 2010 (in Richard, 2010)

in the United States, there has been a decline in publicly funded youth programs with free and inclusive participation policies. As governments face budget crises various social services, including youth sports, have been downsized or eliminated. Some publicly funded programs have survived by imposing participation fees, but most have been eliminated. In response, middle- and upper-middle-class parents have organized private, nonprofit sport clubs and leagues for their children. These organizations depend on fund-raising, membership dues, and corporate sponsorships. They offer opportunities to children from well-to-do families and neighborhoods, but they're usually too expensive and inconveniently located for children from low-income families and neighborhoods.

Private, commercial programs also have become major providers of youth sports as public programs have been eliminated. But they are selective and exclusive, and they provide few opportunities for children from low-income households. The technical instruction in these programs often is good, and they provide closely regulated skills training for children from wealthier families. In addition, some parents hire private coaches for their children at rates of $50 to $200 per hour.

There are two negative consequences of privatizing youth sports. *First,* privatized programs reproduce the economic and ethnic inequalities that exist in the larger society. Unlike public programs, they depend on the resources of individual participants, rather than entire communities. Low-income and single-parent families often lack money to pay for dues, travel, equipment, and other fees. To the extent that income, family wealth, and support systems are less available to members of ethnic minorities, youth sports often create and accentuate ethnic segregation and social-class divisions in communities.

Second, as public park and recreation departments cease to offer programs, they often become

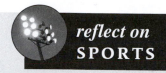

reflect on SPORTS

Sponsorship Matters:
Variations in the Purpose of Organized Youth Sports

The purpose of organized youth sports often varies with the goals of those who sponsor them. Sources and forms of sponsorship differ from one program to another, but they generally fall into one of the following four categories:

1. *Public, tax-supported community recreation organizations.* This includes local park and recreation departments and community centers, which traditionally offer free or low-cost sport programs for children. The programs are usually inclusive and emphasize overall participation, health, general skill development, and enjoyment.

2. *Public-interest, nonprofit community organizations.* These include the YMCA, Boys and Girls Clubs, the Police Athletic League (PAL), and other community-based organizations, which traditionally have provided a limited range of free or low-fee sport programs for children. The goals of these programs are diverse, including everything from providing a "wholesome, Christian atmosphere" for playing sports to providing "at-risk children" with opportunities to play sports and keep them off the streets.

3. *Private-interest, nonprofit sport organizations.* These include organizations such as the nationwide Little League, Inc., Rush Soccer (rushsoccer.com), Pop Warner Football, and local organizations operating independently or through connections with larger sport organizations, such as national federations like USA Swimming. These organizations usually offer more exclusive opportunities to selective groups of children, generally those with special skills from families who can afford relatively costly participation fees.

4. *Private commercial clubs.* These include gymnastics, tennis, skating, soccer, and other sport clubs and training programs. These organizations have costly membership and participation fees, and some emphasize intense training, progressive and specialized skill development, and elite competition.

Because these sponsors each have different missions, the sports programs they fund are likely to offer different types of experiences for children and families. This makes it difficult to draw general conclusions about what happens in organized programs and how participation affects child development, public health, and family dynamics.

When public funds disappear due to tax cuts, one of the first things to be eliminated is youth sport programs—the type in category 1 (above). This has many effects. It limits opportunities for children from low-income families and funnels them into only one or two sports that may survive the cuts. Additionally, it creates a demand for youth sports in the remaining three sponsorship categories. But sponsors in categories 3 and 4 thrive only when they serve people with the money to pay for their programs.

Overall, this means that the opportunities and experiences available to young people are influenced by local, state, and national politics, especially those related to taxation and public spending. At present, youth sport opportunities and experiences are strongly influenced by voters and political representatives who make decisions about taxes and how they are used in local communities. *Do you think that people in your community would vote to increase taxes to support youth sports? If not, what reasons would they give for voting against such a tax?*

brokers of park spaces and rent them to private sport programs. The rental fees are usually reasonable, which means that these private programs benefit from tax-supported facilities without being held accountable for running their programs to benefit the entire community. For example, private programs may not be committed to gender equity or other policies of inclusion that are a key part of public programs.

When privatization occurs, market forces shape who plays youth sports under what conditions. People with resources don't see this as a problem because they have the money to pay for their children's participation and choose the programs they want. But people with few resources face a double bind: They can't pay for their children's participation, and they often are accused of not caring for, controlling, or taking an interest in their children. In this way, privatized youth sport programs disproportionately affect poor people with little political power; therefore, these problems receive little attention from the media and most current politicians.

This point was noted by John Thomas, a director of coaching for United States Youth Soccer, who observed that in all his travels across the United States over the last decade, he'd never seen a travel team with mostly African American girls. In response to this observation, sociologist Paul Kooistra from Furman University in Greenville, South Carolina, suggested that private, fee-based youth sports in the United States are used by some upper-middle-class parents as a tool to "separate themselves and their children from lower social classes and minorities" (Wells, 2008).

Upper-middle-class parents may disagree with Kooistra's statement, but they cannot deny that their children play sports primarily with other children from families that are white and well-off. Poor, working-class, and ethnic minority children are not formally excluded, but they are not on the playing fields. Of course, this has been true of private sport clubs in golf, tennis, swimming, and other sports for over a century, but the privatization of youth sports has re-created a twenty-first century form of ethnic and class segregation in among many populations of young people.

Emphasis on the Performance Ethic

The **performance ethic** *is a set of ideas and beliefs emphasizing that the quality of the sport experience can be measured in terms of improved skills and competitive success.* This ethic is widely emphasized in youth sport programs to the point that *fun* now means improving skills, becoming more competitive, winning, and being promoted into elite

performance categories. "Travel teams" are now an important category in many sports because they separate certain young people from others on the basis of skills. Many parents like this because it enables them to judge their child's progress and prove to themselves and others that they are "good parents" because they have "created talented children."

Private and commercial programs emphasize the performance ethic to a greater degree than do public programs. Their directors and coaches market them as "centers of athletic excellence" to attract parents willing to pay high fees for membership, participation, and instruction. In some cases, the profiles and achievements of successful athletes and coaches who have trained or worked in the program are highlighted to justify costly memberships and dues.

Parents of physically skilled children sometimes define expensive membership fees, equipment, travel, and training expenses as *investments* in their children's future (Hyman, 2012). They also use performance-oriented programs to develop social networks that can provide information about college sports, scholarships, coaches, and elite training programs. Overall, they want their children's sport participation to bring developmental, educational, and eventual occupational payoffs.

Of course, the application of the performance ethic is not limited to organized sports; it influences a range of organized children's activities, and it is changing childhood from a time of exploration and freedom to a time of preparation and controlled learning (Chudacoff, 2007; Elkind, 2007). In this sense, children's sports are part of this larger trend.

Elite, Specialized Sport Programs

The emphasis on performance is also tied to a third trend in youth sports—the development of elite, specialized training programs and leagues. Many private and commercial programs encourage early specialization in a single sport because they have year-round operating expenses that can be paid only if people pay year-round membership fees. If young people played multiple sports and did not pay dues through the entire year, these programs could not to meet expenses or

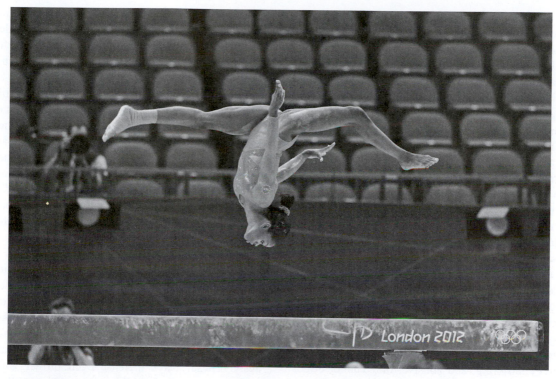

As publicly funded youth sports are downsized or eliminated, private clubs provide participation opportunities. Membership fees in club programs are too costly for most families, and children may not enjoy the emphasis on the performance ethic in these programs. This is especially true in gymnastics where costs and demands for excellence are extreme (*Source:* © Thomas Coex/AFP/Getty Images)

produce profits. Therefore, owners and staff develop clever rationales to convince parents and athletes that year-round participation in a single sport is necessary to stay on track for future success. As parents accept these rationales, "high-performance" teams and clubs grow in number and size.

Commercial clubs for gymnastics, figure skating, ice hockey, soccer, tennis, volleyball, lacrosse, and other sports now advertise that they are dedicated to turning children into headline-grabbing, revenue-producing sport prodigies. Children in these programs even become marketing tools for program managers and symbols of the moral worth of parents, who pay the bills and brag to friends about their children's accomplishments and how much

they have done to "create" successful children. For example, eleven-year-old standout athletes may be used by clubs as marketing hooks to recruit dues-paying members. When this occurs, the adults who work at the club become financially dependent on the performances of eleven-year-olds who they train to succeed in high-profile competitive events, and this can become a recipe for abuse (Donnelly and Petherick, 2004; Hite, 2012; Zirin, 2013a).

Children in high-performance training programs work(out) at their sports for long hours week after week and year after year. They compete regularly, their images and accomplishments may be used to market commercial training programs, they sometimes appear on commercial television and attract paying spectators to events at which they perform, and a few even have product endorsement contracts. All this occurs without government regulation, which might protect the interests, bodies, health, and overall development of child athletes. When the livelihoods of coaches and other adults depend on the performances of child athletes, elite training can become a form of child labor (Donnelly and Petherick, 2004).

Child labor laws in some societies prevent adults from using children to make money, but there are no enforceable standards regulating what child athletes do or what happens to them. Governments in a few countries mandate certain forms of coaching education, but coaches in the United States need no such training to work with children. They can use fear, intimidation, and coercion to turn a few highly talented children into medal-winning athletes without being held accountable to anything but market forces. The results of this situation are sometimes frightening, but many parents and young athletes continue to believe that unless coaches are coercive, controlling, and abusive, they cannot effectively motivate and train successful elite athletes.

As elite programs become more popular, there is a need to have more public discussions about where the line should be drawn to separate abuse from the motivational and training strategies used by some coaches. The argument generally used to avoid this discussion is that the children themselves want to specialize, be pushed, and excel in sports. But these children have not reached the age when they can give legally "informed consent." In addition, we don't allow ten-year-olds to work as actors without regulations just because they like it and their parents approve; there are rules that regulate what child workers can do and how long they can work—even if they enjoy the work.

Increased Involvement and Concerns Among Parents

Youth sports have become serious business in many families. The expectation that parents must control the actions and nurture the dreams of their children 24/7 has made parenthood today more demanding than ever before. Many parents now feel compelled to find the best-organized youth sport programs for their children and then ensure that their children's interests are being met in those programs.

Even though multiple factors influence child development, many people attribute the success or failure of children entirely to their parents. When children are successful in sports, their parents are perceived to be parenting the correct way. When a child succeeds, parents are congratulated, and people want to know what they did to "create" a prodigy; when a child fails, the moral worth of parents is questioned, and people want to know what parents did wrong.

Under these conditions, a child's success in sports is especially important for parents. Youth sports are highly visible activities and become sites where mothers and fathers can prove their moral worth as parents. This greatly increases the stakes associated with youth sports and causes parents to take the success of their child athletes very seriously. These stakes increase even further when parents expect their children to receive college scholarships, professional contracts as athletes, or social acceptance and popularity in school and among peers. When parents think in these terms, the success of their children in youth sports is linked to anticipated social and financial payoffs, and the sponsorship of their children is often seen as an investment for which they expect certain rewards in return.

As the moral, financial, and social stakes associated with youth sport participation have increased, youth sports have become sites for extreme actions among some adults. Parents are increasingly assertive and disruptive as they advocate the interests of their children with coaches, referees, and program managers. A few have attacked and even killed others over sport-related disputes.

As the actions of parents have become more extreme, some sport programs now sponsor parent education seminars combined with new rules and enforcement procedures to control parents at practices and games. These strategies are useful, but their success depends on administering them with an understanding of the cultural expectations that exist for this generation of parents.

As long as parental moral worth is linked to the achievements of their children, and parents feel morally obliged to nurture the sport dreams of their children, parents will be deeply involved in and concerned about youth sports. Furthermore, when parents make major financial sacrifices and invest vast amounts of time in their children's sports, their actions will be difficult to control. As long as the prevailing cultural ideology emphasizes that parents are solely responsible for their children, mothers and fathers will assertively advocate the interests of their children. If they don't, who will? Under these cultural circumstances, many parents conclude that it is their moral obligation to get in the face of anyone standing in the way of their child's success in sports.

Increased Interest in Alternative and Action Sports

As youth sports have become increasingly structured and controlled by adults, some young people seek alternatives allowing them to engage more freely in physical activities on their own terms. Because organized youth sports are the most visible and widely accepted settings for children's sport participation, these unstructured and participant-controlled activities are referred to as alternative sports—alternatives, that is, to organized sports.

Alternative sports, or "action sports," as many now refer to them, encompass a wide array of physical activities. Their popularity is based in part on children's reactions against the highly structured character of adult-controlled, organized sports. For example, when legendary skateboarder Tony Hawk was asked why he chose to skateboard rather than do other sports, he said, "I liked having my own pace and my own rules . . . and making up my own challenges" (in Finger, 2004, p. 84). Similarly, when Sonja Catalano, the president of the California Amateur Skateboard League, was asked

why skateboarding became popular, she explained, "We didn't . . . have any parents. That's what drew a lot of kids. . . . It was their thing" (Higgins, 2007).

When I observe children in action sports, I'm regularly amazed by the physical skills that they develop without adult coaches and scheduled practices and contests. Although I'm concerned about injuries and the informal exclusion of females that often are part of these sports, I'm impressed by the discipline and dedication of young action sport participants who seek challenges apart from adult-controlled sport settings. The norms in these participant-controlled activities vary from one location to another, but most young people use them as guides as they share the spaces used in their sports (Bradley, 2010; Seifert and Henderson, 2010).

Mark Shaw, winner of the first International Mountain Board Championships, explained that action sports often are attractive to young people because the older and more skilled participants teach tricks and give helpful advice to those with less experience. He said, "I look forward to helping young skaters . . . at the park each weekend almost as much as I look forward to skating and my own progression on the board" (2002, p. 3). Many young people find this orientation and the sense of community it creates to be more welcoming than what occurs in organized youth sports.

Participation in alternative and action sports has become so widespread that media companies and corporations wishing to recruit young people as consumers have sponsored competitive forms of these sports and hype them as "extreme" activities. These sponsored events, such as the X Games, the Dew Action Sports Tour, and others sponsored by Oakley, Red Bull, and Lucas Oil, provide exposure and support for athletes, but they alter the activities by making them more structured and controlled. At this point, we need research on the ways that this occurs and its implications for the participation experiences of young people. For example, as coaches and organized competitive programs become more common, these sports cease to be alternatives, and many young people may seek other activities that allow them to be free and creative.

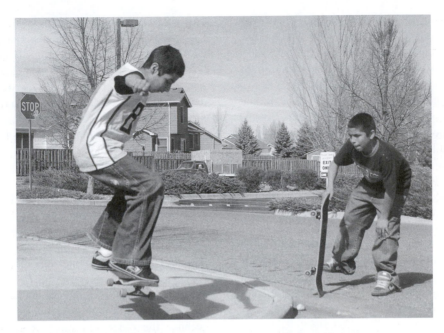

Many young people seek alternatives to adult-controlled youth sports. Skateboarding and BMX biking are popular alternative sports that young people use to express themselves as they learn skills on their own terms. The experience of creating your own sports and playing them on your terms is very different from the experience of playing organized youth sports under the supervision of parents, coaches, referees, and league administrators. (*Source:* © Jay Coakley)

INFORMAL, PLAYER-CONTROLLED SPORTS: A CASE OF THE GENERATION GAP

The structure and culture of childhood have changed dramatically over the past two generations. When I was growing up in the 1950s and 1960s, I spent at least fifteen hours playing in "pickup games" and informal, player-controlled sports for every one hour I played or practiced an organized sport. Few of my sport experiences were ever seen or evaluated by parents, coaches, or referees. They were *my* experiences, and it was up to me to give them meaning because neither parents nor coaches were there to provide their interpretations, praise, or criticisms. I decided if I had fun, played well, succeeded, or failed. My judgments were influenced by peers with whom I played and by my general experiences, but there were no "outside spectators" shaping my perspectives. Further, there were no official statistics, scores, records, game films, or coaches' ratings to influence how I defined, evaluated, and then integrated these experiences into my life.

I played on high school teams in five different sports (over four years) and played other sports during summers. Only in college did I specialize because I had a full, four-year basketball scholarship, and there was a team rule prohibiting involvement in sports that might cause injuries or distract attention from basketball training. However, I golfed, swam, and played in softball, handball, and basketball leagues during summers. Although I played over 130 basketball and baseball games as a college athlete, my parents saw none of them, nor did I expect them to do so.

Two generations later, Maddie, my seventeen-year-old granddaughter has played for eight years on a club travel team organized by a local nonprofit soccer organization. Her team plays two seasons, one in fall and another in spring. About half the games are out of town, and each involves two to seven hours of round-trip driving. Maddie's team also plays in an indoor league between seasons and in three to four major tournaments that require significant travel during the year. Additionally, it is highly recommended that all travel team members play in one or more summer soccer camps.

When I was nine to seventeen years old, and when Maddie's mom was nine to seventeen years old, we were never asked to be so exclusively committed to a single sport. To meet the expectations of her coaches, Maddie has given up opportunities to play basketball, volleyball, karate, and swimming—all of which are sports that she enjoys. My parents could not and would not have supported such intense, specialized sport participation, and I would not have allowed Maddie's mother to specialize this way when she was that age in the 1980s.

Although Maddie has played organized soccer since she was four years old, she's played very few informal sports and pickup games. She lacks time to do so, and her parents, like most parents today, have never felt comfortable allowing her to roam the neighborhood to find other children and create informal games in places that cannot be predicted ahead of time. Even if she did have permission, she would not find peers with whom she could create informal games. This is because parents today fear that their unsupervised children could be exploited by strangers or create trouble of their own doing. Therefore, for every one hour that Maddie has played informal games, she has spent at least twenty hours practicing or playing games on organized teams under the watchful eyes of coaches, referees, and parents. Only a handful of times during thirteen years of playing organized sports has she played an official game without family members in attendance.

Maddie and I typify our respective generations when it comes to youth sports. My experiences were enjoyable, and I think I benefited from them; Maddie, at seventeen years old, says the same thing, even though her experiences have been very different from mine. This raises the sociological question of whether we can make sense of the differences between them. Fortunately, there is research to help us think critically about the changes over the past two generations and the implications that they have for young people and the place of sports in their lives.

Learning from Play: Informal Games and Organized Sports

Informal games exist when young people come together and agree to organize themselves for the sake of having fun. My research indicates that informal games involve *fun* to the extent that they provide action, exciting challenges, and opportunities for personal expression and the maintenance of friendships (Coakley, 1983b). On an individual level, *fun* requires personal involvement in the action of a game and facing game-based challenges that test and extend personal skills. When the players are mixed ages, a seven-year-old playing with older children may have fun without a high level of personal involvement in the action, whereas the older and more skilled players require continuous personal involvement to have fun and they often alter rules to create exciting challenges.

Nearly all informal games are organized to maximize action. When there's plenty of space to play and few available players, the game rules are interpreted and adjusted to keep everyone involved, so that players don't quit and destroy the game. When space is limited and many young people want to play, game rules are enforced more strictly, and those who aren't selected to play are relegated to the sidelines; furthermore, the team winning a game may claim the right to play against a challenger that replaces the losing team. But in all cases, the emphasis is on action and exciting challenges. Action keeps alive a "spirit of play," and challenges require players to focus on testing and extending their skills.

Research shows that informal games help children learn to cooperate and express themselves physically through a wider range of movements than they would try if coaches were evaluating them (Ginsburg, 2007; Henricks, 2006). For example, when Tom Farrey, an Emmy Award-winning journalist at ESPN, investigated why France produces great soccer talent, he was told by André Mérelle, the director of youth soccer development in France, that they emphasize the importance of unstructured play and informal games for French children. Mérelle told Farrey this:

> Everyone wants to win games. That's good. But *how* do you win? If you're too focused on winning games, you don't learn to play well. You get too nervous, because you're always afraid to make errors (in Farrey, 2008, p. 75).

As Farrey talked with Zinedine Zidane, three-time World Player of the Year, Thierry Henry, also rated a top player in the world, and other soccer standouts in France, he concluded that the French developmental approach succeeds because it emphasizes informal play—no uniforms, positions, lined fields, game clocks, league standings, or adults yelling instructions from the sidelines. Without the constraining structures and adult expectations that characterize organized youth sports, young people learn to improvise, feel the joy of intrinsic satisfaction, and develop a playing style and personality that make them unique. This allows them to be creative and claim ownership of soccer, rather than feeling that soccer owns them. As French coaches explained, informal games are the places where children develop a personal "feel" for the game and a vision for what occurs and is possible on the field of play—things that are not learned as readily in organized, adult-controlled games in which the structure and rhythm of play are dictated by rules, coaches, and referees.

Farrey also reports that sport development experts worldwide say that children under eight years old should not play highly organized sports or on (soccer) teams with more than five players. From eight to fourteen years old, games can be increasingly organized, but positional play should not be emphasized. There should be no travel teams and no more than one game per week or thirty to thirty-five games per year. Most important, say the experts, is that all coaches must complete a coaching education course and be regularly recertified through continuing coach education. When coaches learn about child development, they can facilitate participation opportunities through which young people are likely to develop a passion for the sport and the awareness that the sport enables them to be creative and expressive.

Research on Play and Development

Developmental research supports the approach used in French soccer (Balyi et al., 2013; Bloom, 1985; Côté, 2011; Côté and Fraser-Thomas, 2007). When Benjamin Bloom, a noted educational psychologist from the University of Chicago, studied 120 individuals who were recognized world-class talents in classical piano, sculpting, mathematics, Olympic swimming, professional tennis, and neurological research, he concluded that talent development occurred over a long period of time under special conditions. In all cases, the talent development process began with exploration, play, and expressive fun. It did not begin with structured activities organized by other people, early specialization, or childhood commitments to long-term goals. Nor did it begin with pep talks about hard work, sacrifice, dedication, and the need to constantly practice. It began with opportunities to freely and playfully explore an activity and discover that it required creativity and effort. Talent development ultimately depended on whether the young people emotionally bonded with the activity, claimed it as their own, and identified the skills they wanted to master. When this occurred, the young people came to be driven by the feelings of exhilaration that occurred as they met and mastered new challenges.

Bloom found that this process took at least ten years to occur, but when it did, the young people, usually in their mid-to late-teens, were ready to specialize and make the commitments required to excel. At this point, fun merged with the hard work of mastering skills, and this merger fueled the passion and drive that enabled them to achieve excellence.

Bloom's findings have been widely supported by other scholars who study the development of excellence in sports (Côté and Fraser-Thomas, 2007; Ericsson, 2012; Ericsson et al., 2007). For example, reports on the experiences of U.S. Olympians and top collegiate athletes indicate that they attribute their success to being introduced to sports through unstructured play and informal games and having opportunities to play multiple sports through junior high school (SPARC, 2013).

We know that the existence of informal games and sports require and foster creativity, interpersonal skills, and problem-solving abilities among the players (Côté and Fraser-Thomas, 2007; Elkind, 2007, 2008). Creating games requires knowledge of game models, but maintaining them in the face of multiple unanticipated challenges requires keen conflict resolution skills and an ability to develop on-the-spot solutions to problems. Players must understand the basic requirements of an organized activity so they can create games to fit here-and-now circumstances; additionally, they must form teams, cooperate with peers, develop rules, and take responsibility for following and enforcing the rules. These are important lessons, and we need research to explain when and how children learn them in different types of sport experiences and whether the learning that occurs in sports is used by children in their relationships and activities apart from the playing field.

YOUTH SPORTS TODAY: ASSESSING OUR EFFORTS

A few years ago the Citizenship Through Sport Alliance (CTSA) brought together a panel of experts to assess the current state of organized youth sports in the United States. Using their collective knowledge, the panelists created a Youth Sports National Report Card.[2] They also issued grades for twenty-five important elements of existing organized sport programs. The elements were divided into five sets, with each set related to a major topic. The topics and the overall grade for each are

1. Child-Centered Philosophy: D
2. Coaching: C
3. Health and Safety: C+
4. Officiating: B−
5. Parental Behavior/Involvement: D

The panel that assigned the grades consisted of researchers, youth sports leaders, attorneys, youth coaches, and parents. Their goal was to identify where youth sports were succeeding or failing and to alert people to the need for improving the sport experiences of children. The panelists also identified specific problem areas that needed attention. The problem statements emphasized that, in general, youth sports

- Have lost a child-centered focus, meaning that there is too little emphasis on the child's experience and too much emphasis on winning
- Are distorted by overinvested sports parents, who have unrealistic expectations and often undermine for their own child and others the benefits of playing sports
- Fail to adequately train and evaluate youth sport coaches
- Overemphasize early sports specialization that often leads to burnout, overuse injuries, and a hypercompetitive culture focused on travel teams
- Ignore the age-based interests and developmental abilities of children who view sports as a source of fun, friends, physical action, and skill development

---

[2]Grading key for each topic: A = Outstanding; B = Good; C = Fair; D = Poor; F = Failing. Copies of the report cards can be downloaded and used to assess programs in your community and to determine where changes should be made to improve them.

The panel also created a Youth Sports Community Report Card for Parents to enable mothers and fathers to evaluate programs serving young people ages six to fourteen in their communities. A third report card was designed for youth sports leaders to evaluate their programs and identify needed improvements for teams and leagues. These tools were intended to facilitate discussions about the organization of youth sports and how it might be improved to benefit all young people.

Unsurprisingly, the report cards were not widely used and had no significant impact. But this is mostly due to how youth sports are organized in the United States. Most other countries have a central sports authority or governing body, such as a federal ministry of sport, that can exert influence on sport programs nationwide, especially publicly funded youth programs. This makes communication to those programs effective, and it makes policies related to safety, health, and overall development of young people easier to implement and promote.

Youth sports in the United States are a fragmented, disjointed, and uncoordinated array of programs. They are based on diverse adult interests, including profit-making, sustaining jobs for adults, generating local tourism through annual tournaments, identifying sport talent, nurturing the best age-group athletes, introducing children to sports, developing basic sport skills, providing neighborhood-based recreational experiences, training athletes for local high school programs, winning regional and national tournaments, building character and leadership skills, controlling young people identified as "at-risk," keeping kids off the streets, fostering community integration, helping immigrant children learn U.S. culture, creating tough young men, boosting the self-esteem of young women, building new sports like lacrosse or rowing, and achieving many other goals that adults think are worthy.

Of course, all youth programs should not be the same, but because physical inactivity, obesity, and other fitness-related health problems are at crisis levels today, it would be helpful if they followed general principles related to health, well-being, and positive youth development.

To move in this direction, Tom Farrey, an Emmy-winning journalist at ESPN, developed Project Play through the Aspen Institute's Sports and Society Program. Project Play is a bold attempt to re-imagine and re-form youth sports in the United States so that programs are based on good research about child development and the positive consequences of lifelong physical activity. Farrey and his working board of advisors brought together key stakeholders from business, health, sports, education, research, and government to brainstorm how youth sports can better serve the *common good*—the quality of life in the nation as a whole.

The stakeholders agreed that youth sports should be a context for developing **physical literacy**—that is, *the ability, competence, and desire to be physically active for life (Project Play, 2015, p. 8)*. This is done through age-appropriate play, early positive movement experiences, universal access to safe participation opportunities, quality coach education, and support from both public and private sectors.

The stakeholders also agreed that there is a need for a national sports agenda or general policy recommendations that provide guidance to those who organize youth sports. The long-term goal is to link youth sport programs with a nationwide emphasis on physical literacy and lifelong participation in health-producing physical activities.

Canada and other nations have such policies (for example, see http://www.canadiansportforlife.ca/) and are taking them seriously in the face of their own health-related crises, none of which are as extreme as the crisis in the United States, where inactivity and obesity have hit record levels. Although people in other nations sometimes look to the United States when it comes to developing elite athletes in certain sports, they are unlikely to see a model for producing public health. However, there are some recent encouraging moves in that direction, including First Lady Michelle Obama's Let's Move program. And in the realm of traditional sport, USA Hockey has created the American Development Model (http://www.admkids.com), which does an excellent job of outlining for youth hockey coaches an age-appropriate method of teaching hockey and organizing youth programs. The model is based on youth development research, which also was used to create the national Canadian Sport for Life program (CS4L).

Although there are models for organizing youth sports to serve both the common good and the interests of children, it is difficult to convince people to consider those models and implement them in connection with their programs. But the people working with Project Play are focused on doing so.

THE CHALLENGE OF IMPROVING YOUTH SPORTS

Changing youth sports is a formidable task. Many people have vested interests in keeping them as they are, and those who currently control youth sport programs are mostly concerned with increasing their size, promoting the performance ethic more effectively, providing elite training, and taking teams and athletes to state, regional, and national tournaments.

As public programs have been eliminated, youth sport entrepreneurs have come onto the scene. They have developed sport clubs with travel teams and paid coaches. They have built sport-specific programs that control soccer, volleyball, lacrosse, and other teams and leagues in communities across the United States. They sponsor annual tournaments for qualifying teams—or teams that can pay the costly entry fees—and they crown state, regional, and even national champions at all age levels.

> A child's greatest achievements are possible in play, achievements that tomorrow will become her basic level of real action and morality. —Lev Vygotsky (1978)

Cities bid to host these tournaments because they boost the local economy as thousands of youth sport tourist families come to town and spend money during stays of three or more days. Some of these tournaments attract high school and college coaches seeking young talent for their programs, and these coaches are used by the entrepreneurs to entice teams and families to pay the entry fees in the hope that their children will be noticed and recruited.

An extreme example of this approach is illustrated by the partnership formed by ESPN and Walt Disney World Resort, both owned by The Walt Disney Company. These partners hold tournaments year-round for athletes of all ages at their massive sport complex in Orlando, Florida. They host many national youth sport tournaments because families come with teams and often stay for extra days to visit Disney World at $100+ per person per day. Hotels and restaurants also benefit—all in the name of youth sports. This pattern of hosting weekend, postseason, off-season, and preseason tournaments has now spread nationwide, so that youth sports have become a money-making industry more than activities that benefit children. It also means that efforts to make youth sports more child-centered and age-appropriate will meet resistance if they don't support this industry.

The people working with Project Play understand this challenge. But they are motivated by the general sense that in the United States, youth sports are broken: they fail to serve populations with the highest need for physical activity—children who are poor, overweight, disabled, or ethnic minorities. U.S. youth sports also are broken in that many programs and teams have done little to nurture the play element in sports—that is, experimentation, creativity, personal expression, spontaneity, and the intrinsic satisfaction associated with physical movement.

As youth sports have become increasingly organized around the achievement of measurable performance goals, the play element of sport participation

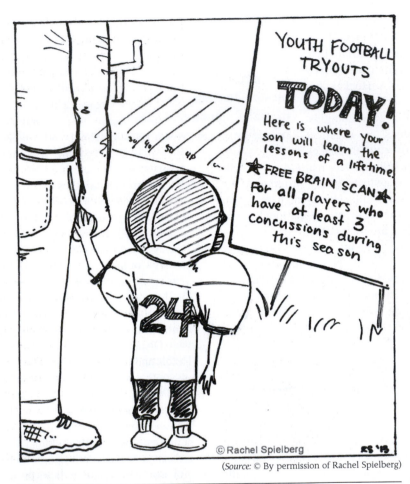

(*Source:* © By permission of Rachel Spielberg)

Information about concussions and injury rates in certain youth sports may lead parents to seek alternative programs that give higher priority to play and creativity than to organization and conquest.

has been marginalized or forgotten. This is a problem because play is the foundation for motivation in physical activities. It is the source of joy and the fuel for good feelings that keep people coming back to physical activities regardless of age, ability, or the likelihood of competitive success. Play is done for its own sake, for the feeling of pleasure that it brings rather than for approval and status. When play is absent or rare in sport experiences, dropout rates are high and the likelihood of returning to sport is low.

This means that part of the task of reinventing youth sports is to reinfuse play into physical activities of all types, including traditional organized, competitive sports. Noted triathlon coach Barry Shepley has observed, "Today kids don't play. They are either totally inactive or they are in a coached, expensive program where they have no time or opportunity to simply play and experiment" (in Richard, 2010). Medal-winning U.S. skier Julia Mancuso explains that memories of childhood play were her source of motivation as she trained and competed in the Olympics and World Cup races: "The only thing that kept me in skiing was all the fun I had when I was little" (Layden, 2010a, p. 34).

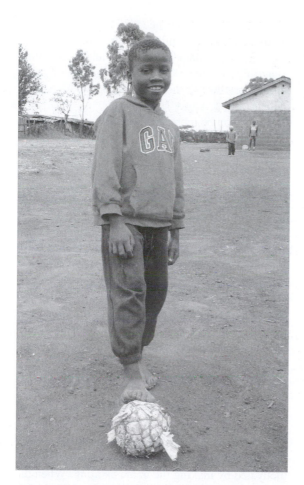

Organized youth sports are a luxury item in most of the world. The parents of this ten-year-old Kenyan boy don't have the resources to nurture his sport dreams. But using his bare feet and a ball of rags bound with twine, he's managed to develop impressive soccer skills. The meaning he gives to kicking this ball likely differs from the meanings that privileged ten-year-old North American boys give to kicking dozens of "official soccer balls" purchased by parents and clubs. (*Source:* © Kevin Young)

Play also is a key factor in achieving excellence in sports. For example, when describing Lionel Messi, reputedly the best soccer player in the world (2011–present), historian and novelist Eduardo Galeano says, "No one plays with as much joy as Messi does—he plays like a child enjoying the pasture, playing for the pleasure of playing, not the duty of winning" (in Longman, 2011c). Messi agrees: "I have fun like a child in the street. When the day comes when I'm not enjoying it, I will leave football (soccer)."

For those interested in attracting and retaining young people in sports of all types, and hopefully producing positive health consequences in the process, the challenge is to develop strategies for facilitating play in sport experiences. This is not an easy task. Externally imposed structures often undermine play. Of course, no policy can make people play. Therefore, the challenge facing Project Play and others concerned about children is to enable and provide incentives to those who manage and coach youth sports to make spaces for play in their programs. If this occurs to at least some degree, parents and children will have alternatives to the costly and often playless programs that are so prevalent today.

The timing for introducing such strategies appears to be good today. Parents are increasingly concerned about the injury rates in youth programs that emphasize the performance principle, and they may be willing to accept changes in existing programs or seek alternative programs that highlight play experiences for young people. At the same time, coaches and program administrators are seeking safer ways to play their sports as well as strategies to retain young people in their programs.

RECOMMENDATIONS FOR IMPROVING YOUTH SPORTS

Recommendations usually focus exclusively on organized youth sports. However, informal and alternative sports also have problems that need to be addressed. Many children opt for these sports because they provide action, exciting challenges, and opportunities for personal expression and maintaining friendships. But they often involve physical risks and various forms of exclusion. This suggests that adults should foster participation opportunities for children interested in joining informal games and participating in action sports. For example, instead of passing laws to prohibit skateboarding or in-line skating, adults could work with young people to design and provide safe settings for them to create their own activities and norms that are inclusive (Donnelly and Coakley, 2003).

The challenge for adults is to be supportive and provide guidance without controlling young people who need their own spaces to create physical activities. Adult guidance can make those spaces safer and more inclusive—for boys and girls as well as children with a disability and from various ethnic and social class backgrounds. The gender exclusion that exists in certain alternative sports is especially problematic and begs for creative solutions that make the cultures of those sports more inclusive.

As the tradition of informal games has nearly disappeared among young people today, there is a need to develop what might be called **hybrid sports** that *combine features of player-controlled informal games and adult-controlled organized sports.* Hybrid sport activities have not been studied, but they come in at least two forms. *First,* there are informal games in which adults provide subtle guidance to children, who create and control most of what occurs as they play games in safe settings that are familiar and accessible to them. *Second,* there are organized sport teams on which parents and coaches encourage un- or semi-structured play during practices and also include children in decision-making, rule enforcement, and conflict resolution processes. As more adults learn that positive youth development requires involvement in unstructured play and informal games, there will be attempts to facilitate them.

Improving Organized Sports

When considering improvements for organized youth sports, programs and teams should be evaluated in terms of whether they are child-centered and organized to match the developmental age of children. This makes children a valuable source of information about needed improvements. If children define fun in terms of action, exciting challenges, personal expression, and reaffirming friendships (see p. 94), it makes sense to organize youth sports so that these aspects of experience are emphasized.

Action can be increased by altering or eliminating certain rules, changing the structure of games, and using smaller teams and playing areas. But many adults resist these changes because they want games to resemble what occurs in elite, adult sports. They say that children must play "the real thing" to learn the sport properly, and they forget that children are more interested in action than mimicking adults and following rules that were never intended to promote a child's fun. Therefore, adults should control their emphasis on rules, order, standardized conditions, predictability, and performance statistics, and abandon tactics that slow and stop action; after all, high-scoring games are fun, even if many adults see them as undisciplined free-for-alls.

Exciting challenges are destroyed by lopsided scores. This is why children often include handicaps, "do-overs," and other adjustments that preserve the excitement of competition when they play informal games. Motivation depends on perceived chances for success, and close games keep children motivated by making the game exciting. When the adults who control youth sports resist changes that affect game scores and outcomes, some people call for "mercy rules" that stop games, or they run game clocks continuously to shorten games with lopsided scores. But this subverts action and excitement for young people, who would alter teams to keep games challenging rather than simply cutting them short. Therefore, adults should use creative rules and strategies to promote exciting and challenging action in youth sports rather than giving priority to winning games, developing a killer instinct in players, and qualifying for postseason tournaments.

Personal expression is maximized when games are organized to allow for creativity and experimentation. Rigid systems of control and specialization

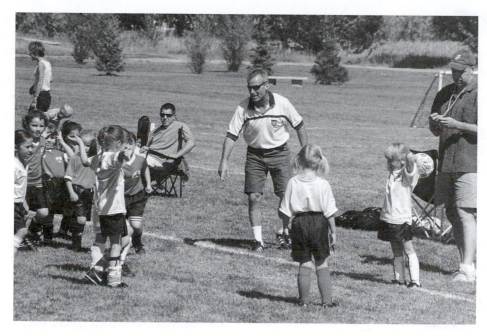

When coaches and parents constantly shout directions during games, it's unlikely that children will feel comfortable engaging in personally expressive actions. This makes it nearly impossible for children to emotionally identify with and claim ownership of a sport. Instead, many of them view organized sports as an adult thing that they'll eventually outgrow—much like braces on their teeth (Farrey, 2008). (*Source:* © Jay Coakley)

by position restrict players' experiences and opportunities to express themselves. Reducing team size increases opportunities for personal involvement and expression. For example, ice hockey games for children under twelve years old should always be played across the width of the rink, thereby allowing three times as many teams to compete at the same time. Basketball could be reorganized so that three-player "first-string" teams play a half-court game at one basket, while second- and third-string teams play at other baskets; a combined score would determine the overall winner. But these strategies require adults to revise their approach to youth sports so that encouraging children to claim ownership of their sport experiences is a high priority.

Reaffirming friendships is central in the lives of children. Organized sports provide contexts for making friends, but friendships are difficult to nurture when children see each other only at adult-controlled practices and games. Additionally, making friends with opponents is seldom considered in organized sports. Therefore, youth teams should be neighborhood- and school-based whenever possible. Pregame warm-ups should mix players from both teams, and players should introduce themselves to the person they line up with as each quarter or half begins. Unless children learn that games cannot exist without cooperation between opponents, they will have no understanding of fair play, why rules exist, why rule enforcement is necessary, and why players should follow game rules. Without this understanding, children don't have what it takes to maintain fair play at the same time that they strive for competitive success. When this occurs, youth sports are *not* worth our time and effort.

summary

ARE ORGANIZED PROGRAMS WORTH THE EFFORT?

Although physical activities exist in all cultures, organized youth sports are a luxury. They require resources and discretionary time among children and adults. They exist only when children are not required to work and when adults believe that experiences during childhood influence individual growth and development. Youth sports have a unique history in every society where they exist, but they characteristically emphasize experiences and values that are central to the dominant culture.

The growth of organized sports in North America and much of Europe is associated with changes in the family and in ideas about children and childhood that occurred during the latter half of the twentieth century. Many parents now see organized sports as the source of important developmental experiences in the lives of their children. The fact that the programs provide adult supervision also makes them attractive to parents who see free time and unstructured activities as opportunities for their children to get into trouble.

Major trends in youth sports today include the privatization of organized programs, an emphasis on the performance ethic, the development of high-performance training programs, and increased involvement among parents. In response to these trends, some young people have turned to informal, alternative, and action sports that they can control on their terms without being controlled and judged by adults.

Children's sport experiences in the United States have changed dramatically over the past two generations. Informal, player-controlled sports were prevalent in the past, whereas organized adult-controlled sports are prevalent today. The decline of loosely structured, informal play and games has influenced the extent to which physical activities are the source of expressive fun among children. This is important in light of research showing that the talent development process in children usually begins with opportunities to freely and playfully explore multiple activities and discover one or more that enable them to be creative and expressive. Unless young people have opportunities to emotionally identify with physical activities, claim them as their own, and decide what they want to learn, excellence is rarely achieved.

The overall benefits of organized youth sports today are limited primarily because they've lost a child-centered focus, neglected the evaluation and training of coaches, and reflect too much the orientations of overzealous parents who have unrealistic expectations. Many programs are costly and designed to favor children who are bigger, faster, and stronger than their peers. This creates access issues that affect children from lower-income families and those whose abilities are average or below. The emphasis on early specialization in a single sport and year-round participation tends to wear out early bloomers, deny access to late bloomers, and exclude those who aren't inclined or selected to be on elite teams.

Youth sports in the United States are driven by the diverse interests of adults who organize teams, leagues, and programs. As a result, they have failed to meet the needs of young people, especially those who are poor, overweight, disabled, and from marginalized ethnic populations. Given the current crises related to physical inactivity, obesity, and other fitness-related health problems, there is a need to rethink the organization and provision of youth sports in the United States. This is a daunting task because there are so many vested interests in preserving youth sports as they are. However, models for reorganizing youth sports do exist, and the current time may be right to develop strategies to encourage and enable people to make changes.

Recommendations for improving youth sports emphasize that there should be action, exciting challenges, and opportunities for personal expression and the maintenance of friendships. This requires more open and flexible structures and less overt control by adults. The goal of such changes is to provide young people with opportunities to learn that cooperation and an understanding of rules and rule enforcement is the foundation of competitive sports played fairly and ethically.

A major obstacle to change is that there are vested interests in maintaining and expanding programs as they are currently organized. Coaching education programs could facilitate critical thinking among those who work most directly with children in these programs, but they tend to emphasize organization and control rather than critically assessing and changing youth sports.

Overall, organized sports for children *are* worth the effort—*if* adults put the needs and interests of children ahead of the organizational needs of sport programs and their own needs to gain status through their association with successful and highly skilled child athletes.

SUPPLEMENTAL READINGS

SPORT MANAGEMENT ISSUES

- You work in the sport and recreation division of a city government. As it faces a budget crisis, you are asked to present arguments for and against privatizing all the city's youth sport programs. List the major points you would include in your presentation.
- You work in the main office of a youth soccer organization that has programs in five states. The actions of players' parents have become increasingly troublesome and extreme in those programs. Coaches want you to tell them why parents are so obnoxious today and what can be done to minimize their troublesome actions. Outline the points you will include in your explanation and recommendations.
- As the director of programs in a park and recreation department, you have an opportunity to hire two people. They will work with you to reform the youth sport programs in the city. Write the job description for these two positions and identify the skills you are seeking in applicants.

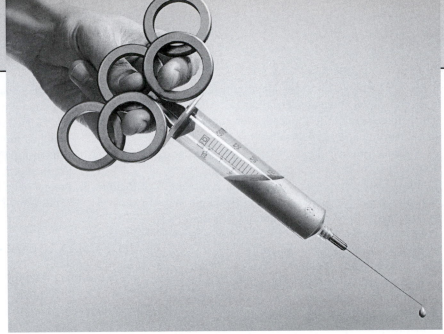

(*Source:* © C. J. Burton/Corbis)

DEVIANCE IN SPORTS

Is It Out of Control?

There's a lot of rule bending going on. It can be a great advantage.

—**College football coach (in Feldman, 2010)**

These individuals and organizations [connected with FIFA] engaged in bribery to decide who would televise games, where the games would be held, and who would run the organization overseeing organized soccer worldwide.

—**U.S. Attorney General Loretta E. Lynch (in Clifford and Apuzzo, 2015)**

Soccer match fixing has become a massive worldwide crime, on a par with drug trafficking, prostitution and the trade in illegal weapons.

—**Brett Forrest, ESPN journalist (2012)**

. . . given that marijuana is a legitimate pain reliever—especially for the migraines that can be a byproduct of head trauma—and is far less dangerous and potentially addictive than, say, OxyContin, it is almost immoral to deny players the right to use it.

—**Howard Bryant, ESPN journalist (2013)**

Chapter Outline

Learning Objectives

- Define deviance and identify challenges faced when studying deviance in sports.

- Explain the absolutist and constructionist approaches to deviance in sports.

- Define the sport ethic, and identify the norms of the sport ethic.

- Distinguish between deviant overconformity and deviant underconformity.

- Identify the athletes most likely to overconform to the norms of the sport ethic.

- Understand the research findings on the major forms of deviance in sports and identify examples that do not involve athletes.

- Explain why performance-enhancing substance use is so prevalent among athletes today.

- Outline the phases in a professional sport career and when performance-enhancing substances become important in that career.

- Understand why the current system of drug testing in sports will not eliminate the use of performance-enhancing substances.

- Outline and evaluate alternatives to the current war on doping in sports.

103

Media stories about drug use, on-the-field rule violations, and off-the-field criminal actions are so common today that deviance is seen by many as out of control in sports. For those who accept the great sport myth these stories create a dilemma: Either they must admit that their belief in the purity and goodness of sport is wrong or they must conclude that sport is being undermined by money, greed, and undisciplined athletes.

Few people are willing to abandon the great sport myth, so they express outrage at offending individuals and insist that they be banned from sport to preserve its essential purity and goodness. In the face of this outrage and the extent to which it is expressed in mainstream media, it is difficult to have a research-based sociological discussion of deviance in sports. But that is the purpose of this chapter.

Our discussion will focus on four questions as we deal with the issue of deviance:

1. What challenges do we face when studying deviance in sports?
2. What is deviance, and how does sociological knowledge about it help us understand sports as a social phenomenon?
3. Are rates of deviance in sports out of control?
4. Why has the use of performance-enhancing substances become such a persistent problem in many sports?

DEFINING AND STUDYING DEVIANCE IN SPORTS

When a softball player punches an umpire after a disputed call, it's a deviant act because it violates a norm. Similarly, when a college football booster hires prostitutes for high school recruits or when an Olympic judge alters scores to ensure a victory for a particular figure skater, we know that deviance has occurred. In each case, norms are violated.

A **norm** is *a shared expectation that people use to identify what is acceptable and unacceptable in a social world.* Norms exist in all social worlds and serve as the standards that people use to identify

deviance. **Deviance** *occurs when a person's ideas, traits, or actions are perceived by others to fall outside the normal range of acceptance in a society.*

Studying deviance is often tricky because norms take different forms, vary in importance, change over time, and differ from one social world to another. **Formal norms** *are official expectations that take the form of written rules or laws,* whereas **informal norms** are *customs or unwritten, shared understandings of how a person is expected to think, appear, and act in a social world.*

When basketball players foul an opponent or shove a referee in anger over a foul call, they violate formal norms that are written in the official rule book. These norms are enforced by "officials" given the authority to sanction or punish violators. When two college basketball players don't face the U.S. flag during the national anthem or don't participate in a pregame team ritual, they violate unwritten, informal norms. In response, fans may deride players who don't conform to flag-related customs, and teammates may refuse to talk with players that don't meet their expectations for togetherness. This means that there are two forms of deviance. **Formal deviance** involves a *violation of an official rule or law, and is punished by official sanctions administered by people in positions of authority.* **Informal deviance,** on the other hand, involves a *violation of an unwritten custom or shared understanding, and is punished by informal sanctions administered by observers or peers.*

These definitions of norms and deviance appear to be straightforward, but there are different ways to interpret norms and identify deviance when studying sports in society.

CHALLENGES FACED WHEN STUDYING DEVIANCE IN SPORTS

Studying deviance in sports presents challenges for four reasons. First, *the types and causes of deviance in sports are so diverse that no single theory can explain them all* (Atkinson and Young, 2008).

For example, think of the types of deviance that occur just among male college athletes: failing to show up for a scheduled practice, violating rules or committing fouls on the playing field during a match or game, taking performance-enhancing substances, hazing rookie team members by demeaning them and forcing them to do illegal things, binge drinking, fighting in bars, harassing women, engaging in group sex, sexual assault, turning in coursework prepared by others, betting on college sports, using painkillers to stay on the field, destroying hotel property during a road trip, taking money from boosters, and going home over a holiday to meet an agent who gives money to their parents.

This list includes only a sample of cases reported for athletes at one level of competition over the past decade. The list would be more diverse if we included all athletes and if we listed examples of deviance by coaches, administrators, team owners, and spectators. Therefore, it is important to study deviance in the context in which it occurs and not expect that a single theory will explain all cases.

Second, *actions accepted in sports may be defined as deviant in other spheres of society, and actions accepted in society may be defined as deviant in sports.* Athletes are allowed and even encouraged to do things outlawed or defined as criminal in other settings. Some things that athletes do in contact sports would be classified as felony assault on the streets. Ice hockey players would be arrested for actions defined as normal during their games. Racecar drivers would be ticketed for speeding and careless driving. Speed skiing and motocross racing would be defined as criminally negligent in everyday life. Even when serious injuries or deaths occur in sports, criminal charges are seldom filed, and civil lawsuits asking for financial compensation are rare and generally unsuccessful when they go to court (Atkinson and Young, 2008; Young 2012).

Coaches treat players in ways that would be defined as deviant if teachers treated students or employers treated employees similarly. Team owners in North American professional sports don't abide by antitrust laws that apply to other business owners. Fans act in ways that would quickly alienate friends and family members in other settings or lead people to define them as mentally deranged.

On the other hand, if athletes take the same drugs or nutritional supplements used by millions of normal citizens, they may be banned from their sports and defined as deviant, even by the people using those products to enhance performance in their non-sport jobs. Athletes who miss practices or games due to sickness or injury often are defined as deviant by coaches and teammates, even though taking "sick days" is accepted as normal in everyday life. College athletes with scholarships violate rules if they hold jobs during the school year, and coaches may punish players who fail to attend class, whereas other students work and cut classes without violating norms. Youth league players may be benched for a game if they miss practice to attend a family picnic, despite the value given to the family outside sports. The fact that norms are applied and enforced differently in sports makes it difficult to use studies of deviance in other contexts to understand what occurs in sports.

Third, *deviance in sports often involves overconformity to norms, rather than rejecting or not conforming to them.* Athletes often go overboard in their dedication to sport and their willingness to do whatever it takes to perform at a level that allows them to stay on the field and do what they love to do. Their attitudes and actions in these cases are *supranormal* in that they overconform to norms widely accepted in society as a whole. Instead of setting limits on what they are willing do as athletes, they evaluate themselves and their peers in terms of their unqualified willingness to go over-the-top and exceed normative limits, even if they jeopardize health and well-being in the process.

This "over-the-top deviance" is often dangerous, but athletes learn to accept it as part of the game they love to play and as the basis for being accepted into the culture of high-performance sports. When this normative overconformity takes

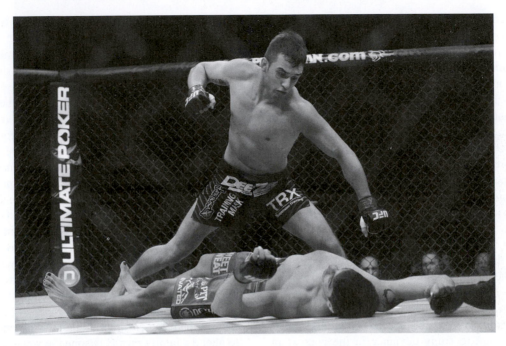

Understanding deviance in sports is a challenge because athletes often do things that are not accepted in other settings. Many actions of mixed martial arts fighters, boxers, football and hockey players, racecar drivers, and wrestlers would be criminal acts off the field. (*Source:* © AP Photo/Jeff Chiu)

the form of extreme dedication, commitment, and self-sacrifice, it brings praise rather than punishment from coaches and fans. It's even used to reaffirm cultural values related to hard work, competition, achievement, and manliness. In the process, people overlook its negative consequences for health, relationships with family and friends, and overall well-being.

This practice of overconformity among athletes makes it difficult to understand certain cases of deviance because they contradict the assumption that deviance always involves *subnormal* or *underconforming* attitudes and actions based on a rejection of norms. However, *supranormal* attitudes and actions also are *abnormal* and deviant (Heckert and Heckert, 2002, 2007; West, 2003). When people don't distinguish between these different forms of deviance, they often define athletes as role models, even though much of what they do is dangerous

to health and well-being and beyond the limits of acceptance in other spheres of life.

Fourth, *training and performance in sports are based on such new forms of science and technology that people have not yet developed norms to guide and evaluate much of what occurs today in sports.* Science and medicine once used only to treat people who were sick are now used regularly in sports. The everyday challenge of training and competition in sports often pushes bodies to such extremes that continued participation and the achievement of performance goals requires the use of new medical treatments and technologies.

Using nutritional supplements is now a standard practice in nearly all sports. As one high school athlete explained, supplements "are as much a fixture in sports participation as mouth guards and athletic tape" (in Mooney, 2003, p. 18). Ingesting substances thought to enhance performance is a taken-for-granted part of being an athlete today—a strategy for living up to the time-honored motto of sport: Citius, Altius, Fortius, which is Latin for "Faster, Higher, Stronger."

A survey of the ads for performance-enhancing substances online (see www.t-nation.com) or in any *Flex, Muscle and Fitness, Planet Muscle,* or *Iron Man* magazine leads to the conclusion that strength and high performance are just a swallow away. Online promotions push protein drinks, amino acids, testosterone boosters, human growth hormone boosters, insulin growth factor, vitamins, energy drinks, and hundreds of other supplements that supposedly will help athletes get the most from their workouts, recover more quickly from injuries, and build a body that can adjust to overtraining and become stronger in the process.

Using the Internet to obtain various substances has occurred since the early 1990s, and this makes it difficult to determine just what actions are deviant and what actions are accepted parts of athletic training; in fact, "normal training" is now an oxymoron because most high performance training involves exceeding boundaries accepted as normal in society as a whole.

Two Approaches to Studying Deviance

When norms are viewed as representing absolute, unchanging truths about right and wrong and good and evil, deviance is identified differently than when norms are viewed as social constructions that people create as they interact with each other and organize their social worlds to meet individual and collective needs.

This truth-based, or **absolutist approach** to deviance *assumes that social norms are based on essential principles that constitute an unchanging foundation for identifying good and evil and distinguishing right from wrong.* According to this approach, all norms represent *ideals,* and whenever an idea, trait, or action departs from an ideal, it is deviant; the greater the departure from the ideal, the more serious the deviance. This approach is illustrated in Figure 5.1, where the broad vertical line signifies a particular ideal, and the horizontal hash line represents increasing deviations from the ideal. The most extreme deviations from the ideal are often described as evil or perverse ideas, traits, or actions. For example, if obedience to the coach is a team norm, any form of disobedience is deviant. The greater and more frequent the disobedience, the more serious the deviance; chronic or consistent deviance would eventually be seen by absolutists as evil or a sign of perverted character.

The absolutist approach has not contributed to a sociological understanding of deviance in sports, but it is often used by fans, media people, and the general public as they discuss rule violations and crimes by athletes and coaches.

It's important for us to understand this approach because it helps us explain how people respond to deviance and why there are so many disagreements when people discuss deviance in sports. For example, if you and I use an absolutist approach but hold

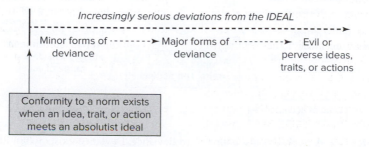

FIGURE 5.1 An *absolutist approach* to deviance: Using ideals as a basis for identifying deviant ideas, traits, and actions.

different ideals, it becomes difficult for us to jointly study deviance. Let's say that my ideal is fair play, and your ideal is achieving excellence as demonstrated through winning. According to my ideal, all violations of game rules would be deviant, whereas you would say that a player was deviant if your team lost because she refused to commit a strategic foul (a "good" or "smart" foul) in the closing minutes of a game. If we don't share the same ideals, we identify *deviance* differently.

Another problem with an absolutist approach is that it leads many people to see deviance as caused by the weak or distorted character of individuals. Therefore they think that controlling deviance always requires more rules, better rule enforcement, and increasingly severe penalties for deviations from the ideal. But this approach undermines creativity and change, creates resistance to rules, and makes people defensive about their own attitudes and actions. When strict conformity to a specific ideal is the only way to avoid deviance, people always wonder if they are doing something wrong.

Despite these problems, many people use an absolutist approach when they discuss deviance in sports. When the actions of athletes don't match their ideals, they define the athletes as deviant. They argue that the only way to control deviance is to "get tough" and eliminate the "bad apples" that lack moral character.

Most sociologists reject an absolutist approach and use a constructionist approach to identify and deal with deviance. A **constructionist approach** assumes that **deviance** occurs when *ideas, traits, and actions fall outside the socially determined boundaries that people use to decide what is acceptable and unacceptable in a society or social world.* This approach is based on a combination of cultural, interactionist, and structural theories in sociology, and it emphasizes the following six points:

1. Norms are socially constructed as people interact with each other and use their values to determine a range of acceptable ideas, traits, and actions. This point is illustrated in Figure 5.2, where the vertical hash marks crossing the horizontal line represent the boundaries that separate what is accepted from what is deviant. This means that conformity does not usually require everyone to think, look, and act exactly alike to avoid deviance, because there is a range of acceptance associated with nearly all norms.

2. Deviance is socially constructed as people negotiate the boundaries of their acceptance. The ideas, traits, and actions that fall outside the range of acceptance are defined as deviant. However, boundary negotiation occurs continuously, and the vertical hash lines that represent normative boundaries move one way or the other over time as norms change.

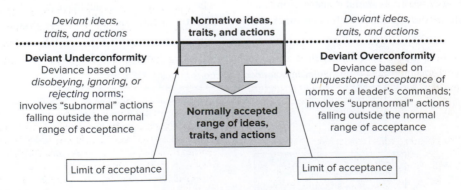

FIGURE 5.2 A *constructionist approach* to deviance: Deviance exists when ideas, traits, or actions go beyond socially negotiated normative limits. Deviance can involve *underconformity* or *overconformity.*

3. The process of negotiating normative boundaries and the range of social acceptance is influenced by power relations in a society or social world. People who possess power and authority generally have the most influence in determining normative limits, because they administer formal sanctions, including both punishments and rewards.

4. Most ideas, traits, and actions in a social world fall into a normally accepted range. Those that fall outside the normal range of acceptance involve either deviant underconformity on the left side of the range *or* deviant overconformity on the right side.

5. **Deviant underconformity** *consists of subnormal ideas, traits, and actions that indicate a rejection of norms or ignorance about their existence*, such as bar fighting, sexual assault, or referring to a person with mental retardation as a "retard." **Anarchy** *is the social condition that exists when widespread underconformity leads to general lawlessness.*

6. **Deviant overconformity** *consists of supranormal ideas, traits, and actions that indicate an uncritical acceptance of norms and a failure to recognize any limits to following norms*, such as playing despite broken bones and torn ligaments or using painkilling drugs to stay in the game. **Fascism** *is the social condition that exists when widespread overconformity is based on unlimited obedience to norms or to the commands of leaders.*

A constructionist approach is useful when studying deviance in sports, especially when it involves the use of performance-enhancing substances and other extreme actions that most people in society define as outside the normal range of acceptance.

Deviant Overconformity in Sports

Research shows that deviant overconformity is a significant problem in sports. When sociologists Keith Ewald and Robert Jiobu (1985) studied men who were seriously involved in bodybuilding or competitive distance running, they found that some of the men engaged in unquestioned overconformity to norms related to training and competition. The men trained so intensely and so often that their family relationships, job performance, and/or physical health deteriorated, yet they never questioned their actions or the norms of their sport cultures.

This study was published nearly thirty years ago, but athletes today are just as likely, if not more likely, to ignore normative limits and do anything it takes to train and participate in sports. Former NFL player Matt Millen explains in this way:

> You have to be selfish, getting ready for a game that only a handful of people understand. It's tough on the people around you. . . . It's the most unspoken but powerful part of the game, that deep-seated desire to be better at all costs, even if it means alienating your family or friends. [Athletes] will do anything to [stay in the game], even if it means sacrificing their own physical or mental well being (in Freeman, 1998, p. 1).

Another player reaffirms Millen with these words:

> I was willing to do anything to be successful, anything. When I got hurt, I just made sure to get myself back into a game as soon as possible. It was do-what-you-have-to-do, and I did it all (in Leahy, 2008, p. W08).

Research has identified many forms of deviant overconformity, including self-injurious overtraining, extreme weight-control strategies, taking untested or dangerous performance-enhancing substances, and playing while injured.[1] When studying deviance in sports, it's important to

---

[1]Many studies identify deviant overconformity, although they may not all use the concept as described in this chapter. These studies (along with detailed media reports) include Beals and Hill, 2006; Beamish, 2011; Brissonneau, 2010; Busch, 2007; Cotton, 2005; Howe, 2004; Ingham et al., 2002; Johns, 2004; Johns and Johns, 2000; Jones et al., 2009; Keown, 2004; P. King, 2004; Leahy, 2008; Liston et al., 2006; Mason and Lavalee, 2011; Pappa and Kennedy, 2013; Peretti-Watel et al., 2004a, 2004b; Pike, 2004, 2005; Schwarz, 2007a, 2007b, 2007c, 2007d; Young and Charlesworth, 2005.

distinguish between those actions based on indifference to or rejection of norms and those actions based on a blind acceptance of norms and a willingness to surpass normal limits of conformity. Such a distinction is identified only by examining the organization and dynamics of sport cultures and the meanings that athletes give to their sport participation. For example, within the culture of high-performance sports, athletes are expected to live by a code that stresses dedication, sacrifice, and a willingness to put one's body on the line for the sake of their sport and their teammates. Following this code to an extreme degree is seen as a mark of a true athlete who is accepted and respected by peers as one of them. This creates a set of conditions in which athletes are likely to *overconform* to norms embodied in the code or ethic of contemporary power and performance sports.

The Sport Ethic and Deviance in Sports

An **ethic** is *an interrelated set of norms or standards that is used to guide and evaluate ideas, traits, and actions in a social world.* Elite athletes and coaches use a **sport ethic** to guide and evaluate attitudes and actions in the social world of power and performance sports. This ethic is formed around four general norms (see Figure 5.3):

1. *Athletes are dedicated to "the game" above all other things.* This norm stresses that athletes must love "the game" and prove it by giving it top priority in their lives, meeting the expectations of fellow athletes, making sacrifices to stay in their sport, and facing the demands of competition without backing down. Coaches' pep talks and locker-room slogans proclaim the importance of this norm. It was explained in these terms by NFL player Brandon Stokley, who said, "I just love it. I can't see myself giving up football because I think I might have something (bad) happen to me or my brain. . . . I am going to live in the here and now and have fun at what I am doing" (in Brennan, 2012).

2. *Athletes strive for distinction.* The Olympic motto *Citius, Altius, Fortius* (faster, higher,

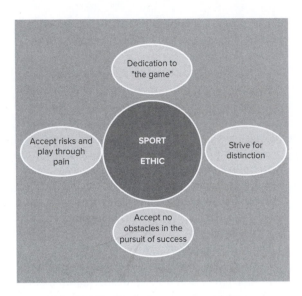

FIGURE 5.3 The four primary norms of the sport ethic.

stronger) captures the meaning of this norm. Athletes are expected to relentlessly strive for improvement by pushing limits and doing whatever it takes to maximize their potential. This norm is highlighted by Justin Wadsworth, the top U.S. Nordic skier in the 30-kilometer race, who pushed his body so hard during the 2002 Olympics in Salt Lake City that he suffered internal bleeding. From his hospital bed he said, "It's pretty special to push yourself that hard," and his coaches and fellow athletes agreed with him (Berger, 2002).

3. *Athletes accept risks and play through pain.* According to this norm, athletes are expected to endure pressure, pain, and fear without quitting. When athletes talk about this, they simply say that "this is part of the game." But in sociological terms, it shows that athletes willingly participate in a **culture of risk** *in which they accept the uncertainty, danger, and consequences of their actions* (Giulianotti, 2009; Howe, 2004; Safai, 2003). As they do this, athletes develop a narrative that normalizes pain and injuries as an unavoidable part of what they do and who they are. This is clearly illustrated in the comments

of X Games athletes who endure pain and injury as they push limits. Levi LaValee, a medal-winning snowmobile athlete, said, "I've been injured so many times . . . [but] every time I'm injured, I can't wait for the moment until I can get back on the sled [and] drive again" (in George, 2013).

For many elite athletes, the endurance of pain comes to be seen as an indicator of inner strength and commitment; eventually, many athletes view pain as a positive—sign that they are alive and doing what they were meant to do. Of course, coaches in most high-performance sports seek athletes who feel this way and then use them as examples of what they expect from everyone on the team.

4. *Athletes accept no obstacles in the pursuit of success in sports.* This norm stresses "the dream" and the obligation to pursue it at all costs. Athletes don't accept obstacles without trying to overcome them. Dreams, they say, are achievable only if you never quit. Champion boxer Lucia Rijker (who starred in the film *Million Dollar Baby*) stated this norm succinctly as she trained for a bout: "I use obstacles as wood on a fire" (in Blades, 2005, p. 96).

Overconformity to the norms of the sport ethic is common in sports even though it is defined as deviant outside of sport and may lead to injuries that irreparably damage the health of athletes.

The danger of this overconformity was explained by Alberto Salazar, a former marathoner and coach for Mary Decker Slaney, a legendary middle-distance runner during the 1970s and 1980s. After multiple injuries and nineteen sport-related surgeries, Slaney attempted a comeback while she lived in constant pain; she trained excessively, hoping to make the U.S. Olympic team. Salazar understood Slaney's overconformity to the norms of the sport ethic, but he also recognized its dangers with this comment:

> The greatest athletes want it so much, they run themselves to death. You've got to have an obsession, but if unchecked, it's destructive. That's what it is with [Slaney]. She'll kill herself unless you pull the reins back (in Longman, 1996, p. B11).

The importance of Salazar's insight, from twenty years ago, has been vividly supported by current research on concussions and brain injuries in sports. When athletes overconform to the norms of the sport ethic by enduring repeated head trauma, they risk permanent brain damage, chronic memory loss, and early-onset dementia that can affect them long before old age. This is in addition to the arthritis and joint injuries that result from intense daily training that pushes their bodies beyond normal limits. This suggests that deviant overconformity is more dangerous than deviant underconformity and is a central problem in sports today. Without critically assessing the culture of high-performance sport, this form of deviance will persist.

Of course, deviant underconformity also is a problem in sports, but when athletes underconform, they are punished immediately. As a result, underconformers are usually pushed out of high-performance sport cultures, whereas overconformers are praised. Additionally, media stories glorify overconforming athletes as role models—as warriors who play with broken bones and torn ligaments, endure surgery after surgery, and willingly submit to injections of painkilling drugs to stay in games. Spectators express awe when they hear these stories, even though they realize that athletes have surpassed the normative limits that are used in society as a whole. But people seldom object to deviant overconformity in sports because it is entertaining to watch and it reaffirms the importance of the sport and values such as dedication, hard work, and achievement. However, they condemn deviant underconformity because it threatens the sport and their values. Therefore, most athletes avoid asking critical questions and setting limits on their conformity to the norms of the sport ethic, even though it creates problems, causes pain, disrupts family life, jeopardizes health and safety, and may even shorten their life expectancy. This illustrates how powerful the sport ethic can be when athletes internalize it and use their own overconformity as a basis for evaluating themselves and sustaining their identity among peers.

Deviant Overconformity and Group Dynamics

Being an athlete is a social experience as well as a physical one. At elite levels of competition, athletes form special bonds with each other, due in part to their collective overconformity to the norms of the sport ethic. When team members collectively dedicate themselves to a goal and willingly make sacrifices and endure pain in the face of significant challenges, they create a social world in which overconformity is "normalized," even as it remains deviant in society as a whole. As they push the envelope together, the bonds between athletes become extraordinarily powerful. Their overconformity sets them apart culturally and physically from the rest of the community, and this leads them to assume that people outside of their sport cannot understand who they are and what they do.

Athletes may appreciate fan approval, but they don't look to fans for reaffirmation of their identity as athletes because in their eyes fans are ignorant of what it takes to perform as no others in the world can perform. Only other athletes understand this, and this makes everyone else peripheral to an athlete's life in sports, even spouses and family members.

The separation between athletes and the rest of the community makes the group dynamics associated with participation in high-performance sports very powerful. Other selective and exclusive groups, usually groups of men, experience similar dynamics. Examples are found in the military, especially among Special Forces units. Former soldiers sometimes talk about these dynamics and the powerful social bonds formed while they faced danger and death with their "teams." These bonds and the desire to remain connected with the select men that have unique and exhilarating experiences can be so strong that group members support increasingly extreme behaviors

You do whatever it takes to play . . . You get hurt, you find a way. . . . You just suck it up and push through, and if you can't, you're out. There's a saying around locker rooms: "No one has ever made the club from the tub." —Dave Pear, former NFL player, disabled (in Leahy, 2008, p. W08)

among themselves. As a result, what happens on the team stays in the team, even when it should be reported to authorities, and even when many team members know it isn't right.

As high-performance athletes strive to maintain their identities and membership in their elite in-group, they often develop the sense that they are unique and extraordinary people. They often hear this day after day from coaches to fans and people on the street. They read it in newspapers and magazines, and they see it on TV and the Internet. And when this sense of being unique and extraordinary becomes extreme, as it often does among high-profile athletes, it can take the form of **hubris**—that is, *pride-driven arrogance and an inflated sense of self-importance that leads one to feel separate from and superior to others.*

The dynamics leading to hubris among athletes are clear. First, they bond together in ways that encourage and normalize deviant overconformity. Second, collective overconformity creates a sense of specialness that separates athletes from the rest of the community at the same time that it inspires awe and admiration from fans. Third, the unique experiences associated with team membership leads athletes to feel a sense of entitlement. Fourth, athletes see people outside their sport culture as incapable of understanding them and their lives, and therefore undeserving of their concern or, in some cases, their respect.

The hubris that emerges on some sport teams can create serious problems, because it leads athletes to believe that general community norms don't apply to them. But this possibility has not been studied, so we don't know if there may be a relationship between the dynamics associated with collective overconformity to the norms of the sport ethic and high rates of deviant underconformity.

Controlling Deviant Overconformity

Deviant overconformity presents special social control problems in sports. Coaches, managers, owners, and sponsors—people who create and enforce rules—often benefit when athletes overconform to the norms of the sport ethic. In their eyes, athletes who willingly put their bodies on the line for the team are a blessing, not a curse. In the eyes of the athletes, their overconformity is proof of their dedication and commitment; and in the eyes of fans and media people it is seen as exciting, a way to win games, and a wonderful boost to media ratings. Therefore, deviant overconformity goes unpunished, even though it often consists of dangerous actions that everyone sees as falling outside normative boundaries. For example, few directors of national federations, such as the USOC (United States Olympic Committee), will tell national team coaches that their athletes are too dedicated to their sports, too focused on achieving distinction, too willing to play in pain, or too concerned with overcoming obstacles to win medals for the United States.

Complicating matters further is the fact that *neither money nor the desire to win is the primary reason that athletes push themselves beyond the normative limits.* Instead, it is their desire to play their sport in a way that sustains the athlete identity around which their entire lives—their relationships, experiences, and everyday decisions and routines—have been organized. Of course, winning, money, and fame are important, but they are secondary to reaffirming the identity that has been at the core of their existence ever since they focused on making it to an elite level in their sport.

Every time people repeat the rhetoric about "winning at all costs" and "money" as explanations for everything that athletes do, they obscure two important things: (1) the deeper meaning and personal issues linked to being an athlete today in societies where sports are highly visible and culturally valued, and (2) the organization of today's high-performance sports, in which athletes must train full time at a level of intensity that precludes other commitments in their lives and makes them dependent on some combination of psychological, physiological, medical, and pharmacological support to be successful (Atry et al., 2013; Beamish, 2011; Brissoneau, 2010; Hoberman, 1992, 2005; Johnson, 2012; Ohl et al., 2015 Waddington and Smith, 2009). The fact that there are very few winners in high-performance sports means that deviant overconformity also occurs on teams and among athletes who will never win Olympic or World Cup medals, be ranked number 1, play in televised games, achieve public fame, receive college scholarships, or sign professional contracts.

One way to control deviant overconformity is to enable athletes to set limits when conforming to the norms of the sport ethic. However, this would not be viewed favorably by most coaches in elite sports. For example, when a fourteen-year-old gymnast is late for practice, her coach immediately sanctions her for violating team norms. But when the same gymnast loses weight and becomes dangerously thin as she strives for distinction and pursues her sport dream, many coaches, parents, and judges don't see deviance as much as they see a dedicated athlete willing to suck it up and pay the price—that is, until stress fractures or anorexia interfere with competition, threaten her life, and put her in the hospital.

Fans also want athletes to exceed normative limits and put their bodies on the line. They see this as exciting and entertaining because it heightens the stakes associated with competition. Fans don't realize that if they accept deviant overconformity, deviant underconformity often follows in its wake. This, in turn, challenges their belief in the great sport myth and leads them to condemn individual nonconformers and call for them to be punished. For these fans it is easier to blame deviance on a few athletes they perceive to be morally corrupt than it is to abandon their belief in the essential purity and goodness of sport. But this will not control deviant overconformity, because it and related ethical infractions among athletes are rooted in the culture of high-performance sports, relationships among athletes, relationships between athletes and all those to whom athletes must answer, and willful neglect on the part of coaches, administrators, and sponsors.

To reduce deviant overconformity, sports would have to be organized primarily around the health and well-being of athletes, with commitment to performance being a secondary concern. It means that "winning at all costs" would be defined as subversive and irrational.

Although many people have seen sports as sites for achieving physical perfection, we have reached a point in many sports where improving on what currently exists requires that athletes train at a frequency and intensity that harms their bodies and requires dependence on technologies to keep them on the field and performing at optimum levels. Transforming high-performance sports into healthy activities is incompatible with how they are organized today, but it is possible to do, if there is the will to do it. Without the will, it is pointless to blame athletes for doing whatever it takes to meet performance expectations today.

RESEARCH ON DEVIANCE IN SPORTS

Media reports of deviance in sports have become daily occurrences. This raises sociological questions: Does deviance occur more regularly in sports than other spheres of life? What are the patterns of deviance in sports? Do athletes have higher rates of deviance than others?

Most research focuses only on deviant underconformity among athletes—that is, deviance grounded in rejecting or ignoring team rules or civil and criminal laws. Deviant overconformity is ignored because it challenges popular acceptance of the great sport myth and the assumptions underlying popular theories of deviance. Additionally, deviance among coaches, managers, team owners, and others connected with sports has seldom been studied in the sociology of sport because it is difficult to collect data from and about people in positions of power. These people have reasons and resources to keep secret the information needed to explain—or, in legal terms, *prove*—what they do.

Cases of sexual assault, rape, and gang rape initiated by male athletes have recently led people to ask if the culture and organization of certain men's sports foster or passively approve of such actions. But most media coverage explains deviance in sports as the result of character weaknesses among athletes and the greed of managers, administrators, and others who financially benefit from sports and the outcomes of sport events. These explanations are so widely stated and accepted that they have become clichés in some societies. But they are oversimplifications of reality and explain little.

Character traits and greed may be related to deviance in sports, but there are important cultural and institutional factors as well, and they must be considered if we wish to understand this issue. These are identified in the following sections.

Deviance on the Field or Related to Sports

Sport-related deviance includes cheating, gambling, shaving points, throwing games or matches, engaging in unfair conduct, harassment and abuse, hazing, administrative corruption, taking illegal performance-enhancing drugs, and other actions that violate rules of sports.

Cheating on the Field of Play   Historical research indicates that cheating, dirty play, fighting, and the use of violence are less common today than in the days before television coverage and mega-salaries (Dunning, 1999; Elias, 1986; Guttmann, 2004; Scheinin, 1994). It also shows that sports today are more rule-governed than in the past and that on-the-field deviance is more likely to be punished and publicly criticized. However, comparing rates of on-the-field deviance among athletes from one time period to another is difficult because rules and enforcement standards change over time. Research shows that athletes in most sports interpret rules very loosely during games, and they create informal norms, which stretch or bend official rules (Shields and Bredemeier, 1995). As one veteran athlete explains, "We players have our own justice system" (Player X, 2009b). But this is not new.

Athletes in organized sports have traditionally "played to the level" permitted by umpires and referees—that is, they adjust their actions according to the way that referees enforce rules during a game. This means they will push the limits of rules as far as particular referees allow them to do so. Players also commit strategic fouls on the field to obtain an advantage over opponents, and players learn what rule violations are likely to be undetected by referees. But these actions are defined by players and fans alike as strategy rather than cheating.

Cheating, Corruption, and Harassment in Sport Organizations

The perception that deviance has increased on and around the field is partly due to a combination of three factors. First, the constant addition of new rules creates new ways to be "deviant." Rulebooks in sport organizations such as the International Olympic Committee, international sport federations, and the National Collegiate Athletic Association (NCAA) have hundreds of rules and regulations today that didn't exist in the past, and every year more rules are added.

Second, the surveillance technologies used today increase the detection of rule violations. For example, slow-motion instant replays enable referees to identify infractions they would have missed in the past. Even text messages, email evidence, photos, and videos from handheld devices have been used to identify deviance that previously would have remained undetected.

Third, personal stakes in the form of status and financial rewards associated with sports are so much higher today that players and others connected with sports have stronger incentives to cheat. This makes everyone concerned with sports more sensitive to the possibility that cheating will occur—and this leads to higher detection rates.

These factors have led to what seems to be an endless parade of cheating scandals in sports. The NCAA and its high-stakes Division I athletic programs provide classic examples of this. Most sport governing bodies, such as the NCAA, are self-policing. But the leaders of those organizations have always accepted the great sport myth to the point that they have not created effective rule enforcement divisions. They felt they didn't need them. Sports, they assumed, were essentially pure and good, and people in sports would regulate themselves because they shared in that purity and goodness. But this assumption is flawed, and it undermines the willingness of leaders to enforce rules and investigate suspected or reported infractions.

A second problem is that the officials at the NCAA and other sport governing bodies often face inherent conflicts of interest. Because they serve at the pleasure of their members, they are not encouraged to create a rule enforcement system that could thoroughly investigate those same members. So they create rules that make them look pure and good to outsiders, but they are ineffective when it comes to enforcement policies and procedures. For example, the NCAA receives self-reports from its members of about 4000 *minor* rule violations each year. With an under-resourced enforcement division that must investigate all these violations, there is little time to fully investigate major violations (Miller, 2012).

Third, the people who run sport organizations lack the experience that would prepare them to administer the systems of rule enforcement needed in today's high-stakes sport cultures. Like people in other spheres of life, people in sports have developed complex ways to cheat and skirt the rules. But the investigators don't have police powers and other investigative resources needed to consistently *prove* that cheating has occurred. This leads to bungled investigations and inconsistent and capricious punishments that weaken the legitimacy of the organizations themselves (Miller, 2012).

Finally, officials in sport organizations have generally been "groomed" for their positions in "good old boy" networks that have never been concerned about transparency and accountability in what they do. This applies to rule enforcement as much as to budgets, travel expenses, hiring procedures, and the everyday business and personnel matters of an organization.

The lack of transparency and accountability creates problems that often escalate into long-term disasters. This was recently seen in connection with sport mega-events such as the men's World Cup and the Olympic Games. Cost overruns, inside deals, and blatant corruption leave large public debts in their wake. Corruption alone reportedly accounted for $30 billion of the $50 billion spent to host the winter Olympics in Sochi, Russia (Zirin, 2013b). Tracking money trails in sports and sport events is difficult. Those who control sports organizations are able to hide and disguise financial transactions because they have not been investigated in the same ways that traditional businesses are investigated.

The takeaway point from this is that we don't know for sure whether cheating is worse now than in the past. However, there is good reason to believe that as the amount of money and other perks associated with sports have increased, there has been a growing problem of **institutional corruption**— that is, *established, widespread, and taken-for-granted processes and practices that, if publicly known, would be seen as immoral, unethical, or illegal to the point of destroying public trust in the organization and its leaders.* But institutional corruption may not always be illegal, meaning that external control is difficult to impose. Identifying institutional corruption is tedious and even dangerous, especially now that literally billions of dollars flow through sport organizations like the IOC, FIFA, and other sport governing bodies and leagues worldwide (Jennings, 2006, 2011; Sugden and Tomlinson, 1998). In each case, the incentives for self-policing are weak and the opportunities for corruption are numerous and lucrative (Thamel and Wolff, 2013).

Research on institutional corruption is scarce. Funding for such research is practically nonexistent, and there are career risks for any academic researcher who publishes evidence of corruption. The researcher will almost certainly be subjected to

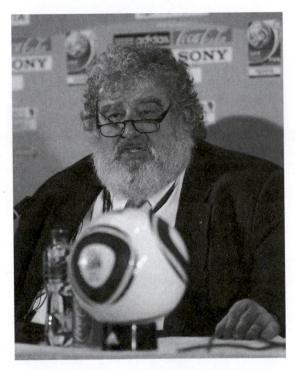

Chuck Blazer, former commissioner of the American Soccer League and vice president of the U.S. Soccer Federation, was arrested by the FBI for allegedly paying himself $15 million in secret commissions while he was CEO and treasurer of the Confederation of North, Central American and Caribbean Association Football (CONCACAF). (*Source:* © ALI HAIDER/epa/Corbis)

a smear campaign by representatives of any organizations implicated in the study, and these representatives often are influential and have more power than any scholars in the sociology of sport. So unless courageous investigative journalists backed by supportive media organizations do such investigations, corruption persists without consequences in certain sport organizations where people have consolidated power and use it to their advantage (Jennings, 2011).

When this occurs in an organization, it becomes a context in which harassment and exploitation are especially likely—again, without consequences for perpetrators. In the United States we saw this in the case of the athletic department at Penn State

University, where a former assistant football coach was able to sexually abuse multiple boys for over a decade as he used the department's facilities without triggering any serious or sustained investigation. Other coaches, including the legendary football coach Joe Paterno, and athletic department and university officials were so concerned with maintaining the money- and status-generating football program that they shirked their legal obligations and overlooked the seriousness of the abuse occurring in their midst. It wasn't until investigative journalists exposed this situation that there was an official response to the deviance of the former coach (Hayes, 2012; Klarevas, 2011; McCarthy, 2012).

The Penn State case is one of many cases of illegal harassment and criminal abuse that have occurred in sport organizations, with administrators and coaches usually the perpetrators (Farrey, 2011). The processes involved in harassment and abuse have been studied meticulously since the 1990s by Celia Brackenridge from the United Kingdom, Kari Fasting from Norway, and their colleagues.[2] The dynamics of these processes vary from one situation to another, but they are most likely to occur in sport organizations where coaches and/or administrators have unquestioned power and control over the careers of others and are not held accountable for anything except sport outcomes. Additionally, the accusations of victims of harassment or abuse may not be believed as perpetrators hide behind the cover of the great sport myth and either escape detection or provide accounts of their actions that are accepted by others.

The only way to break this potential cycle of cheating, corruption, harassment, and abuse is for sport organizations to abandon the practice of

self-enforcement and voluntarily turn all enforcement matters over to an independent outside agency. This transfer would not be without problems, but it would make rule enforcement the job of people who don't have the conflicts of interest that exist when enforcement is handled internally (Miller, 2012). Of course, the independent agency would require adequate funding, and its actions would have to be transparent and competent to establish trust. Additionally, specific forms of training are needed by most management-level people working in sport organizations to make them aware of their responsibilities to athletes and co-workers. Again, this training becomes increasingly effective when athletes and employees have independent authorities to whom they can go with questions and reports about harassment and abuse.

Gambling and Associated Deviance by Athletes and Referees   New technologies help to detect deviance in sports, but they also create new ways to engage in deviance that are difficult to detect (Glanz et al., 2015a, 2015b). Gambling is a classic example of this. Of course, gambling on sports dates back to the first race ever run in the ancient Olympic Gams nearly 3000 years ago. But today it has become pervasive worldwide and is legal in many countries. The existence of gambling websites makes it easy to place bets on nearly any quantifiable aspects of any sport in the world, and this can be done without ever leaving one's home or dorm room in the case of U.S. college students, including athletes.

Betfair.com provides an eBay-like platform that matches up people looking to place a particular bet with one or more others willing to take the other side of the bet. Through this or similar sites people can bet on something as specific as which player will make the assist leading to the second goal in the second half of a World Cup soccer match. Of course, the sites set the "odds" or probabilities that define the bet, and the bettor may take or leave them as they wish. For example, the betting sheets at the "sport books" in Las Vegas casinos at the time of the Super Bowl or the NCAA Men's Basketball Tournament

---

[2]Brackenridge et al., 2008; Brackenridge and Fasting, 2009; Brackenridge et al., 2010a, 2010b; Brackenridge and Rhind, 2010; Fasting et al., 2008; Fasting and Brackenridge, 2009; Fasting, Brackenridge, and Knorre, 2010; Fasting, Brackenridge, and Kjølberg, 2011; Hartill, 2009, and Leahy, 2011.

offer literally hundreds of bets that can be made on various aspects of these events.

Betting on sports in Nevada is legal and very popular, but it is defined as a crime in other states, although some states would like to legalize it. In most of Europe and parts of Asia, betting on sports is legal but regulated by national governments. Worldwide, gambling is a multibillion-dollar business. The major owners of three professional teams are gamblers, and they used their gambling winnings to buy the teams. Some universities in the United Kingdom now offer degrees in "gambling studies," and sport leagues work with bookmakers who alert them to betting patterns that may indicate an attempt to "fix" the outcomes of matches and games or any aspect of a sport event on which bets can be made.

The estimates of money bet on sports are difficult to verify, but Interpol, the global police agency recognized in about 190 countries, estimates that $1 trillion is bet on sports each year, and 70 percent of that total is bet on soccer, with the amount of betting increasing dramatically each year (Assael, 2008; Borden, 2012; Brett, 2012; Hoffer, 2013; Karp, 2011; Millman, 2010a, 2010b; Zaremba, 2009).

Sport federations and other sport governing bodies such as the NFL, the NCAA, and FIFA have explicit rules that prohibit athletes from placing bets on sports, especially their own sports and their own events. Violating these rules brings severe sanctions, including lifetime bans on playing, coaching, or being formally connected with their sport in the future. This is to safeguard the legitimacy of the outcomes of sport competitions, because if people cannot trust that outcomes are achieved fairly, there would be no spectator sports as we know them today.

Despite rules and laws, there have been dozens of match- and game-fixing incidents as online gambling has turned sports betting into a major global industry. When gamblers or the emerging gambling cartels want to increase their chances

of winning, the surest way to do so in sports is to pay players or referees to alter game events or outcomes so that particular bets are won.

Organized crime and very clever, but devious, entrepreneurs have become involved in this industry, so that match fixing today has become an international criminal activity with profits rivaling those for illegal weapons sales, prostitution, and drug trafficking. Cartels in China and Southeast Asia have captured much of this betting activity (Brett, 2012).

In 2013 investigators found evidence of match fixing in more than 600 soccer matches worldwide, with involvement of hundreds of people across fifteen countries (Robinson, 2013). Now that organized crime is involved, this criminal activity is becoming increasingly difficult to investigate and control. The crime organizations operate globally, whereas police forces operate nationally with the exception of Interpol and Europol, which have limited powers and must work with national police forces. Additionally, organized crime doesn't merely bribe players and referees—it threatens them and their families with harm if they do not cooperate.

The ban on sports betting does exactly what Prohibition did. It makes criminals rich. —James Surowiecki, journalist, 2013

Although gambling is becoming an increasing problem, sport organizations also realize that betting on sports is a "hook" that keeps fans watching games until the final minute of play. People who bet on sports also pay for the expensive cable and satellite sports packages for their homes and regularly buy pay-per-view events in mixed martial arts and boxing. There is nothing better than an office pool to keep people watching the NCAA tournament basketball games and the BCS bowl games. People at the NCAA understand this, even though they now try to educate athletes on the dangers of betting on sports (Brown, 2010; Paskus, 2010).

Research by the NCAA shows that college athletes regularly gamble and that golfers are the most likely to gamble and place bets with other golfers—a phenomenon common in golf generally (Paskus and Derevensky, 2013; St. Pierre et al., 2013; Wolken, 2013). This creates potential problems if the athletes have gambling debts and feel that point shaving or match fixing is a way to eliminate debts with a bookie.

During an investigation in 2015, the New York Times and PBS Frontline presented information that exposed the pervasiveness of gambling worldwide and in the United States. Billions of dollars are bet weekly on sports. Bets are placed though offshore gaming sites registered in other countries. Tracking these sites is tedious, and sites can always be replaced to take bets without interruption. Federal laws in the United States, passed in 2006, were intended to ban gambling on sports, but they are ineffective. These laws also allowed fantasy sports—an oversight leading to what has become a multi-billion dollar industry that has merged with gambling interests (Bogdanich et al., 2015). Although the FBI works to police gambling, it has little enforcement power outside the United States. The U.S. Congress can do little to regulate gambling on sports without seriously regulating the Internet, which is unlikely to occur.

As gambling on sports grows, pronouncements coming from professional sports officials in the United States continue to condemn gambling at the same time that team owners invest in fantasy sports companies. The NFL and other leagues say they don't approve of gambling, but they also want revenues related to the gambling industry (Belson and Drape, 2015). Although gambling on sports is unlikely to be a high priority law enforcement target, the profits that it produces fund other criminal activities and create a range of problems for those addicted to gambling (Brett, 2012).

Hazing: Deviance or Team Building?   Hazing has long been an accepted practice as new members enter an established group or organization in which membership increases a person's status in a social world. It is more common in groups of males than groups of females, partly because men are more likely to assume that their groups are linked with high status.

Confusion about hazing often occurs because people don't distinguish between hazing and related processes, such as rites of passage, initiations, and bullying. A **rite of passage** *is an institutionalized cultural ritual that marks a transition from one status to another.* An **initiation** *is an expected, public, and formal ceremony that marks entry into a group or organization.* **Hazing** *is a secret, private, interpersonal process that reaffirms a hierarchical status difference between incoming and existing group members.* Finally, **bullying** *consists of aggressive acts that are meant to intimidate, exploit, or harm another person.* Of these four processes, hazing has been studied the least, mostly because it is private and secretive and involves experiences that people keep private because they are embarrassing.

There are times when hazing in sport teams involves clear cases of deviance, but research indicates that hazing processes are difficult to classify as deviant or as acceptable, for the following reasons (Allan and Madden, 2008; Clayton, 2013):

(a) High school and college athletes are aware of hazing and often expect it when they become new members of a team.
(b) Most athletes who are hazed perceive their own hazing in positive terms or they are ambivalent about their experience and may not conclude that they have been hazed as others define it.
(c) Hazing often involves forms of humiliation, alcohol consumption, isolation, sleep deprivation, and sex acts that athletes keep private.

One way to make sense of these findings is to say that hazing has become normalized for most athletes, at least those who become members of high status teams. Additionally, certain hazing practices have become so normalized that those who experience them don't see them as "out of the ordinary," even though people in the larger community would disagree.

Research on hazing is scarce, but studies by Jennifer Waldron, Vicki Krane, and their colleagues

(Waldron and Kowalski, 2009; Waldron et al., 2011) indicate that hazing contains dynamics that easily get out of hand and can seriously harm people. These dynamics exist largely because hazing is a private, secretive process that reproduces a hierarchical status and power distinction between senior and junior group members. For example, one of the ways to ensure secrecy is to force people to violate important social taboos in ways that they could not admit without being defined as deviant themselves.

In U.S. culture such taboos often are related to sex, so there is a tendency in hazing processes to force people to engage in sexual activity defined as immoral, so they will keep it private. Another guarantee of secrecy is to force people to drink so much that they will not clearly remember what they did or will not be believed if they tell someone about it. This is why hazing often involves forms drinking that put people in danger.

Due to its deviance and danger, hazing creates bonds and a form of vulnerability that coaches can use to control team members. This is why some coaches covertly approve of hazing—it gives them information that can be used to assert power over a team and to demand obedience without destroying team bonds.

My review of the evidence on hazing leads me to conclude that for high school and college students it should be replaced by initiation ceremonies in which new team members have public experiences that mark entry onto the team and signal their right to claim a new identity. In the case of professional teams, information about hazing suggests that it is more controlled and more focused on initiating rookies into a culture of respect for the players that have already "paid their dues" and shown that they deserve to be identified as athletes in this elite context. However, an extreme case of NFL hazing that became public in 2013 led to disclosures that first year players may be subjected to costly and demeaning demands by veteran players on some, but not all teams (Clark, 2013; Gay, 2013; Hochman, 2013; Pelissero, 2013).

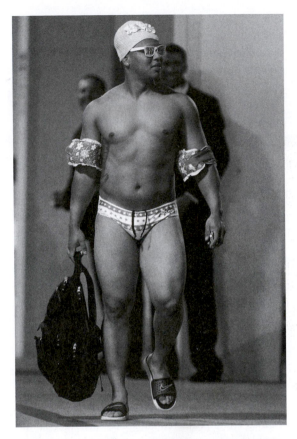

Texas Rangers catcher Luis Martinez was forced by team veterans to wear a costume as part of rookie hazing as the team heads to the bus after the second baseball a game in 2012, in Arlington, Texas. (*Source:* © AP Photo/LM Otero)

From what we know about hazing on professional teams, it can be juvenile and it certainly is designed to reproduce the status and control of senior team members, and it takes different forms than reported cases of high school and college hazing. Gaining access to a team to do research on this issue is difficult, but good studies would help us understand the dynamics and consequences of hazing at all levels of sport.

After this dismal litany of deviance in sports, the following conclusion may seem surprising: there are no historical studies showing that deviant underconformity on and around the field is more common now than in the past. However, cases of institutional corruption and the match-fixing side of gambling constitute significant problems that could jeopardize the future of some sports.

Deviance Off the Field and Apart from Sports

Off-the-field deviance among athletes attracts widespread media attention. When athletes are arrested or linked to criminal activity, they make headlines and become lead stories on the evening news. However, research doesn't tell us if the rates of off-the-field deviance have gone up or down over time or if general rates are higher among athletes than their peers in the general population. The studies that deal with this have focused primarily on three topics: (1) delinquency and sport participation among high school students; (2) academic cheating and excessive alcohol use among high school and college athletes; and (3) particular felony rates among athletes.

Delinquency Rates   Research on high school students shows that delinquency rates among athletes often are lower than rates for other students from similar backgrounds. With a few exceptions, this finding applies for athletes in various sports, athletes in different societies, and both boys and girls from various racial and social-class backgrounds (Hartmann and Massoglia, 2007; McHale et al., 2005; Veliz and Shakib, 2012).

The problem with most of these studies is that they don't take into account three important factors: (1) students who have histories of deviance are less likely than other students to try out and be selected for sport teams; (2) athletes may receive preferential treatment enabling them to avoid being labeled delinquent; and (3) deviance among high school athletes may be obscured by a "facade of conformity"—that is, athletes who conform to norms in public, but violate them in private where detection is rare. This means that many studies may not have valid measures of delinquent actions by

athletes and, as a result, underestimate their delinquency rates.

A study using longitudinal data (1994–2001) collected from a national sample of students in grades seven to twelve found that football players and wrestlers were more likely to be involved in serious fights than young men in other sports or not involved in school sports (Kreager, 2007). This raises issues that are discussed in Chapter 6, "Violence in Sports," but the point in this chapter is that some studies on sport participation and delinquency may overlook patterns of norm violations among certain athletes or analyze data out of context so they can't explain why certain patterns exist.

Even when sport programs are designed as "interventions" for "at-risk youth," we lack a clear theory to explain how and why we might expect sport-based intervention programs to be effective in reducing delinquency or producing other positive effects. Most of these programs have little effect because they do nothing to change the unemployment, poverty, racism, poor schools, and other delinquency-related factors that exist in most neighborhoods where sports for at-risk youth are offered (Coakley, 2011b; Coalter, 2007; Coalter and Taylor, 2010; Hartmann, 2003b; Hartmann and Depro, 2006; Hartmann and Massoglia, 2007).

We know from Chapter 3 (pp. 62–66) that we cannot make generalizations about athletes because sport experiences vary from program to program and because sport participation constitutes only one part of a person's experiences. Therefore, when someone says that "playing sports kept me out of trouble," we should investigate what that statement means in that person's life and then identify aspects of sport experiences that enable young people to see positive alternatives and make good choices in their lives. Until this research is done, our conclusion is that sport participation creates neither "saints nor sinners," although both may play sports.

Academic Cheating   Despite highly publicized cases of college athletes having their coursework completed by "academic tutors," the charge that college athletes generally engage in academic cheating more often than other students, has not been studied systematically (Pennington, 2012a). If we compared athletes with other students, we might find comparable rates but different methods of cheating. An athlete may be more likely to hand in a paper written by an "academic tutor," whereas other students would obtain papers from files maintained at a fraternity house, from an online site, or from a professional writer hired by a parent (Gabriel, 2010; Kristal, 2005). However, when a regular student is caught turning in a bogus paper, the case does not make national news, the student is not rebuked by people around the nation, the reputation of the university is not questioned in the national media, and no faculty members are fired for not policing students effectively—as might occur if the cheater were an athlete.

Do athletes cheat more often because the stakes associated with making particular grades are higher for them than for other students, or do athletes cheat less because they are watched more closely and have more to lose if they are caught? We don't know the answer to this question, and we need studies comparing athletes with other students generally, with other students who would lose their scholarships or job opportunities if they did not maintain minimum grade point averages, and with other students who are members of tightly knit groups organized around nonacademic activities and identities. Only then will we be able to make definitive statements about academic cheating and sport participation.

Alcohol Use and Binge Drinking

Underage and excessive alcohol consumption in high school and college is not limited to athletes. However, research generally indicates that male and female collegiate athletes engage in more alcohol use, abuse, and binge drinking than other male and female students (Bacon and Russell, 2004). Research on high school students shows a similar pattern (Denham, 2011; Hickey et al., 2009; Hoffman, 2006). However, after reviewing dozens of studies on this topic,

my conclusion is that the relationship between sport participation, drinking, and other actions depends on factors such as team culture and the social activities that are a part of that culture. If athletes—male or female, high school or college—create a culture in which weekend parties are frequent, they will be more likely to drink and binge-drink than other athletes and students generally (Hoffman, 2006). Therefore, if being an athlete positions a young person in a culture where party attendance is encouraged or expected, drinking is more likely. However, some sports and teams may have cultures in which weekend social activities do not include parties and other social events at which alcohol may be present. So, the key factor is not so much the sport participation as the culture and social dynamics that come along with membership on a particular team.

Research on this topic is important because alcohol use and abuse is related to other forms of deviance. For example, we don't know if deviant overconformity and the associated group dynamics that exist among college athletes contributes to alcohol use and binge drinking. Slamming drinks and getting drunk with teammates may not be very different, in sociological terms, from playing with an injury to gain approval from peers in a sport culture. When teammates who take risks together and depend on each other say, "Let's do some tequila tonight," do players uncritically overconform by downing multiple shots? Research is needed to see if, why, when, and how often this occurs.

Felony Rates

Widely publicized cases of assault, hard-drug use, and driving under the influence (DUI) in which male athletes are the offenders have made it important to study these forms of deviance. At this point, research is scarce, and existing studies report mixed findings.

Another problem with studies of felony rates is that data on arrest rates for athletes are seldom compared with arrest rates in the general population or in populations comparable to the athletes in age, race/ethnicity, and socioeconomic background. For example, many people were shocked when a study done in the late-1990s reported that 21.4 percent of a sample of NFL players had been arrested at least once for something more serious than minor crimes since the year they started college (Benedict and Yaeger, 1998). However, a follow-up study (Blumstein and Benedict, 1999) showed that 23 percent of the males living in cities of 250,000 or more people are arrested for a serious crime at some point in their lives, usually during young adulthood.

A more recent study of arrest rates from 2000–2013 indicate that rates for NFL players were lower than rates in the general U.S. population for property crimes and public disturbance crimes, but they were higher for violent crimes in six of the fourteen years covered in the study (Leal et al., 2015).

However, when crime rates are compared it must be remembered that professional athletes may be treated differently than their peers in the general population. In some cases, their actions may be so visible that they are held more accountable than others engaging in the same actions. But in other cases, athletes may receive preferential treatment and avoid arrests for actions that would lead to an arrest of others.

In the case of sexual assault the dynamics of filing charges, making arrests, going to trial, and facing a verdict are complex. For example, when Jeff Benedict, a lawyer-social scientist, studied cases involving NBA players during the 2001–2002 season, he found that it was "nearly impossible for a rape victim to file a criminal complaint against an NBA player without being labeled a groupie or a gold digger." He suggested that "it takes a victim nothing less than Snow White to obtain a conviction in a sexual assault case against a celebrity athlete and emerge with a reputation still intact" (Benedict, 2004, p. 29). This issue— the incidence of assault and sexual assault among male athletes—is especially important, and it is discussed fully in Chapter 6, "Violence in Sports" (pp. 163–165).

Race is another issue that must be taken into account when discussing arrest rates for college and professional athletes. An investigation by *USA Today* (Schrotenboer, 2013a) reports that when compared to white NFL players, black players are up to ten times more likely to be stopped by police while they are driving, and when they are stopped they are more likely to have their vehicles searched. Black players interviewed in the investigation said that when they are driving an expensive car in an area where an officer might think they don't belong, they are likely to be pulled over. If they object or give the impression that they are not fully cooperative, they are more likely than whites to be treated as a possible criminal.

This investigation does not prove that police are being unfair, but it certainly raises questions about the data on arrest rates among players when it comes to certain situations and possible crimes.

PERFORMANCE-ENHANCING SUBSTANCES: A CASE STUDY OF DEVIANT OVERCONFORMITY

The use of performance-enhancing substances remains a persistent issue in many sports (Hruby, 2012a, 2012b, 2013a, 2013e; Hughes, 2013; King, 2014; King et al., 2014; Ohl et al., 2015; Sefiha, 2012; Smith, 2015). Media stories about athletes using performance-enhancing substances are no longer shocking. However, most people don't know that drug and substance use in sports has a long history. For centuries athletes have taken a wide variety of everyday and exotic substances to aid their performances, and this has occurred at all levels of competition.

The use of performance-enhancing substances *predates* commercial sports and television, and it occurred regularly when so-called traditional values were widely accepted. Therefore, we must look beyond these factors to explain why athletes use performance-enhancing substances.

Research also suggests that substance use is not caused by defective socialization or a lack of moral character among athletes; in fact, it usually occurs among the most dedicated, committed, and hard-working athletes in sports (Petróczi, 2007). At this point, it appears that most substance use and abuse is tied to an athlete's uncritical acceptance of the norms of the sport ethic. Therefore, it is grounded in overconformity—the same type of overconformity that occurs when distance runners continue training with serious stress fractures; when female gymnasts control weight by cutting their food consumption to dangerous levels; and when NFL players take injections of painkilling drugs so they can put their already injured bodies on the line week after painful week.

Sports provide powerful and memorable experiences, and many athletes are willing to "set no limits" in their quest to maintain participation and gain reaffirmation of their identities as members of a select group sharing lives characterized by intensity, challenge, and excitement (Smith, 2015). Athletes often refer to their desire to win when they are interviewed or when they talk with fans, but for most of them, winning is important because it enables them to continue playing the sport they love to play and to receive identity affirmation from other athletes. These dynamics encourage overconformity to the norms of the sport ethic, and they affect athletes at various levels of sports—from local gyms, where high school players work out, to the locker rooms of professional sport teams; they affect both women and men across many sports, from the 100-meter sprint to the marathon and from tennis to football.

The point here is that athletes use substances like HGH (human growth hormone) for reasons that differ greatly from the reasons that an alienated twenty-five-year-old shoots heroin to get high and escape reality. The alienated twenty-five-year-old rejects society's norms, whereas athletes using performance-enhancing substances accept society's norms about dedication, working hard, ignoring pain, and overcoming obstacles to reach goals. But as they uncritically overconform to these norms, they often go too far and accept without question the idea of using performance-enhancing technologies. This means that athletes don't use performance-enhancing substances (PESs) to escape reality as much as they

use them to survive and succeed in elite sports. Therefore, we need different explanations to understand why athletes use "drugs." The explanations and methods of control used to deal with people who reject norms and use heroin, cocaine, methamphetamines, cannabis, and other so-called "recreational" drugs are not relevant when trying to deal with the issue of PESs in sports.

The Great Sport Myth, Doping, and Lance Armstrong

Most people who watch sports and cover them for the media want athletes to be models of positive character and deeds. When athletes, especially those who are highly visible and talented, say or do things that don't meet this expectation, they challenge believers of the great sport myth (GSM). For example, if I believe that playing sports leads to positive character development and I hear that a person who has played sports for many years violates rules or engages in deviance that contradicts my belief about sport, I can either change my long-held belief in the GSM or I can say that the deviant athlete is "morally corrupt" and unable to learn the lessons that sport teaches. If I have organized part of my life around my belief in the GSM, I find it much easier to condemn the athlete than to give up my belief and admit that I've been wrong about the essential purity and goodness of sport.

This example helps us understand what happened when Lance Armstrong finally admitted that he used substances banned by the IOC and the International Cycling Federation. Many people had turned Armstrong and his life into a fantasy narrative that for them provided absolute proof of the validity of the GSM. When Armstrong confessed, those believers felt betrayed. So they retained their beliefs about sports by vehemently condemning Armstrong as an embodiment of evil.

Exceptions to this response occurred among cancer survivors who never accepted the GSM as a guide for making decisions or making sense of reality. For them, Armstrong was simply a source of hope and comfort in their lives—he

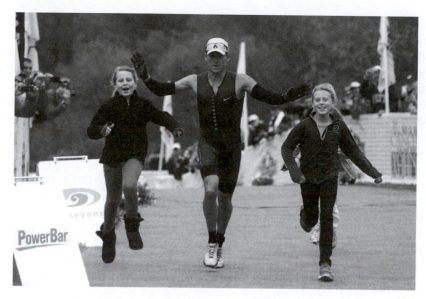

Lance Armstrong completes a half triathlon with his daughters running alongside. After his professional cycling career, he continued to train incessantly for marathons and triathlons, even though he had little chance of winning at his age. During the years when he won seven Tour de France races, he reputedly trained harder and longer than other riders. All but one of the twenty-one riders who placed second through fourth during those years were also found to be "doping." (*Source:* © Elizabeth Kreutz/Corbis)

had survived cancer, worked hard to succeed in cycling, founded the Livestrong Foundation, raised half a billion dollars for cancer research, and used his foundation to support them as they dealt with cancer. These people were less likely to see Armstrong as morally corrupt, even though many were disappointed that he had lied about doping and had treated other people badly in the process. Additionally, they were more likely to realistically understand the role of drugs in contemporary society. They knew that performance-enhancing substances were essential in their own daily lives, because they used them to avoid nausea, restore and build muscle, control pain and depression, and sustain the energy needed to live their lives. On the other hand most GSM believers never made a connection between their own use

of performance-enhancing substances and why an athlete might use them.

Sport Careers and Performance-Enhancing Technologies

The Armstrong case provided a perfect opportunity to ask critical questions about the organization of high-performance sports today, the pervasive use of performance-enhancing technologies by elite athletes, and the ever-increasing demands of training and competition schedules set by sponsors, event organizers, media companies, coaches, and sport organization managers. But this opportunity was lost as people desperately clung to the GSM, heaped condemnation on Armstrong, and discredited everything he had done in his life.

Our discussion here is an attempt to regain this opportunity and discuss research findings that help to explain why the use of PESs persists in many sports despite the efforts of anti-doping agencies that are now part of a powerful multibillion-dollar substance testing and control industry.

Studying the careers of athletes and the contexts in which they train and compete has been the focus of French sociologist Christophe Brissonneau. As a former elite cyclist, he has used his contacts in sports to collect data from athletes, trainers, coaches, and sport medicine professionals. Christophe began to collect data systematically in Europe during the late 1990s. Most recently he received a Fulbright Scholar-in-Residence award to come to the United States and collect data

from and about elite athletes in the NFL and Major League Baseball, among other sports.

After analyzing data collected mostly through in-depth interviews with athletes in cycling, track and field, wrestling, weightlifting, and bodybuilding, Christophe and his colleagues at the University of Paris social science research lab created a model that describes participation in elite sport as a three-part process in a multiphase sport career (Brissonneau and Depiesse, 2006; Brissonneau and Ohl, 2010; Brissonneau, 2010, 2013; Ohl et al., 2015). This model as applied to careers in professional cycling is presented in Figure 5.4.

The model identifies five phases in the overall career of a professional cyclist. In each phase the cyclist experiences socialization in connection with

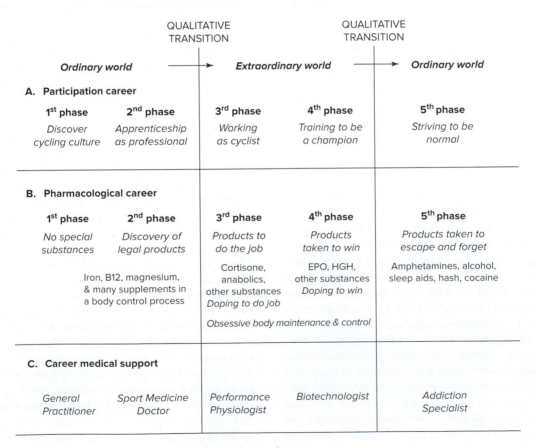

FIGURE 5.4 Brissonneau's model of a professional sport career.

(a) participation, (b) pharmacology, and (c) medical support. The career begins in the ordinary world—that is, the normal, everyday world.

The first phase of the participation career involves discovering the culture of a particular sport—in this case, cycling. At this point, cyclists are amateurs and feel no need to use special performance technologies or performance-enhancing substances, and medical support is provided by a general practitioner during an annual checkup and general health assessment. These cyclists might race in local events, but their lives involve school and family. Cycling during this phase is focused on personal experiences rather than tracking performance, and the goal is primarily to enjoy and learn more about cycling.

In the second phase, cyclists become more serious and set goals; at this point some aspire to become professionals. Depending on the sport and the country, athletes join clubs or become members of competitive programs and teams. Health and recovery from training and competition now become important, as does the need to be more rational and scientific in monitoring and controlling their bodies. This means that specialized sport medicine doctors are sought for support. Performance-enhancing technologies become important because they begin to track and measure their physical attributes, from strength and muscle growth to endurance and the oxygen-carrying capacity of their circulatory systems (heart and lungs).

During this second phase, athletes learn about legal substances that their peers use to fine-tune their bodies for training and racing. Anything that enables them to train more intensely becomes attractive. In the case of cyclists, they begin to see a need for receiving injections of iron and vitamins C, B_6, and B_{12}, among other substances. This marks the initiation of a pharmacological career that often is formally or informally supported by sports doctors, athlete peers, and a larger sport system associated with national teams or elite leagues and organizations that are state-supported in some countries and personally or club-supported in others.

The move from the second to the third phase of an athlete's career is significant, because it involves a qualitative change from the ordinary world of amateur sports to the extraordinary world of professional sports. Sport participation in this phase comes to be defined as a job—sponsors are sought, athletes are paid, training and competition schedules are determined by others, and the pressure to improve performance becomes the sole focus of athletes' lives. Expectations, demands, and personal perspectives change dramatically. The athletes' social world becomes increasingly exclusive and isolated from the ordinary world, and their lives revolve around relationships with elite athletes, coaches, trainers, performance physiologists, team managers, and sponsors. These people are concerned with the cyclist's performance above all else.

During the third phase, training is based on science and rationality. The duration and intensity of training increases dramatically and fatigue becomes the body's enemy. Over time the athletes come to realize that in order to survive and succeed at the professional level, they must do things that in the past they avoided or thought were unwise or unethical. But they also know that for their bodies to function at full capacity, they must use technologies to help them recover from the physical damage done by their training and competition. To ignore these technologies means not doing their job and not being fit for competition. Pharmacological products offer assistance—*if* the athletes are willing to work at the level of intensity needed to take advantage of them. At this point, they go beyond normal boundaries of what is accepted in society at large. To remain at this elite level, the use of these technologies and substances comes to be seen as a necessary part of training, even if they are illegal or banned.

The fourth phase involves an intensification of everything from the third phase. In the case of cyclists this has generally involved a shift from focusing on doing the job to reaching the podium, winning stages in long races, and working with teammates to win races. Athletes feel compelled to use all technologies provided by the biotechnologists who study human performance and control most of their training.

Athletes in this phase of their careers learn that overconforming to the norms of the sport ethic is normal—doing whatever it takes to continue performing at a supranormal level is the standard expectation that they have for themselves and that others have for them. Those unwilling to meet this expectation are seen as letting others down and violating the code that governs the lives of professional athletes. Therefore, athletes train more obsessively and follow year-round training programs designed by personal trainers, nutritionists, and sport scientists. But to remain in their sport and continue to perform at the highest level, they must push their bodies beyond normal limits every day. When this is done for more than fifteen hours per week, it breaks down the body and causes physiological damage. Recovering from this, and from the injuries that are inevitable in training and competition, requires the use of various therapies, technologies, and substances. The harder athletes train, the more they need these things to be competition ready and to sustain their careers.

During the fourth phase, medical support focuses on performance rather than overall health and well-being. This involves using various combinations of substances, legal and/or illegal, to continue training and preparing the body to compete at the highest level. Strategies for doing this are learned from other athletes, but also from sport scientists and sport medicine experts hired by teams, clubs, and sport federations. For athletes to ignore these experts usually puts an end to their high-performance careers, along with their team membership, sponsors, income, relationships with elite peers, and identity as an athlete. For those who have dedicated most of their lives to reaching this point in their sport, refusing to do whatever it takes is seldom a viable option. Some athletes refuse, but we seldom hear about them, because their careers usually end quickly.

The training strategies during the fourth phase are extraordinary. To endure them and maximize the chances of winning, athletes usually try to control everything that affects their ability to perform. This is when doping often becomes normalized as a training strategy. It enables athletes to train harder and longer than their opponents, and it becomes an integral part of the culture that is organized around achieving competitive success (Hruby, 2013a). To refuse to dope under these conditions is especially difficult when athletes now represent teams, sport organizations, sponsors, and their communities or nations (Hoberman, 2005; Johnson, 2012). Additionally, when athletes arrive at this phase, their definition of health has already shifted to focus on competitive success without questioning whether their actions may cause future health problems, such as joint deterioration, arthritis, limited range of motion, and chronic, often debilitating pain that will interfere with rising from bed each morning and engaging in normal physical activities. Additionally, athletes learn to hide their fatigue and injuries because they fear being replaced by other elite performers, and they want to avoid exposing weaknesses to opponents who will exploit them. In fact, athletes who show any weakness in a high-performance sport put in jeopardy their contract, endorsements, sponsorships, and even fan support.

During this fourth phase, sport is not something athletes do—*it is who they are.* Winning is important because it enables them to remain in elite sports, which at this point is the foundation of their lives and identities. To not win is to lose the basis for their primary identity, their relationships, experiences, and everyday routines. Therefore, when overconformity to the norms of the sport ethic is explained only in terms of a "win at all costs" mentality among elite athletes, it obscures the deeper personal meanings that are linked to being an athlete in societies where sports have become a central cultural focus and where being an elite athlete requires total dedication and commitment.

The move from professional sport into the fifth career phase involves another major qualitative change. This is when athletes must re-enter the ordinary world after what may have been a long-term separation. This often creates serious challenges for athletes whose only important identity for many years has been their athlete identity. When being an elite athlete leaves little or no time to develop other skills and identities, athletes stay at the elite level as long as possible. Injuries often are what force them into the fifth phase. But becoming "normal" after many years in the high-intensity, self- and body-focused world of high-performance sports requires significant adjustments (Tinley, 2015a).

Routines are out of sync, and reasons for living seem fuzzy and uncertain. The pleasures of pushing the body to its limits are gone, as is the excitement of competition. The other athletes who have been sources of daily support are no longer there, and people in the ordinary world can't understand the difficulty involved in losing an identity as an elite athlete. Striving to be normal involves renegotiating relationships with family and friends, if they are still available and willing to re-engage. But re-engaging is difficult when pre-sport identities are irrelevant and new identities don't yet exist.

The letdown and confusion experienced during the fifth career phase often lead to a desire to escape the boredom of the ordinary world. Some retired athletes in this phase might use amphetamines to jump-start the day and sleep aids such as Ambien to shut it off. Some also turn to alcohol, cannabis, hashish, and cocaine. The medical support person needed during this phase is an addiction specialist, a psychiatrist, or a clinical psychologist.

The seriousness of problems during this phase depends on many factors. But the difficulties of retirement from elite sports have become more common as the demands and expectations in high-performance sports have escalated since the mid-1980s. When sponsors and television entered the scene, and when training came to be based on rationality and science, expectations for elite athletes intensified. The "off-season" disappeared, there was no time for other jobs or education, and no excuses for poor performances.

Some people find it difficult to accept all the aspects of Brissonneau's model, even though it is based on nearly twenty years of data collected from athletes and others associated with high-performance sports. Of course, not every athlete fits perfectly into this model. There are differences by country, sport, gender, and the place of high-performance sports in specific cultures (Pitsch and Emrich, 2012). But the difficulty in accepting Brissonneau's model is also due to a lack of access to the world inside high-performance sports. The code of the locker room keeps us out and much of the data hidden.

Additionally, athletes and others associated with high-performance sports know or quickly learn that if they publicly use the uncensored discourse from the extraordinary world of elite sports, they would shock people and jeopardize the commercial value of their sports and lose their jobs. Therefore, they use a discourse grounded in the first and second phases of the professional sport career model. This discourse stresses a connection between sports and health and the importance of values, ethics, and the purity and goodness of sports. It uses the language of the great sport myth because people in elite sports know that selling their product to the public is most effective when the integrity of sport is emphasized along with total commitment to purging from its ranks all those who would soil what many believe to be its essential purity and goodness.

Most athletes embrace discourse from the first and second phases because it also represents their beliefs—or what they want to believe. This is not surprising, because others see them as representing the purity and goodness of sports. Sponsors embrace and promote this discourse because it reaffirms their business model as well as the beliefs of its executives, who often claim that their characters were shaped in positive ways back when they played sports. Media people who cover sports and those who work in sport organizations use this discourse to sustain the beliefs on which the popularity of sports has come to depend.

This means that deviance in sports is a political issue as well as a health and cultural issue. What counts as deviance in sports is determined by what will sustain its popularity and support. This also shapes the sanctions and punishments handed out by sport leaders and rules committees. When

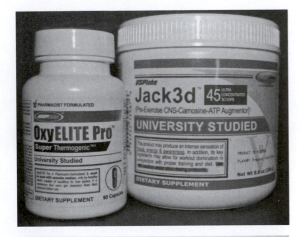

This product may produce an intense sensation of focus, energy & awareness. In addition, its key ingredients may allow for workout domination in conjunction with proper training and diet. Use with caution under strict dosing protocols.

More than half of American adults use "nutritional supplements", spending over $30 billion annually on them. Jack3d allegedly contains, a powerful stimulant, much like amphetamines. People claim that it enables them to work out longer and more intensely. OxyElite Pro warns that it should be used "only by healthy adults capable of handling its true power." Supplements are produced faster than drug-testing organizations can determine if they should be banned. This is partly because the United States does not require Federal Drug Agency approval of supplements before they are marketed and sold. After I took this photo, OxyElite Pro was taken off the market due to its connection with a fatal liver illness. (*Source:* © Jay Coakley)

athletes or low-level employees in sports do or say things that tarnish the perceived integrity of "the game" or allow people to see clearly into the extraordinary world of high-performance sports, they will be sanctioned.

Doping from Inside High-Performance Sports

Controlling the discourse about sport can be tricky. Elite athletes seldom give others a glimpse inside their extraordinary world. However, here are statements about drugs in which athletes do provide us with a brief look inside that world.

> It's professional sports. You do what you need to do to play and, at the end of the season, you get cleaned up [from all the drugs].
>
> —Ryan Zimmerman, MLB player
> (in White, 2012)

> Your first day in the league is the last day you'll ever be 100 percent healthy. (I took Toradol.) That's part of football. You take every legal advantage possible.[3]
>
> —Jamaal Jackson, eight-year NFL veteran
> (in Matz, 2011)

> My body was perpetually feeling bad, as were those of my teammates. Our training staff knew this and would encourage us to get a shot. We were told it would make us feel better. So we lined up for the needle.
>
> —Nate Jackson, five-year NFL veteran
> (in Jackson, 2011)

> It's normal. You drop your pants . . . they give you a shot [of the painkiller Toradol], put the Band-Aid on, you go out and play. It may be stupid, it may be dumb, call me dumb and stupid then, because I want to be on the football field.
>
> —Brian Urlacher, a thirteen-year NFL veteran
> (in NFL Brief, 2012)

---

[3]Toradol is a potent prescription nonsteroidal anti-inflammatory drug (NSAID). Until a few years ago, so many NFL players received injections on game days that they described it as a "cattle call" (Belson and Pilon, 2012). Today team doctors don't administer injections, because NFL players are suing the NFL for damages allegedly caused by the drug. Many athletes continue to use it to enable them to play, but they obtain it on their own.

There's a certain point in your career where you're going through the pounding of the season and getting through that week of practice and trying to get to that next game day. Toradol is part of what gets you back to playing the way you normally can.

—Jim Kleinsasser, thirteen-year NFL veteran (in Wiederer, 2012)

I felt like new money. You get that shot and you feel like you're 18, 19 years old. It's like a sheet of armor. I was a new man.

—A twelve-year NFL player who set records and won a Super Bowl while taking the injections (in Wiederer, 2012)

It does mask pain. But that's the price you pay when you play through injuries. We're a commodity. We're useful only when we're on the field.

—Ronde Barber, seventeen-year NFL veteran (in Matz, 2011)

These statements are about a legal drug, and they come mostly from football players. Players seldom talk candidly in public about illegal or banned substances, but football players felt free to talk more openly about Toradol in 2011 after many had filed a class action suit against the NFL for allowing teams to administer it without following the warnings for the drug or discussing the side effects with players.

The statements also tell us that using drugs to enhance performance is a normal occurrence in the extraordinary world of high-performance sports. This conclusion has been supported in research by Evdoki Pappa and Eileen Kennedy (2013), who interviewed elite track-and-field athletes. They summarize their findings this way:

The athletes give a clear indication that they see doping as a normalized phenomenon . . . Although sporting authorities have banned the use of PEDs, the athletes consider them necessary for their career and for competition at a high level. (pp. 289, 290)

This conclusion does not mean that all elite athletes use illegal substances. But it does mean that using such substances in the extraordinary world of high-performance sports is not seen as an indication of moral corruption and weak character. Therefore, to control doping in sports is a task that may never be fully accomplished, despite the unceasing efforts of the anti-doping industry.

The War on Doping

Drug testing is relatively new in sports (Waddington and Smith, 2009). Prior to the mid-1980s, anti-doping policies existed largely to discourage athletes from dropping dead of overdoses, something that had become too common in certain sports as athletes experimented with a wide range of substances thought to provide a boost to training and performance. But as the money associated with sports has enabled athletes to hide their drug use, anti-doping agencies work to maintain an image of integrity in sports (Aschwanden, 2012). In fact, the stated rationale for the World Anti-Doping Code that guides Olympic sports and is enforced by the IOC, WADA, and USADA is that "doping is fundamentally contrary to the spirit of sport" (WADA, 2009). This rationale is grounded in an absolutist approach in which it is assumed that *any* use of banned performance-enhancing substances violates the ideals represented by sport and is therefore deviant. This approach encourages the demonizing of athletes who use banned substances for any reason (López, 2011).

The war on doping now being waged by WADA and USADA is supported by most people even if they are not sport fans. They feel that the essential purity and goodness of sports have been dirtied by "dopers" and that anything that will purge them from sports should be supported. This approach also allows them to avoid critical questions, such as these:

1. Is it logical to praise athletes as warrior-heroes when they take injections of painkilling drugs to stay on the field, and then condemn them as cheaters when they take steroids, HGH, and other substances that help to heal injuries more

quickly, rebuild muscles damaged by overtraining, or relax and recover after exhausting and tightly scheduled competitions?

2. Does it make sense to condemn athletes for failing to be positive role models for children, when we expect them to put their bodies on the line for the sake of entertainment?

3. Why does drug testing focus on individual athletes rather than the culture of high-performance sports and the complex system in which people other than athletes develop, purchase, supply, administer, and study banned substances to determine how they can be taken without testing positive?

4. How can testing be justified by saying that it keeps athletes healthy and preserves fairness in sports, when it is clear that the sports most watched by fans are not good for a person's health and are not fair when some people have the resources to buy the best training and technology in the world and others don't even know it exists?

5. How can people in the United States, for example, say that athletes using a performance-enhancing substance are morally corrupt and should be banned from their careers, when they are part of a society in which appearance-enhancing, cognitive-enhancing, and performance-enhancing substances are consumed at rates unprecedented in human history?

6. Could the billions of dollars now spent on testing and police-like investigations of the urine, blood, and suspect actions of athletes be better spent on educating and working with athletes in each of the five phases of a sport career so they are fully informed and medically supported when they make choices about using available technologies to aid their training and competition?

7. Is it reasonable to condemn the use of so-called "doping" and at the same time support the Olympic motto "Faster, Higher, Stronger" and demand more record-setting performances, when athletes are now pushing the limits of

human potential and damaging their bodies as they do so?

Asking these and dozens of other critical questions about the current approach to doping control in sports makes many people uncomfortable, so they are seldom asked.

The cat-and-mouse dynamics that have emerged with the current form of drug testing are unlikely to stop. New technologies that improve vision, cognitive alertness, brain function, response time, strength, and speed are being developed at a record pace (Epstein, 2011). Genetic manipulation is close to being possible, if it has not already been done (Epstein, 2010). This suggests that the most reasonable question to ask is this: How can these technologies (including drugs) be integrated into the lives of athletes (and the rest of us) without destroying our health and well-being?

Without asking these questions and changing the current approach to testing, doping scandals will continue to occur. Athletes will be caught, people will express their disgust and demand that the cheaters be punished, and then everyone (other than the punished athletes) will feel good until the next scandal occurs.

When Jörg Jaksche, a former pro cyclist from Germany, was asked what he thought about this approach, he suggested that it will continue because it has no downside for the sponsors of high-performance sports—those whose money drives commercial spectator sports today. He explained (in Gatti, 2013) that the current drug-testing system allows sponsors to "gain all the commercial benefits of the visibility generated by great performances," which often are aided by drugs, and when athletes are caught the sponsors can express surprise and disappointment and "receive the extra benefit of the good publicity gained for being righteous." Overall, he says, "it's a win-win" situation for the most powerful people in sports today, and that's why the current system won't change. But some of us are not so pessimistic and suggest that there are reasonable alternatives to the war on doping.

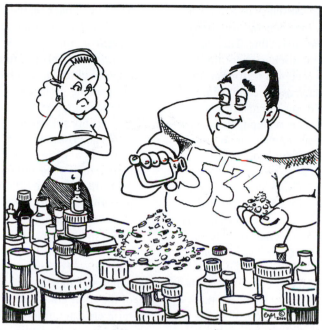

(*Source:* © Frederic A. Eyer)

"Don't worry, most of these are legal and the others won't show up on the drug tests!"

Most athletes today take multiple "nutritional supplements" (Mason and Lavallee, 2012). The industries that produce them are unregulated and often claim that certain products are performance-enhancing.

Alternatives to the War on Doping

A central point in this chapter is that athletes use performance-enhancing substances not because they lack character or are victims of evil or exploitive coaches, but because they (1) uncritically accept and overconform to the norms of the sport ethic and (2) are part of a sport system in which therapies and supplements are needed to recover from intense training and competition schedules over which they have little control. This is why tougher rules and increased testing have not been effective.

Moral panics over drug use and oversimplified solutions will not change the reality of training and competition or the culture of high-performance sports, nor will it stop athletes from using substances that they see as necessary to maintain their identities and continue experiencing the joy and excitement of playing elite sports.

The use of performance-enhancing substances and future forms of cognitive performance enhancement and genetic manipulation cannot be effectively controlled in elite sport cultures as they are now organized. Effective control requires both cultural and structural changes in sports so that athletes, coaches, and others critically assess the sport ethic and control deviant overconformity, or redefine the sport ethic to include new norms. Here are suggestions on where to begin these processes:

- *Critically examine the deep hypocrisy involved in elite power and performance sports.* It isn't possible to effectively control the use of performance-enhancing substances when federations and teams encourage general overconformity to the norms of the sport ethic. Therefore, there's a need for critical discussions of limits on the use of currently accepted performance-enhancing strategies, such as injecting painkilling drugs and massive doses of vitamin B$_{12}$, hydration therapies, playing with pins in broken bones and with high-tech "casts" to hold broken bones in place during competition, and using special harnesses to restrict the movement of injured joints. These practices are common, and they foster a sport culture in which the use of performance-enhancing substances is defined as logical and courageous by athletes.

• *Establish rules clearly indicating that certain risks to health are undesirable and unnecessary in sports.* When sixteen-year-old girls who compete with training-induced stress fractures in elite gymnastics are turned into national heroes and poster children for corporate sponsors, it promote deviants overconformity in sports. This sets up athletes for permanent injuries and disabilities. This is clearly a problem, and sport organizations should refocus on health over performance.

• *Establish a "harm reduction" approach in which athletes are not allowed to play until certified as "well" (not simply "able to compete") by two independent physicians or medical personnel.* This approach differs from current practices in which trainers and medical personnel do what they can to get injured athletes back on the field as quickly as possible (Bennett, 2013). Trainers and physicians should be health advocates paid by someone other than team management. The focus of a player health advocate would be protecting the long-term well-being of athletes. Therefore, instead of testing for drugs, athletes should be tested to certify that they are healthy enough to participate. If drugs damage their health or make it dangerous for them to play, they would not be certified. Only when their health improves and meets established guidelines would they be allowed back on the field. This would be a major step in creating a new sport culture.

• *Establish injury and health education programs for athletes.* This is a first step in establishing a sport culture in which *courage* is defined as recognizing limits to conformity and accepting the discipline necessary to accurately and responsibly acknowledge the consequences of deviant overconformity and sports injuries. Learning to be in tune with one's body rather than to deny pain and injury is important in controlling the use of potentially dangerous performance-enhancing substances.

• *Establish health-based guidelines and codes of ethics for sport scientists, coaches, managers, and those who set training and competition schedules.* Too many sport scientists assist athletes as they overconform to the norms of the sport ethic, rather than helping them raise critical questions about the health risks that come with deviant overconformity. For example, sport science should be used to help athletes understand the consequences of their choices to play sports and help them critically assess *why* they're doing what they're doing and *what* it means in their lives. Using science to encourage or enable athletes to give body and soul to their sports without asking these critical questions is to leave the door open for deviant overconformity, including the use of performance-enhancing substances.

• *Make drug and substance education a key part of health education programs.* Parents, coaches, league administrators, managers, and trainers should participate with athletes in educational programs in which they consider and discuss the norms of the sport ethic and how to prevent deviant overconformity. Unless all these people understand their roles in reproducing a culture that supports substance use and abuse, the problems will continue.

We now face a future without clearly defined ideas about the meaning of achievement in sports. There are new financial incentives to succeed in sports, athlete identities have become central in the lives of many sport participants, and performance-enhancing technologies have become increasingly effective and available. Therefore, we need *new* approaches and guidelines. Old approaches and guidelines combined with coercive methods of control are not effective. Trying to make sports into what we believe they were in the past is futile. We face new issues and challenges, and it will take new approaches to deal with them effectively.

Widespread participation is needed if sport cultures are to be successfully transformed. At present, both nation states and corporate sponsors have appropriated the culture of power and performance sports and used it to deliver messages that foster forms of deviant overconformity for the sake of national and corporate interests. There is no conspiracy underlying this, but it creates a challenge that can be met only through our collective awareness of what needs to be done, followed by collective efforts to do it. Even then changes will be incremental rather than revolutionary, but changes are possible if we work to create them in our sports, schools, and communities.

summary

IS DEVIANCE IN SPORTS OUT OF CONTROL?

The study of deviance in sports presents challenges due to four factors: (1) the diverse forms and causes of deviance in sports cannot be explained by a single theory; (2) the ideas, traits, and actions accepted in sports may be deviant in the rest of society at the same time that things accepted in society may be deviant in sports; (3) deviance in sports often involves accepting norms uncritically and without limits, rather than rejecting them; and (4) training in sports now involves so many new forms of science and technology that we lack norms to guide and evaluate the actions of athletes and others in sports.

People who assume that social reality contains essential truths about right and wrong and good and evil often use an absolutist approach to explain deviance. They believe that unchanging moral truths are the foundation for all norms. Therefore, every norm represents an ideal, and every action, trait, or idea that departs from that ideal is deviant, immoral, or evil. When this approach is used, deviance becomes increasingly serious as the departure from the ideal increases. For example, if using banned substances is contrary to the ideal that sport is pure and good, any use of them at any time or place would be deviant, and if the substance use continued over time, it would eventually be defined as immoral or evil.

Sociologists generally use a constructionist approach to study and explain deviance in sports. This approach, based on a combination of cultural, interactionist, and structural theories, emphasizes that norms and deviance are socially constructed through social interaction. This approach highlights a distinction between deviant underconformity and overconformity. This is important because the most serious forms of deviance in sports occur when athletes, coaches, and others overconform to the norms of the sport ethic—a cluster of norms that emphasizes dedication to the game above all else, striving for distinction, taking risks and playing through pain and injury, and overcoming all obstacles in the pursuit of sport dreams. When limits are not set in the process of conforming to these norms, deviant overconformity occurs and often creates serious problems.

Most sociology of sport research has focused on the deviant underconformity of athletes. Research on deviance among coaches, managers, and others who control sports is relatively scarce, largely because people with power refuse to be studied in ways that might jeopardize their status and influence.

We don't know if cheating in sports is more prevalent today than in the past, but institutional corruption appears to be a growing problem in sport organizations, most of which lack formally enforced mandates to be transparent or accountable.

Institutional corruption is accompanied by dynamics that foster harassment and abuse, including the sexual abuse of athletes by coaches.

Gambling and the forms of deviance that often accompany it are an increasing problem in sports. Recent cases of match fixing in global soccer and other major sports, mostly outside North America, have raised questions about the actions of players and referees who can influence game events and the final scores of matches and games.

Hazing, which also is difficult to study because it occurs in secrecy, often involves dangerous forms of deviance when it occurs among high school and college students who try to preserve secrecy by forcing new team members to violate strong social taboos.

Research indicates that athlete deviance off the field and away from sports is a problem. However, the rates of deviance among athletes do not appear to be higher than rates among their peers who do not play officially organized sports. Exceptions to this involve drinking alcohol, binge drinking, and sexual assault.

The use and abuse of performance-enhancing substances is a widespread common form of deviance among athletes, despite new rules, testing programs, and strong punishments for violators. Because so many people accept the great sport myth and believe that sports are essentially pure and good, they use an absolutist approach when thinking about drugs in sports. Therefore, they see athletes that use banned substances as morally corrupt cheaters who must be purged from sports.

Brissonneau's model of a five-phase professional sports career is based on a constructionist approach, and it explains substance use in connection with the demands and expectations that now exist in high-performance sports and the need for athletes to train in ways that are clearly "beyond normal" to meet them. Because the resulting fatigue, pain, and injuries take a toll on their bodies, athletes depend on specialized medical and pharmacological support to sustain their ability to perform. This normalizes the use of drugs and other technologies that enable them to perform.

Many athletes who are committed to doing whatever it takes to succeed and avoid being cut from their teams, view the use of performance-enhancing technologies as an integral part of training rather than a form of cheating, even though they know it violates rules. This mind-set also explains why athletes take injections of dangerous legal drugs such as Toradol and cortisone to mask pain and stay on the field.

The war on doping waged through the enforcement of current anti-doping policies involves testing athletes' urine and blood, and more recently the investigation of athletes' personal lives. This has created a cat-and-mouse dynamic in which athletes try to stay one step ahead of the testers. Even though this approach to "doping control" is costly and ineffective, it continues to be used because it serves the purposes of sponsors and sport organizations. When there are no positive tests, they can claim to be responsibly safeguarding the purity and goodness of sports, and when there are positive tests, they can express disgust and claim to be morally righteous as they punish the offending athletes.

Alternatives to the war on doping involve asking critical questions about the current organization and culture of high-performance sports and honestly identifying their consequences for athletes. Instead of testing for drugs, a harm reduction approach could be used so that athletes are tested by qualified medical professionals to determine whether they are healthy enough to train and compete. If this were combined with education for athletes and for those who control sports, and if there were guidelines and codes of ethics for sport scientists who develop training programs for athletes, it might be more effective than drug testing as we face a future that will bring many new forms of performance-enhancing technologies.

SUPPLEMENTAL READINGS

Reading 1. Using deviance to create commercial personas in sports

SPORT MANAGEMENT ISSUES

- As a high school teacher and coach you hear that the veterans on the boys' wrestling team are planning to haze new members of their team. In the past, hazing by some of the teams has gotten out of hand, so you report your information to the principal and the athletic director. They ask you to create an alternative to hazing that will help team members bond in positive ways without engaging in demeaning or risky actions. Outline your plan and explain the differences between what you are proposing and hazing as it is defined in the chapter.

- As an athletic director you are concerned with the number of athletes on the track-and-field team who are being treated by your sport medicine staff for injuries due to overtraining. The coach tells you that she demands 110 percent from all her athletes and expects them to train and compete through pain and injury. You could develop a rule that a doctor outside the athletic department must make the decision on whether an athlete will play with pain and injury. Explain what you would do.

- You have an internship with a top professional sport team. You love what you do, and on a few occasions you take modafinil to stay up all night to meet project deadlines. Your supervisor is impressed and offers you a job that all the other interns wanted. You accept the job, pass the company's mandatory drug test, and have a successful first year on the job. Are you a cheater for taking this drug, which is on the WADA banned substance list? Explain why or why not, in a way that is logical.

- You have been hired by the IOC to review and evaluate its current anti-doping approach and suggest alternatives, if appropriate. They have hired you because the current approach has not been well accepted or fully trusted by athletes around the world. Summarize the main points in your review and evaluation, and your suggestions, if any.

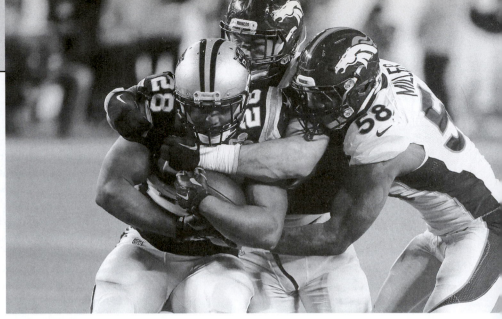

(*Source:* © Jan Kruger/Getty Images)

VIOLENCE IN SPORTS

Does It Affect Our Lives?

I DON'T WANT TO SOUND LIKE I'm bragging, because I'm not, but back [in the 1960s, when I played basketball] the violence was much more intense.

—**Satch Sanders, former NBA player, 1999**

IT'S THE MOST PERFECT feeling in the world to know you've hit a guy just right, that you've maximized the physical pain he can feel. . . . You feel the life just go out of him. You've taken all this man's energy and just dominated him.

—**Michael Strahan, former NFL player (in Layden, 2007)**

". . . fans goad football linebackers into wild acts of aggression on the field, then express shock when those same people get into bar brawls or domestic disputes. Being a fan isn't exactly an exercise in logic."

—**Paul Shirley, journalist (2011)**

We have to make sure we're not creating another Rome where there are gladiators dying on the field depending on whether Caesar gives a thumbs-up or thumbs-down.

—**Tim Ridder, former college football player (in Kelly, 2011)**

Learning Objectives

- Define violence and distinguish it from related behaviors such as aggression and intimidation.

- Discuss historical trends for on-the-field and spectator violence.

- Explain the differences between the four major types of on-the-field violence in sports.

- Know the connections between violence in sports and deviant overconformity, commercialization, and masculinity.

- Understand when and how athletes learn to use violence as a strategy in sports.

- Describe the consequences of violence for athletes and understand the implications of brain trauma for athletes and for certain sports.

- Know the conditions under which athletes may learn to control their violent actions off the field and when their sport experiences may contribute to off-the-field violence, such as assault and sexual assault.

- Distinguish the various forms of spectator violence and identify the ones more common in North America than other parts of the world.

- Identify strategies that could be used to control venue violence and post-event violence.

- Discuss the incidence of terrorism at sport events and explain how and why terrorism influences sport events today.

Concussions and repeated head trauma experienced in football and other sports have recently been connected with serious long-term health problems such as dementia. The high school football team in Steubenville, Ohio, received national news coverage when two high-profile team members were found guilty of raping an unconscious young woman, whom they repeatedly and brutally dehumanized at parties attended by their teammates. A terrorist attack during the 2013 Boston Marathon killed three people and injured 264. And the most rapidly growing spectator sport in the United States in recent years is mixed martial arts, with its often-brutal fights staged in fenced cages.

These and similar cases make violence in sports an important topic to study and understand today. Therefore, the goal of this chapter is to use sociological research and theories to make sense of the origins and consequences of violence in sports. Chapter content focuses on six topics:

1. A practical definition of *violence* and related terms
2. A brief historical overview of violence in sports
3. The incidence and consequences of on-the-field violence among players in various sports
4. The relationship between on-the-field and off-the-field violence among players
5. Violence among spectators who consume media coverage of sports and attend live events
6. The threat and incidence of terrorism at sport events

In connection with the last three topics, I will identify strategies for controlling violence on and off the field.

WHAT IS VIOLENCE?

In sociological terms, **violence** *is the use of excessive physical force, which causes or has obvious potential to cause harm or destruction.* We often think of violence as actions that are illegal or unsanctioned, but there are situations in which the use of violence is socially encouraged or approved. For instance, when violence is tied to a rejection of social norms, it is classified as illegal and punished. However, when violence occurs in connection with enforcing norms, protecting people and property, or overconforming to widely accepted norms, it may be approved and even lauded as necessary to preserve order, reaffirm social values, or achieve important goals. Therefore, violence may be tolerated, or even glorified, when soldiers and police are perceived to be protecting people, or when athletes are perceived to be reproducing accepted ideologies, or pursuing victories in the name of others.

When violence occurs in connection with the widespread rejection of norms, it may be described as anarchy or lawless mayhem. When it occurs in connection with extreme methods of social control or extreme overconformity to norms, it may be defined as morally righteous, even when people are maimed or killed and property is destroyed.

In the case of sports, punching a referee who penalizes you is violence that involves a rejection of norms. It is defined as illegal and punished by teams and sport organizations, even if the referee is not seriously injured. However, it is different when a football player delivers a punishing tackle, breaking the ribs or blowing out the knee of an opposing running back. Such violence involves conformity to norms and is seen as entertaining, highlighted on video replays, and used by teammates and other players as a mark of one's status in football culture. The player might even feel righteous in being violent, despite harmful consequences, and would not hesitate to be violent again. His violence is not punished because it is an effective way to intimidate, control, and dominate others for the purpose of achieving a valued goal. Furthermore, his ability to do violence and endure it when perpetrated by others is used to affirm his identity as an athlete and a football player.

The term **aggression** refers to *verbal or physical actions grounded in an intent to dominate, control, or do harm to another person.* Aggression is often involved in violence, but violence may occur inadvertently or carelessly without aggressive intent. This allows us to distinguish aggressive actions from other actions that we might describe as assertive, competitive, or achievement oriented. For example, a very competitive person may engage in violent actions during a game without the intent to dominate, control, or harm others. This suggests that there is a difference between being aggressive and simply being assertive or striving to win or achieve other goals.

The term **intimidation** refers to *words, gestures, and actions that threaten violence or aggression.* Like aggression, intimidation is used to dominate or control others. These definitions help us understand the research on violence in sports.

VIOLENCE IN SPORTS THROUGHOUT HISTORY

Violence is not new to physical activities and sports (Dunning, 1999; Guttmann, 1998, 2004). Blood sports were popular among the ancient Greeks and throughout the Roman Empire. Deaths occurred regularly in connection with ritual games among the Mayans and Aztecs. Tournaments in medieval Europe were designed to train men for war and often resulted in death and destruction. Popular folk games were only loosely governed by rules, and they produced injuries and deaths at rates that would shock people today. Bearbaiting, cockfighting, dog fighting, and other "sporting" activities during those periods involved treatment of animals that most people today would define as criminally violent.

Research indicates that, as part of an overall civilizing process in Europe and North America, modern sports were developed to be more rule-governed activities than the physical games in previous eras. As sports became formally organized, official rules prohibited certain forms of violence that had been common in many folk games. Bloodshed decreased, and there was more emphasis on

> **Violence is primarily about control. Violence works. It makes people do what they otherwise would not. It governs the thin line between life and death.** —Allan G. Johnson, sociologist, 2013

self-control to restrict the expression of aggressive impulses during competition (Dunning, 1999).

Social historians also point out that rates of violence in sports do not automatically decrease over time. In fact, as actions and emotional expressions have become more regulated and controlled in modern societies, players and spectators view the "controlled" violence in sports as exciting. Furthermore, commercialization, professionalization, and globalization have given rise to new forms of instrumental and "dramatic" violence in many sports. This means that goal-oriented and entertainment-oriented violence have increased, at least temporarily, in many Western societies.

Sociologist Eric Dunning (1999) notes that violence remains a crucial social issue because the goal of modern sports is to create tension rather than eliminate it. Additionally, violent and aggressive sports generally serve, to reproduce an ideology that naturalizes the power of men over women. Overall, historical research shows that sports are

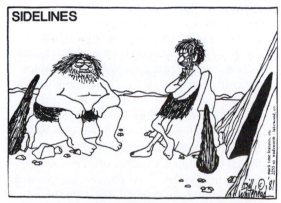

(*Source:* By permission of William Whitehead)

"Now that we've invented violence, we need a sport so we can use it without being labeled as uncivilized."

Violence in sports is not new, but this does not mean that it is a natural or inevitable part of sport participation among men or women.

given different meanings at different times and places and that we can understand violence in sports only when we analyze it in relation to the historical, social, and cultural contexts in which it occurs.

VIOLENCE ON THE FIELD

Violence in sports comes in many forms, and it is grounded in social and cultural factors related to the sport ethic, commercialization, gender ideology, ideas about masculinity, and the strategies used in sports. Violence also has significant consequences for athletes and presents challenges for those who wish to control it. As we discuss these topics, it is useful to consider the different types of violence that occur in sports.

Types of Violence

The most frequently used typology of on-the-field violence among players was developed by the late Mike Smith, a Canadian sociologist (1983; see Young, 2012). Smith identified four categories of violence in sports:

1. *Brutal body contact.* This includes actions common in certain sports and accepted by athletes as part of sport participation. Examples are collisions, hits, tackles, blocks, body checks, and other forms of forceful physical contact that can produce injuries. Most people in society define this forceful physical contact as extreme, although they don't classify it as illegal or criminal. Coaches often encourage this form of violence. As one coach explained: "We expect it, we demand it. . . . Our brand is a physical brand of football . . . you know, pound on these people until they give up" (Frontline, 2011).
2. *Borderline violence.* This includes actions that violate the rules of the game but are accepted by most players and coaches as consistent with

> **Serious sport has nothing to do with fair play. It is bound up with hatred, jealousy, boastfulness, disregard of all rules and sadistic pleasure in witnessing violence: in other words it is war minus the shooting.** —George Orwell, 1945

the norms of the sport ethic and as useful competitive strategies. Examples are the "brush back" pitch in baseball, the forcefully placed elbow or knee in soccer and basketball, the strategic bump used by distance runners to put another runner off stride, the fistfight in ice hockey, and the forearm to the ribs of a quarterback in football. Although these actions are expected, they may provoke retaliation by other players. Official sanctions and fines are not usually severe for borderline violence. However, public pressure to increase the severity of sanctions has grown in recent years, and the severity of punishments has increased in some sports.

3. *Quasi-criminal violence.* This includes actions that violate the formal rules of the game, public laws, and even informal norms among players. Examples are cheap shots, late hits, sucker punches, and flagrant fouls that endanger players' bodies and reject the norm calling for dedication to the game above all else. Fines and suspensions are usually imposed on players who engage in such violence. Most athletes condemn quasi-criminal violence and see it as a rejection of the informal norms of the game and what it means to be an athlete.
4. *Criminal violence.* This includes actions that are clearly outside the law to the point that athletes condemn them and law enforcement officials prosecute them as crimes. Examples are assaults that occur after a game and assaults during a game that appear to be premeditated and severe enough to kill or seriously maim a player. Such violence is relatively rare, and there appears to be growing support for filing criminal charges when it occurs.

Sociologist Kevin Young (2012) has noted that this classification of sport violence is useful but that the lines separating the four types of violence shift over time as norms change in sports and societies.

Furthermore, the classifications fail to address the origins of violence and the relationship of violent acts to the sport ethic, gender ideology, and the commercialization of sports. Despite these weaknesses, these four categories help us understand enables us to the distinctions that people make between various types of violence in sports.

Violence and Overconformity to the Norms of the Sport Ethic

In Pat Conroy's novel *The Prince of Tides* (1986), there is a classic scene in which the coach addresses his team and describes the ideal football player. He uses words that many athletes in heavy-contact sports hear during their careers:

> Now a real hitter is a head-hunter who puts his head in the chest of his opponents and ain't happy if his opponent is still breathing after the play. A real hitter doesn't know what fear is except when he sees it in the eyes of a ball carrier he's about to split in half. A real hitter loves pain, loves the screaming and the sweating and the brawling and the hatred of life down in the trenches. He likes to be at the spot where the blood flows and the teeth get kicked out. That's what this sport's about, men. It's war, pure and simple. (p. 384)

Many coaches don't use such vivid vocabulary because they know it can inspire dangerous forms of violence. However, when athletes think this way, violence occurs regularly enough to become viewed as a problem in certain sports. Journalists describe it, sociologists and psychologists try to explain it, and athletes brag or complain about it. When an athlete dies or is paralyzed by on-the-field violence, the media present stories about violence being rampant knowing that it will increase their ratings.

Although players may be concerned about brutal body contact and borderline violence in their sports, they generally accept it. Even when players don't like it, they may use violence to enhance their status on teams and their popularity among spectators. Athletes who engage in quasi- and criminal violence often are marginalized in sports and may

face criminal charges, although prosecuting such charges has been difficult and convictions have been very rare (Young, 2012).

Violence involving overconformity to the norms of the sport ethic is partly related to the identity insecurities of athletes in high-performance sports. Athletes learn that "you're only as good as your last game," and they know that their identities and status as team members must be regularly reaffirmed through their actions on the field. Therefore, they often take extreme measures to prove themselves, even if it involves violence. Violence reinforces feelings of self-worth by eliciting acceptance from other athletes. Willingly facing violence and

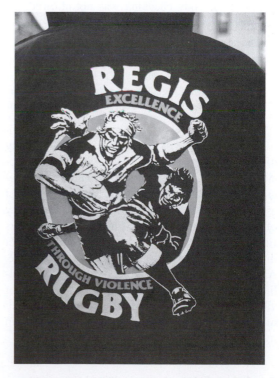

Violence is often connected with overconformity to the norms of the sport ethic. This high school rugby jacket presents violence as part of team culture. By associating violence with excellence, players learn what is expected on the field, even if they do not feel comfortable with brutal body contact and borderline violence. (*Source:* © Jay Coakley)

playing in pain honors the importance of the game and expresses dedication to teammates and the culture of high-performance sport.

It is important to understand that violent expressions of deviant overconformity are not limited to men, even though they are more common among male than female athletes. Women also overconform to the norms of the sport ethic, and when they play contact sports, they face the challenge of drawing the line between assertive physicality and violence. For example, when sociologist Nancy Theberge (1999) spent a full season studying the sport experiences of women on an elite ice hockey team in Canada, she discovered that the women were drawn to the physicality of hockey, even though body checking was not allowed. As one woman said,

> I like a physical game. You get more fired up. I think when you get hit . . . like when you're fighting for a puck in the corner, when you're both fighting so you're both working hard and maybe the elbows are flying, that just makes you put more effort into it (in Theberge, 1999, p. 147).

The experience of dealing with the physicality of contact sports and facing its consequences creates drama, excitement, strong emotions, and special interpersonal bonds among female athletes just as it does among males. Despite the risk and reality of pain and injuries, many women in contact sports find that the physical intensity and body contact in their sports make them feel alive and aware. Although many women are committed to controlling brutal body contact and more severe forms of violence, the love of their sport and the excitement of physicality can lead to violence grounded in overconformity to the norms of the sport ethic.

Commercialization and Violence in Sports

Some athletes in power and performance sports are paid well for their willingness and ability to do violence on the field. However, it would be inaccurate to identify money as the sole cause of violence in sports. Violent athletes in the past were paid very little, and athletes in high schools, colleges, and sport clubs today are paid nothing, yet many of them do violence despite the pain and injuries associated with it (Van Valkenburg, 2012a).

Commercialization has expanded opportunities to play certain contact sports in which violence occurs, and media coverage makes these sports and the violence they contain more visible than ever before. Children watch this coverage and may imitate violent athletes when they play sports, but this does not justify the conclusion that commercialization is the cause of violence on the playing field.

Football players and athletes in other collision and contact sports engaged in violence on the field long before television coverage and the promise of big salaries. Players at all levels of organized football killed and maimed each other at rates that were far higher than the death and injury rates in football today. There are more injuries in football today because there are more players and we are better at diagnosing injuries that would have been officially overlooked in the past. Violence in certain sports is a serious problem that must be addressed, but to say it is caused mainly by commercialization and money is a mistake.

This is an important point because many people who criticize sports claim that if athletes were true amateurs and played for love of the game instead of money, there would be less violence. But this conclusion contradicts research findings, and it distracts attention from the deep cultural and ideological roots of violence in particular sports and societies (Polychroniou, 2013). We could take money away from athletes tomorrow, but violence would be reduced only if there were changes in the culture in which athletes, especially male athletes, learn to value and do violence in sports.

Many people resist the notion that cultural changes are needed to control violence because it places the responsibility for change on all of us. It is easy to blame violence on wealthy and greedy team owners, athletes without moral character, and TV executives seeking higher viewer ratings, but it is more difficult to critically examine our culture and the normative and social organization of the sports that many people watch and enjoy. Similarly, it is difficult for people to critically examine the definitions of *masculinity* and the structure of gender relations that they have long accepted as part of the "natural" order of things, but such critiques are needed if we wish to understand and control violence in sports.

The point in this section is that commercialization has never been the *primary* cause of violence in sports. If violent sports are commercially successful in a community or society, it's because people want to play and watch them. For example, mixed martial arts (MMA) as represented by the UFC— Ultimate Fighting Championship—has become the most rapidly growing media spectator sport in the United States because enough people are willing to participate in it and pay to watch it. UFC event tickets sell out, largely to an under-forty male crowd, at an average of $245 per seat, and they also generate an average of $25 million for pay-per-view subscriptions to events. For some young men, MMA represents the same things that "boxing once did for their fathers and grandfathers: the ultimate measure of manhood, endurance and guts" (Quenqua, 2012). A father in New York explains that his ten-year-old son is an avid fan of UFC because the fighters "are the new superheroes for kids. It's just given them a whole new set of idols" (Quenqua, 2012). According to Joe Rogan, an MMA commentator, the UFC has become popular because people "enjoy violence, especially when it's in a controlled environment" (Bearak, 2011).

Similarly, violent images and words are often used to promote sport events because many marketing people believe that spectators are drawn to events involving violence—or at least the anticipation of it. This also is why some athletes create personas around narratives stressing their willingness to engage in brutal body contact and borderline violence. They want to attract fans who look up to athletes willing to put their bodies on the line for the sake of winning bouts, matches, or games.

Finally, for many athletes in heavy-contact sports, their participation involves a complex and intense mixture of passion, pleasure, violence, anxiety, fear, and pain that creates unique experiences for them. This intoxicating mixture of contradictory elements is linked to the desire to dominate and control others and disrupt an opponent's desire to do the same (Pringle, 2009). Additionally, this process of doing and enduring violence for the sake of the game creates special bonds of mutual respect between athletes. These bonds anchor and reaffirm their identities and infuse special meaning into their lives. The dynamics through which this occurs are difficult for athletes to explain and certainly difficult for "outsiders" to understand. For this reason, many serious participants in sports that are inherently violent say little about what they feel and why they enjoy what they do. They don't expect others to understand, because those of us outside this unique social world live mundane lives that don't involve the rush of pushing the envelope and living on the edge with peers who are the best at what they do. To say that commercialization motivates the actions of players is less accurate than to say that commercialization enables people—mostly men— to play sports in which these experiences are available. Of course, being paid to play a violent sport is not irrelevant, but money is seldom the primary factor that drives the participation of these athletes. For many of them, it is the anticipation of violence that gives their lives meaning.

Gender Ideology and Violence in Sports

Violence in sports is not limited to men. However, research indicates that if we want to understand violence in sports, we must understand gender ideology and issues of masculinity in culture. Sociologist Mike Messner explains:

> Young males come to sport with identities that lead them to define their athletic experience differently than females do. Despite the fact that few males truly enjoy hitting and being hit, and that one has to be socialized into participating in much of the violence commonplace in sport, males often view aggression, within the rule-bound structure of sport, as legitimate and "natural." (1992, p. 67)

In many societies, participation in power and performance sports has become an important way to prove masculinity. Boys discover that if they play these sports and others see them as being able to do violence, they can avoid social labels such as *pussy, girl, fag, wimp,* and *sissy* (Ingham and Dewar, 1999). This learning begins in youth sports, and by the time young men have become immersed in the social world of most power and performance sports, they accept brutal body contact and borderline violence as part of the game as it is played by "real" men. Some even learn to define such forms of violence as exciting because it earns them respect and serves as a basis for creating an identity that makes them unique among their peers.

When women do violence in sports, it may be also seen as a sign of commitment or skill, but it is not seen as proof of femininity (Knapp, 2014; McCree, 2011; Young, 2012). Dominant gender ideology in many cultures links manhood with the ability to do violence, but there is no similar link between womanhood and violence. Therefore, female athletes who engage in violence do not receive the same support and rewards that men receive—unless they wrestle in the WWE, fight in mixed martial arts, or skate on a roller derby team where the sport personas of female athletes are constructed, in part, to shock or titillate spectators (Berra, 2005; Blumenthal, 2004). Boxing and mixed martial arts have recently provided a few female athletes with contexts in which they are rewarded for doing violence, but most women fighters do not feel that doing violence in their sport makes them more of a woman than females who are not fighters.

Despite the recent publicity given to a few women fighters, violent sports are viewed by many people as support for their belief that hierarchical distinctions between men and women are grounded in nature and cannot be altered (Fogel, 2011).

Power and performance sports emphasize sex *difference* in terms of physical strength, *control* through domination, and *status* as a reward for physical conquests. The gender ideology formed around these ideas and beliefs has been central in U.S. culture. The stakes associated with preserving this ideology are so high that male boxers are paid millions of dollars for three to thirty-six minutes of brutalizing one another in the ring. Heavyweight boxers are among the highest-paid athletes in the world because they promote the idea two men facing each other in a violent confrontation is "nature in action," even though the combatants often lose millions of brain cells as they "prove" male superiority.

The irony in this approach is that, if a gender hierarchy were truly fixed in nature, there would be no need for sports to reaffirm "natural" differences between men and women. Gender would simply exist without spending so much time and effort teaching girls and boys how they should perform it. Power and performance sports are used as valuable aids in this teaching and learning process, and the men who play them serve as models of manhood in many countries.

When women participate in violent sports they disrupt the "logic" used to reaffirm traditional beliefs about gender. This causes some people to argue that women should not participate in these sports, and to treat them as jokes, oddities, or freaks of nature when they do.

The participation of women in violent sports often creates a dilemma for people who advocate progressive changes in traditional gender ideology. Although participation contradicts the ideological belief that women are frail and vulnerable, it also reaffirms beliefs that have traditionally disadvantaged women through history. For this reason, some people who support gender equity in sports do not encourage girls and women to participate in violent sports.

The Institutionalization of Violence in Sports

Certain forms of violence are built into the culture and structure of particular sports. Athletes in these sports learn to use violence as a strategy, even though it may cause them pain and injury. Controlling institutionalized violence is difficult because

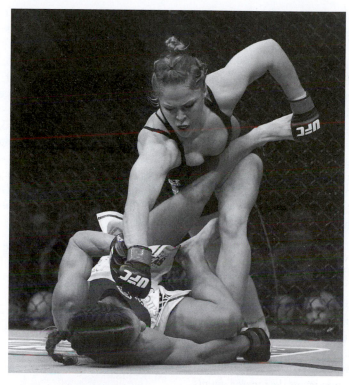

Ronda Rousey punches her opponent in a highly publicized
UFC Championship bout. There is nothing in the genetic make-up
of women that precludes participation in sport violence.
However, women do not use their ability to do violence as a
reaffirmation of their femininity or womanhood.
(*Source:* © AP Photo/Jae C. Hong)

it requires changing the culture and structure of
particular sports—something that most people in
governing bodies are hesitant to do.

Learning to Use Violence as a Strategy in Men's Contact Sports

Athletes in heavy-contact sports
often learn to use intimidation, aggression, and violence as strategies to achieve competitive success
(Shields and Bredemeier, 1995; White and Young,
1997; Young, 2012). These athletes routinely dis-
approve of quasi-criminal and criminal violence,
but they accept brutal body contact and borderline
violence as long as it occurs within the rules of the
game. They may not intend to hurt anyone, but this
does not prevent them putting their bodies and the
bodies of opponents in harm's way.

In boxing, football, ice hockey, rugby, and other
heavy-contact sports, athletes also use intimidation and their willingness to engage in violence to
promote their careers, increase drama for spectators, and enhance publicity for themselves along
with their sports and sponsors. They realize that
doing violence is expected, even if it causes harm
to themselves and others. A classic example of
using violence as a strategy came to light in 2012
when the NFL issued a report summarizing its
investigation of New Orleans Saints coaches and
players who used "bounties"—secret financial

bonuses—to encourage defensive players to injure opposing players seriously enough to take them out of the game (see http://www.nola.com/saints /index.ssf/2012/03/full_nfl_statement_into_bounty .html; ESPN, 2012; Hruby, 2012b; King, 2012). A key statement found in over 20,000 pieces of evidence was a recording in which a Saints defensive coach was heard to say to his players: "We've got to do everything in the world to make sure we kill [49er running back] Frank Gore's head." In the same recording he also said, "Every single one of you, before you get off the pile, affect the head [of quarterback Alex Smith of the San Francisco 49ers]. Early, affect the head . . . touch and hit the head" (Zirin, 2012b).

Players and coaches on the Saints were severely sanctioned by the NFL, partly because the NFL was trying to avoid legal liability by pushing blame for violence on the field to individual players and coaches rather than admitting that the game contains incentives to be violent (Hruby, 2012c).

Violence is also incorporated into game strategies when coaches use players as designated agents

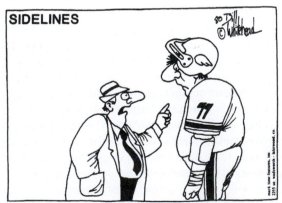

(*Source:* By permission of William Whitehead)

"When are you gonna learn when it's necessary to use unnecessary roughness?"

Physical intimidation and violence are used as strategies in men's contact sports. They have been effective in winning games and building the reputations of players and teams.

of intimidation and violence for their teams. These players are called "enforcers," "goons," and "hit men," and they are expected to protect teammates and strategically assist their teams by intimidating, provoking, fighting with, or injuring opponents. Their violent acts are an accepted part of certain sports, especially ice hockey.

Players who act as enforcers are paid primarily for their ability and willingness to do violence. Every time they maim or come close to killing someone on the ice, court, or playing field, people discuss how to control it. But once violence is built into the culture, structures, and strategies of a sport, controlling it is difficult.

Learning to Use Violence as a Strategy in Women's Contact Sports Information on violence among girls and women in contact sports remains scarce even though more women are participating in them (Knapp, 2014; Young 2012). Participation in collision and heavy-contact sports creates the possibility for violence among female athletes, but few studies explore if and why it occurs.

Women's sports increasingly emphasize power and performance, and they have higher stakes associated with success. As women become increasingly immersed in the social world of elite power and performance sports, they become more tolerant of rule violations and aggressive actions on the playing field, but this pattern is less clear among women than it is among men (Knapp, 2014; Young, 2007a, 2012).

As women compete at higher levels, they often become similar to men in how they embrace the sport ethic and use it to frame their identities as athletes. Like men, they are willing to dedicate themselves to the game, take risks, make sacrifices, pay the price, continue playing despite pain and injury, and overcome barriers in pursuit of their dreams. However, it is rare for them to link toughness, physicality, and aggression to what it means to be a woman in society. Similarly, coaches don't try to motivate female athletes by urging them to "go out and prove who the better woman is" on the field, even though they might urge women to play assertively. Therefore, at this time, women's contact sports are less violent than men's contact sports.

Consequences of Violence on the Field

Spectators often think about sports in a paradoxical way: They accept violence, but the injuries caused by that violence make them uneasy. They seem to want violence without consequences—like the fictionalized violence they see in the media and video games in which characters engage in brutality without being seriously or permanently injured. However, sports violence is real, and it causes real pain, injury, disability, and death, even though it is often hidden from spectators (Bruni, 2012; Layden, 2010b; Le Batard, 2013; McCree, 2011; Muller and Cantu, 2010; Omalu, 2008; Rhoden, 2012a; Shurley and Todd, 2012; Wiedeman, 2013; Young, 2012).

Ron Rice, an NFL player whose career ended when he tackled an opponent, has discussed the real consequences of violence. The brutal body contact of the tackle left him temporarily paralyzed and permanently disabled. He remembers that "before I hit the ground, I knew my career was over. . . . My body froze. I was like a tree that had been cut down, teetering, then crashing, unable to break my fall." Reminiscing about his life as a football player, Rice says that he was "programmed from a very young age to live and think a certain way," to be a warrior who keeps going no matter what (Rice, 2005). He did just that, and today he lives with chronic pain in his neck, wrists, hands, ankles, knees, and back—the toll of doing violence to others and enduring it in return. Rice explained that, "I'm 32 now, . . . These injuries are a part of my life. And I got off easy compared to a lot of these guys" (Rice 2005, p. 83).

Brantt Myhres, a former NHL player, now lives in chronic pain due to the collisions and fights he experienced during his ten-year career. At thirty-seven years old he described his condition in this way:

My back wakes me up. I get on the floor every morning. My left hand has been smashed and broken so many times I'm missing a knuckle. From the concussions, my memory—I have a lapse with my memory at times. It's just little things, and important things. (Branch, 2011b)

Research on pain and injury among athletes helps us understand that violence in sports has real consequences (Young, 2012). Rates of disabling injuries vary by sport, but they are high enough in many sports to constitute a serious health issue. The "normal" brutal body contact and borderline violence in contact and collision sports regularly cause arthritis, concussions, brain trauma, bone fractures, torn ligaments, and other injuries. In other words, the violence inherent in these sports takes a definite toll on the health and well-being of athletes.

Recent discussions of the consequences of violence on the field have focused primarily on football, although there also are concerns about ice hockey, soccer, lacrosse, boxing, and mixed martial arts. Most discussions have been in response to research showing that there is a relationship between head trauma—including concussions and repetitive sub-concussive hits to the head—and the development of chronic traumatic encephalopathy (CTE) and other forms of brain damage (Fainaru-Wade and Fainaru, 2013; Laskas, 2015). CTE is a neurodegenerative disease with symptoms similar to early-onset dementia. These include many types of cognitive impairment related to memory, reasoning, language and communication, problem solving, emotional control, and the ability to focus and pay attention. Evidence of CTE has been found in football players from high school through retired professional players as well as boxers, hockey players, and professional soccer players. Current studies are investigating the incidence and consequences of concussions in youth sports and football at all levels of participation (Belson, 2014; Davenport, 2014; Jordan, 2013; Kerr et al., 2015; Seichepine et al., 2013; Simpson, 2013).

Although the brain is complex and there is much more to learn about head trauma and brain injury in sports, it is clear that the head hits that occur regularly in football can cause brain damage.

This scientific fact has the potential to dramatically alter the sports landscape in the United States. Consequently, researchers are now investigating techniques for identifying brain damage among current athletes, the conditions under which damage is most likely to occur, who is the most susceptible to damage, the ways that damage can be minimized in various sports, and the best treatments for damage that has already occurred.

In the meantime, about 5000 former NFL players and family members sued the NFL in 2012 for failing to inform them of what the league knew about concussions and their impact on players' health (Fainaru-Wada and Fainaru, 2013; Frontline, 2013; Kenny, 2012). The NFL settled out of court with the plaintiffs in late-2013, agreeing to pay $765 million, which included $75 million for baseline medical exams, $10 million for research, and $675 million for compensation to players and their families. The NFL also paid nearly $200,000 for the plaintiffs legal fees. In the agreement, the NFL admitted to no liability for players' problems and the league was allowed to keep secret all its research evidence on concussions. However, the agreement does not stop any of the more than 13,000 other living former players from going forward with individual concussion-relation workers compensation claims in states where such claims can be made.

The NCAA is also being sued by former college players claiming that (a) it has a long established pattern of negligence and inaction related to protecting players from head trauma, (b) it failed to teach proper tackling techniques to avoid head trauma, (c) it failed to implement system-wide procedures for dealing with concussions on the field, and (d) it failed to educate "student-athletes" about head trauma and concussion issues. If the suits filed by former players are combined into a single class, the NCAA will find itself in a legal position similar to what faced the NFL. But the legal issues are more complex in the suits against the NCAA, so it is difficult to predict a likely outcome (Axon, 2013a, 2013b; Harris, 2013).

Most important for the future of football is the fact that parents are increasingly concerned about the safety of the sport for their young children. These concerns are associated with a significant recent decline in football participation among children (Project Play, 2015).

At the same time, school districts, college football conferences and athletic departments, and other sport organizations that sponsor football teams and programs are carefully watching these and other legal cases. The people who run these organizations understand that they may be legally liable for major financial damages if they do not responsibly use current scientific evidence to create policies and procedures that inform and protect young people from sustaining life-changing injuries. This is especially relevant for high schools and youth leagues because their athletes are under the legal age of consent and should not be put in harm's way by those responsible for their safety and well-being.

Growing awareness of research findings that identify the consequences of violence in sports has led the U.S. Congress, about half of all state legislatures, and many sport organizations to develop regulations and protocols to protect young people who play sports—especially those in which there is a possibility for sustaining concussions and regular head trauma. These consist of rules about reporting concussions, dealing with them during events, and treating athletes who have experienced concussions.

These rules and guidelines are certainly needed, but they are useful only to the extent that concussions are either reported by players or diagnosed by qualified medical personnel. However, many athletes, especially males in power-and-performance sports, continue to take pride in not disclosing such injuries or they fear that if they do report them they won't be allowed to play a sport that is important to them and a source of their livelihood (Sifferlin, 2013).

At present it is difficult to accurately identify concussions on the sidelines, and youth, high school, and many college teams don't have the resources to hire neurologists with the training to do so. Sideline concussion tests are useful, although their reliability depends on the qualifications of those administering them and the cooperation of the athletes taking them.

Additional research is under way to improve helmets used in certain sports and to develop other protective technologies. But the brain is difficult to protect whenever there is a forceful impact to or a violent twisting or snapping of the head. The brain is surrounded by fluid that prevents it from routinely coming into contact with the inside of the skull. Existing protective equipment may minimize damage to the skull in the case of a violent impact, but it cannot prevent the brain from slamming into the skull, with cells being damaged in the process. This is why some people argue that the brain cannot be protected and that new technologies give athletes the false impression that they can sustain violent impact to their heads without suffering negative health consequences. Some experts have even said that football should eliminate helmets so that players will take their heads more seriously and protect their brains—a suggestion that has not been tested.

Controlling On-the-Field Violence

The roots of violence on the playing field are deep. They're grounded in overconformity to the sport ethic, commercialization, definitions of masculinity, and competitive strategies.

Brutal body contact is the most difficult type of violence to control. It is grounded in the culture of power and performance sports and its incorporation of dominant gender ideology. Unfortunately, about 90 percent of the serious injuries in these sports occur *within the rules* of the games and contests. This means that many men inevitably pay the price for their destructive definitions of *sports* and *masculinity.*

Efforts to control brutal body contact require changes in gender ideology and the cultures of certain sports. These changes won't occur without persistent and thoughtful strategies to document the dangers of the actions and the language that people use to reproduce violent sport cultures and the gender ideology that supports them. People should

also calculate the cost of injuries due to brutal body contact and other types of violence in terms of medical expenses, lost work time and wages, school days missed, disability payments, family problems, and even reductions in life expectancy. Looking at these statistics will help us understand more fully the connections between sport participation and health.

The recent publicity about concussions and other serious physical and health problems experienced by athletes who play violent sports has initiated a number of moves to control violence on the field and its consequences. Representatives of football, hockey, boxing, and other sports now stress rule changes and tactics to promote safety rather than violence. Media commentators, players, and sport administrators think twice before using words and images that glorify violence on the field. They understand that the commercial success of particular sports is endangered if parents don't encourage children to play them or if young people decide that playing them is not worth the risk of serious injuries (Lavign, 2012; Pennington, 2013; Rhoden, 2012b).

The need to control violence in sports was made clear when U.S. President Barack Obama said, "If I had a son, I'd have to think long and hard before I let him play football." He then added, "Those of us who love the sport are going to have to wrestle with the fact that it will probably change gradually to try to reduce some of the violence" (Foer and Hughes, 2013).

Obama's words, along with previous statements by current and former professional athletes and media coverage of research on sport injuries, especially those affecting the brain, have led people in sport organizations to consider rule changes and new marketing narratives emphasizing safety and concern for the health and well-being of players rather than narratives emphasizing violent action. For example, the NFL has recently spent millions of dollars on commercial messages about their attempts to make football safer for players at all levels of competition (Battista, 2012; see also, http://www.nflevolution.com/). However, as with other sport organizations, it is difficult to determine whether these messages represent effective changes in their sports or if they are mostly public relations hype (Hruby, 2013b).

Rule changes can be helpful, but there is no way to reduce the violence in certain sports without making major structural changes in how the sports are played. For example, a sport like ice hockey can reduce hits to the head with rule changes, and youth programs can eliminate body checking altogether, if they are willing to. But football presents a different set of challenges. Players cannot avoid forceful head impacts as the game is now played. Head impacts will occur regardless of advice on how to tackle or how to strengthen the neck to serve as a shock absorber. After talking with NFL players about the conditions under which violent collisions occur on the field, William Rhoden (2012a), a respected journalist, concluded: "Remove the gore and you kill the game immediately; keep the gore and the game will die a slow death."

Furthermore, people associated with football realize that the vitality and commercial success of their sport depends on recruiting boys and young men onto school and youth teams. If parents don't think the game is safe, they will encourage their children to engage in alternative sports. As with any sport, an inability to attract young people leads to a smaller pool of talent, which usually reduces spectator interest and the vitality of the sport as a part of popular culture.

Spectators have often used violence on the field as an indicator of player commitment and dedication—a sign of their willingness to put their bodies on the line for the sake of team pride and victory. For this reason, brutal body contact and borderline violence have been used by players and perceived by spectators as necessary for achieving victories and championships. How will they react if new rules reduce the amount of violence?

As we learn more about the damage done to the bodies and lives of athletes who engage in violence on the field, more people will raise moral questions

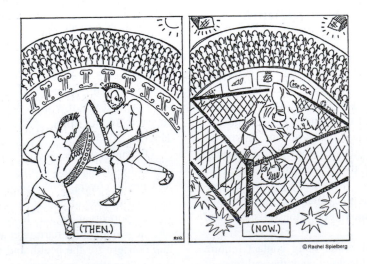

Ultimate Fighting—also known as Mixed Martial Arts, Cage Fighting, and Tough Man Contests—is one of the fastest-growing spectator sports in the world. Is watching men and women being pummeled into submission an appropriate form of entertainment? When does violent entertainment cross the line and raise moral questions? (*Source:* By permission of Rachel Spielberg)

about being entertained by actions that maim, cause lifelong chronic pain, and permanently disable the entertainers. But will people refuse to pay for tickets and media access to the point that football and other violent sports become cultural sideshows rather than part of mainstream U.S. culture? At this point we don't know the answer to this question, but people are asking it more frequently (Krattenmaker, 2013).

VIOLENCE OFF THE FIELD

When athletes in contact sports are arrested for violent crimes, people wonder if their violence off the field is related to the violent strategies they've learned on the field.

An NFL player raised this issue with the following comment:

> When you think about it, it is a strange thing that we do. During a game we want to kill each other. Then we're told to shake hands and drive home safely. Then a week later we try to kill each other again (in Freeman, 1998, p. 1).

It is difficult to do good research on this topic. When people refer to statistical correlations that show a relationship between playing certain sports and high rates of off-the-field violence, it does not prove that playing violent sports causes people to be violent outside of sports. Two other issues must be considered before this conclusion can be made.

First, violent sports may attract people who already feel comfortable about doing violence on and off the field, regardless of what they may learn in their sport. *Second,* off-the-field violence among athletes may be due to unique situations encountered more often by athletes than other people. Athletes known for their toughness on the field may be encouraged, dared, or taunted by others to be tough on the streets. In some cases, they may be challenged to fight because of their reputations in sports. If trouble occurs and athletes are arrested for fighting in these circumstances, it is misleading to say that their actions were caused by what they learned in sports.

Control versus Carryover

Does playing sports teach people to control violent responses in the face of adversity, stress, defeat, hardship, and pain? Or does it create identities, personal orientations, and social dynamics that make off-the-field violence more likely?

French sociologist Loïc Wacquant studied these issues for three years as he trained and gained the trust of the men who worked out at a traditional, highly structured, and reputable boxing gym in a Chicago neighborhood. During that time, he observed, interviewed, and documented the experiences and lives of more than fifty professional boxers. He not only learned the craft of boxing but also became immersed in the social world in which the boxers trained. He found that the social world encompassed by this gym was one in which the boxers learned to value their craft and dedicate themselves to the idea of being a professional boxer; they also learned to respect fellow boxers and accept the rules of sportsmanship that governed boxing as a profession. In a low-income neighborhood where poverty and hopelessness promoted intimidation and violence, these boxers accepted norms that disapproved of fighting outside the ring, they avoided street fights, and they internalized the controls necessary to follow a highly disciplined daily training schedule.

Of course, success in using combat sports of any kind to reduce violence away from the sport depends greatly on the conditions under which sport participation occurs. *If* the social world formed around a sport promotes a mind-set and norms emphasizing non-violence, self-control, respect for self and others, physical fitness, patience, responsibility, and humility (the opposite of hubris), then athletes *may* learn to control violent behavior off the field (Trulson, 1986). Those most likely to learn this seem to be young men who lack structured challenges and firm guidance as they navigate their way through lives in which there are many incentives to engage in violence.

However, heavy contact sports often emphasize hostility, physical domination, and a willingness to use one's body as a weapon. This is consistent with research showing that sport participation, especially for young men in contact sports, is associated with fighting off the field (Kreager, 2007; Wright and Fitzpatrick, 2006). Sociologist Derek Kreager analyzed data from a national sample of 6397 seventh- to twelfth-graders and found that football players and wrestlers were over 40 percent more likely to be involved in fights than male peers who didn't play high school sports. Playing basketball and baseball were unrelated to fighting, and male tennis players had a 35 percent *lower* risk of fighting than male peers who didn't play sports. The likelihood of fighting also increased with the proportion of football players in a young man's friendship network.

In another national study, Wright and Fitzpatrick (2006) found that certain high school sports were associated with status dynamics that created or intensified ingroup versus outgroup differences among young people. Such differences may also account for more fighting.

More research is needed to understand the team cultures created in connection with particular sports, the meanings that athletes attach to their actions, and the place of violence in sport cultures more generally. Sport participation does not automatically teach people to control violence, nor does the violence used in certain sports inevitably carry over to other relationships and settings.

Assaults and Sexual Assaults by Male Athletes

Highly publicized cases in which male athletes are accused or convicted of assault, sexual assault, rape, gang rape, and even murder create the impression that on-the-field violence influences off-the-field actions and relationships, especially relationships with women. Athletes are public figures and may be celebrities, so when they are accused and arrested, we hear and read about it multiple times. This repetition also creates the impression that male athletes are more violent and misogynist than other men.

Violent crimes are committed by male athletes far too often. Furthermore, the victims of these crimes are almost always subject to character assassination and harassment (Macur, 2013). Therefore, there is a need for sport teams and organizations to directly and assertively address this issue. But there's also a need to understand the role of sport participation in violent off-the-field actions and crimes. Without this understanding, the efforts of teams and organizations may not be effective.

Sport sociologist Todd Crosset (1999) has carefully reviewed published research on sexual assaults by male athletes to determine if they are disproportionately involved in violence against women. His findings indicated that male intercollegiate athletes were involved in more sexual assaults than other male students, but the differences were not statistically significant. In his conclusion, Crosset explained that the evidence did not warrant a conclusion that playing sports caused men to engage in violence against women. He also noted that focusing only on athletes when doing research on sexual assault could distract attention from three important points:

1. Violence against women occurs regularly in society and is not simply a "sport problem."
2. Some male athletes have perpetrated sexual assault and rape, but nearly all violence against women is perpetrated by heterosexual men who are *not* currently playing competitive sports.
3. The problem of violence against women must be understood in the context of gender relations in the larger culture if strategies to lower the rates of sexual assault and rape are to succeed.

Combining Crosset's analysis with other research on violence in all-male groups, we can hypothesize that violence against women by male athletes is associated with a sport culture that creates or supports among athletes the beliefs that:

- Violence is an effective strategy for establishing manhood, achieving status as an athlete, and controlling women.
- Athletes should not be held to the same normative standards that apply to others in a community.

- People outside the fraternity of elite athletes do not deserve the respect that athletes reserve for each other.
- Women are celebrity-obsessed "groupies" who can be exploited without consequences.

Research on these factors will help us understand violence against women *in the full social and cultural contexts in which it occurs.*

The importance of being aware of the full context in which sexual assaults occur was seen in a Steubenville, Ohio, case in which two high-profile football team members were found guilty of raping an unconscious sixteen-year-old female student, whom they repeatedly and brutally dehumanized at parties with teammates in attendance. A video of young men at one of the parties contained such shocking and misogynist statements that it attracted nationwide attention and news coverage (Abad-Santos, 2013; Macur and Schweber, 2013; Murphy, 2013).

Although some people said that the culture of football was to blame, a closer look at the situation indicates that many factors were involved, including the place and meaning of high school football in Steubenville; the culture of the town itself; the prevailing local attitudes and beliefs about gender and women who are sexually assaulted; the characteristics and actions of the football coach and other school officials; the social organization of the high school; the separation between the football team and the rest of the community; the hubris, sense of privilege, and powerful group dynamics associated with the bonds between the football players; the use of alcohol by adolescents and a failure of young people at the parties to take responsibility for the safety of the young woman who had too much to drink; and the irresponsible choices of the two young men charged and found guilty in the case.

Future research may clarify the influence of these and other factors, and help to explain why none of the young people witnessing the assault was willing to step in and why men in certain all-male groups appear to lose concern and respect for women to the point of raping them and making fun of the rape.

Finally, the focus on athletes should not distract attention from other sport-related assault issues. For example, sexual assaults, including statutory rape, by coaches have a greater impact in sports and on people's lives than sexual assaults by athletes (Brackenridge et al., 2008; Fasting et al., 2008; Fasting et al., 2004). Research done by journalists at the *Seattle Times* (2003) found that 159 coaches in the state of Washington (where only 2 percent of the U.S. population lives) were fired or reprimanded for sexual offenses between 1993 and 2003. Offenses ranged from harassment to rape, nearly all involved heterosexual male coaches victimizing girls, and about 60 percent of these coaches continued to coach or teach after the misconduct was known. Even though 159 coaches were fired or reprimanded, most reports of misconduct were neither investigated by school authorities nor reported to the police. Even when misconduct was admitted, the incidents were kept secret if the coaches agreed to leave their jobs. Sexual offenses in private sport clubs were especially problematic because clubs seldom regulate coaches' conduct, and most parents trust coaches even when evidence arouses suspicions of misconduct (Willmsen and O'Hagan, 2003).

Crimes of sexual assault go far beyond the realm of sport, but when they are committed by athletes or coaches, they may be reported less often than in other cases, victims may be intimidated by fans and representatives of teams and sport organizations, prosecutors may not file charges, "settlements" may be reached to avoid criminal prosecution, and verdicts may be debated after trials have been held. Even if future research indicates that neither athletes nor coaches have assault rates higher than others, there is a need to address the unique issues associated with sport cultures and the experiences of the victims in these cases.

VIOLENCE AMONG SPECTATORS

Do sports incite violence among spectators? Or do some people use sports as sites for expressing themselves in violent ways? These are important questions because sports capture widespread public attention and spectators number in the billions. To answer these questions we must distinguish between watching sports on television and attending events in person. Further, we must study spectators in context if we wish to understand the emotional dynamics of identifying with teams and athletes, the meanings that spectators give to particular sporting events, and the varying circumstances under which people watch sports (Paradiso, 2009; Young, 2012).

Violence Among Media Viewers

Most people watch sports on television in their homes. They may express emotions and become angry at certain points, but we don't know much about when and why people express anger through violence directed at friends and family members at home. Nor do we know much about violence among people who watch televised sports in public settings such as bars, pubs, and around large video screens in public areas.

Most people who watch media sports outside the home restrict their emotional expressions to verbal comments. When they express anger, they nearly always direct it at the players, coaches, referees, or media commentators rather than fellow viewers. Even when emotional outbursts are defined as too loud or inappropriate, fellow viewers usually try to control the offender informally and peacefully. When fans from opposing teams watch an event at the same location, there often are sources of mutual identification that defuse differences and discourage physical violence, although verbal comments may become heated.

The belief that watching sports is associated with violence has led some people to wonder if watching sports—the Super Bowl, for example—is associated with temporary spikes in the rates of domestic violence in a community or the nation as a whole. During the 1990s, a journalist misleadingly reported that women's shelters were filled on Super Bowl Sunday because of increased domestic violence on that day. Subsequent examination

of his sources and reliable research on this topic proved that he was wrong (Cohen 1994; Sachs and Chu, 2000). Of course, the anger caused by a televised sport event *could* be a factor in particular cases of domestic violence, but the roots of such violence run deep, and to blame it on watching sports overlooks more important factors (Card and Dahl, 2009; Leonard, 2013). Furthermore, we don't know enough about the ways that spectators integrate media sport content into their lives to say that watching sports does anything except provide emotionally focused social occasions.

Violence at Sport Venues

Historical Background Media reports of violent actions at sport events have increased our awareness of crowd violence. However, crowd violence is not new. Data documenting the actions of sport spectators through the ages are scarce, but research suggests that spectator violence occurred in the past and much of it would make crowd violence today seem rare and tame by comparison (Dunning, 1999; Guttmann, 1986, 1998; Scheinin, 1994; Young, 2000).

With the emergence of modern sports, violence among sport spectators decreased, but it remained common by today's standards. For example, a baseball game in 1900 was described by a journalist in this way:

> Thousands of gun slinging Chicago Cubs fans turned a Fourth of July doubleheader into a shoot-out at the OK Corral, endangering the lives of players and fellow spectators. Bullets sang, darted, and whizzed over players' heads as the rambunctious fans fired round after round whenever the Cubs scored against the gun-shy Philadelphia Phillies. The visiting team was so intimidated it lost both games . . . at Chicago's West Side Grounds (Nash and Zullo, 1989, p. 133).

This newspaper account also reports that when the Cubs scored six runs in the sixth inning of the first game, guns were fired around the stadium to the point that gun smoke made it difficult to see the field. When the Cubs tied the score in the ninth inning, fans again fired guns, and hundreds of them shot holes in the roof of the grandstand, causing splinters to fly onto their heads. As the game remained tied during three extra innings, fans pounded the seats with the butts of their guns and fired in unison every time the Phillies' pitcher began his windup to throw a pitch. It rattled him so much that the Cubs scored on a wild pitch. After the score, a vocal and heavily armed Cubs fan stood up and shouted, "Load! Load at will! Fire!" Fans around the stadium emptied the rest of their ammunition in a final explosive volley.

Between 1900 and the early 1940s, crowd violence was common: Bottles and other objects were thrown at players and umpires, and World Series games were disrupted by fans angered by umpires' calls or the actions of opposing players (Scheinin, 1994). Players feared being injured by spectators as much as they feared the "bean balls" thrown regularly at their heads by opposing pitchers.

During the 1950s and 1960s, high school basketball and football games in some U.S. cities were sites for local youth gang wars. Gang members and a few students used chains, switchblade knives, brass knuckles, and tire irons to attack each other. During the late 1960s and early 1970s, some high school games in Chicago were closed to the public and played early on Saturday mornings because the regularly scheduled games had become occasions for crowd violence, much of it related to racial and ethnic tensions in the city.

These examples are mentioned here to counter the argument that violence is a bigger problem today than in the past, that coercive tactics should be used to control unruly fans, and that there is a general decline of civility among fans and in society as a whole. Some spectators are obnoxious and violent today, and they present law enforcement challenges and interfere with the enjoyment of other fans, but there is no systematic evidence that this is a problem out of control.

Violence at Sports Venues as a Social and Cultural Issue Violence that occurs in stadiums and arenas takes many forms. Spectators may verbally or physically attack opposing fans or spectators who represent an adversary outside the stadium, such as a rival gang. There may be invasions of a playing field to express outrage about a referee's decision or a play that is seen as unfair. Bigoted or racist spectators may attack members of a group they define as an enemy. Organized collections of spectators may engage in violent displays to support or oppose decisions made by team administrators, political officials, or other individuals or organizations.

Although scholars in England studied and developed theories about violence at sport events during the 1970s and 1980s, few studies have been published after 1990, and almost no systematic research has been published in the United States apart from work done by sociologist Jerry Lewis (2007). The research done in England provides valuable historical data and thoughtful analyses of the complex social processes in which particular forms of sport violence are located (Armstrong, 1998, 2007; Dunning, 1999; Dunning et al., 1988; Dunning et al., 2002; Young, 2007a, 2007b, 2012). In fact, it has been used as a guide to develop more effective policing strategies in connection with sport crowds worldwide (Kossakowski, 2015; Spaaij, 2008).

For our purposes here, what we know is that sport events do not occur in social vacuums, and when tensions and conflicts are intense and widespread in a community or society, sport events may become sites for confrontations. For example, past spectator violence in the United States was grounded in racial tensions aggravated by highly publicized rivalries between high schools whose students come from different racial or ethnic backgrounds (Guttmann, 1986). In cities where housing segregation created heavily segregated schools, racial and ethnic conflicts contributed to confrontations before, during, and after games.

Research also indicates that nearly all crowd violence involves men. This suggests that ideas about manhood and the expression of masculinity influence crowd dynamics and the actions of spectators. Female fans may become involved in fights, but this is rare. Crowd violence, therefore, is as much a gender issue as it is a racial, ethnic, or social-class issue, and controlling it effectively over the long run requires changes in gender ideology and ideas about masculinity as much as buying expensive surveillance systems and hiring additional police to patrol the sidelines at every event.

Venue Violence in North America   Venue violence does occur in the United States and Canada, but not frequently enough or in patterns that constitute a significant threat to the safety and well-being of spectators. This is partly because North American sports events generally attract diversified crowds in which violent actions are voluntarily held in check most of the time for fear of injuring children or others defined as vulnerable. It also is due

to the tendency among North American fans to see sport events as a realm that is separate from social and political realities outside the stadium. Finally, it is difficult for organized groups of fans sharing strong social or political attitudes to obtain unified blocks of tickets at a major event so they can express feelings through violent displays, as happens with some regularity in certain parts of the world. For these reasons most spectators at North American sport venues limit their expressive actions to loud cheering, stomping feet to make noise, waving objects to show team loyalty, and verbally taunting referees, opposing players, and fans.

Of course, not all sport crowds in the North America are models of good behavior (Young, 2012). Fights do occur, fans say nasty and sometimes hateful things to each other and to referees

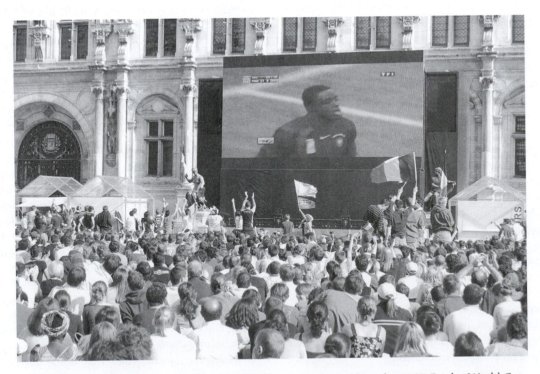

Thousands of diverse fans gathered around public video screens when the 2007 Rugby World Cup was hosted in Paris. These fans, mostly French, with large groups from England, Ireland, Australia, and New Zealand, were expressive, but violence was not observed by the author, who took this photo and talked with people in the crowd. (*Source:* © Jay Coakley)

and opposing players, and they sometimes throw objects onto the playing surface to express their dissatisfaction with the poor play of their team or perceived bad calls by referees and umpires. But most cases of violence inside stadiums and arenas involve individuals or small groups of fans; they are not planned, politically motivated, or executed by large, organized collections of spectators with agendas unrelated to the event. Additionally, such violence would be difficult to initiate, given that spectators are closely "policed" when entering venues, making it rare for them to possess objects that could be used to destroy property or harm others.

Venue Violence Worldwide As you know by now, making sense of what people think, do, and say requires that we understand the context in which people live and give meaning to the reality around them. Therefore, it is not surprising that people give different meanings to their identities as sport fans, the teams they support, and the purpose of attending games and matches. As a result, venue violence occurs in different forms and for different reasons from one country and cultural region to another (Armstrong and Testa, 2010; Braun and Vliegenthart, 2008; Miguel et al., 2008; Spaaij, 2006, 2007; Spaaij and Anderson, 2010). For example, in England during the 1970s and 1980s, young men who came from generations of loyal supporters of their local soccer clubs were alienated and angry when club administrators used new business models and made decisions that ignored the customs and preferences of fans. As they experienced high rates of unemployment and felt that the local and national governments were undermining their way of life, spectators used soccer matches as sites to express their feelings and confront opposing fans and the police in ways that they saw as reaffirming their identities as men. More recently, when so-called "hooligans" stand up against injustices and confront rival supporters, other spectators may understand their actions even though they morally object to their violence (Rookwood and Pearson, 2012).

In a similar manner, soccer venues in parts of Europe, North Africa, Western Asia, and Latin America have become staging areas for young men to collectively express themselves, sometimes in violent and defiant ways. Their violence may express their general sense of alienation, objection to the commercialization of soccer and soccer clubs, nationalist and/or racist attitudes, special political agendas, dissatisfaction with ruling politicians—including powerful dictators, and their disdain for police that use brutality on the streets and, in many cases, enforce the interests of oppressive political regimes. Sport venues—usually soccer stadiums—for these men are places where they have more freedom and opportunities to express themselves collectively than they do on the streets (Dorsey, 2012, 2013a, 2013b, 2013c, 2013d, 2016a; Zirin, 2011a, 2012a, 2013c). Additionally, the stadium, with the help of media coverage and the use of social media, enables them to be seen and heard so that the entire community or nation will know that they exist and are a force to be taken seriously.

It is difficult to make general descriptions or conclusions about venue violence worldwide. But web or YouTube searches for "football ultras," "ultras worldwide," "ultras-tifo," and "football pyro," will provide images of how fans express themselves around the world. In some cases you will see young men behaving badly as they engage in seriously dangerous pyro displays or express chauvinism and racism; in other cases they will be standing up or chanting for justice in the face of repressive political regimes, and in others, delivering powerful political messages through card displays, chants, or orchestrated action. When these expressions are contrary to the social and political positions of other fans in the stadium or officials policing the events, it is difficult to avoid physical confrontations. Depending on the circumstances, these confrontations may involve or precipitate collective violence that can be deadly for people in the stadium. Examples of this have occurred recently in Serbia, Israel, Egypt, Turkey, and in North African countries where rebels have opposed the rule of oppressive regimes.

Research in the sociology of sport indicates that fan cultures in certain regions are organized around nationalist affiliations and feelings, and these are regularly fused with various forms of racism, depending on which populations are perceived as threats or the cause of social and political problems. But nationalism and racism are never limited to stadium crowds alone. They are manifestations of realities in the larger community or society. Inside the stadium they become concentrated and magnified to the point that they cannot be dismissed or ignored. Of course, this is not a new strategy. Political leaders, patriots, sport team owners, and media commentators have used sports and sport venues to deliver political messages of all sorts, progressive as well as reactionary. As research continues, we will learn more about the complex, contentious, and sometimes senseless forms of fan violence as they occur in various regions of the world.

Panics as Venue Violence By far, more people have died and been injured in panics and violent accidents than by any form of intentional spectator violence. The largest number of deaths in a sport-related panic occurred in Lima, Peru, in 1964 during an Argentina versus Peru soccer match to qualify for the 1964 Tokyo Olympic Games. When a well-known fan stormed the field to dispute a referee's call late in the game, he was beaten by police, which caused thousands to rush onto the field, with 300 to 320 people trampled to death in the process.

Similarly, a panic was incited in 2001 at a Premier League soccer match in Accra, Ghana, when police fired tear gas into an unruly crowd. Spectators rushed to exit doors, which had been locked, and 123 people were crushed to death by the force of the crowd (Langton, 2015). Most panics at sport venues follow this pattern: spectators are frightened and rush to limited or locked exits where many are trampled or crushed to death.

Whenever thousands of people gather together for an occasion intended to generate collective emotions and excitement, it's not surprising that crowd dynamics and circumstances influence their actions. This is especially true at sport events, where collective action is easily fueled by what

social psychologists call *emotional contagion*— a process through which social norms are formed rapidly and are followed in a nearly spontaneous manner by large numbers of people. Although this does not always lead to violence, it increases the possibility of violent crowd movements as well as confrontations between collections of spectators and between spectators and agents of social control, such as the police. This also is a factor in post-event violence.

Post-Event Violence

In North America, the most destructive episodes of violence occur in riots after sport events, especially those for which the stakes are high, such as playoff and championship games. Celebratory riots occur among fans of victorious teams, whereas frustration riots occur among fans of teams suffering defeats. But both forms of riots are equally destructive to property, although loss of life is rare.

Celebratory Riots Oddly enough, some of the most dangerous and destructive crowd violence occurs during the celebrations that follow victories in important sport events (Lewis, 2007). Until recently, when middle-class, white college students tore down expensive goalposts after football victories or ransacked seats and threw seat pads and other objects onto the field, it was treated as displays of youthful exuberance and loyalty to the university. However, in the wake of injuries and mounting property damage associated with these incidents, stadium security officials now prevent fans from rushing onto the playing field when games end.

Cases of celebratory violence still occur, but new methods of social control have been reasonably successful in preventing them inside the stadium. But it is a slightly different story outside the stadium, where crowds gather in multiple locations. Local police usually anticipate celebratory crowds around a stadium, but effective control in an entire metro region depends on advance planning and having a requisite number of specially trained officers who can intervene without creating backlash in a crowd.

The use of social media by people in or around a collection of fans who engage in violence to celebrate a victory can aid in identifying and arresting perpetrators of violence, but research is needed to determine whether social media deter violence or fuel it among those who want digital evidence of their celebrations. In the meantime, some cities are using strategically placed surveillance cameras to capture images of perpetrators.

Research done by sociologist Jerry Lewis, author of the book *Sports Fan Violence in North America* (2007), indicates that most celebratory riots are associated with the following six general conditions:

- A natural urban gathering place for fans
- The presence of a "cadre" of young, white men
- Strong identification with the team
- An event with high stakes such as a national or international championship
- A key or deciding game or match in a playoff or championship series
- A close, exciting contest

Although there is no tested theory to explain involvement in a celebratory riot, young men might be seeking reaffirmation of their identification with a winning team and seeking status by engaging in actions that document their presence at a memorable occasion that they can discuss and brag about for the rest of their lives.

Frustration Riots Frustration riots are rare and less common than celebratory riots. Fans of teams that lose a deciding game or match in an important event are more likely to exit the scene of the loss and deal with their disappointment by themselves or with close friends. A notable exception to this pattern was a 2011 post-event riot in Vancouver, Canada, following the loss of the Vancouver Canucks to the Boston Bruins in the deciding game of the National Hockey League Stanley Cup championship series. Hundreds of young people started fires, turned over cars, and broke windows in a downtown area. Property damage was dramatic in terms of its apparent senselessness, and dozens of people were injured, primarily in confrontations with poorly prepared police officers. Unlike riots that occur in connection with political, labor, or civil rights demonstrations, this one was short-lived and people quickly exited the area as the police presence grew.

Police and political authorities initially described the rioters as thugs and professional anarchists with criminal intent, but videos showed that most of them were from local Vancouver families that strongly disapproved of their destructive actions (Mason, 2011). A classic example of this was captured in a photo of a young man trying to set fire to a rag stuffed in the fuel tank of a police car. The car did not blow up, but the young man was identified as a member of Canada's junior men's national water polo team and an academic all-star who had received an athletic scholarship to attend a U.S. university at the end of the summer. After he turned himself in to police, he was suspended from the national team. Research on this event has not been published, but it appeared that this young man and others like him were mimicking what they perceived to be the culture of Canadian hockey as they displayed male rage, tore off their shirts, and yelled as if they were claiming domination through the destruction they caused (Zirin, 2011b).

Controlling Spectator Violence

A prerequisite for effective crowd control strategies is an awareness of factors associated with spectator violence. These include the following:

- Crowd size and the standing or seating patterns of spectators
- Composition of the crowd in terms of age, sex, social class, and racial/ethnic mix
- The importance and meaning of the event for spectators
- The history of the relationship between the teams and among spectators

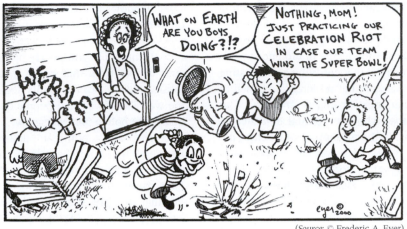

(*Source*: © Frederic A. Eyer)

We need research on so-called celebratory riots. Research on other forms of collective action suggests that celebratory riots may not be as spontaneous and unplanned as many people think.

- Crowd-control strategies used at the event (police, attack dogs, surveillance cameras, or other security measures)
- Alcohol consumption by the spectators
- Location of the event (neutral site or home site of one of the opponents)
- Spectators' reasons for attending the event and their expectations for outcomes
- The importance of the team as a source of identity for spectators (class identity, ethnic or national identity, regional or local identity, club or gang identity)

In other words, there is a combination of background and situational factors that influence the likelihood of spectator violence at a sport event (Spaaij and Anderson, 2010). Over the past forty years, sociologists and law enforcement officials have done a good job of identifying those factors and developing social control strategies that take them into account. But additional things could be done. For example, we know that when spectators perceive violence on the field, they are more likely to engage in violence in the venue. Therefore, it is not wise to promote sport events as violent confrontations between hostile opponents.

Perceived hostility and violence might also be defused if players and coaches make public announcements emphasizing respect for the game and for opponents. The use of competent and professionally trained officials is also important, because when officials maintain control of a game and make calls the spectators define as fair, the likelihood of spectator violence decreases. Referees also could meet with both teams before the event and explain the need to leave hostilities in the locker rooms. Team officials could organize pregame unity rituals involving an exchange of team symbols and displays of respect between opponents. These rituals could be covered by the media so that fans could see that athletes do not view their opponents as enemies. But these strategies conflict with commercial media interests in hyping games as wars without weapons; therefore, we're faced with a choice: promote the safety of fans and players or boost media profits and gate receipts for team owners.

One of the most important preventive measures is to know and respect the needs and rights of spectators. This requires that crowd-control officials be trained to intervene in potentially disruptive situations without escalating the violence. Alcohol consumption should be regulated realistically, as done in many venues worldwide. Venues and the spaces around them should be safe and organized to enable spectators to move around while limiting contact between hostile fans of opposing teams. Exits should be accessible and clearly marked, and spectators should not be herded like animals before or after games. Encouraging attendance by families is important in lowering the incidence of violence.

Being aware of the historical, social, economic, and political issues that often underlie crowd violence is also important. Restrictive law-and-order responses to crowd violence may be temporarily effective, but they will not eliminate the underlying tensions and conflicts that often fuel violence. Policies dealing with oppressive forms of inequality, economic problems, unemployment, political marginalization, racism and other forms of bigotry, and distorted definitions of masculinity are needed. These factors often lead to tensions, conflicts, and violence.

Shaping norms can be difficult, but it's a more effective strategy than moving games to remote locations, hiring hundreds of security personnel, patrolling the stands, using surveillance cameras, scheduling games at times when crowds will be sparse, and recruiting police and soldiers to brandish automatic weapons. Of course, some of these tactics can be effective, but they should be last resorts or temporary measures used only during the time it takes to develop new spectator norms.

TERRORISM: PLANNED POLITICAL VIOLENCE AT SPORT EVENTS

Terrorism and *terrorist* are words that create an emotional response. This is because **terrorism** *is a special form of violence designed to intimidate a target population of people for the purpose of achieving political or social goals.* It can occur anywhere, but it occurs most frequently in divided societies and situations where an oppressed population has an oppositional political agenda. In most cases, it is a strategic response to political repression and feelings of frustration, indignation, and anger (Turk, 2004).

Unlike most warfare, terrorism targets civilians to create pervasive fear in a target population. Therefore, terrorism is seldom random; it is strategically planned so that there will be maximum media coverage. The intent is that coverage will spread and sustain fear and make people feel that the very fabric of their social order is being torn apart. For example, the two terrorists directly responsible for the 2013 Boston Marathon bombings chose the event because it occurred on Patriots Day in Massachusetts and is symbolically linked with the beginning of the American Revolution and the formation of the United States. Also, the marathon is televised live and covered worldwide as a premier sport event. Therefore, news of a terrorist attack at the race would be communicated nationally and globally, and it would be linked to the very foundation of social order in the United States. The pressure cooker bombs used in Boston killed three people and injured 264, some seriously enough to require limb amputations. But the effects this terrorist act went far beyond Boston and marathons.

According to Bill Braniff, the executive director of START—the National Consortium for the Study of Terrorism and Responses to Terrorism, located at the University of Maryland—certain sport events are attractive targets for terrorism because of the following factors (Hruby, 2013c):

- The media are on location.
- The event is communal and seen as representing the values and spirit of a community or society.
- When people seek explanations for the attack, it provides the terrorists opportunity to deliver their political messages.
- The recurring media attention given to a special sport event serves as a regular reminder of the attack and perpetuates fears associated with it.

A marathon is a particularly soft target for terrorism because there is no central security checkpoint for spectators, who can access the race at many points along the 26.2-mile course. But despite this, a study done by START revealed that of the hundreds of marathons held worldwide in the twenty years preceding the 2013 Boston Marathon, only six had been sites for terrorist attacks (START, 2013). Three of these occurred in Northern Ireland (in 1998, 2003, and 2005) where political and social divisions between Protestants and Catholics have a long and violent history. But in each case, bombs were discovered and defused before they could explode.

Another "terrorist" (according to the START Report) attack occurred during a 1994 marathon in Bahrain (in the Persian Gulf) when a few runners were injured by men who allegedly objected to the proximity of the race course to the remains of a mosque and were offended by the shorts and tops worn by female runners. A terrorist attack also occurred in 2006 at a marathon in Lahore, Pakistan, where six buses were burned and four people were injured, including two police officers. The most recent terrorist incident prior to the 2013 Boston Marathon was a 2008 suicide bomb attack at a marathon in Colombo, Sri Lanka, that killed twelve runners and three spectators and injured about 100 others close to the starting line. Finally, in late-2015 there was a failed suicide bomb attempt during a soccer game in Paris's Stade de France. When denied entry to the stadium, the three terrorists blew themselves up, but there were no other fatalities.

This record suggests that terrorists do not usually target sport events. Through the 110-year history of the Olympics there have been two terrorist attacks, one in 1972 when members of a Palestinian terrorist group called Black September entered the Olympic Village in Munich, Germany, went to rooms being occupied by Israeli athletes and coaches, shot and killed a wrestling coach and a weightlifter, and captured nine Israeli athletes. After a 21-hour standoff and a poorly planned rescue attempt, seventeen people were dead—ten Israeli athletes, one coach, one West German police officer, and five terrorists. The remaining terrorists were sought out and killed by Israeli commandos.

The only other terrorist incident at the Olympics occurred at the 1996 Atlanta Games when a former U.S. military explosives expert detonated several bombs that killed two people and injured over 100 to protest against abortion and the "global socialism" that was "destroying" the United States.

The point of these examples is to show that terrorism has occurred at very few sport events. In fact, until the 2013 Boston Marathon, the attack during the 1996 Atlanta Olympics was the only sport-related incident of terrorism in U.S. history. But then came September 11, 2001, and the horrific attacks on the World Trade Center buildings in New York City, the Pentagon outside Washington, D.C., and a hijacked plane that ultimately crashed in Pennsylvania. Over 3000 people were killed and thousands were wounded on that day. The pervasive fear generated by 9/11 and the emerging narratives that imagined future terrorist attacks in vivid details have had a major impact on U.S. culture and on major sport events.

When 9/11 occurred, Salt Lake City was preparing for the 2002 Winter Olympic Games. This led some people—all with different motives—to focus on the Salt Lake Games as the frontline for a possible global war on terror. Large security companies and other companies with security technologies to sell were influential in creating and promoting a new narrative of fear and the need for event organizers to provide comprehensive security no matter the cost (Giulianotti and Klauser, 2012; Hassan, 2012; McMichael, 2012; Schimmel, 2012; Sugden, 2012; Toohey and Taylor, 2012). As a result, the Salt Lake City Olympics and all subsequent Olympic Games have been assumed to be prime terrorist targets, leading organizers to spend increasing amounts of money for security. To question this assumption is nearly impossible in a climate of fear fueled in part by companies wanting to profit from the sales of high-priced security products (Atkinson and Young, 2012; Graham, 2012).

As shown in Table 6.1, security costs for the pre-9/11 Sydney Games were $180 million, or $12,500 per athlete (all data include Olympic and Paralympic athletes). But after 9/11 security costs

Table 6.1 Olympic/Paralympic security costs, 2000–2014 (in U.S. dollars)

Year	City	Security cost	Cost per athlete†
2000	Sydney	$180 million	$12,500
2002	Salt Lake City	$500 million	$131,100
2004	Athens	$1.5 billion	$103,000
2006	Turin	$1.4 billion	$350,500
2008	Beijing	$6.5 billion	$430,000
2010	Vancouver	$1.0 billion	$325,500
2012	London	$1.6 billion*	$114,300
2014	Sochi	NA	NA

Source: Canadian Broadcasting Company News.
*Estimates for London 2012 vary from $800 million to $1.6 billion
†The summer games have at least four-times more athletes than the winter games.

for the much smaller winter games in Salt Lake City were $500 million, or $131,100 per athlete—a more than tenfold increase from two years earlier. This pattern continued with Beijing spending $6.5 billion for security in 2008, or $430,000 per athlete. For London 2012, the security bill was an estimated $1.6 billion, or $114,300 per athlete. Overall, security now constitutes about 12 to 20 percent of the total budget for the Olympics, and the worldwide security industry has gone from being worth $142 billion in 2009 to an estimated $3 trillion in 2014.

Another factor that has boosted security expenses for the Olympics and other sport mega-events is that police and political officials in host cities use the fears of local citizens to buy and install security systems and employ a militaristic command-and-control approach to policing that most people would find unacceptable under other circumstances (McMichael, 2012; Schimmel, 2012). This supports their desire to gentrify the city, move the poor and homeless out, increase property values, and provide services for new urban elite residents seeking upscale housing, restaurants, and entertainment—all in a highly policed and secure environment. At the same time, the new narrative of fear leads people to seek security over privacy and accept a new high-tech approach to policing and social control.

Today, security strategies are part of the everyday routine at major sport venues. Spectators are scanned or searched when they enter venues, and there is strict enforcement of rules governing what may be brought into the venues. However, most security measures are discreet and take place behind the scenes in the form of bomb searches, electronic surveillance, and undercover tactics. When terrorist attacks don't occur, those who support high-tech social control say their system is working; and if a terrorist attack does occur, they argue that even more security technology is needed. In either case, those profiting from fear and uncertainty win. This, of course, makes it increasingly expensive to attend high-profile sport events at the same time that security costs are frequently paid with public money, meaning that the general population pays for the safety and comfort of those wealthy enough to buy tickets. Fear has many consequences.

summary

DOES VIOLENCE IN SPORTS AFFECT OUR LIVES?

Violence is not new to sports. Athletes throughout history have engaged in actions and used strategies that cause or have the potential to cause injuries to themselves and others. Furthermore, spectators throughout history have regularly engaged in violent actions before, during, and after sport events. However, as people define violence in sports as controllable rather than as a fact of life, there's a tendency to view it as a problem in need of a solution.

Violence in sports ranges from brutal body contact and borderline violence to quasi-criminal and criminal acts. It is linked with overconformity to the sport ethic, commercialization, and cultural definitions of masculinity. It has become institutionalized in some sports as a strategy for competitive success, even though it causes injuries and permanent physical impairments among athletes. The use of enforcers is one example of institutionalized violence in sports.

Controlling on-the-field violence is difficult, especially in men's contact sports, because it is often tied to players' identities as athletes and as men. Male athletes in contact sports learn to use violence and intimidation as strategic tools, but we don't know if the strategies learned in sports influence the expression of violence in relationships and situations that occur off-the-field.

Among males, learning to use violence as a tool within a sport is frequently tied to the reaffirmation of a form of masculinity that emphasizes a willingness to risk personal safety and intimidate others. If the boys and men who participate in certain sports learn to perceive this orientation as natural or appropriate, and receive support for this perception from sources inside sports and the general community, then their participation in sports may contribute to off-the-field violence, including assault, sexual assault, and rape. However, such learning is not automatic, and men may, under certain circumstances, even learn to control anger and their expressions of violence by playing heavy-contact sports.

The most important impact of violence in sports may be its reaffirmation of a gender ideology that assumes the "natural superiority of men." This ideology is based on the belief that an ability to do violence is an essential feature of manhood.

Female athletes in contact sports also engage in aggressive and violent acts, but little is known about the connections between these acts and the gender identities of girls and women at different levels of competition. Many women prefer an emphasis on supportive connections between teammates and opponents as compared with the power and performance aspects of sports. Therefore, aggression and violence do not occur in women's sports as often or through the same identity dynamics as they occur in men's sports.

Violence in sports has real consequences. Recent research on the incidence of brain damage caused by concussions and repetitive sub-concussive head hits has made many people aware of consequences that had been purposely hidden or had gone undiagnosed. If further research indicates that permanent and severe damage can be caused by the violence inherent in certain sports, there will be significant changes in the popularity of those sports, especially football. In the meantime, participation in certain sports is connected with regular and sometimes severe injuries and long-term health problems.

The relationship between on-the-field violence and the off-the-field actions of athletes is difficult to untangle. In some cases—and under specific conditions—people may learn, even in violent sports, to control violent actions off the field. In other cases, players may have a difficult time drawing a line between "approved" on-the-field violence and what is appropriate action off the field. Additionally, learning to use violence in a sport may not be as influential as the hubris, sense of entitlement, and all-male group dynamics that often are associated with off-the-field violence among athletes. This may explain why athletes in certain sports seem to have higher sexual assault rates than their peers who don't play sports. But more research is needed on this possibility.

Violence occurs among spectators who view sport events through the media as well as those attending live events. Research is needed to explain the conditions under which violence occurs in crowds watching or listening to media representations of events. Studies at the sites of events indicate that venue violence is influenced by perceived violence on the field of play, crowd dynamics, the situation at the event itself, the overall historical and social contexts in which spectators give meaning to the event, and their relationships with others in attendance.

In some cases, venue violence may be planned to publicly oppose the policies of a political regime or the actions of police; it may be used to attract attention to political issues, injustice, or the existence of a population that seeks public recognition; or it may involve an expression of nationalism, racism, or bigotry directed against disliked groups of people. Venue violence is sometimes dramatic. Usually it involves crowd panics during which people are trampled or crushed to death.

Post-event celebratory riots are the most common form of spectator and fan violence in North America. Frustration riots are much less common, but both types of riots can be prevented or controlled through the use of trained police officers who know how to intervene in such situations without causing backlash and further fueling crowd violence. Controlling any form of spectator violence requires a trained security and police force.

Terrorism at sport events is rare, but the threat of terrorism and the politics of security alters policies, procedures, and the cost of hosting sport events, especially mega-events such as the Olympic Games. The terrorist attack at the 2013 Boston Marathon reminds us that global issues influence our lives, even when we attend our favorite sport events. Just as violence in sports affects our lives, the social conditions in which we live affect violence in sports. The challenge in providing security at sport events is that those responsible for the safety of spectators find that they must limit their security strategies in order to control costs or to protect personal privacy. In some cases, large expenditures on security technology are part of a larger effort to introduce coercive systems of social control and law enforcement.

SUPPLEMENTAL READINGS

Reading 1. Murderball: Violence in wheelchairs
Reading 2. Violence and animal sports
Reading 3. The social psychological dynamics of violence in sports
Reading 4. Sport violence: More barbaric than you think
Reading 5. Fan violence: Ultras in Italy as a case study

SPORT MANAGEMENT ISSUES

- People in sport marketing and management have in the past promoted events in terms of anticipated violence on the field of play. Is this a viable strategy today? Explain why it is or is not.
- Controlling on-the-field violence presents a difficult challenge. Identify strategies for controlling various types of violence, and explain why you have chosen those strategies.
- You are a new program manager in a large public sport and recreation center. The director of the center tells you to design a program through which young people will learn to be less violent in the local neighborhood. Describe the program you would develop, and how it will be organized to meet your supervisor's expectations.
- You are the athletic director at a high school that is hosting an in-state rivalry game between your number-1-ranked football team and the number-2-ranked team in your division. Violence has occurred at past games with this team. Describe the measures you will take to control player and spectator violence in connection with the game.

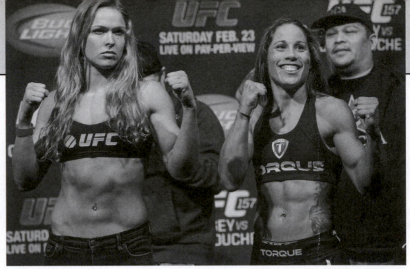

GENDER AND SPORTS

Is Equity Possible?

The biggest milestones are no longer what happens if women are allowed to play; it's how to make it pay so you survive and thrive.

—**Johnette Howard, sport journalist (2013)**

The NFL and the Pentagon walk comfortably together . . . because they present pumped-up versions of masculine invulnerability as admirable qualities.

—**Dave Zirin, sport journalist (2014a)**

. . . the main barriers to . . . gender equity no longer lie in people's personal attitudes and relationships. Instead, structural impediments prevent people from acting on their egalitarian values . . . The gender revolution is not in a stall. It has hit a wall.

—**Stephanie Coontz, sociologist (2013)**

The athletic world remains another intimidating place for many people who aren't heterosexual or have non-conforming gender identities.

—**Maxwell Strachan, sport journalist (2015)**

Chapter Outline

Learning Objectives

- Describe the two-sex classification system, and explain how it impacts the meaning and organization of sports as well as who participates in sports.

- Explain how orthodox gender ideology has influenced sports and how sports have influenced gender ideology.

- Understand the current approach to sex testing and how it is related to orthodox gender ideology.

- Identify reasons for the dramatic increase in sport participation rates among women of all ages since the mid-1970s.

- Identify existing gender inequities in sports and the barriers faced when trying to achieve equity.

- Understand what it means to say that sports and sport organizations today are male-dominated, male-identified, and male-centered.

- Explain how orthodox gender ideology influences lesbians, gay men, bisexuals, and transsexuals in sports today.

- Identify effective strategies to promote gender equity in sports and sport organizations.

I think that female athletes are completely accepted among both the guys and the girls. I mean I have played sports since I was 5 and I have never not been accepted by both the guys and the girls.

This statement by a high school basketball player echoes the feelings of most girls and young women in the United States today (Evans, 2011). Gone are the days when many female athletes endured nasty comments and were taunted by peers. But gender remains important in sports, and gender-related forms of exclusion and discrimination continue to exist. This is why people in the sociology of sport regularly focus on gender and gender relations as they study sports as social phenomena.

This chapter focuses on complex relationships between sports and the way people think and feel about masculinity, femininity, homosexuality, heterosexuality, and other aspects of gender and sexuality in culture and society. The issues discussed are these:

- Why have most sports worldwide been defined as men's activities?
- How have girls and women been excluded or discouraged from playing sports?
- What accounts for recent increases in women's sport participation?
- Do gender inequities remain in sports?
- What barriers interfere with the achievement of gender equity?
- What strategies can produce more progress toward gender equity in sports?

CULTURAL ORIGINS OF GENDER INEQUITIES

In Chapter 1, we saw that **gender ideology** consists of *interrelated ideas and beliefs that are widely used to define masculinity and femininity, identify people as male or female, evaluate forms of sexual expression, and organize social relationships.* The *dominant* gender ideology used in many societies is organized around three ideas and beliefs:

1. Human beings are either female or male.
2. Heterosexuality is normal, and other expressions of sexual feelings, thoughts, and actions are seen as unnatural, abnormal, deviant, or immoral.
3. Men are physically stronger and more rational than women and more naturally suited to possess power and assume leadership positions in the public spheres of society.

Many people question or reject these ideas and beliefs today, but the traditional or orthodox ideology they support has long influenced how people (a) think about and identify themselves and others, (b) form and evaluate relationships, (c) develop expectations for themselves and others, and (d) organize and distribute rewards in social worlds.

Even if we oppose orthodox gender ideology, it is so deeply rooted in our experiences and the organization of everyday life that we unknowingly use it as a cultural guide for making decisions about what we wear and how we talk, walk, present ourselves to others, choose college majors, and think about and plan for our future (Ridgeway, 2011; Risman and Davis, 2013).

Gender ideology varies from culture to culture. In societies where men control most power and resources, people use a gender ideology based on a simple binary (two-sex) classification system. Therefore, they assume that all humans can be classified into one of two **sex categories:** *male or female*. These categories are viewed in terms of physiological and psychological differences. This is why many people refer to males and females as "opposite" sexes, why they believe that the two sexes are naturally different, and why they expect males and females to differ in many ways.

These expectations are the basis for defining **gender,** or *what is considered masculine or feminine in a group or society.* In most societies, gender and gender distinctions are so deeply integrated into language systems, identities, and relationships that people cannot ignore them, even when they don't agree with them. Additionally, gender distinctions are expressed in different ways across social classes, cultural settings, and sports (Adams, 2011; Connell, 2011; Mennesson, 2012; Tagg, 2012; Weber and Barker-Ruchti, 2012).

The two-sex classification system is widely taken for granted. Most people use it as a basis for how they view the world and their place in it. Often they feel confused, uncomfortable, or even angry when they or others don't fit neatly into one of the two orthodox sex categories. This is why so many people find it difficult to think critically about gender and why they become defensive when others do so.

In this chapter, I use the term **orthodox gender ideology** to represent the interrelated ideas and beliefs associated with this two-sex approach. Using the word *orthodox* is meant to show that this view of gender represents a traditional and widely established way of thinking that people view as unchanging "truth" linked to their religious beliefs or an overall sense of right and wrong.[1]

In societies where many people have access to science-based information about sex and gender and have personal experiences to support that information, there is a growing movement, as well as personal inclinations, to question all or part of orthodox gender ideology. As this occurs, some people form new perspectives on gender and what it means for how they see themselves, their relationships, and the organization of social worlds. This is happening mostly among young people whose expanding awareness of human and social variation leads them to feel uncomfortable with an inflexible two-sex classification system that has been used to marginalize and label as immoral or unnatural too many people, including some of their family members and friends. The new ideas and beliefs about gender have not become integrated enough to say that there is an identifiable and widely shared gender-inclusive ideology at this time. But an

increasing number of people are moving in that direction, and this phenomenon is now being studied (Anderson 2002, 2005b, 2008b, 2009b, 2011a, 2011b, 2011c, 2011d; Anderson and McCormack, 2015; Jarvis, 2015; McCormack, 2012).

Even though many people worldwide cling to orthodox gender ideology, it is inconsistent with scientific evidence showing that anatomy, hormones, chromosomes, and secondary sex characteristics vary in complex ways that cannot be divided into two distinct, nonoverlapping sex categories. Noted scientists explain that sex is so biologically and culturally complex that it cannot be forced into two categories if we really want to understand its implications in our lives (Bank, 2012; Fausto-Sterling, 2000a; Harper, 2007; Laqueur, 1990).

Anne Fausto-Sterling, a biologist who has spent her life studying sex and the human body, notes, "There is no either/or; rather, there are shades of difference" (Fausto-Sterling, 2000b, p. 3). In other words, real bodies have hundreds of continuous physical traits that vary on a scale from low to high rather than falling neatly into two separate and opposite categories. Additionally, differences vary and overlap, so that the only way to conclude that there are only two sex categories is to arbitrarily decide what characteristics are most important and then fit them into two separate categories.

This means that the use of a two-category system for classifying all bodies is a reflection of social and cultural ideas rather than biological facts. But the categories have important effects regardless of their biological validity, because using them produces life-altering consequences for people. In fact, when people are born with physical traits that don't fit neatly into one sex category or the other, the gender ideology used by many physicians and parents in the past led them to surgically "fix" genitals and reproductive organs so that infants would appear to be more clearly male or female (Fausto-Sterling, 2000a; Harper, 2007; Quart, 2008). This approach is changing as people realize that bodies are more complex than a two-sex system leads us to believe, and that sex as well as gender is a social construction. Today it is more customary for

---

[1]This choice of terms is inspired by the work of Eric Anderson (2009b, 2011b), who distinguishes orthodox masculinity from inclusive masculinity. His explanation for doing this can be extended to identify orthodox gender ideology and contrast it with inclusive gender ideology, which is increasingly used to think about gender in less rigid and dogmatic terms.

the parents of children with ambiguous anatomical characteristics to wait and let their children make their own decisions about surgeries or other medical treatments when they know how they want to identify themselves and understand the implications of sex identification in society.

Being Out of Gender Bounds

Orthodox gender ideology creates problems when it causes people to have rigid, unbending ideas and beliefs about the ways that males and females are supposed to look, think, feel, and act. Further, it leads to the assumption that heterosexuality is natural and normal and those who have an appearance or express feelings, thoughts, and actions that do not fit into the heterosexual male or female categories are unnatural and abnormal and therefore "out of bounds" in terms of gender (see Figure 7.1).

This approach marginalizes lesbians, gay men, bisexuals, transsexuals, and intersex people (LGBTIs) and leads some people to view them as abnormal, unnatural, or immoral because they exist outside the two orthodox sex categories. This fosters **homophobia,** which is *a generalized fear or intolerance of anyone who isn't clearly classifiable as a heterosexual male or female* (Griffin, 1998).

This fear and intolerance is created when people see others with an appearance or presentation of self that does not make sense to them in terms of the gender ideology they use. As long as the two-sex system is widely accepted, homophobia will exist in some form. For this reason, the achievement of full gender equity depends on transforming that system.

Orthodox Gender Ideology as a Tool to Maintain the Status Quo

Another important aspect of orthodox dominant gender ideology is that it leads people to see males and females as different *and* unequal. For example, Figure 7.1 illustrates that males have greater access to higher levels of privilege, power, and influence than females have. Therefore, men occupy high public positions of power and influence in greater numbers than women do. Of course, this means that some men—*but not all men*—have a strong personal interest in preserving the two-sex system and the ideology it supports. This is why males are more likely than females to "police" gender boundaries and discourage all boys and men from pushing or crossing the line that separates "heterosexual men" from women and from anyone who is "out

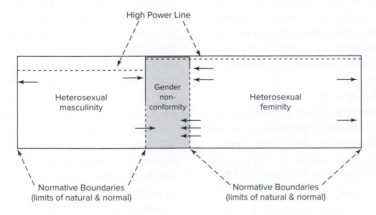

FIGURE 7.1 A two-category classification model: Identifying sex and defining gender in U.S. culture.

of gender bounds" in their view. Maintaining gender distinctions reaffirms orthodox gender ideology and legitimizes disproportionate male power in society.

When boys and men learn to accept orthodox gender ideology, they enforce restrictive normative boundaries for heterosexual masculinity. Additionally, to retain their greater access to positions of power and influence, they must also promote the belief that power and influence are legitimately linked with masculine characteristics and that existing gender boundaries are normal and natural. This is why males are generally more likely than females to intimidate or reject people who push gender boundaries or live outside them. When other males push boundaries, they may be quickly labeled a "sissy," which can put them in a dangerous position among male peers who accept orthodox gender ideology. In a strange way, this is the price that most boys and men must pay to preserve an ideology that leads to the belief that it is natural for men to control sports along with nearly all major sources of wealth and political power in the world.

Women, on the other hand, have less to lose and more to gain in terms of power and influence if they *do* push and blur gender boundaries. This is why some—not all—girls and women take or are given more latitude or permission to exhibit a range of feelings, thoughts, and actions that is wider than the accepted range for boys and men. Of course, they must also be sensitive to gender boundaries if they wish to avoid intimidation or rejection, but girls, at least until their mid-teens, often say that being labeled a "tomboy" is a good thing (Daniels, 2009; Orenstein, 2008).

For the past half century in the United States, orthodox gender ideology based on a two-sex classification system has fostered forms of socialization in which boys learn to limit their sense of personal possibilities more than girls learn to limit their possibilities across a wide range of options. For example, girls and women are more likely to play hockey or take boxing lessons than boys and men are to become figure skaters or take synchronized swimming lessons (Adams, 2011). This is partly

because being female is devalued in mainstream U.S. culture, and because some boys and men feel the need to reject any choices and actions associated with femininity. Therefore, they make choices that perpetuate the notion that men and women are different, with men being more naturally suited for positions involving power, leadership, and control.

Disrupting Orthodox Gender Ideology

Various aspects of orthodox gender ideology are widely challenged today. An increasing number of people worldwide now understand that certain ideas and beliefs produce and perpetuate gender inequalities that are arbitrary, restrictive, hurtful, and far too often brutal in their effects. In Figure 7.1 the arrows that push against the normative boundaries of the heterosexual male and female categories represent efforts to bend, blur, and erase boundaries and escape their constraints. As boundary pushers and gender benders raise critical issues in society, they force others to either defend *or* critically assess prevailing beliefs about *masculinity* and *femininity* and the constraints and inequities created by those beliefs. Therefore, what we see today are cultural struggles between gender defenders and critical gender benders as they try to close or open up spaces in the gender order of society.

When gender defenders are dominant in these struggles, gender benders are more cautious in their self-expression because the personal cost of being gender-nonconforming can be very high. But when gender benders are more dominant, people in society feel less constrained to be gender-conforming and they express a wider range of feelings, thoughts, and actions—which some people think is positive and exciting whereas others think it signals the end of moral order in society. At this point in the United States the gender benders have momentum on their side and people feel freer to challenge the constraints of orthodox gender ideology.

During these struggles most people find it difficult to give up ideas and beliefs that are central to how they make sense of the world, even when those ideas and beliefs sometimes put them at a dis-advantage. For this reason, deeply held ideologies tend to slow the rate and extent of change in any society. For example, we see that many men and some women use their resources to defend and pro-mote orthodox gender ideology because it supports their positions of privilege in the gender order. Therefore, they sponsor media programming, polit-ical candidates, community programs, laws, and informal norms that affirm the foundational ideas and beliefs on which that ideology rests—such as the views that women and men are different and suited for different tasks, and that anyone who is not a heterosexual is abnormal. But the legitimacy of their power and influence is not absolute, and it varies from one social world to another. In many places worldwide that influence is being eroded by science, social action, and the everyday deeds of those who push gender boundaries.

ORTHODOX GENDER IDEOLOGY AND SPORTS

When men created organized sports during the mid-nineteenth century, they were guided by gender ide-ology organized firmly around the three major beliefs that constitute the core of orthodox gender ideol-ogy today. This led them to select physical activities, develop rules, and establish governing bodies that reaffirmed those ideas and beliefs. This was not due to a conspiracy; they just never thought of alterna-tives. In their minds, sports were male territory and sites for establishing and proving heterosexual mas-culinity. Women were too weak and frail to partici-pate. The preferred sports were those that involved physical contact, competition, and conquest.

Although certain ideas and beliefs about gender have changed over time, the legacies of the men who established modern sports and shaped sport cultures remain influential today. For this reason, sports continue to be:

> The inclusion of women at the Olympic Games would be "impractical, uninteresting, unaesthetic, and incorrect." —Baron Pierre de Coubertin, 1912

1. *Male-dominated,* so that ability and perfor-mance qualifications are associated with man-hood and men; therefore, being "qualified" in sports means possessing masculine characteris-tics, or performing "like a man."
2. *Male-identified,* so that what men value is assumed to be valued by all "mankind," mak-ing sports a "man's world" that revolves around men and manhood; therefore, "women's sports" must be identified explicitly, such as "the Women's World Cup" or "the Ladies Professional Golf Association."
3. *Male-centered,* so that men and men's lives are the expected focus of attention; therefore, there are few women and women's sports repre-sented in sport stories, legends, records, events, halls of fame, and media programming (Johnson, 2006, 2013).

This helps us understand that sports are gendered social worlds in which competence is defined in connection with masculine traits, and female bod-ies and traits are viewed as athletically inferior. Therefore, when a female excels in sport, she might be described as "playing like a man," and a female coach, official, or administrator is considered capable when she does her job "like a man would do it." Despite the progress made by women in other spheres of life, sports remain *male-dominated social worlds.*

In *male-identified social worlds,* the values and experiences of men are assumed to be the standards for everyone. Therefore, women in positions of authority are "out of place" and arouse suspicion about how they obtained their power and how they might use it. If women attempt to reduce suspicions by "fitting in" or acting like men, they may be seen as phony or manipulative, and therefore undeserving of their position. This makes it easy to discredit women leaders in sports—people can say that they obtained their positions by unfairly gaining the favor of men, or by being shrewd "stealth femi-nists," or closeted lesbians who don't like men and want to undermine traditional sport cultures. This seriously hinders the careers of women in coaching and administration.

In *male-centered social worlds,* people assume that men are the center of attention. The World Series, Super Bowl, Little League World Series, World Cup, and the Masters (golf tournament) are not described as "men's events," nor are pro football stadiums referred to as "men's sport centers," even though they're all about men and men's culture. In male-centered sports, men are the focus; women and their sports are secondary. Of course, this doesn't mean that women's sports are not important to the players and their supporters. But it does mean that on a general cultural level, they have less significance than men's sports.

Female Athletes as Invaders

Male-dominated/identified/centered sports and sport organizations have never been female-friendly. In the early 1900s, women struggled against tradition, male resistance, and legal prohibitions even to ride bicycles without being arrested and defined as immoral. In fact, the history of girls and women in sports during much of the twentieth century consists of individual and collective efforts to overcome exclusion and discrimination and to persistently claim spaces in which they could do sports.

In the early twentieth century, women began to overcome some barriers and claimed spaces in the "grace and beauty sports" of figure skating and gymnastics (Hart, 1981; Loy et al., 2009). These were considered artistic activities emphasizing coordination and attractive "body lines," so they conformed to emerging ideas and beliefs about femininity at that time in U.S. history. Women also made their way into golf and tennis—individual sports played primarily by privileged white women who were careful to "act like ladies" on the course and court. African American women overcame barriers and participated on some track-and-field teams at segregated high schools and the historically black colleges and universities in regions where black students were not admitted to "white"

state schools. A few of the most talented even made it onto U.S. Olympic teams.

Myths That Discouraged Female Invaders Through much of the twentieth century, medical myths created anxieties about certain forms of sport participation. Girls and women were told that playing strenuous sports would damage the uterus, make child birth difficult, and produce unfeminine bodies. The exclusion of girls from Little League baseball was widely accepted through most of the 1950s due to the myth that being hit in the chest by a baseball or by an opponent sliding into a base could cause breast cancer later in life.

People believed these myths because they were consistent with orthodox gender ideology and the ideas that females were naturally weak and therefore vulnerable to injuries and overexhaustion in sports. Their sport participation was generally limited to activities involving solo performers (figure skating, gymnastics, equestrian events) or competitions in which nets, lane dividers, and other barriers separated opponents (tennis, badminton, swimming, short running races, golf, archery, fencing) and "protected" them from physical contact with each other. Basketball, field hockey, soccer, lacrosse, and other open-field or open-court team sports were labeled unladylike, which is why a women's *team* sport was not included in the Olympics until 1964—and it was volleyball. "Netless" team sports for women were added to the Olympics gradually: in 1976, basketball, team rowing, and team handball; in 1980, field hockey; in 1996, soccer and softball; and in 1998, ice hockey.

Because science has dispelled medical and overexhaustion myths, today's college students dismiss them. But those who lack access to current knowledge in biology and anatomy may still believe gender myths that discourage or exclude girls and women from sport participation. This is especially true in cultures where literacy rates are low and men control information, education, and sports.

In additional to myths, appeals to widely accepted values and norms also discouraged girls and women.

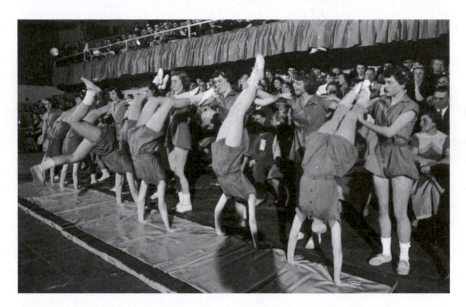

For most of the twentieth century, few schools sponsored competitive teams for girls and young women. Instead, they usually sponsored semi-annual "field days" or "sport nights" during which girls could compete in running races and other field events or give skills demonstrations to parents, as in this photo. Until the 1960s there were widely believed myths that vigorous sports would harm the female body and make it difficult for a woman to conceive, carry, and give birth to children. (*Source:* © Lisa Larsen/Time Life Pictures/Getty Images)

Girls were told that cheering for boys in sports was more appropriate than playing sports. Women were told that the nation depended on them to focus on domestic activities and stay out of the man's world of sports. Those who challenged these restrictions during the late 1940s through the 1960s in the United States were widely perceived as invaders of male territory and made targets of ridicule and condemnation by both males and females who accepted orthodox gender ideology as "natural law."

Although girls and women have continued to push gender boundaries so that most sports in the United States are now open to females, some people continue to believe that females should be banned from the "truly manly" sports of wrestling, football, boxing, and bull riding. Women who are serious about participating in those sports face significant challenges.

Ladies, Not Invaders To avoid being labeled as invaders, girls and women often chose to call themselves "ladies" when they played sports prior to the 1980s. This was done to let men know that they knew "their place" in sports and would not take resources away from the serious sports played by men. This tradition continues today as many female athletes and women's teams are referred to as "ladies."

A similar strategy to avoid being seen as invaders and gender nonconformers was for female athletes to dress and act like stereotypical "ladies" by wearing makeup, dresses, heels, nail polish, and engagement or wedding rings. During competitions they wore skirts, bright hair ribbons, ponytails, and other "heterosexual femininity markers" to make sure they didn't push too hard against normative gender boundaries. The goal was to highlight

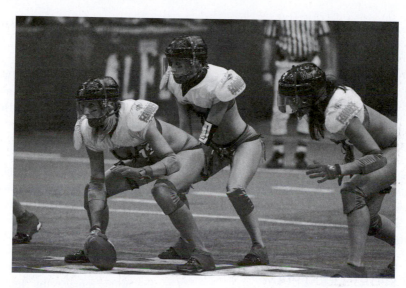

If women play what is culturally defined as a "man's sport," and want people to watch them, they must dress appropriately so that no one mistakes them for seriously pushing gender boundaries. Lingerie football is an extreme example of this. Would these women choose to play like this if there were other opportunities to play football seriously? (*Source:* © Ted Soqui/ /Corbis)

stereotypical femininity *and* downplay any connection to masculinity by hiding their assertiveness and toughness. Even today there are men, a few women, and some sponsors who say that if women athletes want to attract spectators, they should hike up their shorts, tighten their shirts, and look like ladies (Scott, 2012).

Social science researchers referred to this self-presentation strategy as the "female apologetic" when it was used in the past (Adams et al., 2005; Krane et al., 2004). Female athletes today use a "reformed apologetic" that involves proudly expressing their assertiveness, toughness, and rightful place in sport at the same time that they communicate their femininity through clothes, makeup, accessories, and posing with and without clothes in magazines (Hendley and Bielby, 2012). In other words, they push gender boundaries to create more space to be female, but they don't want to erase the boundaries or transform the prevailing gender ideology.

Equipment and apparel companies use this reformed apologetic as a hook for marketing and selling products. There are bikinis in women's beach volleyball; "bunhuggers" (compression shorts) in running and volleyball; "cute" workout clothes; and the pervasive ponytails and bows worn by young white women on soccer and softball teams across the United States (where short haircuts are as rare as players without cleats). The most extreme examples of this are the lingerie leagues in basketball (https://www.youtube.com/watch?v=R8C1l0YTM_4), hockey (now defunct), and football (Conn, 2015; http://www.lflus.com/).

An encouraging exception to uncritical gender conformity occurred in 2012 when women boxers challenged the Amateur International Boxing Association (AIBA) to drop a new rule forcing them to wear skirts "to help spectators distinguish them from men" in the ring (BBC, 2012). Marianne Marston, a leader in women's boxing, expressed the feelings of her peers when she said,

I have more important issues to deal with in women's boxing—the acceptance of women's boxing [and] acceptance of women in boxing gyms—than whether they should wear skirts or not. I think they (AIBA) are saying that women's sport won't get accepted or viewed unless women are feminine, and boxing is not necessarily a sport that attracts particularly a feminine attitude from the women that compete in it. (BBC, 2012a)

Marston and her peers had already challenged the gender ideology used by officials in the boxing federation simply by putting on gloves and stepping into the ring, and they were not about to step backward into skirts.

MAINSTREAM SPORTS REAFFIRM ORTHODOX GENDER IDEOLOGY

Sports have long been sites for reaffirming beliefs about male–female *difference,* celebrating heterosexual masculinity, and legitimizing male power and dominance in nearly all spheres of social life (Paradis, 2012). When these beliefs are challenged, struggles result because many people benefit from them and don't want them changed. But challenges often raise questions that begin to erode traditional beliefs and create new ways of viewing sports and gender at all levels of competition. This is illustrated in the following sections.

Sports Reaffirm Male–Female Difference

Sports remain one of the only activities in contemporary liberal cultures in which sex segregation is expected, accepted, and mandatory in nearly all competitive events. Sex segregation continues because it is assumed that females are physically weaker and less capable than males and therefore must be protected from them (Pappano and McDonagh, 2008a).

Orthodox gender ideology discourages discussions about how and when sex segregation should be eliminated in sports. This contributes to ambivalence, mixed messages, and confusion about female athletes, the realities of biological sex, and

the lived experiences of people for whom gender conformity is not an option.

Using Sex Tests to Maintain the Two-Sex System

A clear example of how sports reproduce beliefs about male-female sex difference is the current International Olympic Committee (IOC) policy requiring women who appear unfeminine to prove that their bodies don't produce and use testosterone like male bodies do. If their bodies naturally produce and utilize too much testosterone, they are disqualified from competition because it is assumed that they have an unfair advantage when competing against other women. Of course, if men produce "too much" testosterone, they are viewed as awesome athletes when they win medals.

This new policy replaces the "fem testing" previously used by sport governing bodies. Female athletes in the 1960s were regularly subjected to exams by medical professionals who would check their genitalia and secondary sex characteristics to document that they were females before they could compete in certain international events (Donnelly and Donnelly, 2013a). Athletes emphatically objected to this, and the test never identified a single gender imposter. But it did lead to unfairly disqualifying women who looked too unfeminine to the judges (Huening, 2009; Karkazis et al., 2012; Simpson et al., 2000). As a result, the international track and field federation as well as the Pan American Games and the Commonwealth Games abandoned such exams in 1967.

In late-1967, the IOC and other sport organizations replaced the exams with a chromosome test that involved scraping cells from the inside of a woman's cheek and analyzing them to identify "Barr bodies" associated with the XX sex chromosomes typical for females. But human bodies are naturally diverse in terms of sex chromosome characteristics as well as genetic, cellular, hormonal, and anatomical characteristics (Fausto-Sterling, 2000a). Therefore, this "Barr body"/chromosome test was clearly invalid and unreliable, but it was used for over thirty years and led to the mistaken disqualification of many women who had no unfair

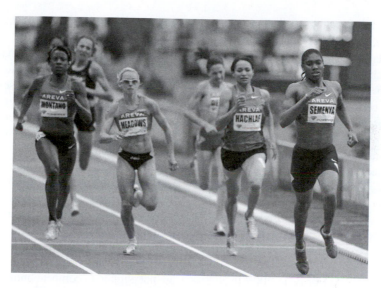

Ms. Semenya (on far right) is running in an 800-meter race in France in 2011 after being suspended by the IAAF for nearly two years while she was examined and tested to determine if she met the IOC requirements to compete as a woman. Women continue to be subjected to such a process if they appear abnormal and "suspicious" to others. But women in high-performance sports are by definition, abnormal, and their bodies often deviate from someone's idea of "feminine." As the leaders of sport organizations cling to orthodox gender ideology, they have difficulty coming to terms with this fact. (*Source*: © CHRISTOPHE KARABA/epa/Corbis)

biological advantage in their sports (Huening, 2009; Karkazis et al., 2012).

By 1991, there was clear consensus among scientists that human bodies do not fit neatly into the two distinct sex categories around which sports were organized; choosing one or more traits to determine if a woman is a *female* would always be arbitrary, subjective, and unfair to some people. Finally, in 1999, the IOC abandoned sex testing and verification. However, the organizers of the 2008 Olympic Games in Beijing set up an "unofficial" gender test lab where they drew blood samples from female athletes who were identified as having a "suspicious" appearance. This received little attention and failed to identify anyone as a gender fraud (Boylan, 2008; Thomas, 2008b). In fact, all the testing over the previous forty years had identified only one case of gender fraud.

Caster Semenya and New Tests   The 2012 IOC gender determination policy and similar policies adopted by other sport governing bodies were developed in response to a 2009 case involving Mokgadi Caster Semenya, an eighteen-year-old woman from South Africa. Ms. Semenya was born and raised a female, always identified herself as female, changed clothes and showered with female teammates, and was treated as a female by everyone she knew. But when she ran a surprisingly good time and won a gold medal in the 2009 800-meter finals of the World Championships, some of her opponents and officials from other nations questioned her sex identification. According to their (cultural) standards, she didn't appear feminine, and they accused her of not being a "real" woman.

Complicating matters was that Semenya is a black African from a family and community with few resources and certainly no professional medical providers, whereas those who questioned her sex were mostly whites from wealthy nations. Many black Africans believed that questions about Semenya were based on a combination of racism and white ignorance about people of color, whose beliefs about gender were not shaped by the global fashion industry and the women it used to represent the feminine ideal (Moyo, 2009; SAPA, 2009; Smith, 2009; see also Cooky et al., 2013).

Semenya's time of 1:55:45 when she won the 800-meter race was fast, but prior to 2009 twelve women from nine nations had posted twenty-five times that were faster (http://www.alltime-athletics.com/w_800ok.htm). Additionally, Semenya had never recorded an indoor time better than any of the top 75 indoor racers in history, her 2009 winning time was more than 2 seconds slower than the world-record time, and there were at least 340 officially recorded 800-meter times that were within 2 seconds of Semenya's 2009 winning time. Therefore, her time was neither abnormal nor record-breaking. But according to some people who viewed the world through the distorting filters of orthodox gender ideology in North America and Europe, she looked "too masculine."

Unlike many eighteen-year-old women in wealthy nations, Semenya did not come from a culture where body management practices involve styling hair, using makeup, whitening teeth, removing most facial and body hair, raising voice pitch, adopting particular gestures and speech styles, wearing "cute" clothing, and having cosmetic surgeries to *appear* feminine. So the International Association of Athletics Federations (IAAF), the governing body for track and field, demanded that she have multiple examinations and tests to identify her "true" sex.

Nearly a year later the officials in the governing body announced that Semenya was who she knew herself to be, and they allowed her to compete again in IAAF events for women. But the controversy that swirled around this young woman and information about her supposedly private test results attracted global media attention that severely humiliated her and pushed her into depression (Levy, 2009; Vannini and Fornssler, 2011). Fortunately, her support system was strong and she made a comeback to run in 2011 and at the Olympics in 2012.

The "female fairness" policy that the IOC and other sport organizations developed in response to Semenya's case was put into use in 2011 and 2012. It involves testing only women who "arouse suspicion" by appearing "too masculine" to compete fairly in women's sport events, which isn't a new approach. What is new is that "suspicious women" are not eligible to compete until they submit to a test for *hyperandrogenism,* a condition that exists when women have *naturally* elevated androgen levels. Androgens are steroid hormones produced by glands in the human body's endocrine system. Although both female and male bodies produce androgens, people mistakenly refer to them as "male hormones" because, among other things, they stimulate the development of secondary sex traits during puberty (deepening of the voice, growth of pubic and facial hair, and muscle and bone growth).

The IOC, with advice from a panel of scientists, decided that it would use testosterone level as *the single biological indicator* of "femaleness" in high-performance sports. Testosterone is naturally produced mainly by the testes and adrenal glands in men, but it is also produced by the ovaries and adrenal glands in women. Therefore, it is *naturally* present in nearly all female bodies, just as estrogens, which aid in protein synthesis, are *naturally* present in all male bodies, even though people mistakenly refer to estrogens as "female hormones."

The IOC and the IAAF ruled that women with hyperandrogenism were eligible to compete only if their testosterone level was below "the normal male range" (IAAF, 2011, p. 12). They also ruled that if a woman's testosterone level was found to be in the normal male range, she could compete *only* if additional tests proved that her body is "androgen insensitive," meaning that it does not process or utilize any amount of testosterone (which could actually put her at a disadvantage in many events). But *if* the tests indicate she is *not* androgen insensitive, she cannot compete as a woman until she has drug treatments to suppress her natural production of testosterone to the point that her testosterone level is well below that of a normal man, which makes her a woman according to the IOC and international sport federations.

Unsurprisingly, access to tests and drug treatments under the supervision of a trusted and experienced physician is not equally available to female athletes worldwide. But the IOC and other sport organizations did not see this as being unfair enough to alter their new "female fairness" policy. According to scientists who don't work for or advise the IOC and other sport organizations, there are many problems with the policy (Karkazis et al., 2012; Robson, 2010; Sailors et al., 2012; Shani and Barilan, 2012; Sullivan, 2012; Viloria and Martinez-Patino, 2012; Wahlert and Fiester, 2012). Among them are the following:

1. Policing femininity isn't easy (or fair) because human bodies cannot be divided into two non-overlapping categories.
2. Basing women's eligibility on appearance invites discrimination, discourages females from participating in elite sports, and encourages women to use gender makeover strategies to look "feminine" as defined in "Western" cultures.
3. The testing and treatment requirements are unfair to women who lack resources or who live in places where "Western" medicine is scarce or unavailable.
4. The policy can have harmful psychological consequences for women who are told they are not "woman enough" to compete in high-performance sports.
5. The policy assumes that testosterone is the only factor that identifies sex, and that varying levels of testosterone create unfairness in women's events. But research has identified more

than 200 *biological* factors that provide advantages to high-performance athletes (Ostrander et al., 2009), and research has shown that neither hyperandrogenism nor testosterone levels accurately predict success in athletic events.
6. The policy claims to be about fairness, but it ignores unfair differences in access to training, quality coaching, equipment, technology, sport medicine, and nutritional foods—which influence performance in women's events more than testosterone does.
7. The policy undermines the inclusion of all intersex and transgendered persons because they will be defined as "suspicious."
8. The policy ignores hormones as a source of unfairness in men's events, even though hormonal variations influence the athletic performances of men.

These problems, along with a long, sad history of women failing gender tests, suggest the need for a new approach to defining sex in sports, one that respects athletes' rights to bodily integrity, privacy, and self-identification, and promotes the inclusiveness that should characterize sports as *human* activities. Many scientists who have studied sex variations recommend that *if a person believes she is female, is raised as a female, is identified as female by those who know her, and is legally recognized as a female in her nation, she can compete as a female* (Dreger, 2012; D. Epstein, 2009; Jordan-Young and Karkazis, 2012; Karkazis et al., 2012). This is not perfect, but it may be more practical and fair than the new policy that requires every National Olympic Committee to "actively investigate any perceived deviation in sex characteristics" for the purpose of maintaining "the essence of the male/female classification."

Alice Dreger, a professor of clinical medical humanities and bioethics at Northwestern University, has argued that it is unfair to eliminate female athletes with relatively high levels of naturally produced testosterone; she uses this analogy:

Men on average are taller than women. But do we stop women from competing if a male-typical height gives them an advantage over shorter women? Can we imagine a Michele Phelps or a [Lebrona James] being told, "You're too tall to compete as a woman?" So why would we want to tell some women, "You naturally have too high a level of androgens to compete as a woman?" There seems to be nothing wrong with this kind of natural advantage. (Dreger, 2009)

Natural physical traits have always contributed to an athlete's ability and performance, but as this statement shows, sports continue to be shaped by the ideas and beliefs that constitute orthodox gender ideology. When women have unique anatomical, mutational, or biochemical advantages, they are seen as deviant and freaks of nature; but when men have them, they are seen as "supermen" and wonders of nature that inspire our sense of human potential.

Sports Celebrate Masculinity

Gender is not fixed in nature. Ideas and beliefs about masculinity and femininity are changeable. For these reasons, it takes never-ending "culture work" to preserve a particular way of thinking about gender and what it means to be a man or woman. This work involves being aware of gender boundaries, voluntarily maintaining them through myths and rituals, and "doing" or "performing" gender in conformity with the prevailing gender ideology. It also involves policing gender boundaries by sanctioning (teasing, bullying, or marginalizing) those who push or ignore the boundaries.

Pushing gender boundaries is risky because the two-sex system usually becomes an embodied aspect of self for most people and influences how they experience the world and identify themselves and others (Fenstermaker and West, 2002; Ridgeway, 2009). This makes sports culturally important in many societies, because sports consist of body movements, norms, thinking processes, and organizational structures that reproduce a form of masculinity revolving around strength, power, and conquest. In the social sciences we often refer to this as **hegemonic masculinity**—that is, the

form of masculinity that is most widely accepted in society. As a result, sports are a primary site where boys learn the language and meanings of manhood in their social worlds and use them as reference points for their identities and everyday "manhood acts" that signify heterosexual masculine selves (Anderson, 2009b; Bridges, 2009; Coles, 2009; Connell, 2008; Cooley, 2010; Drummond, 2010; Fair, 2011; Gregory, 2010; Hickey, 2008; Hirose and Kei-ho Pih, 2010; Lee et al., 2009; Light, 2008a; Messner, 2011; Schrock and Schwalbe, 2009; Wellard, 2012).

The celebration of masculinity is vividly presented through the bodily performances of popular male athletes. In many societies today, "great athletes are now kings of the human jungle [and] male athletes have displaced soldiers as the masculine ideal" (Kuper, 2012, p. 14). For example, male athletes who train and sacrifice their bodies for the sake of victory are described as "warriors," and their achievements in power and performance sports are used as evidence of men's aggressive nature, their superiority over women, and their right to claim social and physical space in social worlds. Sociologist Doug Hartmann (2003a) explains:

> [Sport] makes male advantages and masculine values appear so normal and "natural" that they can hardly be questioned. Therein may lie the key to the puzzle connecting men and the seemingly innocent world of sports: they fit together so tightly, so seamlessly that they achieve their effects—learning to be a man, male bonding, male authority, and the like—without seeming to be doing anything more than tossing a ball or watching a Sunday afternoon game. (p. 20)

Hartmann helps us understand how sports reproduce an orthodox ideology that privileges men and favors a form of manhood that clearly separates heterosexual men from women and LGBTIs in the gender order. This is why many men resist changes in rules that would "sissify" their sport by restricting violence or reducing injuries, although the incidence of brain injures is leading some men to rethink their commitment to this dangerous form of masculinity.

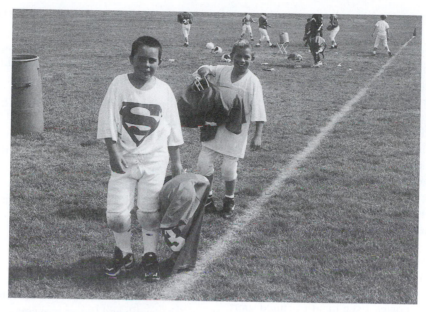

Orthodox gender ideology is reproduced in many men's sports. Some of those sports provide a vocabulary and a set of symbols and stories that erase diverse and contradictory masculinities and present a homogenized manhood in which the heroic warrior is the model of a real man. For boys this can inspire fantasies in which playing the role of warrior and superhero is the substance of being a man. (*Source:* © Jay Coakley)

Sports Legitimize Male Power and Dominance

In 1994, Mariah Burton Nelson, a former Stanford basketball player and an author, wrote a controversial book titled *The Stronger Women Get, the More Men Love Football.* Her point was that strong women, including strong female athletes, threaten people who uncritically accept dominant gender ideology and take football and other heavy-contact sports as "proof" that men and women are different, with men being naturally superior to women. Interestingly, since 1994, women have clearly become stronger in society and sports; at the same time, football, perceived in the United States as the most "manly" sport, has become ever more popular.

With the fading of the symbolic value of traditional markers of masculinity—such as being the sole breadwinner in a family, mentoring sons to success in the labor market, and working in "male jobs"—certain sports have become sites where masculine identity is learned, demonstrated, proved, and acknowledged by others. This is why many men and some women object when women play heavy-contact sports. Watching women wrestle on high school and college teams and watching them play hockey, wrestle, and box in the Olympics, causes these people enough discomfort that they demean and make jokes about those women, trivialize their sports, and express moral or safety concerns about the females who participate in them.

This also is why some people pay high prices to see championship boxing bouts between men, and why male boxers are the world's highest-paid athletes in terms of single-event pay and pay per minute of active competition or game time. In fact, no athletes come close to the boxers' pay per minute.

For example, in a 2012 bout Floyd Mayweather received $32 million, or nearly *$890,000 per minute* over twelve 3-minute rounds, and in 2011 he received $25 million, or *$2.1 million per minute* in a four-round bout. Even Aaron Rogers, who earned $22 million for the 2015 season as quarterback of the Green Bay Packers, makes about $40,000 per minute for his time on the field.

Although playing sports empowers many girls and women as individuals, sport as an institution remains gendered in ways that reaffirm heterosexual male power (McDonald, 2015). A clear example of this is that men control much of the power in women's sports, whereas women control practically no power in men's sports. Girls and women have participation opportunities, but they play sports in contexts where it appears that men are better than women when it comes to being leaders and wielding power. Even in unstructured sport settings, boys and men claim physical space and leadership roles as girls and women almost always resign themselves to being followers rather than leaders (Parker and Curtner-Smith, 2012). Until this gendered form of organization is changed, women will not have equal access to power in business, politics, and other spheres of life.

PROGRESS TOWARD GENDER EQUITY

The single most dramatic change in sports over the past two generations has been increased participation among girls and women. This phenomenon has occurred mostly in wealthy postindustrial nations, but there also have been increases in many developing nations. To remind people in the United States that this change is recent, President Obama noted in 2012 that "it wasn't so long ago that something like pursuing varsity sports was an unlikely dream for young women in America. Their teams often made do with second rate facilities, hand-me-down uniforms, and next to no funding" (Obama, 2012, p. 11).

Recent progress toward gender equity was evident during the 2012 Olympics in London, where for the first time in Olympic history:

- There were no male-only sports (boxing was the last all-male sport).
- Every nation's athletes included women.
- The U.S. team had more women than men.
- An African American woman won a gold medal in all-around gymnastics.
- A female Saudi athlete wore a hijab in judo.

These and other forms of progress have resulted from the following factors:

- New opportunities
- Government legislation mandating equal rights
- The global women's rights movement
- The health and fitness movement
- Increased media coverage of women in sports

New Opportunities

New opportunities account for most of the increased sports participation among girls and women since the mid-1970s. Prior to that time, many girls and women did not play sports simply because there were no teams and programs for them. Today, access to sport participation varies, with white girls and women in middle- and upper-income families having greater access than their peers who are less well-off and living in predominantly ethnic minority neighborhoods. Despite this variation, new teams and programs have inspired and supported interests that were ignored in the past.

> To this generation [of young men], mixed martial arts has come to represent everything that boxing once did to their fathers and grandfathers: the ultimate measure of manhood, endurance, and guts. —Douglas Quenqua, *New York Times* journalist (2012)

Government Legislation Mandating Equal Rights

Many girls and women would not be playing sports today if it weren't for local and national legislation mandating equal rights (Brown and Connolly, 2010). Policies and rules requiring equal opportunities and treatment for females are primarily the result of persistent political actions advocating gender equality (Brake, 2010). For example, the U.S. Congress passed Title IX of the Educational Amendments in 1972 only after years of lobbying by feminists and other concerned citizens. Title IX law declared that *no person in the United States shall, on the basis of sex, be excluded from participation in, be denied the benefits of, or be subjected to discrimination under any educational program or activity receiving federal financial assistance.* The penalty for not following this law is that an educational institution could lose some or all of the funds it receives from the federal government. See Reflect on Sport, "Title IX Compliance" for an explanation of gender equity.

This law made sense to most people when it was applied to education in the classroom, but when it was applied to sports, many people criticized and resisted it. The men who controlled athletic programs in high schools and colleges thought that sharing half of all sport resources with women was outrageous and subversive. Their resistance delayed the enforcement of Title IX for seven years and undermined enforcement of the law through much of the 1980s and between 2005 and 2009. Even today, opposition to Title IX remains strong, but after more than forty years, all court decisions have upheld its legality and its enforcement guidelines.

Initially, those objecting to the law claimed that mandating equity was unfair because boys and men were naturally suited for sports, whereas girls and women were not. In fact, in 1971, there were 3.7 million boys and only 295,000 girls playing high school sports—that is, boys outnumbered girls on teams by 12.5 to 1. Similarly, out of every dollar spent on high school sports, boys received 99 cents and girls received a penny. Overall, the men who ran these programs assumed that these differences actually proved their orthodox ideas about gender and

> There is arguably no piece of progressive legislation that's touched more people's lives than Title IX, which allowed young women equal opportunity in education and sports.
> —Dave Zirin, sport journalist (2012)

demonstrated that Title IX contradicted the laws of nature.

At the college level, it was much the same. In 1971, there were 180,000 men and 32,000 women on intercollegiate teams; 1 of every 10 male college students and 1 of every 100 female students played intercollegiate sports. Women's sport programs received only 1 percent of university athletic budgets, even though student fees and state taxes paid by women were used to fund intercollegiate athletic programs. For many years women subsidized men's college sports with no benefit for themselves.

The impact of Title IX in school sports is clear. Between 1971 and 2014, the number of girls playing varsity high school sports increased from 295,000 to 3.2 million—an increase of more than 1000 percent! Instead of 1 of every 27 high school girls playing on teams, today 1 in 3 play on teams. Similarly, the number of women on college teams increased from 32,000 to over 200,000—an increase of more than 600 percent! Today, about 5 percent of all female college students play intercollegiate sports.

As opportunities for girls and women have increased, the number of boys on high school teams increased from 3.7 million to 4.5 million, and the number of men on college teams increased from 180,000 to 270,000. Another important outcome of Title IX is that many boys and men have learned to see and respect women as athletes—something that rarely occurred prior to the 1990s.

The Global Women's Rights Movement

The global women's rights movement over the past half century has emphasized that girls and women are enhanced as human beings when they develop their intellectual *and* physical abilities. This idea has inspired a wide range of sport participation, even among girls and women who in the past never would have thought of playing sports.

The global women's movement has also influenced changes in the occupational and family roles

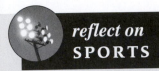

Title IX Compliance
What Counts as Equity?

Title IX compliance requires that a school meet any one of three equity tests:

1. *Proportional participation test*—meaning that the proportion of women on sports teams is similar to the proportion of women enrolled as full-time under-graduate students.
2. *History of progress test*—meaning that a school can document that it has a clear history and continuing practice of expanding its sports programs for female athletes.
3. *Accommodation of interest test*—meaning that a school can prove that it has fully and effectively accommodated the sport participation interests of female students currently enrolled and potential future students in nearby high schools.

Tests 2 and 3 were often used to comply during the early years of enforcing Title IX. But eventually schools had to present concrete numbers to pass test 1 or have exceptional reasons for continuing to claim compliance under tests 2 and 3.

National sport participation numbers for 2015 showed that there were 1.23 million fewer girls than boys playing on high school sport teams (http://www.nfhs.org/ParticipationStatistics/ParticipationStatistics). In NCAA universities, there were nearly 62,000 fewer women than men on teams. In 2015, 43 percent of NCAA athletes were women and 57 percent of NCAA athletes were men.

Participation inequity in universities has become an increasingly serious and contentious matter, as the average student body is now 57 percent female and 43 percent male. In 2005, the George W. Bush admin-istration altered the criteria for complying with the *accommodation of interest test* to appease those who continued to believe that the *proportional participa-tion test* was unfair to men. Instead of demanding mul-tiple indicators to prove that a school met the interests of its female students, the new criteria required only that an email or web-based survey be conducted to identify interests in playing sports. Proponents of Title IX objected to this change, and the Obama adminis-tration reversed course and went back to demanding multiple indicators to show that interests were being met (Brake, 2010; Lederman, 2010).

of women and enabled some of them to acquire the time and resources they need to play sports. When women's rights expand and male control over women's lives and bodies is weakened, more girls and women choose to play sports. Additional changes are needed, especially in poor nations and among low-income women in wealthy nations, but participation opportunities today are far less restricted than they were two generations ago.

The Health and Fitness Movement

Since the mid-1970s, research has made people more aware of the health benefits of physical activ-ity (CDC, 2011; World Health Organization, 2013). This has encouraged girls and women to seek opportunities to play sports. Although much of the publicity associated with health and fitness cam-paigns is tied to the prevailing feminine ideal of being thin and heterosexually attractive, there have been campaigns promoting the *development of phys-ical strength and competence.*

Within ever-shifting cultural limits, well-defined muscles are increasingly accepted as appropriate for women of all ages (Dworkin and Wachs, 2009; Ross and Shinew, 2008; Sisjord and Kristiansen, 2009). Traditional ideas about body image remain strong, as illustrated by fitness fashions and marketing images of women's fitness (Kennedy and Markula, 2010), but many women today reject or temporarily ignore those ideas and focus on physical strength and competence in sports rather than aspiring to look like airbrushed and "photoshopped-to-be-thin" models.

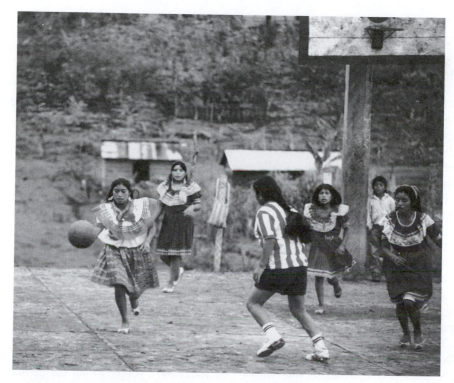

The global health and fitness movement has had a significant impact on creating possibilities for women to participate in sports. However, in some parts of the world, women have played certain sports as part of general community activities. This is the case in Chiapis, Mexico, where the first thing built in a village may be a basketball court that will be used by women and men. In this image, an organized team from the region is playing an informal team from a village. (*Source:* © Tim Russo, Latin America for Free Speech Radio News)

Overall, the health and fitness movement has made many people more aware of the tensions between public health and the companies that produce sporting goods and apparel. Although more girls and women are aware that these companies use insecurity and dissatisfaction with self to promote consumption, they are constantly bombarded with messages and images that stress gender differences and use unreal body images to market products. This often creates mixed message for girls and women: they are encouraged to participate in sports, but the encouraging messages reproduce aspects of orthodox gender ideology that have created past and current inequities in sports. Of course, parents, teachers, physical educators, and those who promote public health offer alternatives to commercially driven messages and images. As these alternatives have influenced the everyday lives of girls and women, sport participation has increased.

Increased Media Coverage of Women in Sports

Women's sports are covered far less often and in less detail than men's sports, but social media and expansion of traditional media now enable girls and women to see and read about the achievements of female athletes in a wide range of sports (Beaver, 2012; Kearney, 2011; MacKay and Dallaire, 2012; Pavlidis and Fullagar, 2013). For example, *espnW* (http://espn.go.com/espnw/) isn't a heavily promoted website, but for those seeking information about women in sport it provides a full range of news, stories, images, and videos. Such exposure encourages girls and women by publicly legitimizing their participation and providing alternatives to media content that portrays women in powerless or sexually objectified terms. When girls see women who are physically strong and competent athletes, it becomes easier for them to envision themselves as athletes and define sports as human activities rather than male-only activities (Daniels, 2009). However, we need research on when and how this occurs.

Media people who make decisions about sports programming realize that they can use women's sports to attract a female audience that they can sell to sponsors. This raises another issue that needs to be studied: Do girls and women who consume mediated women's sports prefer narratives and images that challenge dominant gender ideology, or does such coverage make them uncomfortable? Additionally, do various narratives and images influence girls and women to participate in sports or to abandon ideas and beliefs that might limit their choice of sports, how seriously they play them, and how they integrate sport participation into their lives?

Important today, however, are the new media that increasingly enable girls and women to create their own coverage by posting stories and images online. For example, MacKay and Dallaire (2012) discovered that a Montreal-based group of sportswomen created a "Skirtboarders" blog that presented coverage highlighting alternative femininities and portraying skaters as a polygendered collection of females who revise and poke fun at the paradoxes and socially imposed limitations that come with orthodox gender ideology. This approach, increasingly used by women athletes, provides opportunities for women to present their sport on their terms to all those who follow them online. However, we need more research on the effectiveness of this approach and how it might be expanded to reach more girls and women and show how various forms of sport participation can be integrated into their lives.

GENDER INEQUITIES REMAIN

Anti-discrimination laws combined with the women's rights movement and other factors have produced dramatic increases in sport participation among girls and women. But equity is far from being achieved in the United States and worldwide. The primary areas in which inequalities remain are participation, support for athletes, and access to positions of power (Brake, 2010; Burton, 2015; Cox and Pringle, 2011; Donnelly and Donnelly, 2013b; Donnelly et al., 2015; Erhart, 2011; Grainey and Timko, 2012; Laine, 2012; Sabo and Snyder, 2013; Thomas, 2011; Travers, 2011).

Participation Inequities

Today most people in the United States and many other nations agree that girls and women should have opportunities to play sports. But there continue to be disagreements about the sports they should play and the funding and other resources that should support their participation. These disagreements perpetuate gender inequities worldwide (Donnelly and Donnelly, 2013b; Goldsmith, 2012; Henry and Robinson, 2010; Laine, 2012; Sabo and Snyder, 2013; Smith and Wrynn, 2010). Female athletes remain underrepresented in U.S. high school, college, and professional sports; in most sports and competitions involving teams worldwide, including the Olympics and Paralympics; and in nearly all informal and alternative sports globally.

High School and College Sports in the United States Gender inequities remain in many high schools and colleges, and there is little chance that these schools will be investigated or penalized for violating Title IX. The Office for Civil Rights (OCR) is charged with enforcing Title IX, but it also handles, for the entire United States, all cases

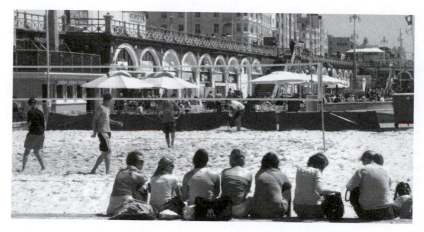

Personal attitudes about gender have become more progressive and less constraining. However, the application of these attitudes in everyday life often lags behind. For example, men are more likely to claim spaces for sports (Kidder, 2013), and women are often left to sit and watch them as seen here at Brighton Beach in England. Additionally, the long-established rules in most sports favor the skills of men and often lead women to be marginalized when they play in mixed-sex games. (*Source:* © Jay Coakley)

of discrimination related to age, race, and disability. Therefore, it lacks resources to investigate more than a few Title IX complaints about gender inequities in sports. Even though reported Title IX violations have been widespread over the past four decades, no school has lost federal funding for violating the law. Noncompliant schools are usually asked to investigate themselves and report back to the OCR, but this process is slow and produces mixed results, with some schools making changes and others resisting or delaying changes for years or indefinitely.

Universities face compliance challenges, but budget crises provide a convenient excuse for not changing athletic programs in ways that would be met with strong protests from those who have a vested interest in men's sports (Pearson, 2010).

A 2011 investigation by reporters at the *New York Times* indicated that even before the budget crisis, dozens of universities had manipulated sport participation data to avoid OCR investigations. Coaches and school officials would count women athletes two and three times by listing

them on rosters for multiple teams, even though teams were the same, such as the indoor and outdoor track teams (Thomas, 2011a). Officials also listed on rosters women who had never tried out for the teams or were cut before seasons began. Some universities counted as women the men who practiced with women's basketball and volleyball teams. In a highly publicized Title IX case, Quinnipiac University did all these things, plus they counted cheerleaders as athletes, even though the cheer team had no budget and no competition schedule that would provide "genuine varsity athletic participation opportunities" (Moltz, 2010, 2011; Sander, 2010).

High schools are seldom investigated for gender inequities in sport participation, even though there were well over 1000 complaints filed from 2010 through early 2012 (Bryant, 2012). In 2010 the National Women's Law Center filed complaints against twelve U.S. school districts where the percentage of female athletes was significantly lower than the percentage of female students according to district data (Nadolny, 2010). The difference was 33 percentage points for Chicago public high

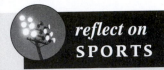

reflect on SPORTS   # Face Off with Football

Many high schools and colleges fail to meet equity goals because of the size and cost of football teams. When a men's football team has 80 to 120 members, awards eighty five scholarships, employs up to ten coaches, and has high operational costs, there is little chance for a women's sport program to match the men's program in terms of budget and number of athletes. Despite this, university officials resist cutting the size and budgets of football teams—even though at least 70 percent of all Division I (that is, "big-time") football programs have more expenses than revenues each year.

This management decision puts many athletic directors in a position where they must save money by dropping men's teams such as wrestling, gymnastics, and diving. When men on these teams become angry, they blame Title IX rather than the management priorities that make football untouchable. But these men don't challenge football, because the culture and structure of the entire athletic department often revolves around it. Defining the loss of men's teams in terms of a men-versus-women conflict makes more sense to many men than challenging the sport (football) that reproduces the gender ideology that many of them have used to form their identities and achieve social status since they were young boys.

When football is the "cultural and structural centerpiece" in schools and communities, gender equity is chronically out of reach. Ironically, some of the best-funded intercollegiate women's sport programs exist in the few dozen universities where big-time football teams enjoy large payouts from bowl games and media rights revenues. The other universities—over 400 of them—have football teams that don't play in lucrative bowl games. These teams incur major financial losses and depend on support from boosters whose identities are deeply grounded in football and the ideologies it reproduces. These ideologies aren't compatible with achieving gender equity, and it is important to understand their impact on the distribution of power and resources in sports.

The point here is that until the status and organization of football is changed, high schools and universities will fail to meet gender equity requirements for participation or access to power in athletic programs.

· ·

schools. Similar complaints were filed against numerous districts nationwide. Nine hundred high schools were named in a complaint filed in California alone.

This flood of complaints occurred in 2009 because people had not filed for the past eight years, knowing that the Bush administration would not investigate them. But despite the Obama administration's commitment to enforce Title IX, there were so many complaints that the OCR dismissed nearly all of them due to a lack of resources to investigate them. With a budget crisis facing the federal government as well as local schools and school districts, there continues to be a strong likelihood that gender inequities will remain or increase simply because there are not enough resources to fully enforce Title IX.

Professional Sports The most glaring gender inequality occurs at the professional level, where women's sports struggle to exist. The WNBA, founded in 1996, is the most successful professional team league for women, but it is floundering financially (Sally Jenkins, 2013). The league has never been profitable, and six of the twelve teams are now owned and supported by NBA teams as the twentieth season (2016) begins. The league's total payroll in 2014–2015 was less than the individual salaries of forty nine NBA players. No WNBA player could earn more than $107,000 for the 2014–2015 season, although bonuses were paid for personal awards, making the playoffs, and winning the WNBA championship. It is also interesting that women playing in leagues outside the United States can make much more than they can in the WNBA. For example, standout player Brittney Griner made twelve times more playing one season in China than she made during her first year in the WNBA.

Women's Professional Soccer (WPS) began operations in 2009 but shut down before the 2012 season, and the Women's United Soccer Association, launched in 2000, closed in 2003 with over $100 million in losses. There are "semiprofessional" women's leagues in volleyball, football, and other sports, but most lose money or operate as nonprofits, and players seldom are paid unless there are cash prizes for winning well-sponsored tournaments.

The Ladies Professional Golf Association (LPGA) and the Women's Tennis Association are long-standing professional organizations. They sponsor tournaments worldwide, but their total annual prize money is considerably smaller than for men's golf and tennis. Interest in these tournaments has declined recently among U.S. spectators and corporations because golfers from Japan, South Korea, China, and Taiwan now win many of the tournaments and because tennis players from the United States now are rarely ranked among the top twenty or even the top 100 in the world.

Olympic and Paralympic Sports   The data in Figure 7.2 and Table 7.1 illustrate that women

in the modern Olympic Games have always had fewer events and participants than men have had. The International Olympic Committee (IOC) had no women members from 1894 to 1981 (87 years), and did not approve a 1500-meter run for women until the 1972 Games in Munich. It was not until 1984 in Los Angeles that women were allowed to run the marathon. Women waited until 1988 and 1996 to run the 10,000- and 5000-meter races, respectively. Wrestling and boxing were not approved until 2004 and 2012, respectively.

The Paralympic Games have an even more dismal record on gender, although some progress occurred recently. Table 7.2 shows that in the Paralympic Winter Games for both 2006 and 2010, male athletes outnumbered female athletes by 4 to 1. This ratio was nearly the same for delegations sent by the United States in those years. At the 2012 Olympic Games in London, the U.S. Olympic team had equal numbers of men and women for the first time in history, whereas only 41 percent of the Paralympic team were women—94 out of 227 athlete. For the Paralympic Games as a whole, women constituted 35 percent of registered athletes. This issue will be discussed more fully in Chapter 10.

Informal and Alternative Sports   Informal games and alternative sports often have gender dynamics

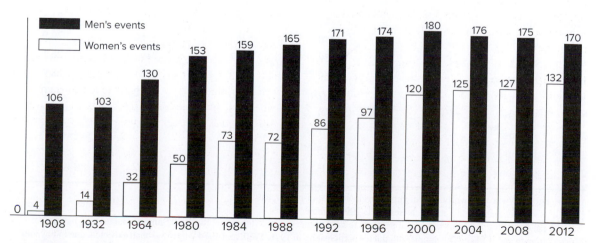

FIGURE 7.2 Number of women's and men's events in selected Summer Olympic Games, 1908–2012.

Table 7.1   Male and female athletes in the modern Summer Olympic Games, 1896–2012

Year	Place	Countries Represented	Male Athletes	Female Athletes	Percent Female
1896	Athens	14	241	0	0.0
1900	Paris	24	975	22	2.2
1904	St. Louis	12	645	6	0.9
1908	London	22	1971	37	1.8
1912	Stockholm	28	2359	48	2.0
1916		Olympics scheduled for Berlin canceled because of World War I.			
1920	Antwerp	29	2561	63	2.5
1924	Paris	44	2954	135	4.4
1928	Amsterdam	46	2606	277	9.6
1932	Los Angeles	37	1206	126	9.5
1936	Berlin	49	3632	331	8.4
1940		Olympics scheduled for Tokyo canceled because of World War II.			
1944		Olympics canceled because of World War II.			
1948	London	59	3714	390	9.5
1952	Helsinki	69	4436	519	10.5
1956	Melbourne	72	2938	376	11.3
1960	Rome	83	4727	611	11.4
1964	Tokyo	93	4473	678	13.2
1968	Mexico City	112	4735	781	14.2
1972	Munich	122	6075	1059	14.8
1976	Montreal	92	4824	1260	20.7
1980	Moscow	81	4064	1115	21.5
1984	Los Angeles	140	5263	1566	22.9
1988	Seoul	159	6197	2194	26.1
1992	Barcelona	169	6652	2704	28.9
1996	Atlanta	197	6806	3512	34.0[*]
2000	Sydney	199	6582	4069	38.2
2004	Athens	201	6262	4329	40.9
2008	Beijing	205	6450	4746	42.4
2012	London	205	6098	4362	41.7

Source: http://www.mapsofworld.com/olympics/trivia/number-of-participants.html.

[*]Twenty-six countries sent only male athletes to the 1996 Summer Games.

Note: These data show 112 years of gradual progress toward gender equity. At this rate, the 2020 Summer Games may have equal numbers of men and women. The number of athletes participating in 1976, 1980, and 1984 was lower than expected, due to boycotts.

Table 7.2   Female and male athletes at recent Paralympic Games, all nations and U.S. delegation

Recent Paralympic Games*	Number of Females (%)	Number of Males (%)	Total Number of Athletes
2012 Summer Games–London 164 nations	1513 (35%)	2756 (65%)	4269
2010 Winter Games–Vancouver 44 nations	121 (24%)	381 (76%)	502
2006 Winter Games–Turin, Italy 39 nations	99 (21%)	375 (79%)	384
2012 Summer Games–London U.S. delegation	94 (41%)	133 (59%)	227
2010 Winter Games–Vancouver U.S. delegation	13 (26%)	37 (74%)	50
2006 Winter Games–Turin, Italy U.S. delegation	11 (20%)	45 (80%)	56

Source: Smith and Wrynn, 2010; International Paralympic Committee; www.teamusa.org.
*Data for China are unavailable

that create access challenges for most girls and women. These activities are nearly always male-dominated/identified/centered. Boys and men usually control the spaces in which they occur and the norms used to acknowledge the identity claims of participants. This discourages girls and women, who must have exceptional skills to be given a chance to participate and be accepted as an athlete by their male peers. In some cases, entry into these activities is "sponsored" by influential male participants who convince others that a particular girl or woman should have a chance to demonstrate her skills as an athlete.

Compared to men, women's access to sport participation opportunities is also limited by the time constraints they face in connection with household chores, child care, and other family responsibilities. Men are more likely than women to compartmentalize their lives, put job and family issues on hold, and take time to work out or play sports (Taniguchi and Shupe, 2014). In the case of married couples, even when both people work full time, women often "subsidize" the sport participation of their male partners by dedicating more of their time to household and family responsibilities.

Title IX law does not apply to informal activities, so changes come slowly. The methods and dynamics of excluding or restricting the participation of girls and women in alternative and informal sports have received little attention in the sociology of sport. However, we do know that various forms of marginalization and exclusion account for significant inequities across most of them (Laurendeau and Sharara, 2005; Wheaton, 2013). At the same time, many boys and men assume that they have priority when using spaces, facilities, or resources.

Research also shows that alternative sports are organized around the values and experiences of boys and young men (Honea, 2007; Laurendeau, 2008; Laurendeau and Sharara, 2008; Rinehart and Syndor, 2003). Observing nearly any skateboard park reaffirms this point. Girls and young women are usually spectators—"skate Bettys" ("groupies" with boards), or they're cautiously assertive participants who work harder than male peers to be taken seriously as athletes (Beal and Weidman, 2003). Additionally, when females do claim space for themselves in bowls or ramp areas, they do so on terms set by the males.

Many so-called extreme sports focus on facing one's fears, taking risks, and pushing normative limits. The boys and young men in these sports say that inclusion is based on skill, guts, and aggressiveness, not gender. However, the vocabulary used in these activities highlights the need to possess "big *cahones*" and the willingness to go "balls to the wall" to be accepted (Meadows, 2006; Roenigk, 2006). Therefore, females must "have balls"—that is, enough skill and guts to attempt and occasionally accomplish creative and dangerous tricks that boys and men deem to be crucial in the identity-claiming process. This vocabulary and the associated norms privilege males and puts females at a disadvantage.

The consequences of the male-dominated/identified/centered culture and organization of alternative sports are seen in media-created, corporate-sponsored versions such as the X Games, Street League Skateboarding Pro Tour, the Maloof Money Cup, and the Dew Tour. Patterns vary from one sport to another, but including women is not usually a high-priority goal in extreme sports.

In response to the masculinized cultures in most alternative sports, some women have created new sports or revised others so they are organized around their own experiences and goals. A good example of this is the rapidly growing flat-track roller derby. The Women's Flat Track Derby Association (WFTDA) in 2016 had about 369 member leagues and 76 apprentice leagues worldwide. As one participant—a young lawyer from Houston—described it,

The roller derby of today is . . . an empowering sport for female athletes. It's also a sisterhood. This is not a sport for dainty girls. Most of the girls are extremely muscular and have some heft to prevent them from being knocked down. . . . (Murphy, 2012)

Roller derby team cultures are organized around the values and experiences of women (Beaver, 2012;

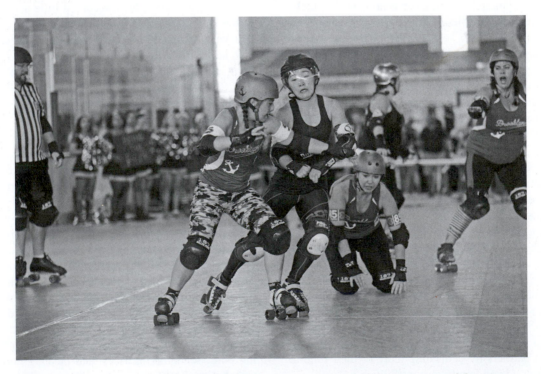

Roller derby teams are becoming widespread as women seek new sport experiences and form new sport cultures. The athletes on these teams embrace a wide array of ideas and beliefs about femininity; many reject a two-category model of gender. Derby bouts are sites where alternative definitions of femininity are presented to spectators. (*Source:* © Bryan Winter/Sports Illustrated/Getty Images)

Donnelly, 2013; Gieseler, 2014; Murphy, 2012; Pavlidis and Fullagar, 2013, 2015). They emphasize inclusion and bring diverse women together in supportive relationships. Attending one of the WFTDA "bouts" shows they have a very different "feel" than male-dominated alternative sports.

Support for Athletes

Female athletes in many U.S. high schools and colleges receive less sport-related support than boys and men receive. This pattern also exists in sport-sponsoring organizations worldwide. Historically, inequities have existed in the following areas:

- Access to facilities
- Quality of facilities (playing surfaces, weight training, locker rooms, showers, and so on)
- Availability of scholarships*
- Program operating expenses
- Provision and maintenance of equipment and supplies
- Recruiting budgets*
- Scheduling of games and practice times
- Travel and per diem expenses
- Opportunity to receive academic tutoring*
- Numbers of coaches assigned to teams
- Salaries for administrators, coaches, trainers, and other staff
- Provision of medical and training services and facilities
- Publicity and media coverage for women's teams and events

Inequities in some of these areas remain a problem in many schools, but they are a greater problem in community programs, where they often go undetected unless someone digs through data from many sources to identify them.

Most people today realize that a lack of support subverts sport participation among girls and women. For well over a century, men built their programs, shaped them to fit their interests and values, generated interest in participation, marketed

them to spectators, and sold them to sponsors. During this time, public funds and facilities, student fees, and private sponsorships were used to fund, promote, and expand programs for boys and men. Few sports for girls and women have enjoyed the support received in the past by sports for boys and men. Today publicly funded, neighborhood-based sport programs have nearly disappeared, and private programs exclude many girls and women who would enjoy local park and recreation funded sports that boys enjoyed from the 1950s through the early 1980s.

Access to Positions of Power

Gender inequality is most glaring when it comes to who holds positions of power in sports. As the visibility and importance of sports for girls and women has increased, most of the positions of power in those sports have been taken by men, and women seldom hold positions of power in men's sports. Data at all levels of competition show that women are severely underrepresented in coaching and administration jobs, especially at the highest levels of power in sports.

Men today coach the majority of women's teams, they occupy the top positions of power in women's sport programs, and they make most of the decisions that impact girls and women in sports. At the same time, women have no noticeable power in men's sports and struggle to gain access to power in women's sports. A forty-year longitudinal study by Vivian Acosta and Linda Carpenter (2012) documents these gender trends for college coaching and administration positions in NCAA institutions:

- When Title IX became law in 1972, women coached 90 percent of women's teams in the NCAA; by 1978 the proportion dropped to 58 percent; in 2016 it was about 43 percent.
- Between 1998 and 2012, there were 2928 new NCAA teams for women; of the head coaches hired for those teams, 1962 (66 percent) were men and 966 (33 percent) were women.
- In 1998, there were 188 woman serving as athletic directors in NCAA institutions (19 percent

These apply primarily to U.S. colleges and universities.

of all ADs); this number grew slightly to 215 (20 percent) in 2012 (men held this position in 807 institutions in 1998 and in 843 institutions in 2012).

- The athletic departments that had female athletic directors in 2012 also had higher proportions of women coaches, and the proportion of female coaches and administrators is lowest in Division I and highest in Division III.
- Only 9.8 percent of all NCAA institutions had a female full-time sports information director in 2012, and 30.7 percent of these schools had a female head athletic trainer (most of these schools are in Division III).
- Since 1971, women constituted between 2 and 3.5 percent of head coaches for men's or gender-combined teams in swimming, cross-country, or tennis.

Table 7.3 presents longitudinal data on the proportion of women's teams with female head coaches for ten popular women's intercollegiate sports from 1977 to 2012. Only soccer had a higher proportion of women coaches in 2012 than in 1977.

Eight of the other nine sports showed at least a 13 percentage point decline in female head coaches. If nearly 80 percent of the administrators and head coaches of all NCAA athletic departments and intercollegiate teams were women, men would be outraged, demand affirmative action programs, and file lawsuits. Up until now, women have been far less demanding as they face limited access to power positions in sports.

The exclusion and underrepresentation of women in coaching and administration exists worldwide (Fagan and Cyphers, 2012; Henry and Robinson, 2010; Laine, 2012; Smith and Wrynn, 2010). The IOC, the world's most powerful sport organization, had *no* women members for eighty-five years (1896 to 1981) and it has never had a female president. In 1996, the IOC promised that in the Olympic movement, women would make up 20 percent of its decision-making boards by 2005. But in 2013, this goal remained far out of reach: Women made up 19 percent of IOC members (20 of 105 total members), but the fifteen-member executive committee has only two women (13 percent). Only two of the twenty-five

Table 7.3   Percentage of female head coaches in the ten most popular women's sports in all NCAA schools, 1977–2012

Sport	1977*	1987	1997	2008*	2012	Percentage Point Change, 1977-2012
Basketball	79.4	59.9	65.2	59.1	59.5	−19.9
Volleyball	86.6	70.2	67.8	55.0	53.3	−33.3
Cross-country	35.2	18.7	20.7	19.2	21.2	−14.0
Soccer	29.4	24.1	33.1	33.1	32.2	+2.8
Softball	83.5	67.5	65.2	64.7	62.1	−21.4
Tennis	72.9	54.9	40.9	29.8	29.9	−43.0
Track and field	52.3	20.8	16.4	18.0	19.2	−33.1
Golf	54.6	37.5	45.2	38.8	41.6	−13.0
Swimming/diving	53.6	31.2	33.7	24.3	26.2	−27.4
Lacrosse	90.7	95.1	85.2	84.6	85.1	−5.6

Source: Carpenter and Acosta (2008) and Acosta and Carpenter (2012); see http://www.acostacarpenter.org/.
*Data for specific sports prior to 1977 and for 2007 are not available.

Table 7.4 Women in National Olympic Committees and International Sport Federations, 2010

	National Olympic Committees	International Sport Federations
Women on executive boards	18%	18%
Women presidents	4%	3%
Women secretaries general	9%	4%

Source: Henry and Robinson, 2010.
Note: Data are based on responses received from 110 of the 205 National Olympic Committees—a 54% response rate, and from 70% of the International Federations.

IOC Commissions are chaired by women, and most women in the IOC serve only on the Women and Sport Commission, which has less power than other commissions. Table 7.4 shows that in 2010 only nine of the 205 National Olympic Committees were headed by women; many of those committees had no women members. The same was true for the International Sport Federations, where men have always occupied all positions of power. Even the influential board of the 2012 London Organizing Committee for the Olympic Games (LOCOG) had only one woman (Princess Anne) among its nineteen members.

Coaching numbers worldwide show that few women coach women's or men's national teams, and women coaches are very rare in professional leagues outside of North America.

The major reasons for the underrepresentation of women in coaching and administrative positions include the following (Henry and Robison, 2010):

• Women are not considered for half of all coaching and administration jobs—that is, coaching men or managing men's programs—due to the mistaken belief that women can't meet expectations in men's sports.

• Men use well-established connections with other men in sport organizations to help them obtain jobs in both women's and men's sports; and compared with men, female applicants for coaching and administrative jobs have fewer strategic connections and networks to obtain jobs.

• Job search committees are primarily composed of men who use evaluative criteria based on orthodox gender ideology, which means that they perceive female applicants as being less qualified than male applicants.

• Many women have not had the support systems and career development opportunities that many men have had.

• Women might not choose careers in coaching and administration, knowing that they would face special challenges working in sport organizations that are male-dominated/identified/centered and where they may be judged more harshly than men are judged.

• Women are more likely to experience sexual harassment, which sets them up to fail or discourages them from remaining in coaching and administration jobs.

These factors affect opportunities *and* aspirations. They influence who applies for jobs, how applicants fare during the hiring process, how coaches and administrators are evaluated, who enjoys coaching, and who is promoted into higher-paying jobs with more responsibility and power (Bruening and Dixon, 2008; Laine, 2012).

People on job search committees seek, interview, evaluate, and hire candidates that they think will succeed in male-dominated/identified/centered organizations. After assessing objective qualifications, such as years of experience and win–loss records, search committee members subjectively assess such things as a candidate's abilities to recruit and motivate players, raise money, command respect in the community (among boosters, fans, sport reporters), build toughness and character among players, maintain team discipline, and "fit into" the athletic department or sport organization.

None of these assessments occurs in a vacuum, and some are influenced by gender ideology in addition to past-performance records. Although people on search committees do not agree on all things, many think in terms that favor men over women. This is because coaching and other forms of leadership often are seen as consistent with traditional ideas about masculinity: a good coach is one who "coaches like a man"—a taken-for-granted principle in male-dominated and male-identified sport cultures.

Under these conditions, women are hired only when they present compelling evidence that they can do things as men have done them in the past. In sport programs and athletic departments where women are scarce, there often is pressure to recruit and hire women so that charges of discrimination can be deflected. Then when women are hired, people often say that the committee "had to hire women." But a more accurate statement would be: "We so blatantly discriminated against women in the past that we would have faced charges of gender discrimination if we didn't hire women now."

When women are hired, they are less likely than men to feel welcome and fully included in sport organizations. Therefore, they often have lower levels of job satisfaction and higher rates of job turnover. This causes some people to conclude that women simply don't have what it takes to survive in sports. But this conclusion ignores the fact that job expectations in sports have been developed over the years by men who have had wives to raise their children, provide emotional support to them and their teams, host social events for teams and boosters, coordinate their social schedules, handle household finances and maintenance, make sure they're not distracted by family and household issues, and faithfully attend games season after season. If female coaches and administrators had an opportunity to build programs and coach teams under similar conditions, job satisfaction would be higher and turnover would be lower.

Finally, some sport organizations have records of being negligent in controlling sexual harassment and responding to complaints from women who wish to be taken seriously in the structure and culture of sport organizations and programs. This means that people in the programs must critically assess the impact of male-dominated/identified/centered forms of social organization on both males and females. Unless this assessment takes place and changes are made, gender equity will never be achieved in coaching and administration.

BARRIERS TO EQUITY

Progress toward gender equity has been significant, but it has stalled since the early-2000s and there continue to be inequities in several important spheres. As strategies are developed to eliminate those inequalities, it is essential to be aware of barriers that will be encountered along the way. These include the following:

1. Budget cuts and privatization of sport programs
2. Resistance to government regulations
3. Few models of women in positions of power
4. A cultural emphasis on "cosmetic fitness" for women
5. Trivialization of women's sports
6. Male-dominated/identified/centered sport organizations

Budget Cuts and the Privatization of Sports

Gender equity is often subverted by budget cuts. Compared with programs for boys and men, programs for girls and women are more vulnerable to cuts because they are less well-established and have less market presence and revenue-generating potential, and less administrative, corporate, community, and institutional support. As relatively new programs they also have development and promotional costs that programs for boys and men no longer have. Therefore, to cut funds equally from sport teams and programs for everyone has a greater negative impact on programs for girls and women. Programs for boys and men are less vulnerable because they've had more than a century to develop legitimacy, institutional support, loyal fans, and sponsors.

As public, tax-supported sport programs are cut, opportunities to play sports become privatized, which also has a disproportionately negative impact on girls and women, especially in low-income areas. Public programs are accountable to voters and regulated by government rules mandating equal rights and opportunities. But private programs are accountable only to the market, meaning that they respond to the needs of dues-paying participants and private sponsors rather than a commitment to gender equity. "Free-enterprise sports" are great for people with money. But they are neither "free" nor "enterprising" when it comes to providing opportunities for girls and women with few financial resources. Commercial programs serve only those who can buy what's for sale, so they are rare in low-income and many ethnic minority areas.

When sport programs are cut in public schools, booster organizations are more likely to step up and provide funds and facilities for boys' sports, such as football, than for girls' sports. Neither boosters nor private providers are required to follow Title IX law, because they receive no support from the federal government. When these resource providers are not committed to gender equity, girls and women lose opportunities.

Resistance to Title IX and Gender Equity

Those who benefit from the status quo often resist government legislation that mandates change. This has been the case for the entire history of Title IX. People today continue to argue that Title IX represents unwarranted government interference in local sport programs, that equity will never be achieved because girls and women are not naturally attracted to sports, and that trying to achieve equity only hurts boys and men (Gavora, 2002; Knudson, 2005). This type of resistance to government legislation has a long history in the United States, and it will not disappear any time soon.

Resistance also occurs among those who are simply opposed to gender equity. For example,

research by Hardin et al. (2012) found that even some sports information directors at Division I universities had negative attitudes toward Title IX and gave women's teams little coverage in their press releases and other information about university sports.

Few Models of Women in Positions of Power

During the years after Title IX became law, women's sports became more visible and important. As this occurred they were taken over by existing men's programs looking to extend their power and influence (Grundy and Shackelford, 2005; Suggs, 2005). During this process, many women lost their jobs as men were hired as coaches and administrators for women's teams and programs. The men who took these jobs were less likely than women to mentor, recruit, and support women seeking jobs in sports. And women coaches often felt pressure to hire male assistant coaches to avoid the perception that they preferred women and disliked men.

As young female athletes observed this, they were less able to envision themselves as future leaders in sports. In their experiences, positions of power automatically went to men and the abilities and contributions of women were valued less than those of men. This remains a barrier to achieving gender equity.

Discussions of this issue often overlook the fact that sex discrimination is illegal in every U.S. public school. This applies to recruiting and hiring new employees in all departments. But nearly every athletic department in those schools discriminates against women when they hire coaches and administrators for men's teams and programs (Sullivan, 2012). They don't even pretend that women candidates would be taken seriously as they interview and hire men. As they do so, they violate national nondiscrimination laws. Men would certainly complain if the same thing occurred when hiring coaches and administrators for women's teams and programs.

Cultural Emphasis on "Cosmetic Fitness"

Girls and women receive confusing cultural messages about body image and sport participation. Although they see powerful female athletes, they cannot escape images of fashion models whose bodies are shaped by food deprivation, cosmetic surgery, and digital modifications. They hear that physical power and competence are important, but they see rewards going to women who appear young, vulnerable, and nonathletic. They are advised to be strong but thin, fit but feminine, in shape *and* shapely. They see attractive athletes packaged and presented as fashion models rather than strong, skilled performers. And they often conclude that even when you're a good athlete, being hot is what really matters.

Cultural messages promoting appearance and beauty clearly outnumber those promoting the pleasure of playing sports. People in marketing departments know that females consume more products when they are insecure about their appearance. Therefore, even ads that show women doing sports are carefully staged to make female consumers feel insecure rather than confident about their bodies. This marketing strategy is so powerful that some females avoid sports until they are thin enough to look "good" and wear "cute" clothes; others combine their sport participation with pathogenic weight-control strategies to become dangerously thin or undernourished.

Overall, the tensions between cosmetic fitness and being physically strong and skilled keep girls and women out of sports, focused on using sports to burn calories so they can eat without guilt, or focused on disciplining themselves through intense training after they've gained weight. Additionally, young women seeking cosmetic fitness sometimes drop out of sports if they gain weight while they train, and others drop out after achieving weight-loss goals. Cultural messages about cosmetic fitness are here to stay, and they continue to be a barrier to gender equity in sports—unless they are critically assessed as subversive tools that foster insecurity and drive consumption.

Trivialization of Women's Sports

The most visible and popular sports in society are based on the values and experiences of men. They usually emphasize skills and evaluative standards that disadvantage women, especially at the elite level. For example, women play football, but they don't hit as hard as men do. They play basketball, but they don't dunk like men. They play hockey, but they don't check or fight like men. They do sports, but they don't do them like men do them.

This logic is grounded in orthodox gender ideology and it is often used to explain why women's sports have lower attendance rates than men's sports and what might be done to boost attendance. For example, in 2012 the international governing body (FIBA) that controls women's professional basketball in Europe told players that they were required to wear shorter shorts to reveal more of their legs. A male executive from FIBA explained that the players are "beautiful athletes and there's no reason not to show it" (Scott, 2012). When Diana Taurasi, a star player in Europe and a former All-American at the University of Connecticut, refused to follow the new rules, she was fined $2600 a game through the eighteen-game season—a total of $47,000, which amounted to half of her salary for the season.

The men at FIBA assumed that the players' sex appeal could attract spectators, recruit sponsors, and boost television rights fees. They did not understand that this strategy had failed in the past (Kearney, 2011). Nor did they know that research by Mary Jo Kane showed that sexualized images of female athletes often lead young people to see the athletes as hot, but they don't increase their interest in women's sports. Kane's conclusion was that "sex sells sex, not women's sports" (Kane, 2011). But many people don't believe this because it doesn't mesh with their orthodox gender ideology.

Male-Dominated/Identified/Centered Sport Organizations

Sports remain closely linked with orthodox forms of masculinity. Males have long used sports as sites to establish their identities as men and gain status in the larger community. The cultures created around sport programs and teams were created to nurture and reaffirm a shared sense of manhood. This gave boys and men a sense of agency—that is, a feeling that they had control over their selves and how others perceived them.

When girls and women finally had opportunities to play sports, the numbers of females playing sports grew exponentially. But their participation has not yet matched male participation rates. The standard explanation for this persistent inequity is that girls and women "just aren't as interested in sports as much as boys and men are." But a more accurate statement would be this: *Compared to boys and men, girls and women experience fewer positive vibes and less support in sports and sport cultures that have been created by and for men for the sake of learning about masculinity*

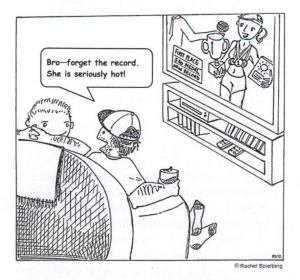

Amy Wamback, former captain of the U.S. Women's Soccer Team, said that teammate Alex Morgan would benefit women's soccer because she had "the mainstream popularity of being the pretty girl" and attracted attention from fifteen- to twenty-five-year-old men. However, research shows that it is the skills of female athletes, not their looks, that sustain interest in women's sports. (*Source*: By permission of Rachel Spielberg)

and reaffirming a shared sense of manhood associated with feelings of power and control.

The point here is that persistent gender inequities are not due to a lack of interest among girls and women as much as they are due to sports and sport organizations that do not directly reflect girls' and women's lived experiences in the same way that they reflect and reaffirm the lived experiences of boys and men.

Research shows that when programs and teams are organized to enable girls and women to control and claim ownership of sports on an organizational and institutional level, gender equity becomes more achievable (Cooky, 2004, 2009). This reminds us that in addition to influencing identity, cultural expectations, and social interaction, gender is embedded in the logic of organizations and institutions (Messner, 2011; Risman and Davis, 2013). It is this organizational and institutional dimension of gender that now slows progress toward equity in sports. In other words, we can change our attitudes and personal relationships to be more inclusive and less constrained by orthodox gender ideology, but until we change the taken-for-granted gender logic that structures so much of sport and sport organizations, full gender equity will not be achieved. When the logic of gender that shapes cultural and organizational processes in sports is based on the values and experiences of men, these processes privilege men more than women and lead women to feel less welcome and less personally accepted in all aspects of sports than their male peers feel.

GENDER EQUITY AND SEXUALITY

Sports have long been associated with male heterosexuality and have been sites for the expression of homophobia and the performance of heterosexual masculinity as a cultural ideal. The history and sociology of sport have clearly documented these patterns and how they have impacted the lives of lesbians, gay men, bisexuals, transsexuals, and intersex persons (LGBTIs). However, in certain regions of the world, including much of northern and western Europe, Australia, New Zealand, and

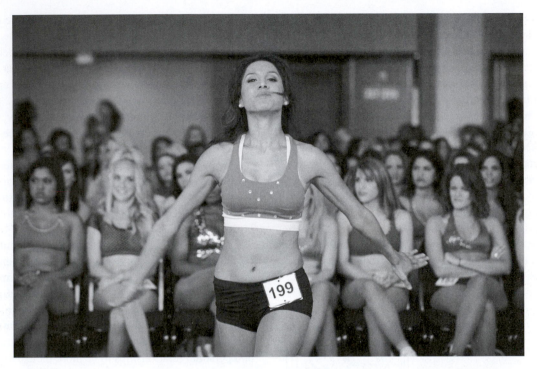

The gendered choices faced by athletes are also faced by women who apply for cheerleading and dance teams in men's professional sports. The bodies of these women are being assessed to see if they meet the criteria of the "judges" for an NBA team. If they do, they will be allowed to try out. In the process, the women view one another in objectified ways, as this photo illustrates. If these women had the power to choose how they are included and represented in sports, would they choose this? (*Source:* © Michele Eve Sandberg/ZUMA Press/Corbis)

North America, there have been changes that are based on a rejection or qualification of orthodox gender ideology (Pew Global Attitudes Project, 2013). As a result, sports have become a less supportive context for homophobia. Examples include the following:

- Players using homophobic slurs have been criticized by other players, reprimanded by team and league officials, and portrayed negatively in mainstream media.
- Both male and female athletes have publicly supported LGBTI rights and marriage equality, and have occasionally been among the most vocal and visible supporters of LGBTI rights.

- Sport organizations, groups of athletes, and Outsports.com have discussed strategies that might be used by athletes if and when they decide to come out (Branch, 2011b).
- The National Hockey League (NHL) and its Players' Association (NHLPA) in early 2013 became the first major men's sport organization to issue a formal statement condemning anti-LGBTI bigotry and promising support for players who come out.
- Major League Soccer has suspended and fined players for using homophobic slurs.
- The Ultimate Fighting Championship (UFC) suspended a mixed martial arts fighter and mandated that he do community service for

the LGBTI community as a result of his transphobic comments about a fighter who had undergone male-to-female gender reassignment surgery.

- The coverage of and response to Jason Collins, the first gay man in a major men's spectator sport (basketball), to come out was positive and supportive with very few exceptions (Collins, 2013). The same occurred when Robbie Rogers came out and rejoined the Los Angeles Galaxy in Major League Soccer (Witz, 2013) and when Steven Davies, a cricket player in England, came out in 2011 (Davies, 2011). There was even public support for Orlando Cruz, a Mexican boxer, who came out in 2012 (Eberle, 2012).
- More than a dozen U.S. states now have rules to enable transgender students to compete on teams that correspond with their gender identities rather than the sex designation listed in their school records. The NCAA has a policy supportive of transgender participation, and other sport organizations, including the IOC, LPGA, USGA, and many Olympic sport federations, now have policies that specify the conditions under which transgendered athletes may participate (Griffin and Carroll, 2012; Griffin and Taylor, 2011).
- The high-profile women athletes who have come out recently have received little news coverage because it has been thirty five years since Martina Navratilova came out in 1981, and coming out today is accepted to the point that it is no longer a major news story.

This list should not be taken to mean that LGBTIs face no challenges or live free of the sting of homophobia and significant forms of discrimination. Men in elite sports are not knocking the door down coming out, and fears about the negative consequences of coming out remain strong in both men's and women's sports. More serious fears are felt by bisexuals and transgendered people, and people with intersex characteristics are not making public announcements about their sexuality.

Homophobia continues to exist. It is based on the notion that homosexuality is abnormal, deviant, or immoral—out of normative boundaries according to orthodox gender ideology. It fuels prejudice, discrimination, harassment, and violence directed toward those identified or believed to have identities or sexual orientations that are something other than heterosexual.

When LGBTIs play sports, many remain careful to keep their sexual identities private or disclosed only to select friends and family members. They either have mixed or confused feelings about themselves or they fear possible negative responses from others. But as more people come out publicly, it normalizes gender nonconforming identities. Still, the anticipated challenges of coming out can be overwhelming, so most LGBTI athletes remain closeted, pass as heterosexual, selectively reveal their identity only to trustworthy others, or choose sports in which they are less likely to confront homophobia.

Lesbians in Sports

Acceptance of gender-nonconforming athletes is greater in women's than in men's sports. But even today, homophobia discourages some females from playing certain sports and from appearing "too masculine" or "too unfeminine" if they do play sports. Additionally, it still causes some parents to steer daughters away from teams, programs, and sports that they believe attract lesbians or have lesbian coaches.

When girls and women fear the label of *lesbian* or fear being associated with lesbians, they may avoid certain sports, limit their commitment to sports, de-emphasize their athletic identities, or emphasize a "presentation of self" that explicitly portrays heterosexuality. For example, some young women in the United States avoid cutting their hair short because it could elicit "homophobic teasing" from peers. At the same time, homophobia prompts lesbian athletes to keep their identity secret even though it limits their relationships with teammates and leads to loneliness and isolation (Sartore and Cunningham, 2010).

Pat Griffin's groundbreaking book *Strong Women, Deep Closets: Lesbians and Homophobia in Sports* (1998) provides clear evidence that "sports and lesbians have always gone together" (p. ix). She notes that this evidence has been ignored in the popular consciousness, largely because of cultural myths about lesbians. Although most myths have been challenged and discredited, some people continue to believe them. For example, some think that lesbians are predatory and want to "convert" others to their "way of life," which is judged to be immoral and depressing. When lesbian athletes, coaches, and administrators perceive that people think this way, they often feel undervalued and experience a sense of isolation (Norman, 2012). When heterosexual peers believe these myths or even wonder about their veracity, they fear or avoid lesbian athletes and coaches; when coaches and administrators believe them, they're less likely to hire and promote lesbians in coaching and sport management.

The homophobic statement "No bow, Lesbo" is still used on some women's teams and accounts for what has become a standard practice of girls and young women wearing cute bows with their ponytails when they play games (Soffian, 2012). In college sports there are still heterosexual coaches who describe their teams as "wholesome" and being grounded in "family values" to indicate that they are anti-lesbian; and they may infer that competing programs don't have the same values—implying that their coaches or some players are lesbian. Such expressions of homophobia have discouraged many young women from pursuing careers in coaching, especially at the college level where recruitment competition can be intense.

Some women's sports and teams are characterized by a "don't ask, don't tell" culture in which lesbians hide their identity to play the sports they love without being harassed or marginalized. However, this strategy has costs, and it slows changes that might defuse or erase homophobia. Overall, a "don't ask, don't tell" approach affects both heterosexual women and lesbians, all of whom restrain their actions to avoid suspicions or being labeled as lesbians.

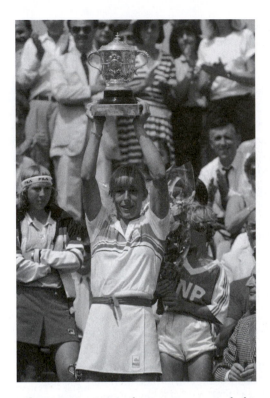

When Martina Navratilova came out as a lesbian in 1981, she was a top-ranked tennis player. The response to her was vicious and personal. She lost millions in endorsement deals and faced challenges from other players, fans, the media, and the general public. But she initiated a sport-based conversation about sexuality that continues today. Additionally, she opened the door for many to follow her, including–over thirty years later–a few men in professional sports. (*Source:* © Jean-Yves Ruszniewski/ TempSport/Corbis)

Pat Griffin encourages people to be open and truthful about sexual identity, but she explains that lesbians must be prepared to handle everything from hostility to cautious acceptance when they come out. She points out that handling challenges is easier when (a) friends, teammates, and coaches provide support; (b) there are local organizations that challenge homophobia and advocate tolerance; and (c) there is institutionalized legal protection and support for gays and lesbians in organizations, communities, and society.

Gay Men in Sports

Changes related to attitudes about homosexuality have not been as significant in men's sports as in women's sports. The culture of many men's sports continues to support a vocabulary of homophobia. However, heterosexual male athletes have in recent years been generally supportive of teammates who come out to them. This has led sociologist Eric Anderson and others (Anderson, 2009b, 2011a, 2011c; Jarvis, 2013) to conclude that there is a more inclusive form of masculinity emerging among young men, a form that rejects the rigidity of orthodox gender ideology (Adams and Anderson, 2011). But Anderson and others note that homophobia remains a serious threat in men's sports and discourages nearly all gay athletes, coaches, and administrators from coming out, especially in highly visible elite sports where it would attract widespread media attention and could seriously disrupt the person's life and interfere with meeting expectations as a player or manager.

Playing certain sports remains a rite of passage for boys to become men. Male athletes in power and performance sports remain models of heterosexual manhood in most societies today. Therefore, there is much at stake in maintaining silence about gay men in sports, discouraging them from revealing their identities, and policing gender boundaries in and through men's sports. This preserves the integrity of existing normative gender boundaries, the glorified status of male athletes, and male access to power and influence in society.

A seldom discussed consequence of homophobia is that it creates a context in which boys and men resist or feel ashamed of their feelings of affection toward other men. When this occurs, they may mimic violent caricatures of masculinity to express their manhood—or it may force male athletes to express their connections with each other through head-butts, belly bashers, arm punches, forearm crosses, fist bumping, and other ritualistic actions that disguise intimacy. These "man gestures" may make boys and men feel good, but they also keep them in the "act like a man box," which limits possibilities in their lives (Glickman, 2011).

Intersex and Transgender Persons in Sports

What happens to people born with a combination of male and female sex traits or those who have a gender identity or behavior that falls outside stereotypical norms (for example, transgender) or does not match the gender they were assigned at birth (for example, transsexual)? This population consists of an estimated 120 million intersex people worldwide and many times that number who identify themselves as "trans" in some way (Fausto-Sterling, 2000a). Where do they fit in sports mostly organized around a rigid two-sex system?

> Instead of having sport based on sex, we're basing it on ability. We're moving away from the idea of sex-based sport. —Kristen Worley, transgender Canadian cyclist (Findlay, 2012)

Although intersex and "trans" women and men have been ignored or routinely excluded from nearly all organized sports, recent policy changes have allowed transsexuals to participate in sports if they meet certain conditions related to standard medical practices and hormone therapy (Cavanagh and Sykes, 2006; Griffin and Carroll, 2012; Randall, 2012; Torre and Epstein, 2012).

The IOC policy approved in 2004 states that trans athletes may compete in their chosen gender category if they undergo sex-reassignment surgery and have had two years of approved medically supervised hormone therapy—either testosterone suppression for a male-to-female transition or testosterone supplementation for a female-to-male transition.

The IOC policy is relatively restrictive compared to the NCAA policy, which does not require surgery because it is prohibitively expensive for college students and sometimes takes a few years to complete—and genitalia have no influence on sport performance. Additionally, NCAA policy states that only one year of testosterone suppression is needed for trans women to be eligible to compete in women's sports; and trans men have a medical exemption to take testosterone under approved medical supervision so they can compete with men without violating drug rules, but they are not eligible to compete in women's sports.

Trans athletes push gender boundaries, but intersex people born with "a reproductive or sexual anatomy and/or chromosome pattern that doesn't fit typical definitions of male or female" create confusion for those using orthodox gender ideology (Griffin and Carroll, 2012, p. 50). The policies developed in the wake of the controversy over Caster Semenya attempt to deal with this by forcing athletes to make a choice that is medically unnecessary—which means that they will be challenged through lawsuits.

Taken collectively, these policies illustrate how difficult it is to develop regulations so that human bodies will fit into sports that are organized around a rigid two-sex classification system (Pieper, 2012). Even more difficult, is renegotiating the meaning of sex to eliminate the traditional normative boundaries that separate females and males into nonoverlapping categories. Gender activists refer to "the queering of sport" as the process of renegotiating or eliminating the two-sex system and becoming fully gender-inclusive. The dynamics of this process have been studied by Ann Travers and her colleagues at Simon Fraser University in British Columbia (Travers, 2006, 2013b; Travers and Deri, 2011). Travers spent over four years observing and interviewing participants in lesbian softball leagues throughout North America. In the process, she investigated tensions around the inclusion of transgender and transsexual persons on teams. Initially she found that many players in the leagues used the two-sex system to identify themselves and others, even though nearly all of them rejected parts of orthodox gender ideology. Therefore, many were uncertain or uncomfortable about allowing a person to play in a "lesbian-women's league" if that person could not be clearly classified as female. In particular, this affected those just beginning the transition from male-to-female and those close to completing the transition from female-to-male.

Most players in the league used a hormone-centered perspective to determine if a person was female enough to play without raising questions about fairness. As a person's testosterone and strength declined, she was accepted in the league, but as testosterone and strength increased it was difficult to know when a person should drop out and play on a men's team. When players were making a female-to-male transition, some others were upset that the person had chosen to identify and live as a man instead of remaining a lesbian, and those making the transition felt unfairly abandoned after they had spent much of their lives working for lesbian rights and sustaining supportive lesbian communities and networks.

As Travers and Deri (2011) observed and analyzed these dynamics, they noted "how deeply complicated it is to attempt to re-negotiate sexed boundaries." But they also noted that it was possible to shift away from organizing sport around a rigid two-sex system. This shift is a work in process, and whether or how it will continue is uncertain. The next challenge for the softball league might be how to include those who reject gender as an identity category because it imposes unnecessary limits on who they can be, how others treat them, and how they live their lives.

STRATEGIES TO ACHIEVE EQUITY

Achieving gender equity requires action by people possessing the critical awareness needed to transform gender ideology and how we do sports, so that participation is accessible and meaningful regardless of gender. This is a complex and challenging task (Packard, 2009). There are practical and effective ways to accomplish it, but they involve both women and men and a willingness to critically assess how we do sports today.

Using the Law and Engaging in Grassroots Activism

In societies where laws mandate equal gender opportunities, as in the case of Title IX in the

United States, those laws must be consistently enforced over time. If this does not occur, backsliding into past inequities is likely, due to the continuing male-dominated power structure in most sport organizations. Even though nearly everyone in the United States supports the idea of gender equity, those who control sport organizations often resist changes because they are likely to lose some power in the process (Gregory, 2009). Additionally, many head coaches who have grown up in the post–Title IX era have little understanding of the meaning of gender equity, how to achieve it, and how it relates to their jobs (Staurowsky and Weight, 2011). This means that legal action is one strategy, but certainly not the only or most important strategy, for achieving gender equity (Love and Kelly, 2011). Most effective are grassroots actions that identify inequities and support needed changes. Such actions include the following:

- Confront discriminatory practices in your athletic department and become an advocate for female athletes, coaches, and administrators.
- Insist on fair and open employment practices in the entire organization, including the athletic department.
- Keep a record of equity data and have an independent group issue a public "gender equity report card" every three to four years for your athletic department or sport program.
- Learn and educate others about the history of gender discrimination in sports and how to recognize the subtle forms of discrimination that operate in sport worlds that are male-dominated, male-identified, and male-centered.
- Object to practices and policies that decrease opportunities for women in sports, and inform the media of them.
- When possible, package and promote women's sports as

revenue producers, so there will be financial incentives to increase participation opportunities for women.

- Recruit female athletes into coaching by establishing internships and training programs.
- Use women's hiring networks when seeking coaches and administrators in sport programs.
- Create a supportive work climate for women and establish policies to eliminate sexual harassment in the athletic department.

These actions involve a combination of research, public relations, advocacy, political participation, and education. They're based on the assumption that equity will be achieved only through persistent struggle, effective political organization, and changes that enable girls and women to play sports on their own terms rather than exclusively on terms set by boys and men with power and influence.

Boys and Men Benefit from Gender Equity

When discussing gender, people often focus on girls and women and overlook the fact that ideas and beliefs about gender have major relevance for boys and men, whose lives may be negatively affected by hegemonic masculinity (Brand and Frantz, 2012). This is true in sports, the military, work occupations, and on the streets, where men are seriously injured, killed, and put in situations that damage their health and well-being at alarming rates.

Gender equity in sports is not just a woman's issue. It also involves creating options for boys and men to play sports based on pleasure and participation more than power and performance. The widely accepted belief that the actions of boys and men are driven by testosterone, innate aggressive tendencies, and a need to dominate others creates havoc in everyday life, and it

> One thing standing in the way of further progress for many men is the same obstacle that held women back for so long: overinvestment in their gender identity instead of their individual personhood. Men are now experiencing a set of limits—externally enforced as well as self-imposed. —Stephanie Coontz, social historian (2012)

promotes heavy-contact sports as primary molders of manhood. But those sports don't fit the interests and body types of most boys and young men, who would benefit if resources and attention were not so disproportionately dedicated to football in high schools and colleges. In fact, most adult males never play tackle football, primarily because they know it is not healthy to do so. Offering opportunities to learn and enjoy sports that can be played throughout life would be a sounder educational choice, and such opportunities could be available if those who control education were not so influenced by dominant gender ideology and the myths of masculinity developed a century ago.

Sports currently privilege men over women, but they also privilege some men over other men. When men realize that certain sports perpetuate attitudes and orientations that often undermine their relationships with one another and with women, they are more inclined to view sports critically and become agents of change. Men who want to move beyond expressing their fondness for each other by teasing, pranking, hazing, mock fighting, and getting memorably drunk at the next football game have good reason to join with those women concerned with critically assessing dominant sport forms in their society. In the process they will learn how to work, play sports, and live with men and women in mutually supportive relationships. The alternative is to remain stuck in the mud of hegemonic masculinity, blame women for problems, and seek refuge by watching bigger, stronger, faster men play sports in which they hurt each other.

Research indicates that growing numbers of young men today, including those who play sports, are more critical of hegemonic masculinity than was common in previous generations. Studies by Becky Beal (1995), Belinda Wheaton (2004), Eric Anderson (2015), and Hamish Crocket (2012) each found that there are growing numbers of male athletes who use "alternative," "ambivalent," "inclusive," and "moderated" masculinities, to identify and assess themselves and male peers. Although this was often an individual or small group/team phenomenon, these young men did not view themselves or others through the lens of orthodox gender ideology. Instead, they avoided violence, expressed their emotions, demonstrated compassion, and nurtured relationships on and off the field that blurred rigid divisions between masculine and feminine. As more boys and men do this, there will be more social and cultural space for inclusive masculinity as well as various forms of gender-inclusive ideology. This makes gender equity more achievable, and opens up possibilities to create sports that provide people of all ages and abilities with more welcoming and satisfying experiences.

Empowering Girls and Women Through Sports

Sport participation offers girls and women opportunities to connect with the power of their bodies and reject notions that females are naturally weak, dependent, and powerless. It helps them overcome the feeling that their bodies are objects to be viewed, evaluated, and consumed. The physical skills and strength often gained through sport participation help some girls and women feel less vulnerable, more competent and independent, and more in control of their physical safety and psychological well-being (Kane and LaVoi, 2007; Ross and Shinew, 2008; Weiss and Wiese-Bjornstal, 2009).

However, empowerment does not occur automatically when a girl or woman plays sports, nor does a sense of personal empowerment always lead to actions that push the normative boundaries of heterosexual femininity or promote gender equity in sports or other spheres of life. Feeling competent as athletes does not guarantee that women will critically assess gender ideology and gender relations or work for equity in sports or society. Those who play at elite levels often avoid becoming "boat rockers" critical of the gender order (Cole, 2000b; Cooky, 2006; Cooky and McDonald, 2005; J. S. Maguire, 2006, 2008; McDonald, 2015).

The reasons for this lack of action and activism include these:

1. Many female athletes feel they have much to lose by promoting civil and human rights

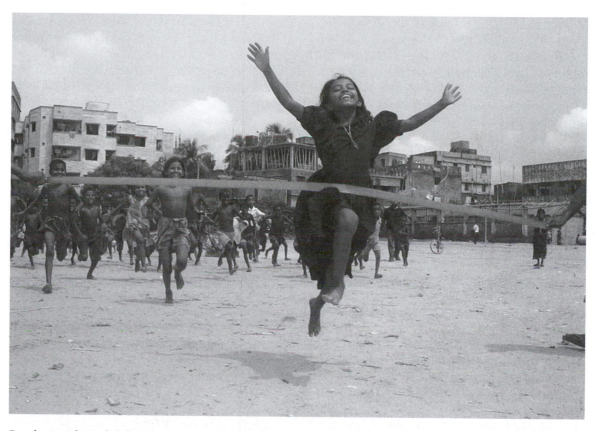

Developing physical skills often improves health and provides girls and women with a sense of empowerment. This is true for Reshma, a seven-year-old in Dhaka, Bangladesh. However, if the culture and social structure in Bangladesh are organized to systematically prevent females from gaining power in society, Reshma's joy and sense of empowerment from winning this race will be temporary and difficult to convert into the power to make needed institutional changes as an adult (see Musto, 2013). (*Source:* Photo courtesy of The Hunger Project; www.thp.org/)

issues for women, because others might identify them as ungrateful or tag them with labels such as *radical, feminist,* or *lesbian.*

2. The corporate-driven "celebrity feminism" promoted through media sports today focuses on individualism, attractiveness, and consumption rather than the everyday struggles faced by ordinary girls and women who want to play sports but also require child care, health care, a decent job, and safe access to sport facilities.

3. The "empowerment discourses" in women's sports emphasize *individual* self-empowerment through physical changes that enhance self-image and self-esteem; they do not emphasize social or cultural changes at an institutional level, which is where gender equity must be achieved.

4. Female athletes, even those with high media profiles and powerful bodies, have little control over their own sport participation and little political voice in sports or society as a whole.

Similarly, women hired and promoted into leadership positions in major sport organizations are expected to promote power and performance sports in society. The men who control sport organizations are not usually eager to hire women who put *women's issues* on the same level as *sport issues.* Of course, not all female leaders become uncritical cheerleaders for power and performance sports, but it takes effort and courage to critically analyze sports and use one's power to change them.

Changing the Way We Do Sports

Gender equity involves more than just pushing boundaries to make space for new ways to define and perform masculinity and femininity. It also requires erasing normative boundaries so that sports are fully gender-inclusive—for LGBTIs *and* heterosexual males and females. This process has begun, but much more needs to be done before it is achieved (Bartholomaeus, 2012; Packard, 2009).

When people talk about gender equity, they usually focus on how to increase opportunities for girls and women to play competitive sports in the same way that boys and men play them. The standard policy position is that the best way to serve girls and women is to provide the same programs and opportunities that boys and men have. But research has shown that this approach does not effectively attract most females or keep them involved (Flintoff, 2008).

The reasons for this are many. First, compared with boys, girls are less likely to see themselves as having sport skills, so they are less likely to take advantage of sport participation opportunities.

Second, the discourse that pervades competitive sports at nearly all levels is and always has been heavily masculinized and is full of military terms and metaphors that appeal more to boys than girls.

Third, men are more likely than women to be coaches and managers in these programs, which leads girls and women to question who is really valued in sports. Additionally, many girls see

during their first competitive sport experiences that "Dad knows sports" and "Mom knows how to pack a lunch."

Fourth, sports are so sex-segregated that many females see them as representing ideas and beliefs that sustain aspects of orthodox gender ideology that are questioned outside of sports. When high schools and colleges fail to sponsor sex-integrated sports, they miss an opportunity to challenge those ideas and beliefs.

Fifth, when males and females play together, males usually assume leadership roles even when they may not be the best leaders. This might make boys and men feel good, but it doesn't make playing sports much fun for girls and women.

Of course, there are notable exceptions to each of these points, and that is partly why many girls and women *do* play sports today. But equity isn't achieved through "exceptions." Nor is it sustainable when sport providers say that "girls just aren't interested" when girls fail to show up for or stay involved in sports that are just like the sports that the boys play. It takes work to critically assess sport programs in terms of gender equity and look beyond the girls and women who learned to love sports and remain in them because they overlook, passively accept, or actively endorse the hypermasculinized discourse, organization, and culture that often characterize them. When sports reproduce orthodox gender ideology, and when orthodox gender ideology is embedded in the logic and structure of sports and sport organizations, those who feel constrained by that ideology will not feel welcome.

From a practical (and pragmatic) standpoint this means that there is a need for new and creative sport programs, discourses, and images that enable more people to see space for themselves as participants. To some degree this has been done in small, exclusive schools where there are no varsity sport teams

> For women, pain and injury are simply the price of playing elite sport; for men, they are badges of masculinity . . . Sports is a gendered institution, whose values, symbols, and core audience are masculine, even with the rise of women's sports and women athletic stars.
>
> —Judith Lorber, professor emerita, City University of New York (2007)

but there are sport participation opportunities for all students. It has also been done in the Gay Games, the lesbian softball leagues studied by Travers and Deri (2011), and in community-based programs where men and women have collectively created welcoming sport cultures and meaningful sport experiences that begin to erase constraining normative boundaries tied to the two-sex system (Atencio and Beal, 2011; Beaver, 2012; Crocket, 2012; MacKay and Dallaire, 2012). Research will help us understand if and when these new approaches are really moving close to gender equity.

In the long run, achieving gender equity requires a dual approach: creating new and different sports as well as expanding opportunities and creating for women and gender nonconformers access to power positions in established sports. Changes are more likely if people currently in positions of power can envision and create alternatives for the future, and if those who already envision new forms of sport gain access to power and resources so they can make their visions a reality.

All of us contribute to achieving gender equity when we critically assess how we talk about and do sports. After all, there is no need for all sports to represent the perspectives of men who are fascinated by domination and conquest. Full equity means that all people have a wide range of choices when it comes to organizing, playing, and giving meaning to sports.

summary

IS EQUITY POSSIBLE?

Gender equity in sports is integrally tied to ideology, power, and structural issues. Although ideas and beliefs about masculinity and femininity are fluid and subject to change, the prevailing gender ideology in many societies remains organized around the assumption that there are essential differences between females and males, that exceptions to heterosexuality are abnormal, and that men are physically stronger and more rational than women. This orthodox ideology is questioned today, but it has shaped the current culture and organization of sport.

Sports today are sites at which this gender ideology is reaffirmed *and* resisted. However, because most sports are based on a two-sex model, the impact of resistance is limited. Even when women achieve excellence in sports, it occurs in a context in which ideas and beliefs about male–female differences and the "natural" physical superiority of men over women are reaffirmed. Gender inequities persist because sports have traditionally been organized to be male-dominated, male-identified, and male-centered. This makes them very difficult to change, and at the same time they provide a less welcoming context for girls and women than for boys and men.

Orthodox gender ideology also leads to the marginalization of lesbians, gay men, bisexuals, transgender, and intersex persons in sports. The culture and organization of sports today celebrate primarily a form of masculinity that leaves little space for those who do not conform to it. This means that sports often are sites where people must push gender boundaries to increase normative spaces for themselves and to be acknowledged as athletes.

Despite orthodox gender ideology, sport participation among girls and women has increased dramatically since the late 1970s. This change is the result of new opportunities, equal rights legislation, the women's movement, the health and fitness movement, and increased publicity given to female athletes. But full gender equity is far from being achieved, and future increases in participation rates will not be automatic.

The reasons to be cautious when anticipating more changes in the future include budget cuts and the privatization of sports participation opportunities, resistance to government policies and legislation, backlash in response to changes favoring women, a relative lack of female coaches and administrators, a cultural emphasis on cosmetic fitness among women, the trivialization of women's sports, and the existence of homophobia.

More women than ever are playing sports and working in sport organizations, but gender inequities continue to exist in participation opportunities, support for athletes, jobs for women in coaching and administration, and informal and alternative sports. Even when sport participation gives women a feeling of personal empowerment, the achievement of full gender equity is impossible without a critical analysis of the gender ideology used in sports and society. Critical analysis is important because it guides efforts to achieve equity and it shows that there are reasons for men to join women in trying to achieve equity.

Historically, gender ideology and sports have been organized around the values and experiences of heterosexual men. Real and lasting gender equity depends on changing the dominant definitions of masculinity and femininity and the way we do sports. Useful strategies include developing new sports and sport organizations and changing existing sports. Changes also depend on using new ways to talk about sports. Until there are significant changes in gender ideology and the logic embedded in sports and sport organizations, full gender equity will not be achieved.

SUPPLEMENTAL READINGS

Reading 1. Definition and explanation of sexual terms used in Chapter 7
Reading 2. A continuing struggle: Women's professional basketball in the United States
Reading 3. Reasons for men to police gender boundaries: Preserving access to power
Reading 4. Using myths to exclude women from sports
Reading 5. Links to South African newspaper coverage of Caster Semenya
Reading 6. "The stronger women get, the more men love football"

Reading 7. History, impact, and current status of Title IX
Reading 8. Building muscles: Pushing boundaries of femininity?
Reading 9. Lost between two categories: The girl who didn't fit

SPORT MANAGEMENT ISSUES

- You've been asked to address the directors of international federations for Olympic sports. They want you to identify for them the major areas in which gender equity has not been achieved and how they might move more quickly toward the achievement of equity. List the main points you would include in your address.

- You have just been appointed chairperson of a special committee charged with studying gender equity in your university's sport programs. You must develop a research design and present it to the rest of the committee members. Outline the kinds of data you will collect to assess whether equity has been achieved. What do you expect to find at your university?

- As an assistant athletic director you have been asked to recommend changes to produce full gender inclusion in athletic department culture. The existing culture has been created by heterosexual men over the years as they occupied positions of power and made all major decisions about the organization of the department. Discuss the major issues that will be covered in your recommendations and the major strategies to creating full inclusion.

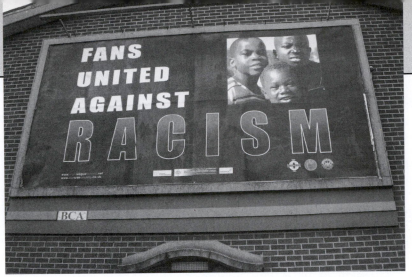

(*Source:* © Michael Boyd, Irish Football Association)

RACE AND ETHNICITY

Are They Important in Sports?

It is American culture that is principally responsible for the perpetuation of the concept of race well after its loss of scientific respectability by the mid-20th century.

> —Justin E. H. Smith, philosopher, Concordia University, Montreal (2013)

Native American mascots and other stereotypes persist because most Americans remain thoughtless, lacking the resources, knowledge, and skills to think critically about them.

> —C. Richard King, author of *Redskins: Insult and Brand* (2016)

There is no [big-time college] football team without black labor. . . . [no] million dollar coaching salaries . . . [no] weekly economic boon . . . bringing in millions in revenue to hotels, restaurants, and other assorted businesses without black labor.

> — Dave Zirin, independent sport journalist (2015a)

South Asian American men are not usually depicted as ideal American men. . . . To combat such stereotypes, some use sports as a means of performing a distinctly American masculinity. . . . [B]asketball, for these South Asian American players is not simply a whimsical hobby, but a means to navigate and express their identities in 21st century America.

> — Stanley Thangaraj, author of *Desi Hoop Dreams* (2015)

Learning Objectives

- Understand the concepts of race, ethnicity, and minority group, and distinguish between them.

- Explain why race is a social construction and how racial categories are based on social meanings rather than a valid biological classification system.

- Explain how and why race and racial ideology have been linked with sports in the United States.

- Explain why scientists and others have searched for sport performance genes in bodies with dark skin and why this is a misleading and futile exercise.

- Explain the author's sociological hypothesis about the relationship between skin color and athletic performance.

- Identify factors that have influenced sport participation among African Americans, Native Americans, Latinos and Latinas, and Asian Pacific Americans.

- Explain why the use of Native American images for team names, logos, and mascots has been a contentious issue in the United States.

- Understand the expressions of racism and bigotry in European sports and the factors that currently influence those expressions.

- Identify the major challenges related to race and ethnic relations in sports today, and explain how they are different from the challenges faced throughout most of the twentieth century.

Sports involve complex racial and ethnic issues, and their relevance has increased as global migration and political changes bring together people from diverse racial and ethnic backgrounds. The challenges created by racial and ethnic diversity are among the most important ones that we face as we live, work, and play together in the twenty-first century (Edwards, 2000).

Ideas and beliefs about race and ethnicity traditionally influence self-perceptions, social relationships, and the organization of social life. Sports reflect this influence and are sites where people challenge or reproduce racial ideologies and existing patterns of racial and ethnic relations in society. As people make sense of sports and give meaning to their experiences and observations, they often take into account their beliefs about skin color and ethnicity. The once-popular statement, "White men can't jump," is an example of this.

Not surprisingly, the social meanings and experiences associated with skin color and ethnic background influence access to sport participation, decisions about playing sports, the ways that people integrate sports into their lives, and the organization and sponsorship of sports. People in some racial and ethnic groups use sport participation to express their cultural identity and evaluate their potential as athletes. In some cases, people are identified and evaluated as athletes, coaches, or media commentators based on the meanings given to their skin color or ethnic background. Sports also are cultural sites where people formulate or change ideas and beliefs about skin color and ethnic heritage.

This means that sports are more than mere reflections of racial and ethnic relations in society: they're sites where racial and ethnic relations perpetuated and changed. Therefore, the depth of our understanding of sports in society depends on what we know about race and ethnicity in various social worlds.

This chapter focuses on the following topics:

1. Definitions of *race* and *ethnicity,* as well as the origins of current ideas about race

2. Racial classification systems and the influence of racial ideology in sports
3. Sport participation patterns among racial and ethnic minorities in the United States
4. The dynamics of racial and ethnic relations in sports worldwide

DEFINING *RACE* AND *ETHNICITY*

Discussions about race and ethnicity are confusing when people don't define their terms. In this chapter, **race** refers to *a population of people who are believed to be naturally or biologically distinct from other populations.* Race exists only when people use a classification system that divides all human beings into distinct categories, which are believed to share genetically based physical traits passed from one generation to the next. Racial categories are developed around the meanings that people give to real or assumed physical traits that they use to characterize a racial population.

Ethnicity is different from race in that it refers to *a cultural heritage that people use to identify a particular population.* Ethnicity is not based on biology or genetically determined traits; instead, it is based on cultural traditions and history. This means that an **ethnic population** is *a category of people regarded as socially distinct because they share a way of life, a collective history, and a sense of themselves as a people.*

Confusion sometimes occurs when people use the term *minority* as they talk about racial or ethnic populations. In sociological terms, a **minority** is *a socially identified population that suffers disadvantages due to systematic discrimination and has a strong sense of social togetherness based on shared experiences of past and current discrimination.* Therefore, *not all* minorities are racial or ethnic populations, and *not all* racial or ethnic populations are minorities. For example, whites in the United States often are identified as a race, but they would not be a minority unless another racial or ethnic population had the power to subject them to systematic discrimination that would collectively disadvantage whites as a population category in American society. Similarly, Polish people in Chicago are considered an ethnic population, but not a minority. Mexican Americans, on the other hand, are an ethnic population that is a minority because of past and current discrimination experienced by people with Mexican heritage.

African Americans often are referred to as a race because of the meanings that people have given to skin color in the United States; additionally, they are referred to as an ethnic group because of their shared cultural heritage. This has led many people to use *race* and *ethnicity* interchangeably without acknowledging that one is based on a *classification of physical traits* and the other on *the existence of a shared culture.*

Sociologists attempt to avoid this conceptual confusion by using the term "race" only when they refer to the social meanings that people have given to physical traits such as skin color, hair texture, facial characteristics, stature, and others. These meanings, they say, have been so influential in society that shared ways of life have developed around them. Therefore, many sociologists today focus on ethnicity rather than race, except when they study the social consequences of widespread ideas and beliefs about skin color in particular.

This information about race confuses many people who have been socialized to take for granted that race is a biological reality. To be told that race is not a biological fact but a social creation based on the meanings given to skin color is difficult to accept. But it begins to make sense when they learn why the concept of race was created and how ideas and beliefs about race were used to gain political and economic power around the world.

CREATING RACE AND RACIAL IDEOLOGIES

Physical and cultural diversity is a fact of life, and people throughout history have categorized one another, often using physical appearance and cultural characteristics to do so (AAA, 2006a, 2006b, 2006c). However, the idea that there are distinct, identifiable races is a recent invention. Europeans developed it during the seventeenth century as they explored the world and encountered people who looked and lived unlike anything they'd ever known. As they colonized regions on nearly every continent, Europeans created classification systems to distinguish the populations they encountered. They used the term *race* very loosely to refer to people with particular religious beliefs (Hindus), language or ethnic traditions (the Basque people in Spain), histories (indigenous peoples such as New World "Indians" and "Aborigines"), national origins (Chinese), and social status (chronically poor people, such as Gypsies in Europe or the Untouchables in India).

More specific ideas about race emerged during the eighteenth century in connection with religious beliefs, scientific theories, and a combination of political and economic processes (Fredrickson, 2003; HoSang et al., 2012; Omi and Winant, 1994, Winant, 2001, 2004, 2006, 2015). Over time, people in many societies came to use the term *race* to identify populations they believed were naturally or biologically distinct from other populations. This shift from a descriptive to a biology-based notion of race occurred as light-skinned people from northern Europe sought justification for colonizing and exercising power over people of color around the world.

Intellectuals and scientists in the seventeenth though twentieth centuries facilitated this shift by developing appearance-based racial classification frameworks that enabled them to "discover" dozens of races, subraces, collateral races, and collateral subraces—terms that many scientists used as they analyzed the physical variations of people in colonized territories and other regions of the world (see http://www.understandingrace .org/history/science/early_class.html).

Faulty "scientific" analyses combined with the observations and anecdotal stories told by explorers led to the development of **racial**

ideologies—*interrelated ideas and beliefs that are widely used to classify human beings in categories assumed to be biological and related to attributes such as intelligence, temperament, and physical abilities.* The racial classification models developed in Europe were based on the assumption that the appearance and actions of white Europeans were normal and that all deviations from European standards were strange, exotic, primitive, or immoral (Carrington, 2007; Carrington and McDonald, 2001). In fact, Europeans captured dark-skinned people to put them in exhibitions at which they were displayed to demonstrate that they were naturally inferior to light-skinned Europeans (AAA, 2006c). In this way, the "whiteness" of northern Europeans became a standard against which the appearance and actions of *others* ("*those* people") were measured and evaluated. In other words, the regions that were white-dominated also became white-identified and white-centered in a social and cultural sense.

From the eighteenth through much of the twentieth century, people from northern and western Europe used these racial ideologies to conclude that people of color around the world were primitive beings driven by brawn rather than brains, instincts rather than moral codes, and impulse rather than rationality. This way of thinking, they believed, gave them "moral permission" to colonize and subsequently exploit, subjugate, enslave, and even murder dark-skinned peoples without guilt or sin in religious terms (Carrington, 2007; Carrington and McDonald, 2001; Fredrickson, 2003; Hoberman, 1992; PBS, 2006; Smedley, 1997, 1999, 2003; Winant, 2001, 2004, 2006). Some also used racial ideology to define people of color as pagans in need of spiritual salvation. These people worked to "civilize" and save the souls of dark-skinned "others" to the point that white historians identified people of color as "the white man's burden."

Over time, these racial ideologies became widely accepted, and white people used them to connect skin color with other traits including intelligence, character, physical characteristics and skills and, in the United States, they were used to

strip humanity from "black, red, brown, and yellow" people.

Racial Ideology in the United States

Racial ideology in the United States is unique. It emerged during the seventeenth and eighteenth centuries as proslavery colonists developed moral justifications for enslaving Africans and treating them inhumanely. By the early nineteenth century, many white people believed that race, represented primarily by skin color, was a mark of a person's humanity and moral worth. Africans and Indians, they concluded, were subhuman and incapable of being civilized. By nature, these "colored peoples" were socially, intellectually, and morally inferior to light-skinned Europeans—a fact that was accepted without question by most light-skinned Euro-Americans (Morgan, 1993; PBS, 2006; Smedley, 1997). This ideology came to be widely shared for three reasons.

First, as the need for political expansion became important to the newly formed United States, the (white) citizens and government officials who promoted westward territorial expansion used racial ideology to justify killing, capturing, and confining "Indians" to reservations.

Second, after the abolition of slavery, white Southerners used the "accepted fact" of black inferiority to justify hundreds of new laws that restricted the lives of "Negroes" and enforced racial segregation in all public settings; these were called Jim Crow laws (DuBois, 1935).

Third, scientists at prestigious universities, including Harvard, did research on race and published influential books and articles claiming to "prove" the existence of race, the "natural superiority" of white people, and the "natural inferiority" of blacks and other people of color (St. Louis, 2010).

The acceptance of this ideology was so pervasive that the U.S. government established policies to remove Native Americans from valued lands, and in 1896, the U.S. Supreme Court ruled to legalize the segregation of people defined as "Negroes." The opinion of the court was that "if one race be inferior to the other socially, the Constitution of the United States cannot put them on the same plane" (U.S. Supreme Court, *Plessy* v. *Ferguson,* 1896). This ruling, even more than slavery, has influenced race relations from 1896 until today because it legitimized hundreds of laws, political policies, and patterns of racial segregation that connected whiteness with privilege, full citizenship, voting rights, and social-intellectual-moral superiority over people of color in the United States (Nobles, 2000).

As patterns of immigration changed between 1840 and 1920, people came to the United States from Ireland, southern Europe (Italy, Greece, Sicily), China, Japan, and Israel. At the same time, racial ideology was used to link whiteness with one's identity as an American. Therefore, the question of who counted as white was often hotly debated as immigrant populations tried to claim American identities.

Through the late 1800s and early 1900s, Irish, Jewish, Italian, Japanese, Chinese, and all Eastern European and Western Asian populations were considered to be nonwhite and, therefore, unqualified for U.S. citizenship or running for a federal political office. As some members of these ethnic populations objected to being classified as "colored" and denied citizenship, they took legal cases all the way to the Supreme Court to prove that they had ancestral links to "real" white people. It took some of these people many years to establish or prove their whiteness because whites with Western and northern European backgrounds carefully maintained racial ideology to preserve their privilege in U.S. culture and society.

These cases confused the Supreme Court because the justices differed on how to define "white." For example, in one case the court ruled that even though a Japanese man was light-skinned, he was not a true Caucasian, so he could not become a citizen. But in another case the court ruled that even though a man had ancestors from the Caucasus region, his dark skin disqualified him for citizenship (Dewan, 2013).

Today we are witnessing changes in the form of white and black racial categories as the idea of race is modified in connection with (a) new patterns of immigration from Asia, Latin America, and the Caribbean; (b) new expressions of anti-immigrant attitudes; and (c) the racialization of Latino and new Asian immigrant populations (Kretsedemas, 2008). But this has not changed the traditional belief that whiteness is a pure and innately special racial category and this has, through recent history, created a deep cultural acceptance of racial segregation and inequality and strong political resistance to policies addressing the racial and ethnic inequities that remain part of American society (Kochhar et al., 2011).

The Problem with Race and Racial Ideology

Research since the 1950s has produced overwhelming evidence that the concept of *race* is not biologically valid (Fox, 2012; Graves, 2002, 2004; Omi and Winant, 1994; PBS, 2006; Smith, 2012). This point has received powerful support from the Human Genome Project, which demonstrates that external traits such as skin color, hair texture, and eye shape are not genetically linked with patterns of internal differences among human beings. We now know that there is more biological diversity within any so-called racial population than there is between any two racial populations, no matter how different they may seem on the surface (AAA, 1998; PBS, 2006; Williams, 2005).

Noted anthropologist Audrey Smedley (2003), explains that the idea of race has had a powerful impact on history and society, but it has little to do with real biological diversity among human beings. This is because the concept of *race* identifies categories and classifications that people use to explain the existence of social differences and inequalities in social worlds. In this sense, race is a myth based on socially created ideas about variations in human potential and abilities that are assumed to be biological.

This conclusion is surprising to most people in the United States because they've learned to "see" race as a fact of nature and use it to sort people into what they believe are biology-based categories. They've also used ideas and beliefs about race to make sense of the world and the experiences of various people. Racial ideology is so deeply rooted in U.S. culture that many people see race as an unchangeable fact of nature that cannot be ignored when it comes to understanding human beings, forming social relationships, and organizing social worlds.

To put biological notions of race aside requires a major shift in thinking for many people. This complicates the world and changes our sense of how it is organized and how it operates. But when we move beyond traditional racial ideology in the United States, we see that definitions of race and approaches to racial classification vary widely across cultures and over time. Thus, a person classified as black in the United States may not be considered "black" in Brazil, Haiti, Egypt, or South Africa, where approaches to racial classification have been created under different social, cultural, and historical circumstances. For instance, golfer Tiger Woods is classified as a black person in the United States, Asian in Japan, and Thai in Thailand where his mother was born.

Definitions of race have also varied from one U.S. state to another through much of the twentieth century. This created confusion because people could be legally classified as black in one state but white in another. To add more confusion, definitions within states changed over time as social norms changed (Davis, 2001). These cultural and historical variations indicate that race is a social construction instead of a biological fact.

Another problem with *race* is that racial classification models force people to make clear racial distinctions on the basis of *continuous traits* such as skin color and other physical traits possessed to some degree by all human beings. Height is an example of a continuous physical trait: All humans have some height, although height measurements vary along a continuum from the shortest person in the world to the tallest. If we wanted to classify all human beings into particular height categories, we would have to decide where and how many lines we should draw along the height continuum. This could be done only if the people in charge of drawing the lines could come to an agreement about the meanings associated with various heights. But agreements made in one part of the world would likely vary from agreements made in other parts of the world, depending on social and cultural factors that influenced the relevance of height. Therefore, in some societies a 5-foot, 10-inch-tall man would be classified as tall, whereas other societies might define "tall" as 6 feet, 5 inches or more. To make classification matters more complicated, people sometimes change their ideas about what they consider to be short or tall. Additionally, evidence clearly shows that the average height of people in different societies changes over time as diets, lifestyles, and height preferences change, even though height is a physical, genetically based trait (Bilger, 2004). This is why the Japanese now have an average height nearly the same as Americans, and northern Europeans have surpassed Americans in average height (Komlos and Lauderdale, 2007).

Like height, skin color also is a continuous physical trait. As illustrated in Figure 8.1, it varies from *snow white* at one end of the spectrum to *midnight black* on the other, with an infinite array of shades in between. When skin color is used to identify racial categories, the lines drawn to identify different races are based on the meanings given to skin color by the people doing the classifying. Therefore, the identification of races is based on social agreements about where and how many racial dividing lines to draw; it is not based on objectively identifiable biological division points.

Racial classification in the United States was traditionally based on the "one-drop rule." This meant that any person with a black ancestor was classified as "Negro" (black) and could not be considered a white person in legal terms even if he or she appeared to be white, although some people with black ancestors "passed" as white. This approach to racial classification was based on decisions that white people made in an effort to perpetuate slavery, maintain the "purity" of the "white race," discourage white women from forming

Snow white   Midnight black

Skin color continuum

Skin color is a continuous trait that varies from snow white to midnight black with an infinite number of skin tones in between. As with any continuous trait,° we can draw as many "racial category lines" as we choose and locate them anywhere on the skin color continuum. We could draw two lines or thirty, depending on our ideas about "race." Our decisions about the number and location of lines are determined by social agreements, not biological facts. Over the past four centuries, some people have drawn many lines; others have drawn few; and scientists today draw none, because they no longer try to classify human beings into distinct races.

°Continuous traits are such things as height, weight, nose width or length, leg length or leg length to body height ratio, number of fast or slow twitch muscle fibers, brain size or weight—any trait that varies continuously from low to high or from a few to many.

FIGURE 8.1 Racial ideology: Drawing lines and creating categories.

sexual relationships and having children with black men, deny interracial children legal access to the property of their white parent, and guarantee that white men would retain power and property in society (Davis, 2001). The uniquely American one-drop rule was based on a social agreement among white men, not on any deep biological significance of "black blood" or "white blood."

The problem with using the one-drop rule to define race is that "mixed-race" people are erased in history (and sports). It also creates social and identity confusion. For example, when golfer Tiger Woods was identified as "black," he declared that he was *Cablinasian*—a term he invented to represent that he is one-fourth Thai, one-fourth Chinese, one-fourth African American, one-eighth Native American, and one-eighth white European (Ca-bl-in-asian = *Ca*ucasian + *Bl*ack + *In*dian + *Asian*). However, when people use the one-drop rule, they ignore diverse ancestry and identify people as black if they are not "pure" white. This is why mixed-race persons in sports are described as black, even though a parent or multiple grandparents are white, Asian, and/or Latino (Middleton, 2008).

To say that race is a social construction does not deny the existence of physical variations between

human populations. These variations are real and some are meaningful, such as those having medical implications, but they don't correspond with the skin-color–based racial classification model widely used in the United States. Additionally, scientists now know that physiological traits, including particular genetic patterns, are influenced by the experiences of individuals and the long-term, collective experiences of specific populations. Therefore, a population that has lived for centuries in a certain mountainous region in Africa may have more or less of a specific trait than a population that has lived for centuries in Norway, but this does not justify classifying these populations as different races due to skin color.

Even though race is not a valid biological concept, its social significance has profoundly influenced the lives of millions of people for three centuries. As people have developed ideas and beliefs around skin color, the resulting racial ideologies have become deeply embedded in many cultures. These ideologies change over time, but they continue to exert a powerful influence on people's lives.

The primary problem with *race* and racial ideologies is that they have been used for three centuries to justify the oppression and exploitation of one population by another. Therefore, they've fueled and supported **racism,** defined as *attitudes, actions, and policies based on the belief that people in one racial category are inherently superior to people in one or more other categories.* In extreme cases, racial ideology has supported beliefs that people in certain populations are (1) childlike beings in need of external control; (2) subhuman beings that can be exploited without guilt; (3) forms of property that can be bought and sold; or (4) evil beings that should be exterminated through **genocide,** or *the systematic destruction of an identifiable population.*

Another problem with race and racial ideologies is that they foster the use of **racial stereotypes,** or *generalizations used to define and judge all individuals who are classified in a particular racial category.* Because stereotypes provide ready-made evaluative frameworks for making quick judgments and conclusions about others, they're widely used by people who don't have the opportunity or aren't willing to learn about those who have experiences influenced by popular beliefs about skin color. Knowledge, when used critically, undermines racial stereotypes and gradually erodes the ideologies that support them and the racism that often accompanies them.

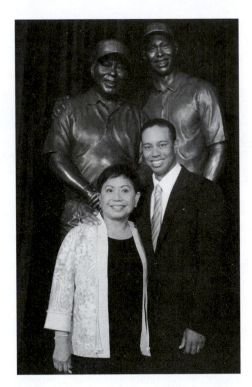

Tiger Woods is only one-fourth African American, yet he is often identified as black because of the way race has been defined by most people in the United States. His mother, Kultida Woods, shown here, is half Thai and half Chinese. (*Source:* © AP Photo/Damian Dovarganes)

Race, Racial Ideology, and Sports

None of us is born with a racial ideology. We acquire it over time as we interact with others and learn to give meanings to physical characteristics such as skin color, eye shape, the color and texture of hair, or even specific bodily movements. These meanings become the basis for classifying people into racial categories and associating categories with particular psychological and emotional characteristics, intellectual and physical abilities, and even patterns of action and lifestyles.

This process of creating and using racial meanings is built into the cultural fabric of many societies, including the United States. It occurs as

we interact with family members, friends, neighbors, peers, teachers, and people we meet in our everyday lives. And it is reproduced in connection with general cultural perspectives as well as images and stories in children's books, textbooks, popular films, television programs, video games, song lyrics, and other media content. We incorporate these perspectives, images, and stories into our lives to the extent that we perceive them to be compatible with our experiences. In this sense, race is much like gender: it consists of meaning, performance, and organization (see Chapter 2, pp. 39–41).

The influence of race and racial ideologies in sports has been and continues to be significant in the

United States.[1] Through the nineteenth and much of the twentieth century when African Americans engaged in clearly courageous acts, many whites used racial ideology to conclude that such acts among blacks were based on ignorance and desperation rather than *real* character. Some white people went so far as to say that black people, including black athletes, did not feel pain in the same way that white people did and this permitted black people to engage in superhuman physical feats and endure physical beatings, as in the case of boxers (Mead, 1985).

Many white people concluded that the success of black athletes was meaningless because blacks were driven by simple animal instincts instead of the heroic and moral character that accounted for the achievements of white athletes. For example, when legendary boxer Joe Louis defeated a "white" Italian for the heavyweight championship of the world in 1935, the wire service story that went around the world began with these words:

> Something sly and sinister and perhaps not quite human came out of the African jungle last night to strike down [its opponent] . . . (in Mead, 1985, p. 91)

Few people today would use such blatantly racist language in public, but traditional ideas about race continue to exist and there is ample evidence of racist feelings in online comments and responses. Therefore, when eight "black" athletes line up in the Olympic finals of the 100-meter dash or play in an NBA All-Star game, many people talk about "natural speed and jumping abilities," and some scientists study dark-skinned bodies to discover the internal physical traits that will explain why they outperform white athletes.

On the other hand, when white athletes do extraordinary physical things, dominant racial ideology leads people to conclude that it is either expected or a result of fortitude, intelligence, moral character, strategic preparation, coachability, and good organization. Therefore, few people want to study white-skinned bodies when all the finalists in multiple Olympic Nordic (cross-country skiing) events are "white." When white skiers from Austria and Switzerland—countries half the size of Colorado, with one-twentieth the population the United States—win World Cup championships year after year, people don't say that they succeed because their white skin is a sign of genetic advantages. Everyone already knows why the Austrians and Swiss are such good skiers: They live in the Alps, they learn to ski before they go to preschool, they grow up in a culture in which skiing is highly valued, they have many opportunities to ski, all their friends ski and talk about skiing, they see fellow Austrian and Swiss skiers winning races and making money in highly publicized (in Europe) World Cup competitions, and their cultural heroes are skiers. But this is a cultural explanation, not a biological one.

When athletes are white, racial ideology focuses attention on *social* and *cultural* factors rather than biological and genetic factors. This is why scientists don't do studies to identify hockey genes among white Canadians, weight-lifting genes among white Bulgarians, or swimming genes among white Americans. Dominant racial ideology prevents people from seeing "whiteness" as an issue in these cases because it is the taken-for-granted "normal," standard against which "others" are viewed. When dominant racial ideology serves as the cultural foundation of a white-dominated, white-identified, and white-centered society, the success of white athletes is the benchmark against which the actions and achievements of others are assessed and interpreted. At the same time, the success of black athletes is seen as an invasion or a takeover—a "problem" in need of an explanation focused on dark-skinned bodies.

When people don't ask critical questions about their own ways of viewing race and ethnicity, it will influence their explanations of human performance in sports. These explanations are based on three things: (1) the facts people choose to examine; (2) the ways that people classify and organize those

[1](Bass, 2002; Carrington, 2013; Cashmore, 2008, 2012; Cooley, 2010; Cooper, Gawrysiak, and Hawkins, 2013; Doidge, 2013; Elling and van Sterkenburg, 2008; Hallinan and Jackson, 2008; Hannah, 2011; Hartmann, 2012; Hawkins, 2010; Hylton, 2008; King, 2010; Leonard, 2011; Leonard and King, 2010, 2011; Lomax, 2008; Montez de Oca, 2011; Rowe, 2010; Seung-Yup Lim, 2012; Sailes, 2010; St. Louis, 2010; Sze, 2009; Thangaraj, 2012; Withycombe, 2011; Yep, 2012.)

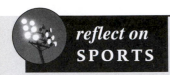

"Jumping Genes" in Black Bodies
Why Do People Look for Them, and What Will It Mean If They Find Them?

When people seek genetic explanations for the achievements of black athletes, sociologists raise questions about the validity and purpose of the research. Let's use the search for "jumping genes" to explore whether these questions are justified. Our questions about research on this issue are based on two factors: (1) many current ideas about the operation and effects of genes are oversimplified and misleading, and (2) jumping is much more than a simple physical activity.

OVERSIMPLIFIED AND MISLEADING IDEAS ABOUT GENES

Most people have great hopes for genetic research. They see genes as the building blocks of life that will enable us to explain and control everything from food supplies to human feelings, thoughts, and actions. These hopes have inspired studies seeking genes for violence and intelligence as well as genes that enable people to sprint fast, run record-setting marathons, and jump high. Genes, in the minds of many people, constitute the "magic bullets" that will enable us to understand the world and everyone in it.

According to Robert Sapolsky (2000), a professor of biology and neurology at Stanford University, this notion of the "primacy of the gene" fosters deterministic and reductionist views of human actions and social problems. The actions of human beings, he explains, cannot be reduced to particular genetic factors. Even though genes are important, they do not work independently of the environment. Research shows that genes are activated and suppressed by many environmental factors; furthermore, even the *effects* of genes inside the human body are influenced by numerous environmental factors, including the body itself (Cloud, 2010; Coop et al., 2009).

Genes are neither autonomous nor the sole causes of important, real-life outcomes associated with our bodies and what they do. The influence of genes is regulated by chemicals that exist in cells as well as chemicals, such as hormones, that come from other parts of the body. These chemicals and hormones are influenced, in turn, by a wide range of external environmental factors. For example, when a mother rat licks and grooms her infant, her actions initiate biochemical processes that activate genes regulating the physical growth of the infant rat. Therefore, geneticists have concluded that the operation and effects of genes cannot be separated from the environment that switches them on and off and influences their effects in the body (Davids et al., 2007).

The point is this: Genes do not exist and operate in environmental vacuums. This is true for genes related to diseases and genes related to jumping. Furthermore, we know that physical actions such as jumping, running, and shooting a basketball all involve one or more clusters of multiple genes. To explain overall success in a sport such as basketball or soccer requires an investigation of "at least 124 genes and thousands, perhaps millions, of combinations of those genes," and this would provide only part of an explanation (Farrey, 2005). The rest would involve research on why people choose to do certain sports, why they're motivated to practice and excel, how they're recognized and identified by coaches and sponsors, and how they're able to perform under particular conditions.

This means that discovering "jumping genes" would be exciting, but it would *not* explain why one person jumps higher than another, *nor* would it explain why people from one population jump, on average, higher than people from other populations. Furthermore, no evidence shows that particular genes related to jumping or other complex sport performances vary systematically with skin color or any socially constructed ideas about race and racial classifications (PBS, 2006, episode 1).

JUMPING IS MORE THAN A PHYSICAL ACTIVITY

Jumping is much more than a mechanical, springlike action initiated by a few leg muscles. It is a total body movement involving neck, shoulders, arms, wrists, hands, torso, waist, hips, thighs, knees, calves, ankles, feet, and toes. Jumping also involves a timed coordination of the upper and lower body, a particular type of flexibility, a "kinesthetic feel," and a total body rhythm. It is an act of grace as much as power, a rhythmic act as much as a sudden muscular burst, an individual expression as much as an exertion, and it is tied to a sense of the body in harmony with space as much as overcoming resistance through physical force.

Athletes in different sports jump in different ways. Gymnasts, volleyball players, figure skaters, skateboarders, mogul skiers, BMX bikers, wakeboarders, basketball players, ski jumpers, high jumpers, long jumpers, triple-jumpers, and steeple-chase runners all jump, but their techniques and styles vary greatly from sport to sport and person to person. The act of jumping among people whose skin color and ethnic heritage have been given important social meanings is especially complex because race and ethnicity are types of performances in their own ways (Clammer, 2015). In other words, performing race and ethnicity often involves physical expressions and body movements that are grounded in the cultural–kinesthetic histories of particular populations and stereotypes about them.

Noted scholar Gerald Early (1998), explains that playing sports is an *ethnic performance* because the relevance and meaning of bodily movements vary from one cultural context to another. For example, jumping is irrelevant to the performances of world leaders, CEOs of major corporations, sport team owners, coaches, doctors, and college professors. The power, influence, and resources that these people possess do *not* depend on their jumping abilities. The statement that "white men can't jump" isn't defined as a racial slur by most whites, because jumping deficiencies have not stopped them from dominating the seats of power worldwide (Myers, 2000). Outside of a few sports, jumping ability has nothing to do with success, power, or wealth. As Public Enemy rapped in the 1998 film, *He Got Game,* "White men in suits don't *have* to jump."

To study the physical aspects of jumping, sprinting, and distance running is important because it helps us understand human biology more fully. But this research will not explain why people in some social and cultural populations jump high in certain sports and not others, or don't jump at all. Such explanations must take into account the historical, cultural, and social circumstances that make jumping and running important in some people's lives and why some people work hard to develop jumping and running abilities. There certainly are genes related to jumping, but it's wrong to assume that they operate independent of environmental factors, are connected with skin color in physical terms, or correspond with the racial categories that people have

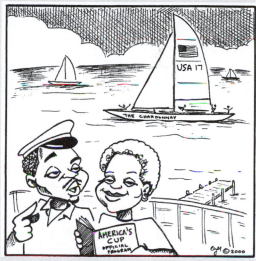

(*Source:* © Frederic A. Eyer)

"Of course, white folks are good at this. After 500 years of colonizing the world by sea, they've been bred to have exceptional sailing genes!"

This statement is laughable when made about whites. However, similar statements about blacks have been used by scientists as a basis for hundreds of studies over the last century. As a result, racial ideology has influenced the process of knowledge production as well as everyday explanations of social worlds and the actions of individuals.

constructed for social and political purposes. Knowledge about genes is important, but it will never explain the complex physical and cultural performance of slam dunks choreographed by NBA players with varying skin color from more than thirty-seven territories and nations (in 2015). Nor will it explain the amazing vertical leaps and hang times of European, Brazilian, Chinese, and Japanese volleyball players who have won so many international events. Nor will it tell us why whites always win America's Cup yacht races and nearly every "big air" event in action sports. But when people see the world through a racialized lens, they miss most of what they don't expect to see.

facts; and (3) the theories people use to analyze and interpret the facts that they have classified and organized. Therefore, if people are not critically self-reflective as they observe, analyze, and explain the actions of human beings, racial ideology will influence the process of producing knowledge. This is highlighted in the box " 'Jumping Genes' in Black Bodies" on pages 234–235.

Racial Ideology and a Sense of Athletic Destiny Among African American Men   Does racial ideology influence the ways that African Americans interpret their own physical abilities and potential as athletes? This is a controversial question. Research combined with statements by athletes and coaches suggests that many young African Americans, especially men, grow up believing that the black body is superior when it comes to physical abilities in certain sports (May, 2008; Steele, 2010). This belief inspires some young people to believe it is their biological and cultural destiny to play certain sports and play them better than others. This inspiration is intensified when young black men and women feel that their chances of gaining respect and material success are dismal in any realm other than a few sports (Bimper and Harrison, 2011; Harrison et al., 2011; May, 2008, 2009b; Shakib and Veliz, 2012; Singer and May, 2011; Smith, 2007).

Figure 8.2 outlines a hypothesized sociological explanation of the athletic achievements of African American male athletes. The top section of the figure shows that racial stereotypes about the innate physical abilities of black people have been a part of U.S. history and culture. When these stereotypes are combined with restricted opportunities in mainstream occupations and heavily sponsored opportunities to develop skills in certain sports, many black youngsters are motivated to play those sports. Over time they come to believe that it is their destiny to excel in those sports, especially relative to whites (see the middle section of Figure 8.2). When this sense of destiny is widespread and strong, it creates a context in which young black men work hard to develop their skills and frame their achievements

in terms of race as well as personal motivation (see the bottom section of Figure 8.2).

Does this sociological approach explain the notable achievements of African American men in basketball, football, track, and boxing? This is a difficult question to answer, but historical evidence indicates that a perceived collective sense of biological or cultural destiny can dramatically influence the achievements of an entire population. Three centuries ago, white men from the small island nation of England felt that it was their biological and cultural destiny to colonize and rule other parts of the world. This belief was so powerful that it led them to conquer over one-half the world as they formed the British Empire! This dwarfs the achievements of blacks in certain sports today. Further, it is clear that British colonization was driven by a combination of historical, cultural, and social factors; it was not due to British genes. Overall, when social worlds are organized to foster a sense of destiny among particular people, it shouldn't be surprising when those people achieve notable things in pursuit of what they believe they can accomplish.

The Challenge of Escaping Racial Ideology in Sports   The most effective way to defuse racial ideology is for people to understand each other's history and heritage and to depend on each other to achieve their goals. However, when ethnic segregation exists, as it does in U.S. residential housing and schools, there is a tendency for black males to be "tagged" in a way that subverts their success in claiming identities that don't fit expectations based on racial ideology. For instance, if black high school students play on sport teams *and* participate in the school's honors program, other students and teachers are more likely to identify the black males as athletes rather than honors students, whereas black females are identified in connection with both statuses. At the same time, if Asian and white students (male and female) are in the honors program *and* on school teams, they are more likely to be identified as honors students rather than athletes. This tendency to

When these three social and cultural conditions are added together:

A long history of racial ideology has emphasized
"black male physicality" and innate, race-based physical abilities among black people

+

A long history of racial segregation and discrimination has limited
the opportunities for black men to achieve success and respect in society

+

The existence of widespread opportunities and encouragement
to develop physical skills and excel in a few sports

There are two intermediate consequences:

Many black men and women, especially young men, come to believe
that it is their biological and cultural destiny to become great athletes

+

Young black men are motivated to use every opportunity
to develop the skills they need to fulfill their destiny as athletes

The resulting hypothesis is this:

This sense of biological and cultural destiny, combined with
motivation and opportunities to develop certain sport skills,
leads some black men and women, especially those with certain physical
characteristics, to be outstanding athletes in certain sports

FIGURE 8.2 A sociological hypothesis to explain the achievements of black male athletes.

differentially identify students in connection with race has been consistently documented in research (Evans et al., 2011; May, 2008, 2009; Shakib and Veliz, 2012; Withycombe, 2011).

As two black male college athletes noted, "Everyone around perceives us being [on campus] only for our physical talents," and "Everything is white [on campus], only sports [are] for blacks" (Harrison, 1998, p. 72). This is not a new phenomenon and it continues to exist with little change (Bimper and Harrison, 2011; el-Khoury, 2012; Harrison et al., 2011; Hodge et al., 2008; Melendez, 2008; Singer, 2008). But its consequences are frustrating for black men who want to expand their social identities beyond sports, or who don't play sports and don't want to be identified with them.

When these identity dynamics occur, relationships in schools may be organized so that black male students are academically marginalized. We need to know more about the conditions under which this marginalization occurs and how it affects those involved. At this point, many people say that black students, especially young men, avoid and devalue an academic identity, but this factor is less important than the perceptions of people and their tendency to acknowledge certain identities and skills and ignore others.

These identity dynamics can undermine the positive consequences of sports in the lives of many black students, because it frames their achievements in sports in racial terms and reduces the significance of other achievements and potential.

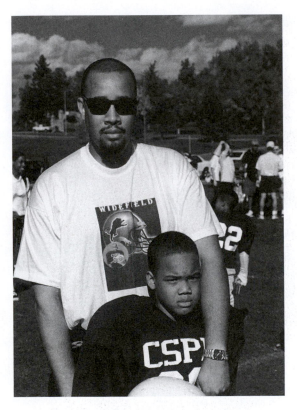

Many African American men grow up taking sports, especially basketball and football, very seriously. By age eleven this boy has learned not to smile when presenting himself as an athlete. His father reminded him to look serious and tough for this photo because it represented an identity that should be taken seriously. (*Source:* © Jay Coakley)

Racial Ideology and Sport Choices Among Whites Research also shows that choices and achievements in sports are influenced by racial ideology and the stereotypes it supports (Allen et al., 2011; Harrison and Lawrence, 2004; Harrison et al., 2011; Steele, 2010). The influence of ideology is subtle, but it continues to influence people's lives and the organization of the social worlds in which choices are made.

Black girls and boys in certain areas of the United States might think twice before taking up a sport that is identified by their peers as "white," for fear of being labeled a "wannabe white." Similarly, white girls and boys in certain areas might choose to play soccer or lacrosse because the school football and basketball teams have mostly black players.

Research is needed to determine the conditions under which sport participation choices are influenced by racial ideology, but doing this research can be tricky because these choices quickly become taken for granted and built into physical environments. Therefore, people are more likely to see them as "personal preferences" rather than as reflections of a pervasive racial ideology that shapes the social and physical environment as well as people's choices (Harrison, 2013).

Racial Ideology, Gender, and Social Class

Racial and gender ideologies are interconnected in U.S. sports. For example, the implications of racial ideology for black men are different from those for black women. This is partly because the bodies of black men in U.S. culture have been viewed and socially defined differently than the bodies of black women.

Over the past three centuries, but especially during the last century, many whites in the United States grew up fearing the power of black male bodies, feeling anxious about their sexual capacities and being fascinated by their movements. Ironically, this consequence of racial ideology has enabled some black men to use their bodies as entertainment commodities, first on stage in music and vaudeville theater and later on athletic fields. Black female bodies, on the other hand, were seen in sexualized terms or as the nurturing nanny—neither of which made them valuable entertainment commodities in sports (Collins, 2005; Corbett and Johnson, 2000).

This means that racial and gender ideology create slightly different challenges for black female athletes. For example, Donna Daniels, an African American studies scholar, suggests that the norms for physical appearance among females in predominantly white cultures have been racialized so that black female athletes exist in a realm outside the normal range of acceptance. To gain acceptance, they

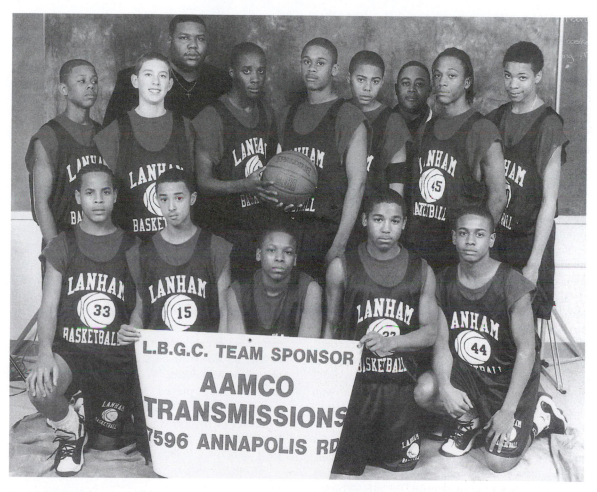

Racial ideology operates in diverse ways. In some cases, it influences whites to avoid the sports in which blacks have a record of excellence. This way of thinking did not influence the white teen on this team, nor does it influence whites in Europe and Australia where racial ideology does not discourage them from playing basketball and learning to run and jump as NBA players do. (*Source:* © Pat Miller)

must carefully "monitor and strategize about how they are seen and understood by people who are not accustomed to their physical presence or intellect, whether on the court, field, or peddling a product" (2000, p. 26). If they're not careful, there's a danger that people will interpret their confidence and intelligence as arrogance and cockiness or as an indication that they are "too black."[2] Therefore, some black women learn to present themselves to others in ways that tone down their toughness and make them appear amicable and nonthreatening—much

---

[2]This was experienced by Michelle Obama as the wife of Senator and President Barack Obama. Some people identified her as "too black" and a "typical angry black woman." Her confidence and intelligence were viewed by many as arrogance and cockiness, which made it necessary for her to be especially diplomatic in how she presented herself in public.

like Oprah Winfrey—lest they face chronic marginalization in the cultural mainstream (Withycombe, 2011).

This point was poignantly illustrated when radio and talk show host Don Imus saw the strength and toughness of the black women on the Rutgers University basketball team and could find no other words to describe them except "some rough girls from Rutgers . . . some nappy-headed ho's." As for Rutgers' opponents, Imus said, "The girls from Tennessee—they all looked cute." Then the show's executive producer said that the game pitted "the jigaboos versus the wannabes." To Imus and his producer, both of whom were fired for their on-air conversation, the appearance of the women from the Rutgers team was "too black," and outside of their normal range of acceptance.

This was reminiscent of ways that the media in the 1990s pathologized the bodies of Venus and Serena Williams as exotic yet repulsive, animalistic yet supremely athletic, unfeminine yet erotic. These stories are put into a historical context in the Reflect on Sports box, "Vénus Noire."

This type of response among potential fans was anticipated by the marketing people at the WNBA. When they first promoted the league, they presented ad after ad highlighting black players who had modeling contracts or newborn babies (Banet-Weiser, 1999; A. Solomon, 2000). When lip gloss and cute infants were not used, the ads depicted nicely groomed black players in nurturing and supportive roles, especially with children.

Studies of black women playing sports or coaching in college suggest that they often feel a special sense of isolation on predominantly white campuses (Borland and Bruening, 2010; Carter and Hart, 2010; St. Louis, 2010). This is primarily due to dealing with the double jeopardy of racial and gender ideology. Compared with their male peers, black females are more likely to be patronized, lack access to power and the people who wield power in athletic departments, and have fewer mentors and sources of social support in the schools or departments in which they play or work. As a result, they often depend heavily on their families for guidance

and support (Carter and Hart, 2010)—and it may be that black families are more likely to offer and provide this support for their daughters than for their sons. When all these factors are combined, black female athletes and coaches face formidable challenges as they negotiate their way in sports, especially on predominantly white campuses.

SPORT PARTICIPATION AMONG ETHNIC MINORITIES IN THE UNITED STATES

Sports in the United States have long histories of racial and ethnic exclusion. Men and women in all ethnic minorities traditionally have been underrepresented at all levels of competition and management in most competitive sports, even in high schools and community programs. Prior to the 1950s, the organizations that sponsored sport teams and events seldom opened their doors fully to African Americans, Latinos, Native Americans, or Asian Americans. When members of ethnic minority groups played sports, they usually played among themselves in games and events segregated by choice or by necessity (Giles, 2004; Miller and Wiggins, 2003; Niiya, 2000; Powers-Beck, 2004; Ruck, 1987).

Sport Participation Among African Americans

Throughout much of the twentieth century, white people in the United States consistently avoided playing with and against black people. Black people of all ages were systematically excluded from participation in white-controlled sport programs and organizations because many white people believed that they didn't have the character or fortitude to compete with them. As a result of various aspects of racial ideology, participation opportunities for young black girls and boys were limited to only a few sports—usually those that their segregated schools could afford to provide. Even today, 44 million black Americans are underrepresented

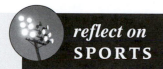

reflect on
SPORTS

Vénus Noire
A Legacy of Racism After 200 Years

The legacy of past racist beliefs about the black female body was resurrected again in December 2012 when Danish tennis player Caroline Wozniacki stuffed bulky towels over her sports bra and into the back of her tennis skirt to portray her caricature of Serena Williams during a match with Maria Sharapova in Brazil. Wozniacki probably did not know what that meant for her friends, Serena and Venus Williams. For them it was a naïve act of racism and a reminder of how they have been compared to "Hottentot Venus," a South African woman whose real name was Saartjie Baartman.

Baartman was captured by British colonizers in 1810, brought to Europe, and displayed in exhibitions, World Fairs, and "freak shows" as an example of the primitive character of black Africans (AAA,

2006c; Hobson, 2005; Holmes, 2007; Kechiche, 2005; A. Little, 2012; Martin, 2009; Maseko, 1998; Webster, 2000).

Baartman was a member of the Hottentot people, who had a genetic trait causing them to retain fat cells in their breasts and buttocks. Through the rest of her life Baartman was exhibited to whites as an animal-like creature. Her genital region evoked special curiosity because white people at that time were fascinated by what they believed to be the innate hypersexuality of the black female body.

After Baartman died, the anthropologist who had sold her to a carnival showman years before repossessed her body for an inhumane postmortem in which he removed her brain and cut off, dissected, and examined her genitals

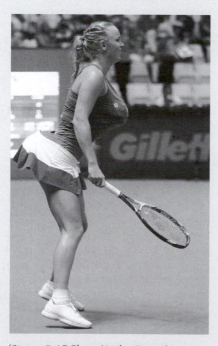

(*Source:* © AP Photo/Andre Penner)

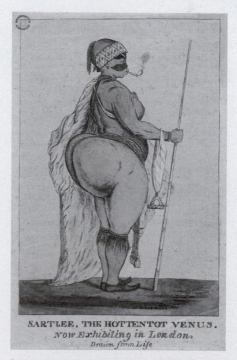

SARTLEE, THE HOTTENTOT VENUS.
Now Exhibiting in London.
Drawn from Life

(*Source:* City of Westminster Archives Centre)

When Caroline Wozniacki mimicked Serena Williams in public she unwittingly revived a global legacy of racist beliefs about black female sexuality. For those who know racial history, this stunt was reminiscent of what happened to Saartjie Baartman, who is caricatured in this racist image that is 200 years old.

Continued

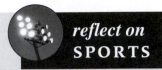

Vénus Noire (*continued*)

in hopes of contributing to white knowledge about black female bodies and brains.

This widespread fascination with Baartman's assumed hypersexuality marked an early chapter in a continuing 200-year-old story of the beliefs that white people have had about the black female body (see Burton, 2012). Throughout much of the story, those beliefs were emotionally charged with a complex combination of desire and repulsion grounded in the racism of the day (Hobson, 2005).

To illustrate the indirect impact of that story we can go back to the mid-nineteenth century, when beliefs about Baartman's body reaffirmed the use of a bustle and corset to accentuate the buttocks ("booty" today) and breasts while thinning the waist. In England and other parts of Western Europe this "look" represented idealized female sexual identity—a way to be sexy while covering every inch of the body with layers of Victoria Era clothing. Anyone who has watched Disney's animated "princess" films depicting women of this era is familiar with this "bustle and corset look."

Of course, history books have told only the racially censored white interpretation of the "bustle and corset" fashion. But Venus and Serena Williams know the African interpretation—as did Nelson Mandela, who, as the globally respected former president of South Africa, finally in 2002, succeeded in convincing the French government to return Baartman's body to her homeland to be buried there.

White journalists covering the match in which Caroline Wozniacki pulled her stunt represented it as "fun and games." Anita Little, a young journalist writing for *Ms.* magazine called it a case of "accidental racism." But as an African American woman, Little knows that such accidents damage black women and reinforce a 200-year-old story about white superiority and black inferiority that has shaped recent human history. For Serena Williams, this accidental racism was probably interpreted in terms of that longer story combined with the fifteen years of nasty and racist comments about her body—comments naively reaffirmed by someone she considered a friend.

Now that you know a small part of one chapter in that 200-year-old history, what would you tell Caroline Wozniacki to do the next time she sees Serena Williams in private? *Regarding the larger picture, what does that history say about perceptions of female bodies today, especially those of black women?*

in or absent from most sports at most levels of competition. This fact is often overlooked because a few of the most popular spectator sports involve high proportions of black athletes. People see this and don't realize that black men and women are absent or nearly absent in thirty-nine of forty-four men's and women's sports played in college, most of the dozens of sports played at the international amateur level, and all but five of the dozens of professional sports in the United States. There is a similar pattern in Canada and in European countries with strong sporting traditions.

The exceptions to this pattern of exclusion stand out because they *are* exceptions. The underrepresentation of blacks in most sports is much greater than the underrepresentation of whites in basketball, football, and track and field. Additionally, there are proportionately many more white students who play basketball and football in high school and college than there are black students who play tennis or golf at those levels. Finding black drivers at an Indy-car or NASCAR race is difficult or impossible; drivers, support personnel, and nearly 100 percent of the spectators are white, but the races are never described as white events (King, 2007c; Kusz, 2007b).

In a *white-centered* cultural setting where the lives of whites are the expected focus of attention, whites don't think about the whiteness of these sports. And in *white-dominated, white-identified*

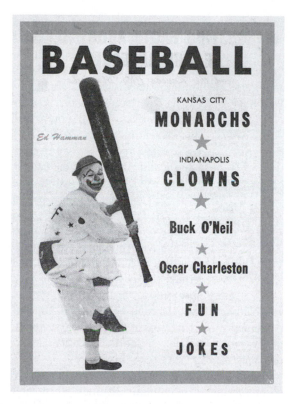

Black athletes were not taken seriously by most white people through much of the twentieth century. To earn a living playing sports, they often had to present themselves in ways that fit the racial (and racist) stereotypes held by white people. The Indianapolis Clowns baseball team and the Harlem Globetrotters basketball team joked around and behaved in childlike ways so that white people would pay to watch them. Racism restricted cultural space for black men and women to be entertainers, and they faced near-total exclusion in other spheres of social life, including mainstream sports. (*Source:* Library of Congress)

settings where the characteristics of whites are used as the standards for judging qualifications, most white people never think that they might have an advantage when it comes to fitting in or being hired and promoted. At the same time, blacks and other ethnic minorities must be careful not to be too black or too ethnic if they wish to succeed in these settings.

Throughout U.S. sports history, the participation of black females has been severely limited and has received little attention, apart from that given to occasional Olympic medal winners in track events. As noted previously, research shows that black women are keenly aware of the need to "tone down" their toughness and confidence lest they "threaten" white people who don't know them or understand race relations in the United States.

In the case of black girls, a study by ethnomusicologist Kyra Gaunt (2006) shows that games in urban girl culture traditionally combine songs, chants, handclapping, footstomping, and rhythmic movement—a combination that doesn't fit with widely used definitions of sport (Cole, 2006). Many of these games, including traditional double-dutch, involve complex physical challenges combined with a body-conscious physicality and embodied musicality traceable to African origins.

Overall, rates of sport participation in middle- and upper-middle-income white communities in the United States are much higher than those in most predominantly black communities, especially those where resources are scarce. Racial ideology causes many people to overlook this fact. They see only the black men who make high salaries in high-profile sports and assume that blacks have "taken over" sports, that racial discrimination no longer exists, and that the nation is now color blind. Overall, this is how dominant racial ideology erases people and problems that cause discomfort for the racially privileged (Harrison, 2013; Lee-St. John, 2006).

Sport Participation Among Native Americans

There are 5.2 million "American Indian and Alaska Natives" in the United States and about 1.7 million live on or very close to 324 federally recognized reservations. Although the U.S. census counts Native Americans as a single demographic category, they comprise dozens of diverse cultural populations and come from 566 federally recognized "Indian tribes," according to the Bureau of Indian Affairs. The differences between many of these populations are socially significant. However, most non-Native Americans tend to erase these differences by referring generally to "Indians" and envisioning stereotypical habits and dress—long hair, feathers, buckskin, moccasins, bows and arrows, horseback riding, war-whooping, tomahawk-chopping, and half-naked, even in cold northern states.

Native American sport participation patterns are diverse. They vary with cultural traditions, socioeconomic status, and whether people live on or off reservations. For example, participation patterns are heavily affected by a poverty rate of 30 percent and up to 50 percent on reservations—over twice the poverty rate in the United States as a whole (about 15 percent in 2014).

Many sports in traditional Native American cultures combine physical activities with ritual and ceremony. Although individual Native American athletes have done well and set records over the past century, public recognition has often been limited to those few standouts on the football and baseball teams from reservation schools. For example, when Jim Thorpe and his teammates at the Carlisle School, a segregated government training school, defeated outstanding college teams in 1911 and 1912, they attracted considerable attention (Bloom, 2000; Oxendine, 1988). But apart from a few teams and individual athletes in segregated government schools, Native American sport participation has been limited by high rates of poverty and poor health, a lack of equipment and facilities, and little support from those who control sports.

Native Americans who can play intercollegiate sports often fear being cut off from their cultural roots and support systems. For those who grow up learning their culture, there often is tension between the larger U.S. or Canadian culture

> If you want [your mascot] to be a savage—use your own picture. . . . How would you feel if the team was called the Washington Darkies? —Former Colorado senator Ben Nighthorse Campbell, the only Native American senator in U.S. history (in Zirin, 2013c)

and their way of life. These tensions increase when they encounter negative representations of their culture in the form of teams named Indians, Redskins, Redmen, and Savages and mascots and logos that mimic stereotypes of "Indians." Watching or playing sports under such conditions involves losing control of one's identity (King, 2016). It is depressing to see a distorted or historically inappropriate caricature of a Native American on the gym wall or floor (!) of a school where students have no knowledge of local or regional native cultures. For Native Americans this means that they must (1) swallow cultural pride; (2) repress anger against insensitive, historically ignorant non-Native Americans; and (3) suspend hope of being understood in terms of their identity and cultural heritage. Reflect on Sports, "Identity Theft," on pages 246–247 discusses this issue.

Native American athletes also face the challenge of preserving their cultural identities when their orientations don't fit with the culture of the power and performance sports sponsored by most schools. Through the years, some white coaches who have worked in reservation schools have tried to strip students of cultural traditions that emphasize cooperation and replace them with Euro-American orientations that favor competition. When Native Americans don't give up their cultural souls voluntarily, coaches simply avoid recruiting them. This is a problem that affects many Native American high school students who play basketball, a popular sport on reservations and one in which young Native Americans often excel (Longman, 2013b).

Fortunately, Native American sport experiences do not always involve dramatic cultural compromises. Some Native Americans play sports in contexts in which their identities are respected and supported by others (King, 2004a, 2004b; Longman, 2013b; Schinke et al., 2010). In these cases, sports provide opportunities for students to learn about the cultural backgrounds of others. In other cases, Native Americans adopt Euro-American ways and play sports without expressing any evidence of their cultural heritage; that is, they "go along with" the dominant culture, even if they don't agree with or accept all of it. And there are cases in which Native Americans redefine sport participation to fit their cultural beliefs—a strategy used by many ethnic minorities who play sports developed by and for people in the dominant culture (Brenner and Reuveni, 2006; Maguire, 1999).

Sport Participation Among Latinos and Latinas

The 55 million Latinos in the United States include people from diverse cultures.[3] They may share language, colonial history, or Catholic religious beliefs, but their cultures, histories, and migration patterns vary greatly. Mexican Americans constitute the largest Latino/a group (63 percent), followed by Puerto Ricans (9 percent), Cubans (4 percent), Central and South Americans (15 percent), and other Hispanic people (9 percent).

When dealing with sports in the United States, it's useful to distinguish between three categories of Latinos: (1) U.S. born and naturalized citizens; (2) Latin Americans working as athletes in the United States; and (3) workers and their family members who are in the United States without legal approval. The role of sports varies greatly in the everyday lives of people in each of these three categories.

Native-Born and Naturalized Citizens with Latino Heritage Because much of the southwestern United States (California, Texas, Nevada, Utah, most of Arizona and New Mexico, and parts

[3]*Latino* is the term often used by people from Latin America to identify themselves as a single population with shared political interests and concerns. It was created as an alternative to *Hispanic,* a term invented by the U.S. Census Bureau to refer to people of any race who have "Spanish/Hispanic/Latino origin." I use *Latino* because it is more socially and politically meaningful than *Hispanic,* which is mostly a demographic term.

of Colorado and Wyoming) was part of Mexico prior to the mid-nineteenth century, the ancestors of Latinos were living in this region long before 1620 when European pilgrims docked the *Mayflower* in Plymouth Harbor. Therefore, Latino people have played major roles in establishing communities, schools, businesses, churches, hospitals, and sport programs in the Southwest, which is home to 25 percent of the total U.S. population. Unsurprisingly, they've also played and been successful in the same sports as others in the Southwest (Mendoza, 2007).

The exceptions to this pattern involve people who emigrated from Mexico and other parts of Latin America during the twentieth century to work in low-status jobs in U.S. industry and agriculture. Many people in this category are naturalized citizens or children who were born in the United States. They frequently maintain family connections in Mexico and generally experience various forms of ethnic discrimination. Work patterns, poverty, segregation, general discrimination, and cultural traditions have influenced their sport involvement. Scarce time, resources, and little access to facilities and teams have restricted participation (Swanson et al., 2013). These patterns are similar to the ones that exist among Latinos and Afro-Caribbeans in Canada (Joseph, 2012).

When anthropologist Doug Foley (1990a, 1990b, 1999b) studied "Mexicano-Anglo relations" associated with high school football in a small Texas town, he found that working-class Mexican males (*vatos*) rejected sport participation but used Friday night football games as occasions for publicly displaying their Mexican identities and establishing social reputations in the community. Foley also described how the Mexicans protested a high school homecoming ceremony that marginalized Mexicans and gave center stage to Anglos (that is, white people with European ancestry). Additionally, the Mexican-American football coach resigned in frustration when faced with the bigotry and contradictory expectations of powerful Anglo boosters and school board members.

Foley concluded that despite being a site for resistance against prevailing Anglo ways of doing

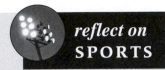

reflect on SPORTS

Identity Theft?
Using Native American Names and Images in Sports

Using stereotypes to characterize Native Americans is so common that most people don't realize they do it. When people take Native American images and names, claim ownership of them, and then use them for team names, mascots, and logos, sports perpetuate an ideology that trivializes and distorts the diverse histories and traditions of native cultures. No other ethnic population is subject to this form of cultural identity theft. As sportswriter Jon Saraceno (2005) exclaims, "Can you imagine the reaction if any school dressed a mascot in an Afro wig and a dashiki? Or encouraged fans to show up in blackface?" (p. 10C).

To understand this issue, consider this story told by the group, Concerned American Indian Parents:

> An American Indian student attended his school's pep rally in preparation for a football game against a rival school. The rival school's mascot was an American Indian. The pep rally included the burning of an Indian in effigy along with posters and banners labeled "Scalp the Indians," "Kill the Indians," and "Let's burn the Indians at the stake." The student, hurt and embarrassed, tore the banners down. His fellow students couldn't understand his hurt and pain.

This incident occurred in a public school in 1988, twenty years after the National Congress of American Indians initiated a campaign to eliminate stereotypes of "Indians" in U.S. culture. In 1970, over 3000 schools were using Native American images, names, logos, and mascots for their sport teams. Many of these changed their names and mascots when they realized that it wasn't right to use the identities of other human beings to represent and promote themselves. However, a number of schools and a few professional teams still engage in this form of identity theft as they call themselves "Indians," "Savages," "Warriors," "Chiefs," "Braves," "Redskins," "Red Raiders," and "Redmen" and have mascots that cross-dress as Indians by donning war bonnets and paint, brandishing spears and tomahawks, pounding tom-toms, intoning rhythmic chants, and mimicking religious and cultural dances.

Some schools continue to display "*their* Indian" on gym walls and floors, scoreboards, and products they sell for a profit. They say that they're engaging in a

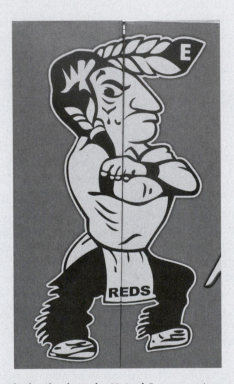

Many high schools in the United States continue to cling to ownership of "their" Indian names, logos, and mascots, despite objections from Native Americans. Some school officials, coaches, parents, and students say that their intent is to "honor their Indian," but they put his caricatured image on their gym floors and benches where people step and sit on them—actions unlikely to be accepted when honoring culturally important historical figures, such as Abraham Lincoln or Ronald Reagan. This [cartoon] image is used by a public high school in Colorado calling themselves the "Fightin' Reds." (*Source*: © Jay Coakley)

"harmless" tradition that "honors" the "Indians" from whom they've taken images and identities. But Native

Americans point out that they are not honored by people who don't listen to them or respect their cultures.

What if the San Diego Padres' mascot were a fearsome black-robed missionary who walked the sidelines swinging an 8-foot-long rosary and carrying a 9-foot-long plastic crucifix? And what if he led fans in a hip-hop version of the sacred Gregorian chant as spectators waved little crucifixes and rapped the lyrics of their chant? People would be outraged because they know the history and meaning of Christian beliefs, objects, and rituals.

If more Americans knew the histories, cultural traditions, and religions of the 566 Native American tribes and nations in the United States today, would they be as likely to use Native American team names and allow naïve students to dress in costumes made of items defined as sacred in the animistic religious traditions of many Native Americans? Would they allow fans to mimic sacred chants and perform war-whooping, tomahawk-chopping cheers based on racist images from old "cowboy and Indian" movies?

Most public school officials and state legislators now realize that it's cruel and inconsiderate to misrepresent people whose ancestors were massacred, ordered off their lands at gunpoint, and confined to reservations by U.S. government agents. They also realize that romanticizing a distorted version of the past by taking the names and images of people who currently experience discrimination, poverty, and the negative effects of stereotypes is a careless act of white privilege and hypocrisy. Therefore, some states and school districts now have policies banning such practices.

In 2003, the National Collegiate Athletic Association (NCAA) recommended that all universities using American Indian names, mascots, or logos review their practices and determine if they undermined the NCAA's commitment to cultural diversity. In 2005, the NCAA banned the display of Native American names, logos, and mascots on uniforms and other clothing and at NCAA playoff games and championships. But NCAA officials made an exception for Florida State University (FSU), whose officials claimed they had permission from the Seminole Tribe in Florida (but *not* the Seminole Nation of Oklahoma) to use the Seminole name and logo image in an honorable way (Staurowsky, 2007). "Honorable" for FSU means having a white European American student paint his face, put on a headband and a colorful shirt, carry a feather-covered spear, and ride into the football stadium on a horse named Seminole. And fans can honor *their* "nole," as they call "their Indian," by buying products adorned with the painted and feathered "Seminole face." These products include floor mats, welcome mats, stadium seats, paper plates, and other things that fans use to sit, stand, and wipe their feet on. This is a strange way to show honor, but it makes money for the university and keeps the wealthy white boosters happy, even if it mocks the courses in their history department and makes the FSU diversity policy a symbol of hypocrisy.

The insensitivity of people at FSU is not an isolated case (Davis-Delano, 2007; King, 2016; Williams, 2007). For example, in 1999, a panel in the U.S. Patent and Trademark Office ruled that "Redskins," "Redskin-ettes," and the logo of a feathered "Redskin" man as used by Washington, DC's NFL team "disparaged" Native Americans. The panel canceled six exclusive trademarks, ending the NFL's exclusive ownership of the "Redskins" name and logo. But in 2003, a federal district court judge overturned the panel's ruling because Native Americans had not objected back in 1967 when all NFL trademarks were registered. Although this decision is under appeal, the NFL still controls its "Redskins"—located in the capital city of the government that broke all but 1 of over 400 treaties with Native Americans (Dorgan, 2013). This case symbolizes the history of oppression endured by Native Americans.

However, in 2013, there were additional efforts to convince the owner of the Washington team to change its name, but he said he would NEVER do so. But that only increased the pressure being put on him and on the NFL, which claims to value racial and ethnic diversity (King, 2016; TheDailyCaller, 2013; Zirin 2013c, 2013d).

things in the town, high school football ultimately perpetuated the power and privilege of the local Anglos. As long as Mexicanos saw and did things the Anglo way, they were accepted. But when they raised ethnic issues they were ignored, opposed, or marginalized.

There's a need to update Foley's work and to do research in urban areas as well as smaller towns. We know little about sports in the lives of young people who are first-, second-, and third-generation Latinos in the United States. There are anecdotal accounts of young people who overcome barriers to play on school teams or at the professional level, but in-depth, community-based research is lacking.

Similarly, there's been little research on Puerto Ricans in northeastern states, especially New York, and Cubans in southeastern states, especially Florida. Among those who are second- or third-generation residents of the United States, sport participation patterns match the patterns of those with similar family incomes and levels of education. For example, the relatively poor Puerto Ricans in New York City and other urban areas on the eastern seaboard have sport participation patterns matching other populations with scarce resources. Boxing, baseball, and soccer are among the most popular sports. The relatively wealthy Cubans who came to the United States after Castro and the communist party came to power in 1959 have sport participation patterns that match their socioeconomic counterparts. More recent Cuban immigrants have patterns closer to those of recent immigrants from Mexico—boxing, soccer, and baseball among the men and softball and basketball among the women.

Research on Latinas in the United States indicates that diverse ethnic traditions and gender norms influence their sport participation (Acosta, 1999; Jamieson, 1998, 2005, 2007; Sylwester, 2005a, 2005b, 2005c). First-generation Latinas may lack parental support to play sports. Parents often control their daughters more strictly than they control their sons, and daughters are expected to do household tasks such as caring for siblings, assisting with meal preparation, and cleaning house—all of which

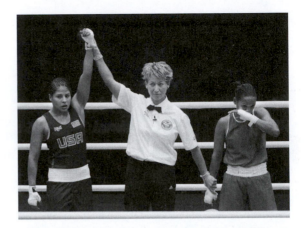

Marlen Esparza, the daughter of a Mexican immigrant father, grew up in Houston. After having trouble in school, she took up boxing and at sixteen-years-old became the youngest woman to win a national Golden Gloves championship, which she won six consecutive times along with a world championship in 2006. In 2012, she became the first woman in the United States to qualify for a spot in boxing at the Olympics in London, where she won a bronze medal. (*Source:* © DENNIS M. SABANGAN/epa/Corbis)

interfere with playing sports in households where meeting expenses is a struggle and transportation to practices and games is unavailable or costly.

Second- and third-generation Latinas face fewer parental constraints, and many parents are willing to use family resources to fund their daughters' sport participation. However, talented high school players often remain hesitant to play intercollegiate sports if it means going to a college far from home where there is little support for their Latina identities and traditions. Katherine Jamieson's (1998, 2005, 2007) research describes the unique identity management experiences of Latina intercollegiate athletes who must bridge a cultural divide as they live, study, and play with others who know little about merging cultural identities and managing relationships in two cultural spheres. But this research also needs to be updated, because ethnic relations are constantly emerging social phenomena.

Young Latinas today are more likely than their peers in past generations to see athletes who look like them. There's some media coverage showing Latinas in golf, softball, and soccer, but most inspiration comes from older sisters and neighbor girls who play sports. Research on the experiences of Latinas is important because it helps us understand the dynamics faced by young women caught up in the experience of immigration and making their way in a new society. At this point, we know little about the experiences of younger Latinas as they combine family life with school, sports, and jobs, and about adult Latinas who play sports in local leagues. Women playing in local leagues often use their participation to maintain regular contact with relatives and friends in the United States and Mexico, which makes soccer and softball especially important in their lives.

Latin Americans Working as Athletes in U.S. Sports   For well over a century boys and young men from poor families in Cuba, Puerto Rico, the Dominican Republic, Mexico, and Venezuela have dreamed about playing professional baseball in their home countries or the United States (Burgos, 2007; Regalado, 2008).

Between 1880 and the late 1930s, players from Latin America—often from Cuba—played on white U.S. professional teams and Negro League teams. Although they faced strong discrimination on white teams, they learned that they could negotiate team membership by using their Spanish names to claim they were Latino, not "black." White players and management often accepted this in the interest of including highly skilled players on their teams, even when the Latino players were dark-skinned. Therefore, Latino players quietly passed through "the color line" and disrupted the "one-drop" racial classification model that was used in Major League Baseball. Additionally, many white, black, and Latino players had played in ethnically mixed Latin American leagues in the decades prior to the desegregation of MLB (Burgos, 2007).

These factors, according to historian Adrian Burgos (2007), helped erode resistance to desegregation and made it easier for Branch Rickey to convince his co-owners of the Brooklyn Dodgers to make Jackie Robinson a team member in 1947. This means that breaking the color line in baseball was a multi-ethnic process rather than a single event in black-white relations (Lapchick, 2010). Latino players had long been involved in weakening the color line and demonstrating that the definition of race used in the United States was arbitrary and inconsistent. In fact, during the early twentieth century, some African Americans were known to learn Spanish and take Spanish names so they could pass as Cubans or Dominicans and play on U.S. teams.

Latinos constitute 25 percent of the players in MLB today and about 40 percent of all minor league players; 85 percent of Major League players born outside the United States come from Latin America. This is part of a century-long process through which players learned skills in community and professional leagues in Latin America, and more recently, in baseball training academies, mostly in the Dominican Republic (Klein, 2006). Baseball has long been seen as the ticket to take a young man out of poverty, enabling him to support his extended family and make contributions to his local community.

When scouts for MLB teams realized that there was so much baseball talent in the Dominican Republic, they built training academies to gain access to the young players and then assess, develop, and control them. This began in the 1970s and continues today, although Dominicans with ties to their communities have now developed their own academies so they can "broker" players to academies sponsored by Major League teams (Klein, 2006). In this way, the Dominicans have regained partial control over their own talent so that Major League teams don't just take the best players and, as they do so, destroy local leagues and teams. The success of the academies is seen through the 95–100 Dominicans who currently play on MLB teams; in fact, over the years, seventy MLB players have come from San Pedro de Macorís, a city of 200,000 people, and in 1990 it was the birthplace of five of the twenty-six starting shortstops in the major leagues (Dannheisser, 2008).

Once Latino players sign contracts with MLB teams, they face significant cultural adjustments and language problems and the strain of living in a society where few people understand their cultural backgrounds (Bretón and Villegas, 1999; Burgos, 2007; Klein, 1991, 2006). This is partly why 90 to 95 percent of Latino players who sign contracts never make it beyond the minor leagues. Even those lucky enough to make minor league teams often are cut after a year or two, and rather than return home as "failures," they often find ways to remain in the United States as undocumented workers at low-wage jobs. Overall, this is a typical pattern in the lives of young men recruited by teams seeking relatively cheap baseball talent from Latin America and the Caribbean (Breton, 2000, p. 15), but their stories remain untold in U.S. and Canadian media.

Since the 1970s, the proportion of Latin American players has increased in U.S. professional leagues because they constituted a pool of cheap baseball labor. Established Latino stars are well paid, but young players have signed for a fraction of the money paid to new players born and trained in the United States. For example, a vice president of a MLB team said that it costs less to sign five Latin American players than one player from the United States. This "boatload approach" to signing these players has begun to change now that Latino "agents" are advocating the interests of many new players and as MLB teams have fewer visas they can give to non-citizen players because of new immigration and homeland security policies (Klein, 2006).

One of the problems now faced by Latino players is that they are more likely to test positive for drugs than players raised in the United States (Gordon, 2007). Since 2005 when MLB initiated its new drug-testing policy, most of the Latinos who have tested positive have spoken little English; have not known all the substances on the by MLB; and have come from countries where medical care is scarce and taking vitamins, supplements, and over-the-counter drugs is common (Gordon, 2007; Jenkins, 2005; LeBatard, 2005). Many drugs are less regulated in Latin America than in the United States, and some, including anabolic steroids, are available over the counter. The cheapest and most accessible steroids are those used by ranchers and farmers to increase the growth of their animals. Therefore, when young baseball players are desperate to escape poverty and hunger and hope to support their families, they may take these drugs despite risks to their health.

On the positive side of things, Latino players today enjoy the benefits of a visible and growing Latino culture in the United States, a growing Spanish-language media, a shared identity with many other players, and increased salaries that give them financial leverage that players in previous eras never had. Stereotypes continue to exist, but they are not as widely held as in the past, and when they are used in public, they are more likely to be challenged.

Undocumented Workers and Their Family Members We know little about sports in the lives of undocumented Latino workers and their families, who number in the millions. Sport involvement patterns are likely to vary with their income, education, and the number of years they've been in the United States. In some cases, sports are used as a means of assimilating into and expressing familiarity with U.S. culture and developing relationships with non-Latinos. In other cases, workers and their families often use weekend soccer, baseball, and softball games to come together and exchange information about jobs, friends, and family in Mexico, transferring money home, obtaining medical care and housing, and other things crucial to survival and maintaining support that can be helpful when a crisis strikes—a regular occurrence for many of these workers and their families.

A Need for Research Knowledge about the sport experiences of Latinos and Latinas is important because they are the fastest-growing ethnic population in the United States. Physical educators, coaches, and sport administrators need research that helps them to provide services and opportunities that meet the needs of Latinos. For example, the economic success of professional soccer in much of the United States depends on being sensitive to the interests and orientations of Latino athletes and spectators. Latinos are eager to have their cultural heritage recognized and incorporated into sports and sport experiences in the United States and into the awareness of their fellow citizens. In the public sector, there's a growing need for inclusive programs that provide participants from diverse backgrounds with opportunities to learn about the heritage, personal orientations, and experiences of their Latino peers.

Existing research indicates that sports are related to ethnicity in three ways: (1) they can be used to break down social and cultural barriers, discredit stereotypes, and facilitate assimilation; (2) they can be used by ethnic groups to preserve and extend ingroup relationships that support ethnic identities and make it possible to effectively bridge the gap between their native culture and dominant U.S. culture; and (3) they can be used to maintain segregated lifestyles that prevent people from having experiences and gaining knowledge that often leads to intergroup understanding, tolerance, and cooperation.

Sport Participation Among Asian Pacific Americans[4]

There are just over 16 million Asian Pacific Americans (APAs) in the United States. The legacy of wars and the global migration of labor has brought people from many Asian Pacific cultures to the United States. Most live on the West Coast and in cities where particular jobs have been plentiful. However, the heritage and histories of APAs are very diverse, representing at least twenty nations and dozens of cultures. This diversity is often ignored in media coverage and research that focuses on "Asians."

Although people with Chinese and Japanese ancestry have long played sports in their own communities (Chen, 2012; Niiya, 2000; Yep, 2009, 2010, 2012), the recent success and popularity of APA athletes has raised important issues about ethnic dynamics in sports. For example, the popularity of Jeremy Lin (Taiwanese/Chinese) in the NBA; Japanese and Korean baseball players, and a number of Samoan, Tongan, and Hawaiian players in the NFL; along with golfers Tiger Woods (Chinese and Thai) and Se Ri Pak (Korean); speed skater Apolo Anton Ohno; and figure skaters Kristi Yamaguchi (Japanese) and Michelle Kwan (Chinese), highlights the extent to which many Asians and Asian Americans have embraced sports played in the United States.

The popular all-star baseball player Ichiro Suzuki attracted so many Japanese spectators to Safeco Field in Seattle that signs in the stadium are now posted in both Japanese and English—although we don't have good information on the impact of Suzuki and other APA players on ethnic relations in the stadiums and communities where they play and live.

Historical research shows that certain sports have provided APAs with opportunities to challenge and discredit stereotypes about their lack of height and strength, their introverted "nature," and their singular dedication to intellectual development (Lapchick, 2007; Liang, 2007; Regalado, 2006; Yep, 2009, 2010, 2012). Yun-Oh Whang, a native Korean and a professor of sports marketing, acknowledged this point when he said:

> Asian Americans put huge value on education. [Therefore, it] is common that coaches and teachers at schools presume that an Asian American kid belongs in the science lab, not on the football field. This is why it is so important that Asian American athletes have to rise to the top and show the general public that Asian Americans can also achieve excellence in sports (in Lapchick, 2007).

[4]At this point in time, the literature related to North America focuses primarily on Asians whose ancestry is from Pacific Rim nations and cultures. This excludes people from countries in South Asia, including India, and in Western Asia, including Persian Gulf countries and cultures (or "The Middle East" from a British geographical standpoint). The literature in Europe, especially research done in Britain, focuses more on ethnic populations from South and Western Asia (Fleming, 2007; Fleming and Tomlinson, 2007; Long et al., 2007).

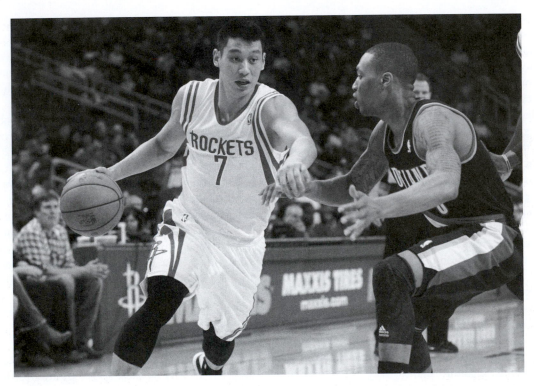

When Jeremy Lin came off the bench to propel the New York Knicks to a successful 2011-2012 season, his accomplishments created a "Linsanity" among basketball fans worldwide, especially in Taiwan and China, each of which claimed him as a native son because his mother and father are from Taiwan but his paternal grandparents are from mainland China (Chiang and Chen, 2013). Lin, who played for the Charlotte Hornets in 2016, initiated a socially important national discussion about Asian Americans and their contributions to U.S. culture and society. (*Source:* © Song Qiong/Xinhua Press/Corbis)

Playing sports also has been a way for some APAs to gain greater acceptance in schools and local communities. This is especially true for recent immigrants who seek assimilation. However, sociologist Christina Chin (2010; 2012; 2015) found that third- and fourth-generation Japanese American parents have used Japanese youth sport leagues to network and build relationships with other Japanese families. The league provides a context in which their children can meet and befriend Japanese American peers, including cousins and members of their extended family. The lack of recent immigrants from Japan and the current tendency of many families to choose housing to be close to jobs or good schools, means that children who are recent immigrants have had few opportunities to meet peers from Japanese families. This hasn't bothered the children as much as it does their parents, who value preserving important aspects of Japanese culture and passing them on to the next generation.

One of the league's founders explained that he started the sport program to provide an activity through which children could meet "other Japanese and give them the opportunity to eventually someday marry if they want to. . . . We weren't trying to say you have to marry Japanese, like some parents. I just wanted to expose them . . . to other Japanese" (Chin, 2012, p. 112). In addition to the matchmaking possibilities, the league also provides parents with a setting in which they can join with their Japanese American peers to become involved in their local communities. So they use the youth sport leagues to solidify relationships with other Japanese American families, perpetuate cultural values among their children, and form networks to support their involvement in the larger community.

Christina Chin's research shows that the experiences and sport participation patterns of APAs often vary depending on their immigration histories. Chinese Americans and Japanese Americans whose families have lived in the United States for four or more generations have different experiences from those of first- and second-generation Americans from Vietnam, Thailand, Cambodia, Laos, the Philippines, Malaysia, and Indonesia. Researchers must be sensitive to these differences and the ways that they influence sport participation patterns and experiences. Gender and social-class variations among APAs also are important areas for study.

A relatively exceptional pattern exists in the case of young men from the Samoan Islands (American Samoa and Western Samoa, including Tonga) who come to the United States to play football (Feldman, 2007; Garber, 2007a, 2007b; T. Miller, 2007). With a population the size of Anchorage, Alaska (260,000 people), these islands are the birthplace of thirty NFL players in 2015, plus more than 200 college football players. Universities also recruit many players from neighboring Tonga Island, which has a population the size of Peoria, Illinois (115,000). The sport traditions on all of these islands tend to involve rugby and cricket more than American sports, but young men from low-income families have defined football as their ticket to upward mobility, much as

the young men from the Dominican Republic see baseball. At this point, research is needed on the conditions under which this and other patterns occur.

Currently, we also need to know more about the ways in which images of Asian and Asian American athletes are taken up and represented in the U.S. media and in the minds of Americans. Research is also needed on the dramatic rise in popularity of various martial arts in the United States. Karate, judo, taekwondo, and other sports with Asian origins have become especially popular among children, but we don't know if participation in these martial arts has increased children's knowledge and awareness of Asian cultures, influenced ethnic relations in elementary schools, or discredited anti-Asian stereotypes among children and others who participate in these sports. It may be that these sport forms become so Americanized that their Asian roots are lost or ignored by participants—but we don't know.

> With [NBA player Jeremy] Lin, Asian Americans have found a role model who combines both the traditional Asian values of our parents with the Western traits needed to excel. "Linsanity" [may] make . . . corporate executives . . . take a second look at an Asian American for a leading role, as the Knicks did with Jeremy. —Anthony Youn, author of *In Stitches* (2012)

RACE, ETHNICITY, AND SPORT IN A GLOBAL PERSPECTIVE

Sociologist Mauro Valeri, director of Italy's Observatory on Racism and Anti-Racism in Football (Soccer), collected data on racist incidents in Italian soccer from 2000 to 2009. After analyzing the data, he concluded that racism has become part of the structure of soccer in Italy. Although his research focuses on one country, his conclusion applies to many others. As global migration patterns change the demographic profiles of cities and nations, and as soccer teams and fans become more racially and ethnically diverse, the stereotypes and racism that have often been dormant are renewed as people encounter others with unfamiliar customs and cultures.

Valeri's (2010) analysis led him to identify three primary expressions of racism in soccer:

1. **Direct racism** in which fans insult players for ethnic, racial, or religious reasons. Examples of this include spectators who throw bananas and make monkey sounds when players with African ancestry take the field. In some cases this racism is even directed at players on the home team, as spectators have always seen their club and team as direct representations of their local or national culture, which for them is tied to ideas about race and ethnicity. Racist chants and songs sung by groups of fans are so offensive that black players and their teammates have walked off the field to forfeit matches in protest, and referees have threatened to penalize the home team if officials do not control the racist expressions of spectators.

2. **Indirect racism** in which fans use chants or banners that promote a bigoted or discriminatory political agenda having no direct connection with soccer or players. These agendas often call for restricting immigration from certain countries, policing certain immigrant groups, or prohibiting ethnic forms of clothing or customs in public.

3. **Racism on the field** in which negative racial, ethnic, or religious comments are made by and to players, coaches, and referees. An example of this is players using bigoted slurs to demean opponents or referees. As these slurs have become public, soccer officials have created new anti-racist policies and fined players and referees who violate them. But the slurs continue and some fans cheer the players who make them.

Valeri found that each of these forms of racism increased significantly over the decade he collected data and they continue today.

This pattern of expressing racist ideas and beliefs at sport events

> **Every professional footballer should be able to play competitive football in the knowledge that references to the color of his skin will not be tolerated.** —English Football Association Commission (Fox Sports, 2011)

has become a persistent problem in many countries, especially in Europe where immigration policies are less strict than in other parts of the world (Massao and Fasting, 2010). Although these policies reflect a desire to have access to cheap immigrant labor, many citizens see the immigrants as threatening their cultural values, their quality of life, and the political stability of their cities and country. Some local citizens have turned to right-wing populist political candidates whose campaigns and policy positions include inflammatory rhetoric about certain racial, ethnic, or religious populations.

Because sport teams are sponsored by clubs with members from the local population, sport events often become sites for the expression of this rhetoric. This differs from North America, where fans don't identify so closely with the management of teams, don't see stadiums as sites for overt political expression, and are more controlled in the public expression of racist and bigoted comments.

As people around the world respond to changing global forces and conditions that push them away from certain geographical regions and pull them toward others, racial and ethnic relations become important social, political, and economic issues. When people have not had to deal with social and cultural diversity as a regular fact of life, they often resist coming to terms with rapidly growing immigrant populations that have unfamiliar customs and cultures that they see as strange, disruptive, or immoral. At the same time, the new immigrants often find it difficult to adjust to local customs and culture and resent the discrimination they face as they try to make a living. There is no end in sight for these migration processes as regional economies and job opportunities go through boom-and-bust cycles and as communications and transportation technologies make it easier for people to move around the globe in the hope of supporting themselves and their families.

Sports are clearly involved in these global push-and-pull processes. Teams and athletes regularly vacate locations where they cannot survive or meet expectations for success; at the same time, they are attracted to locations where success is more likely, even when the spectators are of a different ethnicity. Teams now recruit athletes and coaches worldwide, elite athletes move wherever they have the best opportunity to make a living, and coaches and managers follow opportunities without giving much thought to national borders—unless visa requirements create barriers they cannot overcome. Wealthy individuals and corporations that have made huge profits from global expansion and financial deals now shop for professional teams worldwide and may own teams in three or four different countries across multiple sports. Additionally, nations now bid to host global sport events so they can increase tourism and investments among diverse noncitizens.

Soccer players in Africa and parts of Latin America now look to European leagues and clubs for professional contracts, just as Latin American and some East Asian baseball players look to the United States. The United States is also a priority global destination for young people seeking high school and college athletic scholarships so they can attend school as they develop sport skills and earn degrees that will enable them to survive in a global economy. As China and India grow economically, they too will become sources and destinations for athletes seeking opportunities to play their sports at a professional level, and this will create new ethnic relations issues in sports.

These global processes now force people to deal with racial and ethnic issues for which they are unprepared and which they are often unwilling to consider. Sports are regularly described as sites for creating social integration, but it is clear that this does not occur automatically; in fact, the opposite often occurs when they sports become sites for the expression of racial, ethnic, and religious conflict and prejudices. This has led to efforts among some people—in and outside of sports—to create programs designed to defuse racial and ethnic conflict and make sport venues "racist-free zones"

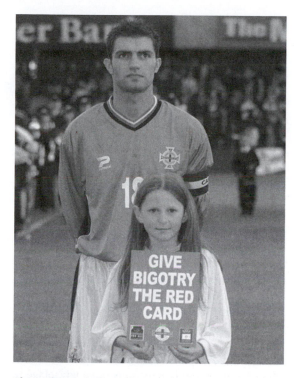

The Irish Football Association (IFA) in Northern Ireland was a pioneer in using sport to strategically intervene in the lives of young people to bridge social divisions related to race, ethnicity, and religion. They began in the early 1990s and have revised their approach as they learned what succeeded and what didn't. Their success is due to the continuity of leadership and IFA support—things that similar efforts in other countries often lack. In response to increased racial incidents in recent years, many anti-racism organizations now exist in Europe. (*Source:* © Michael Boyd, Irish Football Association)

in their communities and in sport leagues that cross national borders (Kassimeris, 2008, 2009; Llopis-Goig, 2013).

There also is a need for teams and leagues to sponsor carefully planned efforts to facilitate more tolerant forms of racial and ethnic relations. In some cases, diversity courses are needed for everyone from owners to athletes. To work in sports today and have positive experiences, people must do their homework and learn about the cultural perspectives of players, coaches, spectators, and even club and team owners from unfamiliar ethnic backgrounds. In this sense, as people in sports become more effective in facilitating amicable racial and ethnic relations, the better off their lives, teams, organizations, and communities will be.

From a sociological perspective it is interesting that as global migration creates a need for teams and sport organizations to become more ethnically and culturally inclusive, the growing inequality in many nations is leading to the creation of local sports and sport organizations that are more ethnically and culturally homogeneous. However, it is naïve for people in these homogeneous programs to assume that they can avoid facing the racial and ethnic issues that exist in the rest of the world.

Regardless of where they grow up, nearly all aspiring athletes will be required to deal constructively with ethnic differences on their teams and in their sport organizations. Coaches and team officials now must go beyond simply dealing with ethnic diversity and turn it into a competitive advantage if they wish to keep their jobs. Cultural and language issues present never ending challenges that call for creative solutions to bring athletes and other personnel together in ways that help the team succeed.

THE DYNAMICS OF RACIAL AND ETHNIC RELATIONS IN SPORTS

Racial and ethnic relations in the United States are better today than in the past, but more changes are needed before sports are a model of inclusion and fairness. The challenges today are different from the ones faced twenty years ago, and experience shows that when current challenges are met, new social situations are created in which new challenges emerge. For example, once racial and ethnic segregation is eliminated and people come together, they must learn to live, work, and play with each other despite diverse experiences and cultural perspectives. Meeting this challenge requires a commitment to equal treatment, *plus* learning about

the perspectives of others, understanding how they define and give meaning to the world, and then determining how to form and maintain relationships while respecting differences, making compromises, and supporting one another in the pursuit of goals that may not always be shared. None of this is easy, and challenges are never met once and for all time.

Many people think in unrealistic terms when it comes to racial and ethnic relations. They believe that opening a door so that others may enter a social world is all that's needed to achieve racial and ethnic harmony. However, this is merely a first step in a never-ending process of nurturing relationships, producing an inclusive society, and sharing power with others. Racial and ethnic diversity brings potential vitality and creativity to a team, organization, or society, but this potential does not automatically become reality. It requires constant awareness, commitment, and work to achieve and maintain it (Adair et al., 2010; Cunningham, 2007a, 2007b 2009; Cunningham and Fink, 2006; Fink and Cunningham, 2005).

The following sections deal with three major challenges related to racial and ethnic relations in sports today: (1) eliminating racial and ethnic exclusion in sport participation; (2) dealing with and managing racial and ethnic diversity by creating an inclusive culture on sport teams and in sport organizations; and (3) integrating positions of power in sport organizations.

Eliminating Racial and Ethnic Exclusion in Sports

Racial and ethnic diversity is most likely to exist in a sport under the following six conditions:

1. When those who control teams personally benefit if they recruit and play the best players regardless of skin color or ethnicity.
2. When athlete performance can be measured in concrete, objective terms so that racism and prejudice are less likely to influence judgments about skills.

3. When an entire team benefits from a good performance by a teammate, regardless of the teammate's skin color or ethnicity.
4. When excellence on the playing field does not give a player more power and authority on a team or control over players from the dominant racial or ethnic group in society.
5. When friendships and off-the-field social relationships between teammates are not required for team success.
6. When all athletes are controlled by coaches, managers, administrators, and owners from the ethnically dominant group in society.

These six characteristics limit the threats that cause fear and create resistance to racial and ethnic desegregation. Therefore, when the white men who controlled professional teams and revenue-producing college teams in the United States realized that they could benefit financially from recruiting ethnic minority players without giving up power and control and without disrupting the existing structure and relationships in their sports, they began to do so.

Desegregation occurs more slowly in sports that lack the characteristics listed above. Golf, tennis, swimming, and other sports played in private clubs where social interaction is much more personal and often involves male–female relationships have been slow to accept racial and ethnic diversity. As social contacts become increasingly personal, people are more likely to enforce various forms of exclusion. This is why informal forms of racial and ethnic exclusion still exist in many private sports clubs and why there are so few African Americans, Latinos, and Asian Pacific Americans in professional golf and tennis or in club-based sports such as lacrosse.

The most significant forms of racial and ethnic exclusion today occur at the community level where they are hidden behind the fees and other resources required for sport participation. People can claim to have ethnically open sport programs when in reality their location, fees, and lack of public transportation preclude ethnically inclusive participation.

As public programs are dropped and sports are offered primarily by commercial providers, patterns of exclusion reflect race and ethnicity to the extent that race and ethnicity influence residential location and income. This type of exclusion occurs regularly in the United States and is difficult to eliminate because market forces do the dirty work of segregation without race or ethnicity even being mentioned. Developing strategies to undermine these dynamics and make sports more inclusive is one of the most difficult challenges we now face worldwide.

Dealing With and Managing Racial and Ethnic Diversity in Sports

History shows that, after Branch Rickey signed black player Jackie Robinson to a contract with the Brooklyn Dodgers in 1946, many new challenges confronted Rickey, Robinson, the Dodgers organization, players throughout the league, other baseball teams in the National League, and spectators attending baseball games. Rickey had to convince his partners in the Dodgers organization and other team owners that it was in their interest to abandon their practice of segregation. Robinson had to endure unspeakable racism from opponents, spectators, and others. To control his anger and depression, he needed support from Rickey, his coach, teammates, and his wife, Rachel.

As thousands of African American fans wanted to see Robinson, the Dodgers and other teams had to change their policies of racial exclusion and segregation in their stadiums. Teammates on the Dodgers were forced to decide if and how they would support Robinson on and off the field. The team's coach had to manage interracial dynamics he knew nothing about: Who would be Robinson's roommate on road trips, where would the team stay and eat in cities where hotels and restaurants excluded blacks, and what would he say to players who made racist comments that could destroy team morale? These questions had never been asked in the past because Major League Baseball had excluded black players.

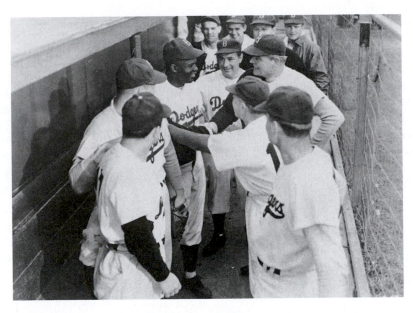

Eliminating racial barriers to sport participation is as important today as it was when Jackie Robinson joined the Brooklyn Dodgers in 1947. After the desegregation of Major League Baseball, there were new challenges associated with managing intergroup relations on teams and integrating positions of power in sport organizations. These challenges continue to exist. (*Source:* Library of Congress #LC-USZ62-119883)

White baseball fans who had never met a black person now faced the prospect of sitting next to one if they wanted to attend a game. Black fans, who were uncomfortable with white people, faced a similar challenge. Stadium managers faced the challenge of serving food to people with different tastes and traditions; white, working-class service workers had to serve black customers—a totally new experience for them. Journalists and radio announcers had to decide how they would represent Robinson's experiences in their coverage—would they talk about racism on the field and in the clubhouse and about the way Robinson handled it, or would they ignore race, even though it was relevant to the game?

These are just a few of the new challenges created when MLB was desegregated. And as these challenges were met, new ones emerged. For example, as other black players were signed to teams, players began to racially segregate themselves in locker rooms. Black players could not buy homes in segregated white areas of the cities where they played, and when they challenged records set by whites, they received death threats. Stadium security became an issue, some teams became racially divided, and black players often felt marginalized because all coaches, managers, trainers, and owners were white men.

Even the positions of black and white players fit patterns shaped by racial ideology. Black players, expected to be fast and physically gifted, were assigned to the outfield in baseball and defensive back in football—positions believed to call for speed and quick reactions—whereas white players, expected to be smart, played positions believed to require intelligence, leadership, and decision-making skills, such as pitcher and catcher in baseball and quarterback and offensive guard in football. These position placements, or "stacking" patterns, as they've been called in the sociology of sport, prevented most blacks from playing the positions at which they would be identified as good candidates for coaching jobs after they retired. This is related to a challenge that has become chronic in most sports: the lack of black CEOs, general managers, and head coaches.

This example illustrates that challenges related to race and ethnicity are an ever-present part of our lives; they will exist as long as skin color and ethnicity influence people's lives and are viewed as socially important. This is not new, nor is it unique to sports. Managers and coaches must now be ready and able to work effectively with players from multiple cultural and national backgrounds, meld them into a team, defuse and debunk players' racial and ethnic stereotypes, and facilitate respect for customs and lifestyles they've not seen before. Even determining the food to be served in pregame meals now requires creative management strategies.

Athletes and coaches must learn new ways to communicate effectively on ethnically diverse teams, and marketing people must learn how to promote racially and ethnically diverse teams to predominantly white, Euro-American fans. Ethnic issues enter into sponsorship considerations and products sold at games, and ethnic awareness is now an important qualification for those who handle advertising and sponsorship deals. For example, the success of professional soccer in the United States depends partly on attracting ethnic spectators to games and television broadcasts. Spanish-speaking announcers are crucial, and deals must be made with radio and television stations that broadcast in Spanish.

Teams in the NFL and NBA now face situations in which 70 to 80 percent of their players are black, whereas 90 to 95 percent of their season ticket holders are white. Many people are aware of this issue, but it's rarely discussed because Americans have a "civic etiquette" that keeps these issues "off the table" in public settings (Eliasoph, 1999). But if the challenges related to race and ethnicity in sports are to be met, changes in this etiquette are needed so that open and honest discussions can occur.

Integrating Positions of Power in Sport Organizations

Despite progressive changes in many sports, positions of power and control are held primarily by white, non-Latino men. There are exceptions to this pattern, but they do not eliminate pervasive and persistent racial and ethnic inequalities related to power and control in sports.

Data on who holds positions of power change every year, and it is difficult to obtain consistent information from sport teams and organizations. Fortunately, Richard Lapchick, director of The Institute for Diversity and Ethics in Sport (TIDES) and his colleagues at the University of Central Florida, regularly publish *Racial and Gender Report Cards* for the NCAA and many professional sports. They contain data on the racial and ethnic composition of players in major professional team sports and an analysis of the number and types of jobs held by women and people of color in major professional and university sports organizations. The report cards cover everyone from owners and athletic directors to office staff, athletic trainers, and radio and television announcers.

The recent report cards on professional leagues and teams show that white men are overrepresented in the top power positions in the major professional sports played in the United States. Blacks are overrepresented among players in a few sports, but they generally play under the control and management of white men.

Patterns are similar in most sport organizations at nearly all levels of competition. Overall, data suggest that full inclusion in terms of sharing power is far from being achieved. In fact, the movement of women and ethnic minority persons into power positions in sports has stalled recently. Without constant attention and effective strategies, power remains in the hands of white men whose backgrounds position them to obtain leadership roles.

Overall, people do not give up racial and ethnic beliefs easily, especially when they come in the form of well-established ideologies rooted deeply in their cultures. Those who benefit from dominant racial ideology generally resist changes in the relationships and social structures that reproduce it. This is why certain racial and ethnic inequities remain part of sports.

Sports may bring people together, but they do not automatically lead them to adopt tolerant attitudes or change long-standing practices of exclusion in the rest of their lives. For example, white team owners, general managers, and athletic directors in the United States worked with black athletes for many years before they ever hired black coaches or administrators. It often requires social and legal pressures to force people in positions of power to act more affirmatively in their hiring practices. In the meantime, blacks and other ethnic minorities remain underrepresented in coaching and administration.

Although there is resistance to certain types of changes in sports, some sport organizations are more progressive than others when it comes to improving racial and ethnic relations. However, good things do not happen automatically, nor do changes in people's attitudes automatically translate into changes in the overall organization of sports. Challenging the negative beliefs and attitudes of individuals is one thing; changing the relationships and social structures that have been built on those beliefs and attitudes is another. Both changes are needed, but neither will occur automatically just because sports bring people together in the same locker rooms and stadiums.

The reports cards published by Lapchick and TIDES and similar studies on hiring practices done by the Black Coaches and Administrators association have kept a bright light shining on the racial and ethnic composition of major sport organizations in the United States. This light creates heat that makes decision makers uncomfortable if they are not making progress toward full racial and ethnic inclusion. Public scrutiny is an effective strategy because progress comes only when those in power work to bring about change. It has never been easy for people to deal with racial and ethnic issues, but if it is done in sports, it attracts public attention that can inspire changes in other spheres of life.

The racial and ethnic diversity training sessions used over the past two decades have produced some changes, but promoting positive changes in ethnic relations today requires leaders who are trained specifically to create more inclusive cultures and power structures in sport organizations. This means that training must go beyond athletes and include everyone from team owners and athletic directors to mid-level management, coaches, and people in marketing, media, and public information. When training programs are directed primarily toward employees, the employees won't take them seriously if they don't see their superiors making a personal commitment to them.

Even people who are sensitive to ethnic diversity issues require regular opportunities to renew and extend their knowledge of the experiences and perspectives of others who have different vantage points in social worlds. This means that effective training requires information and approaches organized around the perspectives of underrepresented ethnic populations. This is crucial because progressive change takes into account the interests of those least likely to be heard or to hold positions of power.

summary

ARE RACE AND ETHNICITY IMPORTANT IN SPORTS?

Racial and ethnic issues exist in sports, just as they exist in other spheres of social life. As people watch, play, and talk about sports, they often take into account ideas about skin color and ethnicity. The meanings given to skin color and ethnic background influence access to sport participation and the decisions that people make about sports in their lives.

Race refers to a category of people identified through a classification system based on meanings given to physical traits among humans; *ethnicity* refers to collections of people identified in terms of their shared cultural heritage. Racial and ethnic *minorities* are populations that have endured systematic forms of discrimination in a society.

The idea of race has a complex history, and it serves as the foundation for racial ideology, which people use to identify and make sense of "racial" characteristics and differences. Racial ideology, like other social constructions, changes over time as ideas and relationships change. However, over the past century in the United States, dominant racial ideology has supported the notion that there are important biological and cognitive differences between people classified as "black" as opposed to "white," and that these differences explain the success of black athletes in certain sports and sport positions.

Racial ideology influences the ways that many people connect skin color with athletic performance. At the same time, it influences participation decisions and achievement patterns in sports. Race, gender, and class relations in American society combine to create a context in which black males emphasize a stylized persona that adds to the commodity value of the black male body in sports and enables some black athletes to use widely accepted ideas about race to intimidate white opponents in sports.

Sport participation patterns among African Americans, Native Americans, Latinos, and Asian Pacific Americans each have unique histories. Combinations of cultural, social, economic, and political factors have influenced those histories. However, sport participation in ethnic minority populations usually occurs under terms set by the dominant ethnic population in a community or society. Minority populations are seldom able to use sports to challenge the power and privilege of the dominant group, even though particular individuals may experience great personal success in sports.

Racial and ethnic issues affect sports worldwide. Europe currently faces challenges as increased migration has created tensions between native-born citizens and immigrants. As a result, previously dormant racist attitudes are now being expressed in connection with sports, especially soccer. This has created new challenges for sport teams and organizations worldwide. Racist and bigoted actions by spectators, athletes, coaches, and referees have increased since the beginning of this century and now are a significant problem for which there must be local and sport-related solutions.

The fact that some sports have histories of racially and ethnically mixed participation does not mean that problems have been eliminated. Harmonious racial and ethnic relations never occur automatically, and ethnic harmony is never established once and for all time. As current problems are solved, new relationships and new challenges are created. This means that racial and ethnic issues require regular attention if challenges are to be anticipated accurately and dealt with successfully. Success also depends on whether members of the dominant ethnic population see value in racial and ethnic diversity and commit themselves to dealing with diversity issues alongside those with different ethnic backgrounds.

Sports continue to be sites for racial and ethnic tensions and problems. But despite this, they also can be sites for challenging racial ideology and transforming ethnic relations. This happens only when people in sports plan strategies to encourage critical awareness of ethnic prejudices, racist ideas, and forms of discrimination built into the culture and structure of sport organizations. This awareness is required to increase ethnic inclusion, deal with and manage ethnic diversity, and integrate ethnic minorities into the power structures of sport organizations. Without this awareness, ethnic relations often become volatile and lead to overt forms of hostility.

SUPPLEMENTAL READINGS

Reading 1. Knowledge about race today (from PBS, "Race: The Power of an Illusion")

Reading 2. Media coverage of Joe Louis

Reading 3. Racial ideology in sports

Reading 4. Native Americans and team mascots

Reading 5. Samoan men in college and professional football

SPORT MANAGEMENT ISSUES

- The athletic department in your predominantly white university has asked you to develop a campaign for the campus and community that will make it possible for African American students, especially young men, to be seen by teachers and students as students who take their education seriously. The ultimate goal is to change campus culture to support the student identities of African American students, especially those on sport teams. Where would you begin and what would be the focus of your program?

- You have been hired as the athletic director for a school district in Colorado. One of the high schools in the district has the nickname "Redmen," and the school's mascot is a caricature of a male Indian who dances and chants on the sidelines holding and waving a plastic tomahawk. A group of Native Americans from the local area tells you they are offended and asks you to convince people at the school to drop the name, the mascot, and team cheers that mimic Indian religious chants. Explain what you will do to respond to the group and to facilitate an educational solution for this issue.

- Your town has recently had a large influx of immigrants from Mexico and a few Asian countries. The editor of your local newspaper writes an editorial in which he suggests that the high school's varsity sport program is an effective tool for establishing good intergroup relations in the town. You read it and conclude that he has not thought of the challenges faced when trying to use sports in this way. You write a letter to the editor in which you explain these things to the readers of the paper. What does your letter say?

- Data clearly suggest that it is difficult to integrate positions of power in sport organizations. As a sport management consultant you have been hired to offer recommendations to enhance racial and ethnic diversity in a suburban school district on the West Coast. Describe your three primary recommendations, and explain why you made them.

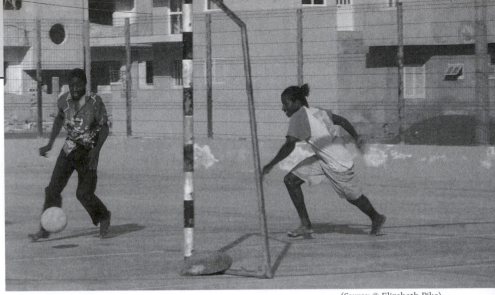

(*Source:* © Elizabeth Pike)

chapter 9

SOCIAL CLASS

Do Money and Power Matter in Sports?

Children remain the poorest age group in America. . . . 37 percent of Black children and 32 percent of Hispanic children are poor, contrasted with 12 percent of White non-Hispanic children.

—**Children's Defense Fund (in Hassler, 2015)**

. . . 26 percent of parents hope their child who plays high school sports will be able to do so professionally. The views of the parents vary by socioeconomic status. . . . 44 percent of parents with a high school education or less hope their children become a professional athlete, compared to 9 percent of parents who have graduated college.

—**NPR et al., 2015**

Richer kids are roughly twice as likely to play after-school sports. They are more than twice as likely to be the captains of their sports teams. . . . Poorer kids have become more pessimistic and detached.

—**David Brooks,** *New York Times* **columnist (2012)**

We're moving toward an America that none of us have ever lived in, in which being affluent or being poor is inherited. . . . The most important decision any kid makes [today] is choosing their parents.

—**Robert Putnam, Professor of Public Policy, Harvard University (in Rinaldi, 2015)**

Social Class and Class Relations

Sports and Economic Inequality

Social Class and Sport Participation Patterns

Global Inequalities and Sports

Economic and Career Opportunities in Sports

Sport Participation and Occupational Careers Among Former Athletes

Summary: Do Money and Power Matter in Sports?

Learning Objectives

- Define social class, class ideology, and class relations, and explain how they are manifested in sports today.

- Identify who has power in sports today, and the interests that are served by that power.

- Critically assess the argument that professional sports franchises benefit everyone and create jobs in a city.

- Explain how class, gender, and ethnic relations come together and influence sport participation patterns in society.

- Explain why sports in the future are likely to be less diverse in terms of ethnicity and social class.

- Describe the ways in which social class impacts sport spectators today.

- Outline the economic and career opportunities that exist in sports today, especially for women and ethnic minorities.

- Identify the conditions under which sport participation is most likely and least likely to lead to upward mobility and occupational success.

- Understand the reality of college scholarships today. Assess the significance of athletic scholarships for occupational success.

People like to think that sport is the great equalizer, that it transcends issues of money, power, and economic inequalities. They see sports as open activities in which success comes only through individual ability and hard work. However, all organized sports depend on material resources, and those resources must come from somewhere. Therefore, playing, watching, and excelling in sports depend on resources supplied by individuals, families, governments, or private organizations.

More than ever before, it takes money to play sports and develop sport skills. Tickets are expensive, and spectators often are divided by social class in the stadium: The wealthy and well connected sit in luxury suites and club seats, whereas fans who are less well off sit in other sections, depending on their ability to pay for premium tickets or buy season tickets.

Today, it takes money to watch sports on television as satellite and cable connections come with ever-increasing monthly subscriber fees, expensive sport packages, and pay-per-view costs. This means that sports and sport participation are closely linked with the distribution of economic resources in society.

Many people believe that sports are a new path to economic success for people from all social classes. Rags-to-riches stories are common when people talk about athletes. However, these beliefs and stories distract attention from the ways in which sports reflect and perpetuate existing economic inequalities.

This chapter deals with matters of money and wealth, as well as larger sociological issues related to social class and socioeconomic mobility. Our discussion focuses on the following questions:

1. What is meant by *social class* and *class relations?*
2. How do social class and class relations influence sports and sport participation?
3. Are sports open and democratic in the provision of economic and career opportunities?
4. Does playing sports contribute to occupational success and social mobility among former athletes?

SOCIAL CLASS AND CLASS RELATIONS

Understanding social class and the related concepts of social stratification, socioeconomic status, and life chances is important when studying social worlds. Economic resources are related to power in society, and economic inequalities influence many aspects of people's lives.

Social class refers to *categories of people who share an economic position in society based on their income, wealth (savings and assets), education, occupation, and social connections.* People in a particular social class also share similar **life chances**—that is, *similar odds for achieving economic success and power in society.* Social classes exist in all contemporary societies because life chances are not equally distributed across all people.

Social stratification refers to *structured forms of economic inequalities that are part of the organization of everyday social life.* In other words, in comparison with people from upper social classes, people from lower social classes have fewer opportunities to achieve economic success and power. Children born into wealthy, powerful, and well-connected families are in better positions to become wealthy, powerful, and well-connected adults than are children born into poor families that lack influence and social networks connecting them with educational and career opportunities.

Most of us are aware of economic inequalities in society. We see them all around us. We know they exist and influence people's lives, but there are few public discussions about the impact of social class on our views of ourselves and others, our social relationships, and our everyday lives. In other words, we don't discuss **class relations**—the *ways that social class is incorporated into the organization of our everyday lives.* We often hear about the importance of equal opportunities in society, but there are few discussions about the ways that people in upper socioeconomic classes use their income, wealth, and power to maintain their positions of advantage in society and pass that advantage from one generation to the next. Instead, we hear "rags-to-riches" stories about individuals who overcame poverty or a lower-class background to become wealthy, stories about "millionaires next door," and stories about CEOs who are "regular guys" with annual incomes of $10 million or more.

Ignored in the media and popular discourse are the oppressive effects of poverty and the limited opportunities available to those who lack economic resources, access to good education, and well-placed social connections. Those stories are too depressing to put in the news, claim executives for the commercial media—people don't like to hear about them, and they lower audience ratings. However, social-class differences in the form of socioeconomic inequalities are real; they have real consequences for life chances, they affect nearly every facet of people's lives, and all of this is clearly documented by valid and reliable data (Duncan and Murnane, 2011; Ferguson, 2013; Kochhar et al., 2011; Lardner and Smith, 2005; Reardon and Bischoff, 2011; Stiglitz, 2012; Wilkinson and Pickett, 2010).

People in the United States often shy away from critical discussions of social class and class relations because they're uneasy about acknowledging that equality of opportunity is largely a myth in their society (Stiglitz, 2012). This is especially true in regard to sports and sport participation—a sphere of life in which most people believe that money and class-based advantages don't matter.

The discussion of social class and class relations in this chapter is grounded in a critical approach that identifies who benefits from and who is disadvantaged by the ways that sports are organized and played. The focus is on economic inequality, the processes through which inequality is reproduced, how it benefits wealthy and powerful people, and how it affects sports and the lives of people associated with sports.

SPORTS AND ECONOMIC INEQUALITY

Money and economic power exert significant influence on the goals, purpose, and organization of sports in society. Many people believe that sports and sport participation are open to all people and that inequalities related to money, position, and influence have no effect on the organized games we play and watch. However, formally organized sports could not be developed, scheduled, or maintained without economic resources. Those who control money and economic power use them to organize and sponsor sports. As they do so, they give preference to sport forms that reflect and maintain their values and interests. As a result, sports emerge out of a context in which inequality shapes decisions and the allocation of resources. In the process, sports reproduce the very inequalities that so many people think are absent in them.

The wealthy aristocrats who developed the modern Olympic Games even used their power to establish a definition of *amateur* that favored athletes from wealthy backgrounds. This definition, which excluded athletes who used their sport skills to earn a living, has been revised over the years so the Olympics now include those who are not independently wealthy. However, money and economic power now operate in different ways as elite-level training has become privatized and very costly in many countries.

Elite and powerful people have considerable influence over what "counts as sport" and how sports are organized and played in mainstream social worlds. Even when grassroots games and physical activities become formally organized as sports, they don't become popular unless they can be used to reaffirm the interests and ideologies of sponsors with resources. For example, ESPN organized and televised the X Games to fit the needs of corporate sponsors that buy advertising time to promote their products to young males.

Even informal games require facilities, equipment, and safe play spaces—all of which are more plentiful in upper- and upper-middle-income neighborhoods. Low-income neighborhoods generally lack what is needed to initiate and sustain informal activities; families don't have large lawns at their homes, they don't live on safe cul-de-sacs without traffic, and there is a short supply of well-maintained neighborhood parks. This is why social class and class relations must be taken into account when we study sports in society and try to explain the patterns of sport participation we see around us.

The Dynamics of Class Relations

To understand the dynamics of class relations, think about the ways that age relations operate in sports. Even though young people are capable of creating and playing games on their own, adults intervene and create organized youth sport programs. These programs emphasize the things that adults think are best for their children. As noted in Chapter 4, adults have the resources to develop, schedule, and maintain organized sports that reflect their ideas of what children should be doing and learning. Children often enjoy these adult-controlled sports, but their participation occurs in a framework that is determined by adults and organized to legitimize and reproduce adult control over their lives.

Age relations are especially apparent in youth sports when participants don't meet adult expectations or they violate the rules developed by adults. The adults use their power to define deviance, identify when it occurs, and demand that children comply with rules and expectations. Overall, the adults use their superior resources to convince young people that "the adults' way" is "the right way" to play sports. When young people comply with adults' rules and meet adults' expectations, they're rewarded and told that they have "character." This is why many adults are fond of college and professional coaches who are autocratic and controlling. These coaches reaffirm the ideas that it is normal and necessary for adults to control young people and that young people must learn to accept that control. In this way, sports reproduce a hierarchical form of age relations, with adult power and privilege defined as normal and necessary aspects of social worlds.

Class relations work in similar ways. People with resources sponsor sports that support their ideas about "good character," individual responsibility, competition, excellence, achievement, and proper social organization. In fact, whenever

people obtain power in a social world, they define "character" in a way that promotes their interests. For example, when wealthy and powerful people play sports in exclusive clubs, such as Augusta National (golf club) in Georgia, they use a class ideology that legitimizes their right to do so and establishes their membership in such a club as a privilege they deserve for being winners in society. This also is reflected in the compensation received by CEOs of large corporations: In 1965 they received about eighteen times more than typical workers that year. In 1978 it was twenty-seven times more, in 1995 it was 135 times more, and in 2013 it was over 300 times more (Mishel and Sabadish, 2013). As top executives took more pay for themselves, the pay for typical workers remained stuck at 1980 levels. This illustrates how power and position often influences class relations.

Over those same years corporate sponsorship of sports has increased exponentially. This, too, is linked to class relations because CEOs seek to sponsor sports that can be presented in ways that reaffirm the existing class structure in society and the ideology that supports it. This is partly why popular spectator sports worldwide emphasize competition, individualism, highly specialized skills, the use of technology, and dominance over opponents. When these values and cultural practices are widely accepted, average people are more likely to believe that the status and privilege of the wealthy and powerful are legitimate and deserved.

Sports that emphasize partnership, sharing, open participation, nurturance, and mutual support are seldom sponsored because people with power don't want to promote values that reaffirm equality and horizontal forms of social organization in society.

As the globalization of money, commercial trade, and financing opened up in the late 1970s, class relations in many societies changed to increase the income, wealth, and consumption gaps between the poor and the powerful. These economic changes enabled those who were connected with the flow of capital around the world to increase their power and wealth (Saez and Piketty, 2006; Stiglitz, 2012). As a result, the gap between

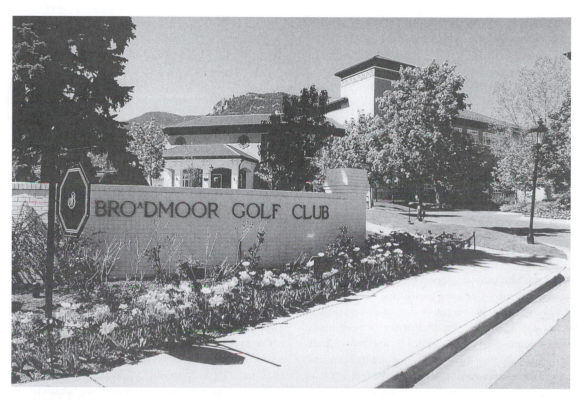

BROADMOOR GOLF, TENNIS CLUB & SPA
Members and Guests Only

The belief that wealth and power are achieved through competitive success implies that being wealthy and powerful is proof of one's abilities, qualifications, and overall moral worth. Exclusive sports clubs reaffirm this belief and reinforce the idea that the class privileges enjoyed by wealthy and powerful people are deserved; and the clubs are sites for establishing relationships used to perpetuate mutually beneficial privileged status. (*Source:* © Jay Coakley)

the rich and the poor expanded in terms of income, wealth, and political influence.

Class Ideology in the United States

Sociologists define **class ideology** as *interrelated ideas and beliefs that people use to understand economic inequalities, identify their class position, and evaluate the impact of economic inequalities on the organization of social worlds.* Dominant class ideology in the United States has long been organized around two themes: the American Dream and a belief that the United States is a meritocracy.

The **American Dream** is *a hopeful vision of boundless opportunities for individuals to succeed economically and live a happy life based on consumption.* It focuses attention on individual aspirations and often blurs an awareness of social class differences in material living conditions and differential life chances among categories of people. The uniquely American belief that "you can be anything you want to be" never acknowledges that a person's class position influences life chances or that life chances influence patterns of social and economic mobility in all social classes. Therefore, Americans often dream about what they hope to be in the future rather than critically examining their current economic circumstances and the ways that class relations affect their lives. The belief that "you can be anything" also discredits poor and low-income people by associating poverty with individual failure, laziness, and weakness of character.

The American Dream is usually connected with a belief that the United States is a **meritocracy**—*a social world in which rewards go to people who deserve them due to their abilities, qualifications, and recognized achievements.* Believing that the United States is a meritocracy helps people explain and justify economic inequalities. It supports the assumption that success is rightfully earned and failure is caused by poor choices and a lack of ambition.

Sustaining a belief that the United States is a meritocracy depends on related beliefs that individual ability, qualifications, and character are objectively proven through competitive success; that humans are naturally competitive; and that competition is the only fair way to allocate rewards in a society. This is why people with money and power like to use sports as a metaphor for life—it identifies winners like them as deserving individuals who have outperformed others in a natural process of individual competition and achievement.

Figure 9.1 shows that class ideology in the United States consists of interrelated ideas and beliefs about the American Dream, meritocracy, and competition; it illustrates that inequality is a result of people receiving what they deserve; it emphasizes that opportunities exist and that success is achieved only when people develop abilities and work hard; and it justifies inequality as a natural result of competition in a society where merit counts.

One of the outcomes of such an ideology is that competitive success comes to be linked with moral worth. The belief that "you get what you deserve, and you deserve what you get" works to the advantage of people with wealth, because it implies that they deserve what they have and that inequality is a fair and natural outcome of competitive processes. A related belief is that as long as competition is free and unregulated, only the best will succeed and only the lazy and unqualified will fail.

Promoting this ideology is difficult when it conflicts with the real experiences of many

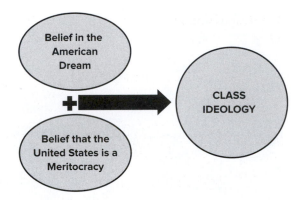

FIGURE 9.1 The two primary beliefs that inform and support class ideology in the United States.

Americans who work hard and haven't achieved success in the form of the American Dream or have seen their success disappear due to factors beyond their control. Therefore, people in the upper classes are most likely to retain their position and status *if* they can create and perpetuate widespread agreement that competition is a natural and fair way to allocate rewards and that the winners in competitive processes deserve the rewards they receive. This, of course, is how sports come to be connected with class relations in society. Sports offer "proof" that inequalities are based on merit, that competition identifies winners, and that losers should work harder or change themselves if they want to be winners, or simply get up and try again. Most important, sports provides a metaphor for society that portrays social class as a characteristic of individuals rather than an economic structure that influences life chances and the distribution of resources in society (Falcous and McLeod, 2012).

Alan Tomlinson, a British sociologist who has studied power and social class for decades, has noted that sport, as it is sponsored and played today, "ultimately serves to reproduce social and economic distinctions and preserve the power and influence of those who control resources in society." As a result, he says, sports today "cannot be fully understood unless this key influence and core dynamic is fully recognized" (2007, p. 4695).

Class Relations and Who Has Power in Sports

Decisions that affect the meaning, purpose, and organization of sports are made at many levels—from neighborhood youth sport programs to the International Olympic Committee. Although scholars who study sports in society identify people who exercise power in various settings, they usually don't rank those with power in and over sports. But this has been done by journalists at *The Sporting News* in the past and more recently at *Sports Illustrated* (Rushin, 2013).

The list of the top twenty most powerful from the 2013 *Sports Illustrated* rankings is shown in Table 9.1. There are no coaches or athletes on the list because they are simply hired hands—workers who serve at the discretion of those who run the business of sport. Therefore, the journalists who did the selecting and ranking focused on who could make decisions that would have a profound influence on the organization and culture of sports. At the same time, they realized that "all power is contextual" and that power depends on the positions of people in the overall business of sports.

Among the top twenty are seven CEOs in major sport organizations, five in media companies, and two from corporate sponsors; there also are four team owners, the CEO of IMG (the largest sports

Table 9.1 The 2013 top twenty in the *Sports Illustrated* "Power 50" list

Rank	Name	Position
1.	Roger Goodell	NFL commissioner
2.	David Stern	NBA commissioner
3.	Philip Anschutz	AEG owner
4.	John Skipper	ESPN president
5.	Bud Selig	MLB commissioner
6.	Stan Kroenke	Kroenke Sports Enterprises owner
7.	Mark Lazarus	NBC Sports chairman
8.	Jacques Rogge	IOC president
9.	Phil Knight	Nike chairman
10.	Hedge Fund Dude	[investment advisor(s)]
11.	Mark Walter	Guggenheim Partners CEO & Dodgers owner
12.	Robert Kraft	Patriots owner
13.	Sean McManus	CBS Sports chairman
14.	Michael Dolan	IMG Worldwide CEO
15.	Eric Shanks	Fox Sports co-president
16.	Sepp Blatter	FIFA president
17.	Mike Slive	SEC commissioner
18.	Adam Silver	NBA deputy commissioner
19.	Jerry Jones	Cowboys owner
20.	Larry Ellison	Oracle CEO

Source: Rushin, 2013; http://gamedayr.com/sports/sports-illustrated-50-most-powerful-people-in-sports/

marketing company in the world), and an anonymous hedge fund advisor who made it possible for many men on the list to accumulate billions of dollars so they could buy teams or exert influence over what occurs in sports. The list is unapologetically U.S.-centric, although it includes four powerful European men; everyone on the list is a white man.

It is clear that white men hold nearly 100 percent of the major power positions in elite sports today. These men have much in common with other economic elites in the United States. Collectively, they benefit from a class ideology that legitimizes the existing status and power hierarchy in American society and supports the idea that the current level of economic inequality, even though it is greater than it has been for a century, is good for the country. This is why they are sincerely committed to a form of sport—elite men's sports—in which competition, conquest, individualism, authority, and consumption are highlighted in everything from media coverage and stadium design to team logos and ads for upcoming games and contests.

Although the power wielded by these and other powerful people in sports does not ignore the interests of common folk in the United States and worldwide, it clearly focuses on the expansion and profitability of the organizations represented by the power holders. Therefore, sports are sponsored and presented to highlight the meanings and orientations valued by economic elites at the same time that they provide exciting and enjoyable experiences to people like you and me.

This relationship between sports and social class explains why many of us in the sociology of sport use a combination of structural and cultural theories to help us understand sports in society. For example, Antonio Gramsci, an Italian political theorist, developed a theory stating that members of the "ruling class" in contemporary societies maintain their power to the extent that they can develop creative ways to convince most people that their society is organized as fairly and efficiently as possible under current social and economic conditions. One of the strategies for doing this is to become the primary providers of popular pleasure and entertainment so that people see the ruling class as sponsors of their joy and excitement. This strategy is especially effective if the ruling class can use

entertaining events to promote particular ideas and beliefs about what should be important in people's lives. In this way, sports and other forms of exciting entertainment become cultural vehicles for establishing "ideological outposts" in the minds of people who are ruled. These outposts can then be used to deliver other messages into the popular consciousness—messages from sponsors and media commentators who reaffirm a class ideology legitimizing current forms of class inequality in society. This critical theoretical approach helps us see the dynamics of class relations and the process of hegemony at work in sports and other spheres of our lives.

SOCIAL CLASS AND SPORT PARTICIPATION PATTERNS

In all societies, social class and class relations influence who plays, who watches, who consumes information about sports, and what information about sports is available in mainstream media. Patterns of sport participation and consumption are closely associated with money, power, and privilege. At a basic level, organized sports are a luxury item in the economies of many nations, and they are most prevalent in wealthy nations where people have discretionary money and time.

Active sport participation, attendance at events, and consuming media sports are positively correlated with a person's income, education, and occupational status. Training at the elite level of sports requires considerable resources. Some costs may be covered by sponsors for those lucky enough to have them, but others must be covered by personal funds. For example, when the record-setting swimmer Dara Torres trained for the 2008 Olympics, she spent about $100,000 per year for her support staff, including a pool coach, a strength and conditioning coach who also is her dietician, two full-time people who stretch her muscles, a physical therapist, a masseuse, and a nanny to care for her daughter (Crouse, 2007). Torres was forty-one years old, but she represents a widely accepted approach to training for elite athletes of any age.

Most elite sports require expensive equipment and training. For example, in any form of motor racing the costs can reach $200,000 per year, *plus* private driving coaches at $5000 per weekend (Cacciola, 2012). Clearly, this influences who can become seriously involved and successful in these sports.

Even the health and fitness movement, often described as a grassroots phenomenon in North America, involves mostly people who have higher-than-average incomes and education and work in professional or managerial occupations. For the most part, people in low-income jobs don't run, bicycle, or swim as often as their high-income counterparts. Nor do they play as many organized sports on their lunch hours, after work, on weekends, or during vacations. This pattern holds true throughout the life course, for younger and older people, men and women, racial and ethnic populations, and people with disabilities: *Social class is related strongly to participation among all categories of people* (Federico et al., 2013; Kahma, 2012; Kamphuis et al., 2008; Stokvis, 2012; White and McTeer, 2012).

> It cost hundreds of thousands of dollars over the years [to pay for his training and competitions]. But I knew I was going to do whatever I had to make sure he followed his dream. —David Ali, father of a 19-year-old boxer on the 2008 U.S. Olympic team (in Ellin, 2008)

Over time, economic inequality in society leads to the formation of class-based lifestyles that involve particular forms of sports (Bourdieu, 1986a, 1986b; Falcous and McLeod, 2012; Kahma, 2012; Mehus, 2005; Stempel, 2005, 2006; Stokvis, 2012; Wheeler, 2012). For the most part, sport participation in various lifestyles reflects patterns of sponsorship and access to participation opportunities. For example, the lifestyles of wealthy people routinely include golf, tennis, skiing, swimming, sailing, and other sports that are self-funded and played at exclusive clubs and resorts. These sports often involve expensive facilities, equipment, and/or clothing, and generally require that people have jobs and/or lives in which they have the control, freedom, and time needed to participate; some people also combine sport participation with their jobs by using facilities that their business associates also

use. This has interesting implications in the United States, where companies pay the club memberships of their top executives and then classify most club expenses as "business deductions" on the corporation's tax returns. Taking these deductions reduces the company's taxes and reduces the tax revenues that fund public sport programs for people who cannot afford golf, tennis, or elite health club memberships. At the same time, executives and their friends and relatives enjoy free perks worth untold billions of dollars, which they refer to as "investments" rather than "welfare."

The lifestyles of middle-income and working-class people, on the other hand, tend to include sports that by tradition are free and open to the public, sponsored by public funds, or available through public schools. When these sports involve the use of expensive equipment or clothing, participation occurs in connection with various forms of financial sacrifice. For instance, buying a motocross bike so his child can ride and race means that a father must work overtime, cancel the family vacation, and organize family leisure around motocross races.

The lifestyles of low-income people and those living under the poverty line seldom involve regular forms of sport participation, unless a shoe company identifies a young potential star and sponsors his or her participation. When people struggle to stretch the family budget, they seldom can maintain a lifestyle that includes regular sport participation. Spending money to play or watch sports is a luxury that most low-income people can't afford.

Homemaking, Child Rearing, and Earning a Living: Class and Gender Relations in Women's Lives

The impact of social class on sports participation often varies by age, gender, race and ethnicity, and geographic location. For example, married

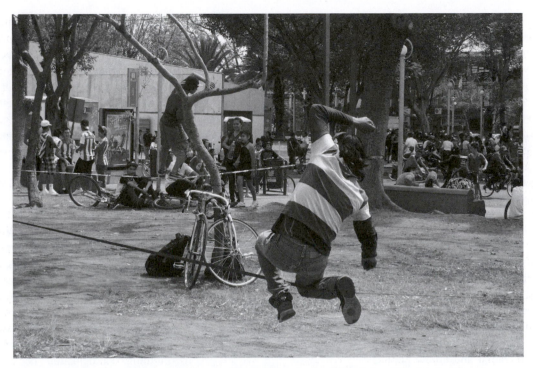

Young people in low-income families usually play sports at public parks and schools. These activities often are creatively arranged, as shown by these slackliners. But they lack the support and consistency characterized by organized sports. Young people in upper- and upper-middle-class families have resources to purchase access to privately owned sport facilities and spaces. This results in different sport experiences and different sport participation patterns from one social class to another. (*Source:* © Basia Borzecka)

women with children are less likely than their male counterparts to have the time and resources to play sports (Taniguchi and Shupe, 2012). To join a soccer team that schedules practices late in the afternoon and plays games in the evening or on weekends is all but impossible when you're the family cook, chauffeur, housekeeper, and homework supervisor.

On the other hand, married men with children are less likely to feel such constraints (Taniguchi and Shupe, 2012). When they play softball or soccer after work, their wives may delay family dinners or keep dinner warm until they arrive home. When they schedule a golf game on a Saturday morning, their wives make breakfast for the children and then

chauffeur one or more children to their youth sport games.

Women in middle- and lower-income families are most constrained by homemaking and child rearing responsibilities. Unable to pay for child care, domestic help, and sport participation fees, these women have few opportunities to play sports. They also lack time, transportation to and from sport facilities, access to gyms and playing fields in their neighborhoods, and the sense of physical safety that enables them to feel secure enough to leave home and travel to places where they can play sports.

When playing a sport requires multiple participants, the lack of resources among some women affects others, because it reduces their prospects for assembling the requisite number of players. This is also true for men, but women from middle- and lower-income families are more likely than their male counterparts to lack the network of relationships out of which sport interests and participation emerge and are sustained over time.

Women from upper-income families, on the other hand, usually face few constraints on sport participation. They can afford child care, domestic help, carryout dinners, and sport fees. They participate by themselves and with friends and family members. Their social networks include other women who also have resources to play sports. Women who grow up in these families play sports during their childhoods and attend schools with well-funded sport programs. They seldom experience the same constraints as their lower-income counterparts, even though their opportunities may not equal those of their upper-income male peers.

> Nothing is more sacred in sports than a level playing field. Too bad it doesn't exist. . . . it now takes more resources—a lot more—to compete at the highest level. —Peter Keating, Senior writer, ESPN (2011)

The sport participation of girls and young women also is limited when they're expected to shoulder responsibilities at home. For example, in low-income families, especially single-parent and immigrant families, teenage daughters often are expected to care for younger siblings after school until early evening when parents return from work. In some cases, schools or teams could organize cooperative child care for students who must care for siblings. This would enable them to play sports or participate in other extracurricular activities. Such cooperative strategies are foreign to individualistically oriented people in the United States and might be rejected as being "socialist." But without arrangements that help them with their child-care responsibilities, such students will typically drop out of sports or never try out.

Boys and girls from higher-income families seldom have household responsibilities that force them to drop out of sports. Instead, their parents drive them to practices, lessons, and games; make sure they are well-fed and have all the equipment they need; and provide access to cars when they are old enough to drive themselves to practices and games.

The implications of social-class dynamics become very serious when health and obesity issues are considered. Limited opportunities to exercise safely and play sports are among the factors contributing to high rates of obesity, diabetes, and heart disease, especially among girls and women from low-income households (Edwards et al., 2013). The availability of facilities, safe spaces, transportation, and sports programs all vary by social class, and girls and women in low-income households experience the effects of social class in different and more profound ways when it comes to involvement in physical activities and sports (Kelley and Carchia, 2013; NPR et al., 2015).

Being Respected and Becoming a Man: Class and Gender Relations in Men's Lives

Many boys and young men use sports to establish a masculine identity, but the dynamics of this process vary by social class. For example, in a qualitative analysis of essays written about sports by fifteen- and sixteen-year-old French Canadian boys in the Montreal area, Suzanne Laberge and Mathieu Albert (1999) discovered that upper-class boys connected their sports participation with masculinity because playing sports, they said, taught them leadership skills, and being a leader was central to their definition of masculinity. Middle-class boys said that playing sports provided them with opportunities to be with peers and gain acceptance in male groups, which fit their ideas of what they needed to do to establish identities as young men. According to working-class boys, playing sports enabled them to display toughness and develop the rugged personas that matched their ideas of

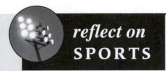

reflect on SPORTS

Public Money and Private Profits
When Do Sports Perpetuate Social Inequality?

The dynamics of class relations sometimes have ironic twists. This is certainly true when public money is used to build stadiums and arenas that are then used by wealthy individuals who own professional sport teams that often bring them large profits. Between 1990 and 2008, over $22 billion of public money in the United States was spent to build these facilities that add to the wealth of powerful individuals and corporations and then subsidize their real estate developments in the area immediately around the facilities.

Furthermore, wealthy investors often purchase the tax-free municipal bonds that cities sell to obtain the cash to build these facilities. This means that while city and/or state taxes are collected from the general population to pay off the bonds, wealthy investors receive tax-free returns, and team owners use the facilities built by taxpayers to make large amounts of money for themselves. When sales taxes are used to pay off bonds, people in low- and middle-income households pay a higher percentage of their annual incomes to build the stadiums than people in higher-income households. This amounts to a case of the poor subsidizing the rich with government approval.

Ironically, the average residents whose taxes build stadiums and arenas usually can't afford to buy tickets to sports events in these venues. One reason for high ticket prices is that corporate accounts are used to buy so many tickets to games that the team owners raise ticket prices to match the demand. Higher prices seldom discourage corporate executives because they claim a portion of the ticket costs as a business deduction, thereby reducing their taxes so they receive an indirect reduction in ticket costs of 18–35 percent. As a result, tax revenues decline and the government has less money to fund sport programs for average taxpayers,

and most of those taxpayers can't afford the expensive tickets. This means that stadiums today seldom are places where social classes mix as they cheer for the same team. In fact, when corporate credit cards are used to purchase blocks of season tickets, as they are in most venues, the only mixing of social classes is between

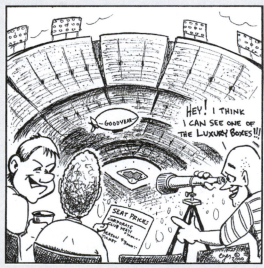

(*Source:* © Frederic A. Eyer)

"I thought they said 'Sport brings everyone together' when they used our tax money to build this place!"

Many stadiums today have policies that create the equivalent of "gated neighborhoods" for high rollers with premium tickets. Stadiums may be built with public money, but they are full of no-trespassing areas for the public. Who benefits from this example of class relations in action?

manhood. In this sense, social class influenced the ways that sports and sport experiences were integrated into the lives of these young men.

Boys in U.S. culture are more likely to make commitments to athletic careers at a young age

when they perceive limited options for other careers and when their family situation is financially insecure (Gregory, 2013b; May, 2009). This means that the personal stakes associated with playing sports are different and often greater for boys from "the haves" and "the have-mores." Meanwhile, team owners misleadingly blame players' salaries for escalating ticket prices.

The dynamics of class relations do not stop here. After contributing public money to build stadiums and arenas, local and state governments often give discounted property tax rates to team owners and their real estate partners who develop areas around the new venues. Property taxes are the main source of revenues for public schools, so urban public schools often have less money as team owners and developers increase their wealth. Meanwhile, professional teams sponsor a few charity programs for "inner-city kids" and occasionally send players to speak at urban schools—all of which garner press coverage that describes team owners and millionaire athletes as great public servants! As school systems fail due to poor funding and teachers complain about this scam, local editorials and letters to the editor accuse educators of wasting public money and demand that they become more frugal.

This method of transferring public money into the private pockets of wealthy individuals has occurred as social services for the unemployed, the working poor, children, and people with disabilities are being cut.

WHAT ABOUT JOBS CREATED BY SPORTS?

Jobs are created whenever hundreds of millions of dollars are spent in a city. But those jobs also would be created if the arenas and stadiums were privately financed. Furthermore, when cities spend public money to build stadiums for professional teams, they create far fewer jobs than could be created by other forms of economic development. Measuring the true cost of job creation is tricky. The type of job created and the economic conditions at the time and place that the job is created all influence costs. However, for the money spent to build a major sport facility, the returns in the form of new jobs are relatively low—the facilities employ relatively few people, the facilities are closed much of the time, and most of the jobs in the facility are seasonal and low paying. Therefore, after reading reports of studies done by independent economists, it appears to me that for each job created by a new stadium, between ten and twenty new jobs could have been created if the same amount of public money had been invested in more strategically chosen development projects. This means that stadiums and large arenas are lousy job creators for the public money spent on them.

WHO ELSE BENEFITS?

Sport team owners are not the only wealthy and powerful people who benefit when stadiums and arenas are built with public money. New publicly financed sport facilities increase property values in urban areas in which major investors and developers can initiate profitable projects. Others also may benefit as money trickles down to the rest of the community, but the average taxpayers who fund the facilities will never see the benefits enjoyed by the wealthy few. Additionally, these developments often require the displacement of housing for people living near or below the poverty line, and this housing is seldom replaced.

Publicly financed sport venues may provide the illusion of unity and generally beneficial development in a city, but they are mostly vehicles for transferring public money to wealthy individuals and corporations. Behind the illusion often exists disunity and class inequality.

low-income households than they are for boys from higher-income households. Similarly, male athletes from poor and working-class households often use sport participation to obtain "respect" in a society where they often lack other means to do so.

Because young men from low-income households often have more at stake when it comes to playing sports, they face more personal pressure than wealthier peers, because they often lack the material resources required to train, develop skills, and be noticed by people who can serve as their advocates. Unless public school athletic programs and coaches can provide these things, these young people—boys and girls alike—have fewer opportunities for moving up to higher levels of competition than their upper-income peers have. The last remaining exceptions to this social-class discrepancy are in football, basketball, and track, which are usually funded in public schools with qualified coaches and enough visibility for some players to be seen by potential mentors and advocates.

Young people from upper-income households often have so many opportunities that they seldom see sports as high-stakes, career-related activities in their lives. For a young person with a car, nice clothes, money for college tuition, and good career contacts for the future, playing sports can be fun, but it's not perceived as necessary for economic survival, gaining respect, or establishing an identity. Therefore, young men from middle- and upper-income backgrounds often disengage gradually from childhood dreams of becoming professional athletes and develop new visions for their futures. For them, playing sports does not hold the same life significance as it does for their peers from working-class and low-income households (NPR et al., 2015).

Fighting to Survive: Class, Gender, and Ethnic Relations Among Boxers

Chris Dundee, a famous boxing promoter, once said, "Any man with a good trade isn't about to get himself knocked on his butt to make a dollar" (in Messner, 1992, p. 82). What he meant was that middle- and upper-class boys and men have no reason to play a sport that destroys brain cells, that boxers always come from the lowest and most economically desperate income groups in society, and that boxing gyms are located in neighborhoods where desperation is most intense and life-piercing (Wacquant, 2004).

The dynamics of becoming and staying involved in boxing have been studied and described by French sociologist Loïc Wacquant (1992, 1995a,

1995b, 2004). As noted in Chapter 6, Wacquant spent over three years training and hanging out at a boxing gym in a low-income Chicago neighborhood. During that time, he documented the life experiences of fifty professional boxers, most of whom were African Americans. His analysis shows that deciding to dedicate oneself to boxing in the United States is related to a combination of class, race, and gender relations.

The alternative to boxing for these young men often was the violence of the streets. When Wacquant asked one boxer where he'd be today if he hadn't started boxing, he said,

> If it wasn't for boxin,' I don't know where I'd be . . . Prob'ly in prison or dead somewhere, you never know. I grew up in a tough neighbo'hood, so it's good for me, at least, to think 'bout what I do before I do it. To keep me outa the street, you know. The gym is a good place for me to be every day. Because when you're in d'gym, you . . . don' have to worry about getting' into trouble or getting shot at (in Wacquant, 2004, p. 239).

Wacquant explains that most boxers know they would not be boxing if they had been born in households where resources and other career opportunities existed. "Don't nobody be out there fightin' with an MBA," observed a trainer-coach at the gym (in Wacquant, 1995a, p. 521). Wacquant notes that these men see boxing as a "coerced affection, a captive love, one ultimately born of racial and class necessity" (1995a, p. 521). When he asked one boxer what he would change in his life, the answer represented the feelings of many men at the gym:

> I wish I was born taller, I wish I was born in a rich family, I . . . wish I was smart, an' I had the brains to go to school an' really become somebody real important. For me I mean I can't stand the sport, I hate the sport, [but] it's carved inside of me so I can't let it go (in Wacquant, 1995a, p. 521).

Overall, these men were simultaneously committed to and repulsed by their trade, and their participation was clearly connected with the dynamics of social class in their lives. Boxing and the gym provided for them refuge from the violence, hopelessness, and indignity of the racism and poverty that framed their lives since birth. They excelled at the sport because being a young, poor, black man in America "is no bed of roses" (Wacquant, 2004, p. 238).

This case of boxing shows that all sport participation is embedded in a particular social and cultural context. For young people from resource-deprived areas and families, sport participation may help them cope with or survive the immediate circumstances of their lives, but it does not automatically provide them with "lifelines" or "hook-ups" that connect them with other social worlds in which opportunities may be more plentiful. Philosopher-boxer Joseph Lewandowski (2007, 2008) points this out in his research on boxing in communities characterized by "social poverty"— that is, there is an absence of *vertical social capital* that connects young persons to real opportunities to move "up and out" of their immediate circumstances, or even to change them. In other words, playing a sport may earn a person respect in the local neighborhood, but this respect comes in the form of horizontal social capital that is useful only in managing current circumstances. For sport participation to pay off, it must also enable a young person to earn vertical social capital that opens doors to real hope and possibility.

Class Relations in Action: Changing Patterns in Sport Participation Opportunities

Publicly funded youth sport programs have been reduced or eliminated in many U.S. communities, and varsity teams in low-income school districts are being eliminated (Kelley and Carchia, 2013). When this occurs, fewer young people from low-income neighborhoods have opportunities to play sports, especially those requiring large fields and safe, functional facilities. This is why basketball remains a primary focus among low-income boys and girls; public schools usually can offer basketball teams and coaches if they have a usable gym that has not been converted into a permanent lunchroom or classroom.

School sport programs in middle- and upper-income areas also may be threatened by financial problems, but they're maintained by "participation fees" paid by athletes' parents. These fees, as high as $250 or more per sport, guarantee that teams across many sports are available for young people lucky enough to be born into well-to-do households. Additionally, when school teams don't meet the expectations of well-to-do parents, they either vote to raise more public funds or use private funds to build new fields and facilities, hire coaches, and run high-profile tournaments that often attract college coaches who recruit athletes by giving them scholarships. Therefore, when tax revolts and political decisions cause public programs to disappear, well-to-do people simply buy private sport participation opportunities for their children.

This highlights the influence of social class in sports. In fact, when it comes to sport participation today, the socioeconomic status of an athlete's family has never been more important, because participation now depends almost exclusively on family resources.

Therefore, we can expect that sport participation, the development of sport skills, and rewards for sport performance will increasingly go to people in households with above-average income and wealth.

When we compare the availability and quality of school and club sport programs by social class, we see that economic inequalities have a major impact on opportunities for sport participation today. With funds being cut and coaches laid off, schools in poor neighborhoods struggle to maintain sport programs while looking for new funding from corporations. But corporations usually sponsor only the sports that promote their brand and products. For example, a shoe company will support basketball because it fits with its marketing and advertising programs. Corporate funders support individuals, teams, and sports that generate product visibility through media coverage and high-profile state and national tournaments. This

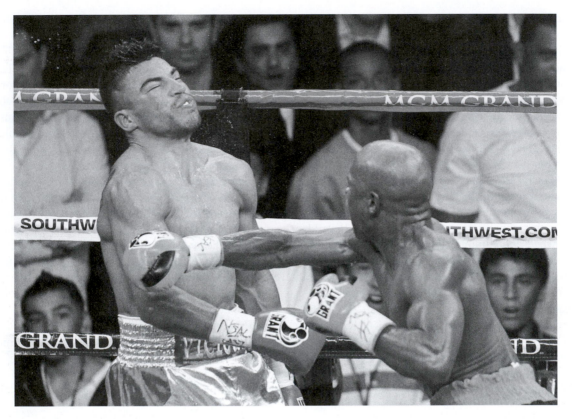

Boxing has long been a sport for men from low-income groups. As a long-time boxing coach says, "If you want to know who's at d' bottom of society, all you gotta to do is look at who's boxin" (in Wacquant, 2004, p. 42). (*Source:* © RD/ Kabik/Retna Ltd./Corbis)

keeps certain sports alive, but only on terms that continue to meet corporate interests.

Tables 9.2 and 9.3 show that the socioeconomic playing field is not level when it comes to race and ethnicity. Black and Latino households are at a significant disadvantage when it comes to financial resources that could be spent on sports and sport participation. In terms of annual income, Latino and black households, respectively, have incomes that are $17,307 and $23,672 less than the annual incomes of white households. The racial and ethnic wealth gaps as shown in Table 9.3 are even more influential when it comes to making financial decisions in a family. When compared with white households, black

households possess $104,033 less wealth, and Latino households possess $102,798 less wealth. Wealth serves as a cushion that provides stability in a household, and it certainly has an impact on family decisions about spending money for sport participation. These income and wealth gaps will influence who has opportunities to develop elite sport skills, receive athletic scholarships, and play sports at elite levels.

Class Relations in Action: The Cost of Attending Sport Events

It remains possible to attend some sports events for free. High school and many college games and

Table 9.2 Median household income in United States by race and Hispanic origin, 2013

Category	Income
All categories	$51,939
Asian households	$67,065
White households (not Hispanic)	$58,270
Latino households (any race)	$40,963
Black households	$34,598

Source: U.S. Census Bureau, Current Population Survey, 1968 to 2014 Annual Social and Economic Supplements.

Table 9.3 Median household wealth in United States by race and ethnicity, 2011

Category	Median wealth*
White households	$111,146
Latino households (any race)	$8,348
Black households	$7,113

Source: Traub and Ruetschlin, 2015
*Household **wealth** consists of all assets in the form of money in the bank; equity in a home, car, or other appraised possessions; and retirement funds in investments or savings.

meets in the United States are affordable for most people, and in some communities the tickets for minor league sports are reasonably priced. But tickets to most major intercollegiate and professional games are beyond the means of most people, even those whose taxes were used to build the venues in which the games are played. The cost of attending these events has increased much more rapidly than the rate of inflation over the past fifteen years.

Table 9.4 shows that the inflation rate between 1991 and 2012 was 69 percent, whereas average ticket prices increased 213 percent, 209 percent, 126 percent, and 154 percent for MLB, the NFL, the NBA, and the NHL respectively, during the same period. Therefore, ticket prices have increased three to four times the rate of inflation—partly due to increased costs at new stadiums and arenas, but mostly due to team owners wanting to attract people who have money to spend on food, drinks, apparel, and everything else they sell. This is why new facilities resemble giant circular shopping malls built around a central entertainment stage. They house expensive luxury suites and separate club seating, where high-income spectators have special services available—waitstaff, hot food menus,

Table 9.4 Escalating ticket prices versus inflation in the United States, 1991–2012

	AVERAGE TICKET PRICE*						21-Year
	1991 ($)	1996 ($)	2001 ($)	2004 ($)	2008 ($)	2012 ($)	Increase (%)
Major League Baseball	9	11	19	20	25	27	213
National Football League	25	36	54	55	67	78	209
National Basketball Association	23	32	51	45	49	51	126
National Hockey League	24[†]	38	48	44	50	61	154[†]

U.S. inflation rate from 1991 to 2012 = 69%[§]

Source: Adapted from data in Team Marketing Report, www.teammarketing.com.
*Ticket prices are rounded to the nearest dollar. Data for the NBA and NHL for 2004–2012 do not include premium ticket costs in the average, and this makes it difficult to do totally accurate long-term comparisons.
[†]This is an estimate because no NHL data were available prior to 1994.
[§]Represents the official rate of inflation as determined by the U.S. government.

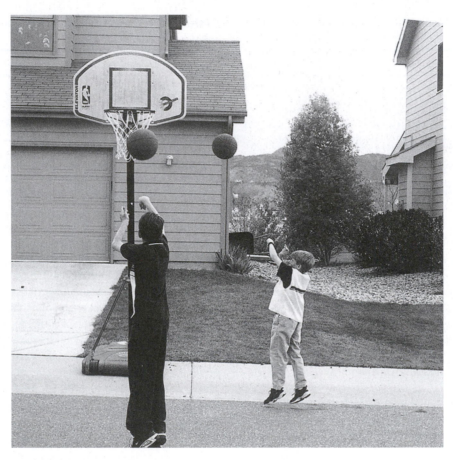

Children in middle-class suburban areas often have safe streets on which to play. The boys in this cul-de-sac have multiple portable basketball goals, and they occasionally play full-court games in the street. They have many sport participation options in their lives, which their families often use as opportunities for sociability. (*Source:* © Jay Coakley)

private restrooms, televisions, refrigerators, lounge chairs, temperature controls, private entrances with no waiting lines or turnstiles, and special parking areas—so that attending a game is no different from going to an exclusive private club.

As tickets become more expensive and spectators are increasingly segregated according to their ability to pay, social class and class relations become more evident in the stands. Spectators may cheer at the same times and experience similar emotions, but this is the extent to which social-class differences are transcended at the events, and the reality of social class and inequality returns as soon as people leave the stadium.

Efforts by some fans wanting to reduce ticket prices seldom develop traction because people in luxury boxes, club seats, and other premium seats don't want to join or be identified with spectators who can't afford high-priced tickets and concessions. Expensive tickets are status symbols for wealthy spectators; they *want* class distinctions to be part of the sport experience, and they are willing to pay—or have their corporations pay high prices so they can conspicuously display their status and have an experience with other wealthy people.

Attendance and seating at many events, from the opening ceremonies at the Olympics to the NFL Super Bowl, are now tied to conspicuous displays of wealth, status, influence, and corporate power. After observing a recent Super Bowl and the events leading up to the game, journalist Dave Zirin (2008a) concluded that "Before it is anything else, before it's even a football game, the Super Bowl is . . . a two-week entertainment festival for the rich and shameless." Those attending the game in 2008 had an average household income of $222,318—nearly five times greater than the median U.S. household (Thomas, 2008a). This is an important point, because efforts to make games affordable to the people whose taxes build the facilities will fail as long as corporations use them as party sites for executives and customers. In 2016, this pattern of mega-events being designed for the wealthy became even more apparent with the Super Bowl. Ticket prices ranged from $4370 to over $10,000 depending on which pre-game party a person wanted to attend. But most of these tickets were purchased using company credit cards and partly deducted as "business expenses."

> The Super Bowl as a live event is primarily a perk for the nation's elite, and an opportunity for companies to sell their products to a coveted demographic of influencers and decision-makers. —Katie Thomas, *New York Times* journalist (2008a)

GLOBAL INEQUALITIES AND SPORTS

When we discuss social class and sports, it is essential to think beyond our own society. Inequalities exist at all levels of social organization—in families, groups, organizations, communities, societies, and the world.

Global inequalities related to per capita income, living standards, and access to developmental resources cause many of the most serious problems that we face today. Research shows that the gap between the richest and poorest people worldwide is growing wider. For example, people in the United States, *on average,* spend about $65 per day to live as they do—and this includes everyone, even newborns. In the forty-eight nations classified as "least developed countries" (LDCs), people spend about 60 cents a day to live as they do. In terms of consumption, an average person in the United States spends per day about 100 times more than nearly half the individuals in the world spend per day.

The meanings given to this global gap between the wealthy and poor differ depending on the ideologies that people use to guide their understanding of world affairs. But apart from ideological interpretations, it is clear that about 40 percent of all people in the world have few resources to use on anything beyond basic survival. They may play games, but they seldom have the resources needed to organize and play sports as we know them. For these people, the sports played in the United States and other post-industrial nations are clearly out of reach. They can't understand how or why boxer Floyd Mayweather made $300 million in 2015, an amount that is more than 600,000 times what someone like them would spend during an entire year. Similarly, the workers who make less than $3 a day producing the balls, shoes, and other equipment and clothing used by most Americans who play sports, would question the fairness of such inequality.

The Olympic Games provide a clear example of the impact of global inequality in sports. Those who follow the Summer or Winter Olympics through mainstream media hear and read that these are celebrations of athlete commitment, dedication, hard work, and sacrifice. Absent in the coverage is recognition that the Games are also a celebration of wealth and inequality. For example, coverage for the 2012 Olympic Games in London, regardless

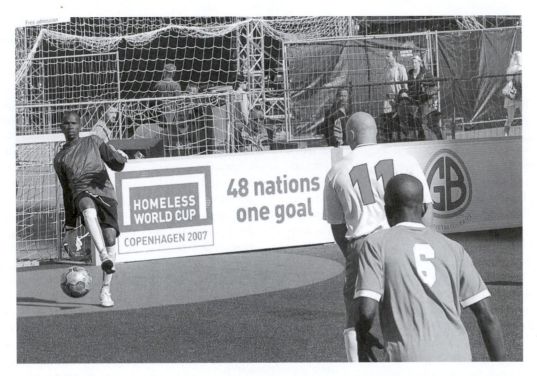

Since 2003, the annual Homeless World Cup has been held in different cities where national teams comprised of homeless people, mostly men, compete during a three-day tournament. This event was initiated by two editors of newspapers that serve homeless people. Their readers sometimes played informal soccer games, so they recruited sponsors and have organized the event each year. In 2015, teams from more than seventy countries competed in Amsterdam. In addition to being a sport event, the tournament is a site for initiating and sustaining political strategies advocating the rights of homeless people worldwide. (*Source:* © Jay Coakley)

of where in the world the coverage occurred, did not mention that 80 of the 204 participating nations had never won an Olympic medal, and another 51 had won fewer than five medals in Olympic history. Many nations had not won a medal for at least forty years. The United States, on the other hand, with its combination of wealth and population size, had won 2,549 medals—many more than any other nation.

Even in wealthy countries, a disproportionate share of medals has always been won by athletes with support from families. Exceptions to this pattern are few. The former Soviet Union, German Democratic Republic (East Germany), China, and Cuba have experienced considerable success. But

in these communist countries, central state planners used public money to train and support an impressive number of medal winners.

Other exceptions are individual athletes who have wealthy corporate sponsors. For example, U.S. hurdler, Lolo Jones, was able to use her talent, face, and physique to attract corporations that wanted to capitalize on the media attention she receives (Longman, 2012b). But even Red Bull, her major sponsor, hedged its investment in Jones by hiring twenty-two scientists and technicians to work with her exclusively from 2005 through 2012. These performance specialists monitored her training runs with forty motion-capture cameras. An Optojump system replicated her feet hitting the track surface on her every stride during 110 meters of hurdling. The Phantom Flex high-speed camera moved astride her and recorded 1500 frames per second as she ran. The resulting analyses of these data and input from other specialists were then used to customize daily training for Jones (McClusky, 2012). This makes the idea of a "level playing field" laughable, despite claims by the IOC and NBC commentators that it is so.

Because athletes are now pushing the performance limits of the human body, they increasingly seek technologies that will bring them success. But these technologies are expensive, especially when they are delivered and managed by physiologists, biomechanists, medical experts, biochemists, strength coaches, nutritionists, psychologists, recovery experts, and statistical analysts who work with coaches to turn scientific findings into training programs. Access to this training costs more than most villages in developing nations produce every four years between the Olympic Games!

Patterns are similar for the Paralympics, where GDP—*gross domestic product,* or the monetary value of all goods and services produced annually—along with the population size of a country are highly correlated with the number of medals won by athletes (Buts et al., 2013). Traveling to the Paralympics is especially costly for Paralympians because they often must bring with them prostheses, wheelchairs, and a person to help them navigate unanticipated barriers. This is why athletes from the nation that hosts the Paralympics win 80 percent more medals than it's athletes won in the previous Paralympic Games. Travel is not a major issue for them, and they know what to anticipate while in the host city. Additionally, host cities and nations make special efforts to make sure that their athletes confront as few barriers as possible.

Athletes from nations with relatively low GDP are extremely unlikely to have access to the training and support required to qualify for and travel to the Paralympics. In countries where poverty rates are high, people with physical or intellectual impairments have little or no opportunity to participate in sports.

ECONOMIC AND CAREER OPPORTUNITIES IN SPORTS

Many people in the United States see sports as a sphere in which people from low-income and poor backgrounds can experience upward social mobility—an affirmation of the American Dream (Green and Hartmann, 2012). **Social mobility** is a term used by sociologists to refer to *changes in wealth, education, and occupation over a person's lifetime or from one generation to the next in families.* Social mobility can occur in downward or upward directions.

On a general level, career and mobility opportunities exist in sports and sport organizations. However, as we consider the impact of sports on mobility in the United States, it is useful to know the following things about sport-related opportunities:

1. The number of paid career opportunities in sports is limited, and the playing careers of most professional athletes are short-term.
2. Professional opportunities for women are growing but remain limited on and off the field relative to men.
3. Professional opportunities for ethnic minorities are growing but remain limited on and off the field relative to whites with European heritage.

These points are discussed in the following sections.

Career Opportunities Are Limited

Young athletes often have visions of playing professional sports, and their parents may have similar visions. But the chances of turning these visions into realities are remote. The odds or chances for a person to become a college or professional athlete are difficult to calculate, and many different methods have been used. For example, we could calculate odds for all high school or college athletes in a particular sport, or for high school or college athletes from particular racial or ethnic groups, or for any male or female in a particular age group of the total population of the United States. Additionally, the calculations could be based on the number of players in the top league in a sport, such as the NHL in hockey, or they could be based on the number of professional hockey players in all major and minor league teams worldwide. The fact that about 80 percent of the players in the NHL come from outside the United States means that it is meaningless to calculate the odds of a U.S. high school hockey player making it to the NHL without taking this into account.

The point here is that all calculations must be qualified, and many estimates reported in the media are inaccurate. The data in Table 9.5 represent calculations made by NCAA researchers in 2012. The footnotes for the table explain the limitations of these calculations and suggest that most of the odds listed in the table are overestimates of the chances of moving from one level of competition to the next in these sports. At any rate, the NCAA calculations indicate that playing at the professional level is a long shot. In fact, if there was a race horse that had similar odds of winning a race, nobody would even think of betting on it.

Additionally, professional sport opportunities are short-term, averaging three to seven years in team sports and three to twelve years in individual sports. This means that, after playing careers end, there are about *forty additional years* in a person's work life. Unfortunately, many people, including athletes, coaches, and parents, ignore this aspect of reality.

Media coverage focuses on the best athletes in the most popular sports, and they often have longer

Table 9.5   Estimated probability of competing in athletics beyond the high school interscholastic level*

Athletes	Men's Basketball	Women's Basketball	Football	Baseball	Men's Ice Hockey	Men's Soccer
HS athlete	535,289	435,885	1,095,993	474,219	35,720	411,757
HS senior athlete	152,940	124,539	313,141	135,491	10,209	117,645
NCAA athlete	17,890	16,134	69,643	31,999	3,891	22,987
NCAA 1st-year roster slots	5,111	4,610	19,898	9,143	1,112	6,568
NCAA senior athlete	3,976	3,585	15,476	7,111	865	5,108
NCAA athlete drafted	51	31	253	693	10	37
Percent HS to NCAA	3.3	3.7	6.4	6.7	10.9	5.6
Percent NCAA to pro	1.3	0.9	1.6	9.7	1.2	0.07
Percent HS to pro	0.03[†]	0.02	0.08	0.5	0.1	0.03

Source: NCAA, 2012.

*The numbers do not include players at non-NCAA schools, players from outside the United States recruited by NCAA schools, players in North American professional leagues who haven't attended high school or college in the United States, or U.S. high school and college players that play professional sports in other countries. Therefore, the odds of a U.S. high school or college athlete making it to the next levels of competition in these sports are lower than these numbers suggest.

[†]How to read the last line: For men's basketball, 3 of every 10,000 high school players will be drafted by the NBA, or 1 of every 3,333. But this does not mean these selected players will make teams. In women's basketball, 2 in 10,000 high school players, or 1 of every 5000 will be drafted; in football it is 8 of every 10,000 high school football players, or 1 of every 1250.

and more lucrative playing careers than others. Little coverage is given to the more typical cases— that is, those who play for one or two seasons before being cut or forced to quit for other reasons, especially injuries or lack of resources to pay for training. We hear about the long careers of popular NFL quarterbacks, but little about the many players whose one-year contracts are not renewed after their first season. The average age of players on the *oldest* NFL team in 2015 was less than twenty-seven years old. This means that few players older than thirty are still in the league. Much more typical than thirty-year-old players contemplating another season are twenty-four-year-olds facing the end of their professional sport careers.

Finally, many professional athletes at the minor league level make less than workers in nonsport occupations. For example, many of the players in minor league baseball and hockey make no more than minimum wage when all their hours of training, completion, and traveling are added together (Hayhurst, 2014). Elementary school teachers have higher salaries than these players, and they also have better working conditions, greater financial security and stability, and a pension plan.

Opportunities for Women Are Growing but Remain Limited

Career opportunities for female athletes are limited relative to opportunities for men. Tennis and golf provide opportunities, but the professional tours for these sports draw athletes worldwide. For women in the United States, this means that the competition to make a living in these sports is great. More than 2100 players competed in Women's Tennis Association (WTA) tournaments during 2015, but only the top 200 players won enough money to fully pay for their expenses on the tour. Of those, only twenty-five were from the United States. In fact, most U.S. players are among the 1300 that had made less than $4000 during the year.

In the Ladies Professional Golf Association (LPGA), only 30 of the top 100 money winners in 2015 were from the United States. Fewer than

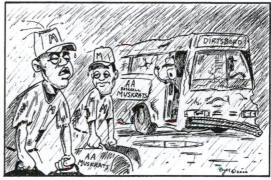

(*Source:* © Frederic A. Eyer)

"Ah, the glamorous life of a spoiled, overpaid professional athlete!"

Only a few professional athletes achieve fame and fortune. Thousands of others play in minor and semipro leagues in which salaries are low and working conditions are poor.

forty women golfers out of the approximately 90 million adult women in the United States make enough prize money to cover their expenses as professional golfers.

There are opportunities in professional basketball, volleyball, soccer, figure skating, bowling, skiing, bicycling, track and field, and rodeo, but the number of professional female athletes in these sports remains low, and only a few women make decent money. For example, when Forbes magazine ranked the top 100 moneymaking athletes during 2015, only tennis players Maria Sharapova and Serena Williams were on the list.

Professional leagues for women now exist in basketball and beach volleyball, but they have provided career opportunities for fewer than 400 athletes at any given time in recent years. The National Women's Soccer League was established in April 2013 as the third attempt to make women's professional soccer a spectator sport. It employed about 185 players on eight teams, with a league salary cap of about $2.7 million. Players' salaries in 2015 ranged from $6842 to $37,800, with most players making less than $15,000 for the season. To assist the league, the soccer federations from the United States, Canada, and Mexico pledged to pay the salaries of players on their national teams—about fifty players in all.

In the WNBA, the pay is a fraction of what men in the NBA make—an average of about $75,000 in 2015, with a league minimum salary of about $34,500. None of the 146 players is allowed to make more than $107,000 for the season. The total salaries for all WNBA players amounted to less than $11 million, which was 44 percent of what Kobe Bryant alone made for the 2015–2016 season. Another way to compare is to say that for every salary dollar that an NBA player makes, a WNBA player makes less than 2-cents, and NBA players outnumber WNBA players about four to one.

Of course, there are opportunities for women athletes to play professional sports in other parts of the world. For example, U.S. national soccer team star Megan Rapinoe has played for a professional team in France, where she made $14,000 a month. Most of the top WNBA players also play on teams in Europe where they often make more than during their seasons in the United States.

What about other careers in sports? There are jobs for women in coaching, training, officiating, sports medicine, sports information, public relations, marketing, and administration. As noted in Chapter 7, most of the jobs in women's sports continue to be held by men, and women seldom are hired for jobs in men's programs, except in peripheral support positions. In the United States, when men's and women's high school or college athletic programs are combined, men become the athletic directors in about 80 percent of the cases. Women in most post-industrial nations have challenged the legacy of traditional gender ideology, and progress has been made in some sports organizations. However, a heavily gendered division of labor continues to exist in nearly all organizations. In traditional and developing nations, the record of progress is negligible, and very few women hold positions of power in any sports organizations.

Job opportunities for women have not increased as rapidly as women's programs have grown. This is partly due to the persistence of orthodox gender ideology and the fact that Title IX does not have precise enforcement procedures when it comes to equity in coaching and administration. Title IX enforcement focuses almost exclusively on athletes, and hasn't had as much impact in other aspects of school sports and no direct impact on sports outside of schools that receive money from the federal government. Therefore, a pattern of female underrepresentation exists in nearly all job categories and nearly all sport organizations.

Opportunities for women in sports may continue to shift toward equity, but many people resist making the structural and ideological changes that would produce full equity. In the meantime, there may be gradual increases in the number of women coaches, sports broadcasters, athletic trainers, administrators, and referees. Changes will occur more rapidly in certain sport industries that target women as consumers and need women employees to increase their sales and profits. But the gender ideology used by influential decision makers *inside* many sports organizations will continue to privilege those perceived as tough, strong, competitive, and aggressive—and men are more likely to be perceived in such terms.

Many women who work in sport organizations continue to deal with organizational cultures that are primarily based on the values and experiences of men. This contributes to low job satisfaction and high job turnover among women (Bruening et al., 2007; Bruening and Dixon, 2008; Dixon and Bruening, 2005, 2007; Dixon and Sagas, 2007; Gregory, 2009). Professional development programs, workshops, and coaching clinics have been developed since the late 1990s to assist women as they work in and try to change these cultures and make them more inclusive. However, full equity won't occur until more men in sport organizations change their ideas about gender and its connection with sports and leadership.

Opportunities for African Americans and Other Ethnic Minorities Are Growing but Remain Limited

The visibility of black athletes in certain spectator sports often leads people to conclude that sports

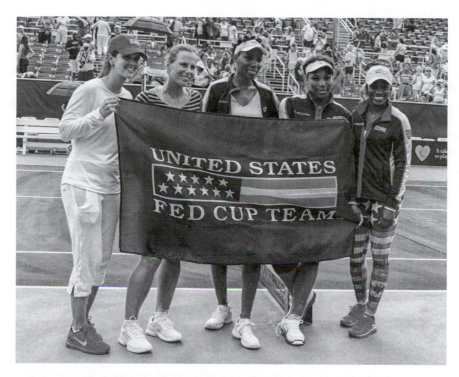

The U.S. team celebrates a victory over Sweden in the Fed Cup World Group playoff tennis matches in 2013. From left to right, team members are Mary Joe Fernandez, Varvara Lepchenko, Venus Williams, Serena Williams, and Sloane Stephens. Their victory guaranteed the United States a place in the coveted 2014 Fed Cup World Group. This photo that includes three black women provides a misleading picture of diversity in U.S. tennis, because they are a total of only five black women who play regularly on the WTA tour, and only one Latina. (*Source:* © Arnold Drapkin/ZUMA Press/Corbis)

offer abundant career opportunities for African Americans. Anecdotal support for this conclusion is provided by successful black athletes who attribute their wealth and fame to sports. However, the extent to which job opportunities for blacks exist in sports has been greatly overstated. Very little publicity is given to the actual number and proportion of blacks who play sports for a living or make a living working in sport organizations. Also ignored is the fact that sports provide very few career opportunities for black women.

African American athletes are involved almost exclusively in five professional spectator sports: boxing, basketball, football, baseball, and track. At the same time, some of the most lucrative sports for athletes are almost exclusively white—tennis, golf, hockey, and motor racing are examples. My best guess is that fewer than 6000 African Americans, or about 1 of every 6660 African Americans, currently make significant incomes as professional athletes in the United States.

This indicates that sports don't provide exceptional upward mobility opportunities and that there are better career opportunities outside of sports—if there are educational opportunities to take advantage of them. Of course, these facts are distorted in media content that presents disproportionately more images of successful black athletes than blacks in other positive roles. If young African Americans use media images as a basis for making choices and envisioning their future, there will be less progress toward achieving racial equality in the United States (Archer et al., 2007; Singer and May, 2011).

Employment Barriers for Black Athletes   When sports were first desegregated in the United States, blacks faced *entry barriers*—that is, unless they had exceptional skills and exemplary personal characteristics they were not recruited or given professional contracts. Racial prejudice was strong and team owners assumed that players, coaches, and spectators would not accept blacks unless they made immediate and significant contributions to a team. Black athletes without exceptional skills were passed by. Therefore, the performance statistics for black athletes surpassed those of whites, a fact that many whites used to reinforce their stereotypes about black physicality.

As entry barriers declined between 1960 and the late 1970s, new barriers related to retention took their place. *Retention barriers* existed when contracts for experienced black players were not renewed unless the players had significantly better performance records than white players at the same career stage. This pattern existed through the early 1990s, but it no longer exists.

Race-based salary discrimination existed in most sports immediately following desegregation, but evidence suggests that it has faded in major team sports. This is because performance can be objectively measured, tracked, and compared to the performances of other players. Statistics are now kept on nearly every conceivable dimension of an athlete's skill. Players' agents use these statistics during salary negotiations, and they have an incentive to do so because they receive a percentage of players' salaries and don't want racial discrimination to decrease their incomes.

Employment Barriers in Coaching and Off-the-Field Jobs   During the 1980s and 1990s, many college and professional sport teams had plantation-like hiring practices—they employed black workers but hired only white managers. Since the mid-1990s, the rate at which blacks have been hired in managerial positions has varied by sport. There's been slow progress in most sport organizations, especially those associated with college and professional football.

To rectify the lack of black coaches, legal pressures forced the NFL in 2003 to adopt the "Rooney Rule," which required teams to interview minority candidates for open coaching positions. Although the impact of this affirmative action policy is not clear, only five of the thirty-two NFL teams had black head coaches during the 2015 season. Over two-thirds of the players are black men, but twenty-seven of thirty-two coaches are white men.

Discriminatory hiring patterns have also been troubling in big-time college football. Although the NCAA claims a commitment to diversity, their progress in achieving it has been slow. In 2007, Keith Harrison, a scholar at the University of Central Florida, completed a thorough study of NCAA hiring practices and concluded that the head football coach position "is the most segregated position in all college sports" (Harrison, 2007). At the start of the 2015–2016 season, there were only thirteen African American head football coaches in the 128 Football Bowl Subdivision (FBS), down from twenty one during the 2013–2014 season; 88 percent of the head coaches were white men. The percentage of black head coaches across all men's and women's sports in NCAA Divisions I, II, and III hovers around 5 percent. Overall, black men and women make up less than 5 percent of the athletic directors at more than 1200 NCAA universities, and in the thirty Division I conferences there is only one black commissioner.

Research indicates that when chief executive officers (CEOs) recruit candidates for top management positions, they favor people with backgrounds and orientations similar to their own, and they often hire people they know or have worked with in the past (Cunningham and Sagas, 2005; Harrison, 2012). Familiar people are "known quantities" and perceived to be predictable and trustworthy. Therefore,

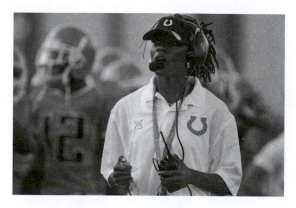

Black women are seriously underrepresented at all levels of coaching. When Natalie Randolph was named head coach of a high school football team in Washington, DC, she and her team took her job seriously, but everyone else saw her as a novelty. For this reason, many jobs in sports are not available to women. (*Source:* © AP Photo/Jacquelyn Martin)

if a team owner or university athletic director is a white male, which is true in nearly all cases, he may wonder about the qualifications of ethnic minority candidates, especially if he lacks exposure to diversity (Roberts, 2007a). He may wonder if he can trust them to be supportive and fit in with his managerial style and approach. If he has doubts, conscious or unconscious, he'll choose the candidate he believes is most like himself. Additionally, black head coaches in professional and big-time college sports appear to be assessed more critically than white head coaches, and when they are fired, they are less likely to be rehired at the same level (Bell, 2013b; Harrison, 2012).

These dynamics, which are seldom identified as "racial" or "ethnic," often exist in sports and other organizations. But they continually reproduce an organizational culture and operating procedures that cause minority men and all women to be underrepresented in positions of power and responsibility.

Opportunities for Ethnic Minorities The dynamics of ethnic relations in every culture are unique (see Chapter 8). Making generalizations about ethnic relations and opportunities in sports is difficult. However, dominant sport forms in any culture tend to reproduce cultural values and the social structures supported by those values. This means three things:

1. Members of the dominant social class in a society may exclude or define as unqualified job candidates with characteristics and cultural backgrounds different from their own.
2. Ethnic minorities often must adopt the values and orientations of the dominant social class if they want to be hired and promoted in sport organizations.
3. The values and orientations of ethnic minorities are seldom represented in the culture of sport organizations.

Latinos, Asian Pacific Americans, and Native Americans are clearly underrepresented in most sports and sport organizations in the United States (Lapchick, et al., 2012). Many Euro-Americans feel uncomfortable with ethnic diversity in situations in which they must trust and work closely with co-workers. Most often, this feeling is caused by a lack of knowledge about the heritage and customs of others and little exposure to ethnic diversity involving meaningful communication. Exceptions to this are found in Major League Baseball and Major League Soccer teams that have many Latino players and a fair representation of Latinos in management. However, neither Asian Pacific Americans nor Native Americans fare very well in any U.S. sport organizations, partly because they are perceived as having

> The boosters of inequity, the true power brokers of college football . . . take comfort in their "white-like-me" hires as a perk of owning the program with their six-figure donations. . . . [But their] contribution to higher education is not enlightenment but enwhitenment. They tailgate for ignorance.
> —Selena Roberts, sports journalist (2007b)

little sports knowledge and experience, regardless of the reality of their lives (Lapchick, 2007, 2008a; Lapchick et al., 2012a).

SPORT PARTICIPATION AND OCCUPATIONAL CAREERS AMONG FORMER ATHLETES

What happens in the occupational careers of former athletes? Are their career patterns different from the patterns of others? Is sport participation a stepping-stone to future occupational success and upward social mobility? Does playing sports have economic payoffs after active participation is over?

Research suggests that, as a group, young people who played sports on high school and college teams experience no more or less occupational success than others from comparable social class and educational backgrounds. This doesn't mean that playing sports has never helped anyone in special ways; it means only that research findings don't allow us to conclude that former athletes have a systematic advantage over comparable peers in their future occupational careers.

Research on this topic becomes out-of-date when the meaning and cultural significance of sport participation changes over time. Such changes are likely to influence the links between playing sports and success in later careers. However, past research suggests that, if playing sports is connected with career success, the reason may involve one or more of the following factors:

- Playing sports under certain circumstances (see the numbered list below) may teach young people *interpersonal skills* that carry over and enable them to succeed in jobs requiring those skills.
- The people who hire employees may define former athletes as good job prospects and give them opportunities to develop and demonstrate work-related abilities, which then serve as the basis for career success.
- Former high-profile athletes may have reputations that help them obtain and succeed in certain occupations, such as sales and service jobs.
- Playing sports under certain circumstances (see the numbered list below) may enable athletes to develop social networks consisting of social relationships that help them obtain good jobs after retiring from sports.

After reviewing much of the research on this topic, I've tentatively concluded that playing sports is positively related to future occupational success and upward mobility when it does the following things:

1. Increases opportunities to complete academic degrees, develop job-related skills, and/or extend one's knowledge about the world outside of sports.
2. Increases support from significant others for *overall* growth and development, not just sport development.
3. Provides opportunities to develop social networks that are connected with career possibilities outside of sports and sport organizations.
4. Provides material resources and the guidance needed to successfully create and manage opportunities.
5. Expands experiences, identities, and abilities *unrelated* to sports.
6. Minimizes risks of disabling injuries that restrict physical movement or require expensive and/or regular medical treatment.

> **A player's career is always a blink in a stare . . . There is a tipping point in a player's career where he goes from chasing the dream to running from a nightmare. . . . It is a downhill run and it spares no one.** —Doug Glanville, MLB player, 1996–2004 (2008)

This list suggests that playing sports can either expand *or* constrict a person's overall development and future career possibilities. When expansion occurs, athletes develop abilities and forms of social and cultural capital that lead to career opportunities and success. When constriction occurs, abilities and social and cultural capital may

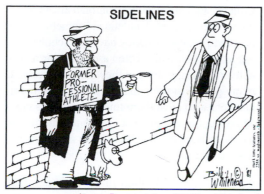

SIDELINES

FORMER PRO-FESSIONAL ATHLETE

(*Source:* By permission of William Whitehead)

Only a few former athletes can cash in on their athletic reputations. The rest must seek opportunities and work just like the rest of us. Those opportunities vary, depending on qualifications, experience, contacts and connections, and a bit of luck. In some cases, former athletes face hard times after their sport careers end.

be so limited that career opportunities are scarce and unsatisfying.

Highly Paid Athletes and Career Success After Playing Sports

Conclusions about sport participation, career success, and social mobility must be qualified in light of the following recent changes related to elite and professional sports in the United States and other wealthy societies:

- An increase in salaries that began in the mid-1970s has enabled some athletes to save and invest money that can be used to create future career opportunities.
- An increase in the media coverage and overall visibility of sports has created greater name recognition than past athletes enjoyed; therefore, athletes today can convert themselves into a "brand" that may lead to career opportunities and success.
- Athletes have become more aware that they must carefully manage their resources to maximize future opportunities.

Of course, most professional athletes have short careers or play at levels at which they do not make much money. When they retire, they face the same career challenges encountered by their age peers, and they experience patterns of success and failure similar to patterns among comparable peers who didn't play sports. This means that playing sports neither ensures nor boosts one's chances of career success.

In Chapter 3 it was explained that retirement from sports is best described as a process rather than a single event, and most athletes don't retire from sports on a moment's notice—they disengage gradually and revise their priorities as they disengage. Although many athletes handle this process smoothly, develop other interests, and move into relatively satisfying occupations, others experience short- or long-term adjustment problems that interfere with occupational success and overall life satisfaction.

The four challenges that retiring athletes face are to (1) reaffirm or reconstruct identities in terms of activities, abilities, and relationships that are not directly related to sport participation; (2) nurture or renegotiate relationships with family and friends so that new identities can be established and reaffirmed (Sheinin, 2009); (3) re-engage with the normal, everyday world in ways that provide a personal sense of meaning (Brissonneau, 2010); and (4) come to terms with the totality of their life in sports (Tinley, 2012, 2015a, 2015b). Meeting these challenges successfully may take time, and it always involves relationships that support nonsport identities.

The fact that athletes today have had to make such a complete commitment to their sports from an early age has often cut them off from the very experiences and relationships they need when they must adjust to life after they stop competing. They have never had an "off season" as athletes had in the past, nor have they had the time or energy to focus on personal development away from the intense seven-day-a-week training and competition schedule. The longer athletes are cut off from nonsport relationships and experiences, and the greater the centrality of their athlete identity, the more difficulty they will have when making the transition out of sport and into non-sport-related social worlds.

Studies also show that adjustment problems are most likely when injuries force an athlete to retire without notice (Empfield, 2007; Swain, 1999; Tinley, 2012; Weisman, 2004). Injuries link retirement with larger issues of health and self-esteem and propel a person into life-changing transitions before they're expected. When this occurs, athletes often need career-transition counseling.

When athletes encounter problems transitioning out of sports into careers and other activities, support should be and occasionally is provided by the sport organizations that benefited from their labor (McKnight et al., 2009). Some sport organizations, including universities and national governing bodies for Olympic sports do this through transition programs focusing on career self-assessments, life skills training, career planning, résumé writing, job search strategies, interviewing skills, career placement contacts, and psychological counseling. Retiring athletes often find it helpful to receive guidance in identifying the skills they learned in sports and how those skills can be transferred to subsequent careers.

Athletic Grants and Occupational Success

Discussions about sport participation and social mobility in the United States often include references to athletic scholarships. Most people believe that these grants-in-aid are valuable mobility vehicles for many young people. However, NCAA data indicate that the actual number of *full* athletic scholarships is clearly exaggerated in the popular consciousness. This occurs for the following reasons:

1. High school students who receive standard recruiting letters from university coaches often tell people they are anticipating *full* scholarships when in fact they receive only partial aid or no aid at all, and they don't disclose this disappointing outcome.

2. College students receiving tuition waivers or other forms of partial athletic aid sometimes lead people to believe that they have full scholarships.

3. Athletic scholarships often are one-year renewable contracts, but when they are not renewed, many people assume that those who had them last year also have them this year and the next.

4. Many people assume that everyone who makes a college team, especially at large universities, has a scholarship, but this is not true.

There were over 13 million full-time undergraduate students in 2012–2013. Table 9.6 shows that 517,849 (about 4 percent) of these students were on intercollegiate teams. Approximately 177,559 athletic scholarships were available for those team members. Some received full scholarships covering tuition, room, meals, and fees, but many received partial scholarships amounting to half or one-fourth of the value of a full scholarship. The average amount of a scholarship in NCAA Division I schools was about $14,270 for men and $15,162 for women in 2013, but these dollar amounts were much lower for athletes in NCAA Division II, NAIA, and NJCAA schools.

When parents and athletes discover that full scholarships are available to only one-third of the athletes playing on college teams, they are shocked. Their shock may turn into disbelief when they remember that they spent $5000 or more a year to keep their son or daughter in a sport from age six to seventeen—a minimum "investment" of $60,000, to say nothing of the time, energy, and long weekends spent driving to and sitting at practices, games, and tournaments—and eating fast food. Even if their son or daughter does receive a scholarship in an NCAA Division I school, he or she will work very hard for 35 to 40 hours per week for all or nearly all of the academic year. Scholarships may be lost due to injuries or coach decisions, and some athletes may quit teams because they don't feel that the scholarship is worth the effort. Additionally, the dollar value of an average scholarship is often far less than parents have "invested" into their child's sport career. This means that spending

Table 9.6   Number of college athletes and maximum number of scholarships available, 2013.

	Total	Men	Women
Total number of college athletes*	517,849	308,171	209,678
Maximum number of athletic scholarships*	177,559	92,658	84,901
Average athletic scholarship per athlete in			
NCAA Division I		$ 14,270	$ 15,162
NCAA Division II		$ 5,548	$ 6,814
NAIA		$ 6,603	$ 6,964
NJCAA		$ 2,069	$ 2,810

Source: http://www.scholarshipstats.com/ncaalimits.html (retrieved, 12-4-15)

* Includes athletes in all three divisions of the NCAA and athletes in schools aligned with the National Association of Intercollegiate Athletics (NAIA) and the National Junior College Athletic Association (NJCAA).

** Each college team has a maximum number of scholarships that can be awarded in any year. However, the actual number of scholarships awarded is less than the maximum due to budget constraints and decisions by athletic directors and coaches.

money to develop a child's sport skills in the hope of seeing a return in the form of a college scholarship makes no financial sense.

Another way to make sense of the data in Table 9.6 is to say that among all full-time undergraduate students only about 2 percent receive some form of athletic aid. In fact, *academic* scholarships amount to many millions of dollars more than the total amount of athletic scholarships, even though many high school students and their parents don't know this.

Class, gender, and race dynamics are strongly connected with athletic scholarships. First, young people in upper-middle-class families (with household incomes of $100,000 per year or more) have resources to develop skills in highly privatized sports such as lacrosse, soccer, volleyball, rowing, swimming, water polo, field hockey, softball, and ice hockey. As a result, they are more likely than athletes in middle- and lower-income families to receive athletic scholarships, although most could afford college without athletic aid.

When Tom Farrey (2008), an Emmy-Award-winning journalist at ESPN, investigated this issue he concluded that "college athletics in general are more the province of the privileged than the poor" (p. 145). Farrey's observation is supported by recent studies. Amanda Paule's (2012) study of the recruiting strategies of college coaches showed that they looked for athletes from upper-income backgrounds who could afford to take a partial rather than a full scholarship, or athletes from very low-income backgrounds who could qualify for need-based aid that came from outside the athletic department. Additionally, because many coaches had small recruiting budgets, they sometimes limited their scouting to camps and tournaments at which young people from middle- and upper-income families were usually overrepresented.

A study investigating the social class and family backgrounds of NBA players led Joshua Dubrow and Jimi Adams (2012) to conclude that white athletes from low-income backgrounds were 75 percent less likely to play in the NBA than athletes from families that were better off. For black athletes, those coming from low-income families were 37 percent less likely to become NBA players than their peers from well-off families.

Second, the college sports that offer high school seniors the best odds for a scholarship include rowing, golf, equestrian events, gymnastics, lacrosse, swimming, fencing, and water polo—all of which are upper-middle-class, suburban, and white (Farrey, 2008).

Despite these studies and what we now know about social class and sport participation, people in the media regularly feature stories that highlight young people who rise from poverty to achieve fame and financial security. This recycles the myth that sports are a path to a better life at the same time that it reaffirms the American Dream, reinforces the image of the United States as a true meritocracy, and promulgates the class ideology supported by those beliefs (Green and Hartmann, 2012).

Third, the only college sports that consistently generate revenues are those in which the majority of players are black men: Division I football and men's basketball. On average, these men come from households with less wealth and income than the households from which most other Division I athletes come. This creates an interesting class- and race-based scenario: Black men from households with little wealth work in their sports to generate revenues that provide scholarships to white athletes from households generally having far greater wealth. White parents, students, and athletes don't think about this pattern of resource distribution, but black football and basketball players are well aware of it.

Overall, when athletic aid goes to financially needy young people who focus on learning and earn their degrees, college sports increase their chances for career success. But this is the exception rather than the rule (Mackin and Walther, 2011; Singer and May, 2011). This does not mean that athletic aid is a problem, but it does mean that it contributes little to overall upward social mobility.

> **"Beneath the thin layer of sport entertainment that makes its way onto television are the bulk of college athletes: Well-off and white."** —Tom Farrey, ESPN journalist (2008)

ways that support their interests by establishing economic arrangements that work to their advantage.

This is why dominant sport forms in the United States and other nations with market economies promote an ideology based on a belief in meritocracy and the idea that people always get what they deserve, and they always deserve what they get.

In the United States this belief combined with belief in the American Dream constitutes a class ideology that promotes favorable conclusions about the character and qualifications of wealthy and powerful people at the same time that it disadvantages the poor and powerless. Furthermore, it leads to the conclusion that economic inequality, even when it is extreme and oppressive, is natural and beneficial for society as a whole.

Class relations also are tied to patterns of sport team ownership, event sponsorship, and media coverage of sports. As public funds are used to build stadiums and arenas, wealthy team owners receive subsidies that expand their income and power. At the same time, economic and political elites, including powerful transnational corporations, sponsor the teams, events, and media coverage that bring people pleasure and excitement. Although fans don't always give sports the meaning that sponsors would like them to, they seldom subject sports to critical analysis and usually don't see sports as perpetuating a class ideology that justifies inequality and public policies that foster inequality. But this is part of what makes sports useful tools for influencing popular assumptions about how the world works.

Sport participation patterns worldwide are connected with social class and the distribution of material resources. Organized sports are a luxury that people in many regions of the world cannot afford. Even in wealthy societies, sport participation is most common among those in the middle and upper classes, and class-based lifestyles often go hand-in-hand with staging and participating in certain sports.

Sport participation patterns also are connected with the intersection of class, gender, race, and

summary

DO MONEY AND POWER MATTER IN SPORTS?

Social class and class relations are integrally involved in sports. Organized sports depend on resources, and those who provide them do so in ethnicity in people's lives. This is seen in the case of girls and women who have low participation rates when resources are scarce and among men who see sports as a means of obtaining respect when they are living on the social and economic margins of society. Boxing provides an example of a sport in which class, gender, race, and ethnicity intersect in a powerful combination. As a result, the boxing gym often becomes a safe space that offers temporary refuge for minority men who live in neighborhoods where poverty, racism, and despair spawn desperate acts of violence among their peers.

The same social forces that bring ethnic minority men to boxing also fuel many variations of *hoop dreams* that captivate the attention of young ethnic minorities, especially black males. These dreams are sources of hope but they seldom come to fruition amid the reality of school and gym closings, school teams being dropped, and a lack of access to the resources required for training and the development of elite sport skills.

Patterns of watching sports also are connected with social class and class relations. This is demonstrated by the increased segregation of fans in stadiums and arenas. Luxury suites, club seating, and patterns of season-ticket allocations separate people by a combination of wealth, power, and access to resources. In the process, inequality becomes increasingly normalized to the point that people are less likely to object to policies that privilege those with the money to buy a spot at the front of the line, or to establish their own line-free VIP entrance to the luxury suites.

Opportunities for careers that hold the hope of upward social mobility exist for some people in sports. For athletes, these opportunities often are scarce and short-lived, and they reflect patterns of class, gender, and ethnic relations in society. These patterns take various forms with regard to careers in sport organizations. Although opportunities in some of these jobs have increased, white men still hold most of the power positions in sport organizations. This will change only when the organizational cultures of sport teams and athletic departments become more inclusive and provide new ways for women and ethnic minorities to participate fully in

shaping the policies and norms used to determine qualifications in sports and organize social relations at the workplace.

Research generally indicates that people who use sport participation to expand their social and cultural capital often have an advantage when seeking occupational careers apart from sports. However, when sport participation constricts social and cultural capital, it's likely to have a negative effect on later career success. The relevance of this pattern varies by sport and is affected by the resources that athletes can accumulate during their playing careers.

Ending athletic careers may create stress and personal challenges, but most athletes move through the retirement process without experiencing excessive trauma or difficulty. Problems are most likely when identities and relationships have been built exclusively in connection with sports. Then professional help may be needed to successfully transition into satisfying careers and relationships in which mutual support encourages growth and the development of new identities. Otherwise, it is possible to become stuck in the "glory days" of being an athlete instead of facing the challenges presented in life after sports.

Athletic scholarships help some young people further their educations and possibly achieve career success, but athletic aid is relatively scarce compared with other scholarships and forms of financial aid. Furthermore, athletic scholarships do not always change the future career patterns of young people because many recipients would attend college without sport-related financial assistance.

In conclusion, sports are clearly tied to patterns of class, class relations, and social inequality in society. Money and economic power do matter, and they matter in ways that often reproduce existing patterns of social class and life chances.

SUPPLEMENTAL READINGS

Reading 1. Social class and the future of high school sports
Reading 2. Home countries of the 100 highest-paid athletes

SPORT MANAGEMENT ISSUES

- You have a job with a multi-state youth soccer
  organization. One of your assignments is to prepare a "Guide for Parents" in which, among other
  things, you tell parents what they can expect for
  their children. You include a realistic discussion
  of the probability that a son or daughter would
  receive a scholarship. However, the head of the
  organization tells you to take it out of the guide.
  Explain what you initially wrote to parents, and
  also explain why the head of the organization
  told you to eliminate it from the guide.

- Your soccer coach tells you and everyone else
  on the university lacrosse team that sports are
  uniquely American activities because they
  embody the American Dream and are organized so that money has no influence on performance. He also says that sports are the best
  way for young people from "disadvantaged"
  backgrounds to get ahead in life. One of your
  teammates doubts the truth of what the coach
  said and asks you to critique his comments.
  Explain what you would tell your teammate.

- One of your classmates is an international
  student from Brazil. When she learns you're
  taking a course on sports, she tells you that
  sports are luxury items that distract people from
  political realities in their lives and use valuable
  resources that should be spent on meeting basic
  human needs. She wants to know what you
  think. List and explain at least five points that
  you will make in your response.

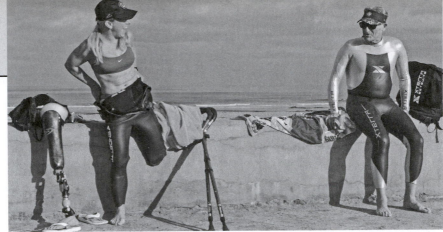

chapter

10

AGE AND ABILITY*

Barriers to Participation and Inclusion?

. . . as a younger person I was never successful. I was never really good at something and when I discovered that at this age group I could win things and get recognition from it, it just really spurred me on.

—Marlene, a 66-year-old Masters swimmer (in Dionigi et al., 2013)

. . . we must demolish the false dividing line between 'normal' and 'disabled' [meaning impaired] and attack the whole concept of physical normality. We have to recognise that disablement [impairment] is not merely the physical state of a small minority of people. It is the normal condition of humanity.

—Allan Sutherland, British author, performer, and activist (1981)

I am a disabled woman interested in sport and I do not know of one disabled athlete who has made a difference in the lives of the people who are disabled in my circle of disabled friends.

—Esther, Disability Rights activist (in Braye et al., 2013)

We're going to see a point in this century where the running times, the jumping heights, in the Paralympics, are all superior to the Olympics. The Paralympics won't constrain technological development . . . [and] will be this exciting human-machine sport like race-car driving. It will make normal human bodies seem very boring.

—Hugh Herr, director, Biomechatronics Group, Massachusetts Institute of Technology (2012)

*Coauthored with Elizabeth Pike

Chapter Outline

What Counts as Ability?

Constructing the Meaning of *Age*

Constructing the Meaning of *Ability*

Sport and Ability

Disability Sports

Technology and Ability

To "*Dis*" or Not to "*Dis*"

Summary: Are Age and Ability Barriers to Participation?

Learning Objectives

- Know the meaning and consequences of ableist ideology, ageism, and ableism.

- Explain the relationship between age and sport participation patterns and why older people are playing sports more frequently today.

- Distinguish between handicaps, physical impairments, and disabilities, and give examples of each.

- Understand the differences between the medical and social models of disability.

- Describe what it means to live in "the empire of the normal" for those who have a disability and want to play sports.

- Explain how the media and gender are involved in the social construction of disability.

- Identify the barriers that impact the sport participation of people with disabilities.

- Understand the dynamics of exclusion and inclusion processes involving sports and people with disabilities.

- Describe the major challenges facing disability sports, especially the Paralympics and Special Olympics.

- Explain the pros and cons associated with the use of new technologies in disability sports.

Are you able-bodied? If so, what makes you so? If not, why not? Will you always be this way, regardless of your age or circumstances?

Trying to answer these questions helps us realize that abilities are variable and impermanent. They change over time, sometimes increasing, sometimes declining. Some abilities may be very important in some situations but irrelevant in others. This means that being able-bodied is a temporary and variable condition.

How *able* must you be to think of yourself as able-bodied? Which abilities matter the most? If you wear contacts to see more clearly, are you able-bodied or merely "passing" as such? Are you disabled if you have a prosthetic knee or hip replacement? What if your legs are amputated below the knees and you can use prosthetic legs to run faster than most of your peers with legs of flesh and bones?

Does age affect how you assess your ability? If at age twenty you are physically stronger, faster, and more coordinated than a four-year-old or a forty-four-year-old, would you consider them disabled? If strength, speed, and coordination have nothing to do with accomplishing a task, what does it mean to be able-bodied?

These questions force us to consider how ability is defined and who defines it. For example, we might ask a person born without sight to talk about ability and learn how she understands it from her perspective. We could compare her ideas and perceptions with those who have 20/20 vision and with those who must wear glasses or contacts to see properly. Similarly, we could ask people who are eight, twenty-two, forty-five, and seventy-years-old to do the same. This would provide a good starting point for discussing the meaning of ability and the extent to which meanings vary from one perspective to another.

Fortunately, others have already done this and given us a basis for discussing how age and ability are linked with sport participation. We will use their research to explore four questions in this chapter:

1. What counts as ability, who decides this, and how do ideologies related to age and ability influence the meaning of disability in sports?
2. How do ideas and beliefs about age and ability influence physical activity and sport participation?
3. What issues do people who are defined as "disabled" face when they seek or take advantage of opportunities to play sports?
4. What are the connections between human beings, technology, and ability in sports?

WHAT COUNTS AS ABILITY?

A primary theme in this book is that our lives and the social worlds in which we live are influenced by **ideologies**—the ideas and beliefs commonly used to give meaning to the world and make sense of experiences. In this chapter, we consider the ways that *age* and *ability* are related to sport participation. This is partly because the body is central to our sense of self and our social identity (Thualagant, 2012). From an early age we learn norms for evaluating and classifying bodies—whether they are tall, short, fit, frail, thin, fat, attractive, unattractive, young, old, athletic, awkward, disabled, and so on. As we learn these norms, most of us maintain, modify, and fashion our bodies as part of a self-identity project.

When sports were first organized during the late 1800s and early 1900s, an emerging social psychological theory at that time stressed that proper physical and character development required young people to participate in organized physical activities (Addams, 1909; Cavallo, 1981; Goodman, 1979; Mrozek, 1983). At the same time, it was widely believed that people older than forty should avoid vigorous activities, including strenuous sports, and not overstress themselves, because they had passed their prime and were facing inevitable and unavoidable physical decline.

Similarly, people with particular physical and intellectual impairments were denied access to sport participation because it was believed that vigorous activity would overexcite them and be dangerous for them and for others around them. As a result, persons defined as *old* or *disabled* according to standards used at the time were marginalized or excluded from physical activities and sports.

Unfortunately, the legacies of these historical practices and standards remain with us. They exist in the form of **ableist ideology** consisting of *interrelated ideas and beliefs that are widely used to identify people as physically or intellectually disabled, to justify treating them as inferior, and to organize social worlds and physical spaces without taking them into account.*

This ideology is common in meritocracies where people are frequently compared and ranked in terms of abilities, qualifications, and recognized achievements. As it informs everyday social interaction, people tend to patronize, pity, pathologize, demean, and sometimes dehumanize those perceived to be incapable of meeting particular standards of physical or intellectual performance. Over time, ableist ideology leads to forms of social organization in which older and disabled people are marginalized and segregated from mainstream settings and activities, especially organized, competitive sports.

Ableist ideology is based on a rejection of physical and intellectual variation as a natural and normal part of human existence. It also ignores the fact that the meanings given to different abilities change from one situation to another and that everyone's abilities vary over time and can change suddenly as a result of injury or disease.

An irony associated with ableist ideology is that those who use it to categorize others as disabled overlook the temporary nature of their own abilities. When people use gender, racial, or class ideologies to claim superiority over others, they usually escape being negatively evaluated by others who use them. But this is not the case with ableist ideology, because others will use it to negatively evaluate those who used it earlier in their lives (Harpur, 2012).

Ableist ideology is also based on the assumption that impairments are abnormalities, disregarding the fact that no mind or body works perfectly in all situations and at all times. We might have an ideal image of a human being without any impairments, but such a person does not exist. Each of us is impaired in some way. This is simply part of the human condition. If we are lucky, we live our lives around our impairments without major inconvenience, we are appreciated for the abilities we have, and we avoid being labeled by others as *subnormal* and *disabled*. When we think of our future, we hope to avoid profound impairments that prevent us from being who we want to be and doing what we want to do.

So if none of us is perfect and everyone who lives long enough is limited by impairments at some point during the lifecourse, how is it possible to divide people into two categories: *able-bodied* and *disabled?* Who decides which impairments count when classifying people as *dis*abled—a term that implies a condition worse than "unable." For example, if a ten-year-old with an impaired left arm and hand uses an adapted ski pole and skis faster and with more control than her friends, should she be classified as disabled? Who makes that decision and for what reason? Likewise, if the same ten-year-old cannot do cartwheels and backflips like her best friend but can tie her shoes one-handed and run a 5-kilometer race faster than her friend, is it appropriate to say she is a disabled runner?

These questions are meant to encourage critical thinking about the meaning of ability and disability and how we distinguish between able-bodied and disabled. They are *not* meant to dismiss or understate the real challenges faced by people with impairments that force them to make substantial and often difficult adjustments in their lives. Some of these challenges may also influence their opportunities and choices, especially when others take a visible impairment to be a mark of general inability. But when and under what conditions does a particular impairment become a disability?

To answer these questions and understand the meaning of ability and disability in sports, it is important to know about the two "isms" that form the foundation for ableist ideology. These are *ageism* and *ableism*.

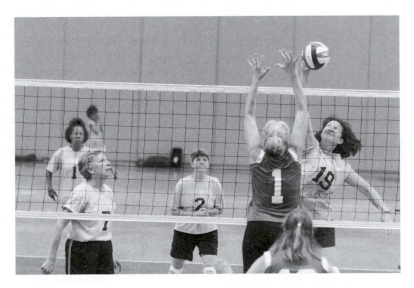

Ageism affects relationships in North America and many parts of Europe today. This leads to age segregation, especially in physical activities and sports. As a result, older people, such as these volleyball players in the 2013 U.S. National Senior Games in Cleveland, Ohio, seldom engage in sports or physical activities with younger people. (*Source:* © Angelo Merendino/Angelo Merendino/Corbis)

Ageism

The term *ageism* was first used in 1969 by Robert Butler, a physician and psychiatrist who was inspired to study how older people were treated in society when his teachers in medical school used rude and sarcastic terms as they talked about older patients and their medical conditions. He grew up with his grandparents, so he was angered by this. As he learned more about the negative attitudes and stereotypes that shaped the treatment of older people in the United States, he defined **ageism** as *an evaluative perspective that favors one age group—usually younger people—over others and justifies discrimination against particular age groups that are assumed to be incapable of full participation in mainstream activities.* According to Butler, this perspective distorted relationships with older people and denied their abilities, both physical and intellectual.

The perspective of ageism rests on the belief that younger people are more capable than and superior to those who have passed through middle age and become old. This belief is so widespread in some cultures that most people take it for granted, joke about older people, and develop a general fear of their own aging. This belief also accounts for much of the age discrimination that has become one of the most frequently reported forms of workplace discrimination in many countries today. Reported cases of age discrimination in U.S. workplaces outnumber race or sex discrimination cases by three to one (Age Concern, 2006; EEOC, 2013). The irony of this in the United States is that when people in the baby-boom generation, born between 1946 and 1964, were young, they were guilty of negatively stereotyping older people, and now that they are in their fifties and sixties, they are fighting against ageism and age discrimination.

Although people in the baby-boom generation saw many of their parents passively accept age discrimination in employment and other spheres of life and even internalize aspects of ageism, many of them now defy ageist stereotypes and blur the normative boundaries that limited their parents' lives. One strategy is to critique the words that others use to describe them. For example, "the elderly," "golden agers," "seniors," "senior citizens," "the aged," and "dear" or "honey"—terms commonly used in the past and occasionally used today—are now seen as patronizing, inaccurate, or based on ageist stereotypes.

Older people is the age identification term preferred by older people today, because it locates age on a continuum along which people are identified as "younger" or "older," depending on the point of reference. This approach challenges ableist ideology and recognizes that aging is a natural process and that everyone remains a *person* at every point along the way. This and other strategies have been effective to the point that attitudes about aging and older people are changing.

> **Being active is no longer simply an option—it is essential if we are to live healthy and fulfilling lives into old age.** —U.S. Department of Health (2004, p. iii)

Ableism

The dominant form of ableist ideology today is also shaped by **ableism**, *an evaluative perspective in which the label of disability marks a person as inferior and incapable of full participation in mainstream activities.* People using this perspective tend to patronize, pathologize, or pity those who cannot meet particular standards of physical or intellectual ability due to a visible or inferred **impairment**—which is *a physical, sensory or intellectual condition that potentially limits a person's full participation in social and/or physical environments.*

Over time, ableism leads to forms of social organization in which people with disabilities are marginalized and segregated from settings and activities created by those who don't currently have a visible impairment that could mark them as **disabled**, that is, as *a person with an impairment that is determined to cause significant functional limitations.*

Thomas Hehir, director of the School Leadership Program at Harvard University, explains that when ableism shapes our decisions, it usually leads us to make "the world unwelcoming and inaccessible for people with disabilities" (Hehir, 2002, p. 13). In the case of schools, says Hehir, ableism leads people, including parents and teachers, to assume that "it is preferable for a child to read print rather than Braille, walk rather than use a wheelchair, spell independently rather than use a spell-checker, read written text rather than listen to a book on tape, and hang out with non-disabled kids rather than with other disabled kids" (Hehir, 2005, p. 13).

In this way, ableism leads people to forget that variations in ability are a normal part of human existence, occur over time for each of us, and exist across multiple ability dimensions. Similarly, it leads people to overlook the possibility that able-bodied persons could become disabled tomorrow due to injury, disease, or other events in their lives. This means that being able-bodied is a temporary condition, and to classify people as *disabled* and *able-bodied* tells us little about people's lives, even though it may be useful for political purposes and to identify special service and support needs for particular people. We know that there are many types of abilities used for many purposes, and even though it might be possible to rank people from low to high on a particular ability in a particular situation or in reference to a specific task, it is impossible to have one ability-based ranking system that is meaningful across all situations and tasks, or across all sports.

So how do we decide when to use a "disability vocabulary" and what are the implications of doing so? This question will be answered in the following sections.

CONSTRUCTING THE MEANING OF *AGE*

Ideas and beliefs about age vary over time and from one culture to another. They even vary from one situation to another, depending on the activities and attributes valued in particular social worlds. In societies characterized by high rates of change, youth is generally valued over age. Being "old" in such societies is associated with being inflexible, out of touch, resistant to change, and possessing outdated knowledge. When this view is combined with beliefs that aging involves physical and intellectual decline, many people develop negative attitudes about becoming older. These attitudes may then become stereotypes of the experience of being older. For example, children in North America often learn that ability is associated with youth and inability is associated with being old. Therefore, a five-year-old girl may describe her grandfather as *old* if he has health-related impairments and does not play with her in physically active ways. At the same time, she may describe her grandmother of the same age as *young*—or *not old*—because she enjoys physical activities and plays soccer with her in the park. Through her relationships and experiences, this five-year-old has learned to equate old age with inactivity and a lack of physical abilities. For her, being physically able and active is a sign of youth.

> We don't stop playing because we grow old; we grow old because we stop playing. —George Bernard Shaw

When this perception of age is widely accepted and incorporated into the general narratives and stories about aging in a culture, it perpetuates negative beliefs about becoming and being old (Pike, 2013). This leads people to reduce physical activity as they age, and it supports the notion that communities should not be concerned about providing publicly funded opportunities for older people to be active and play sports. Under these conditions, those who wish to be active have little social support and few opportunities to play active sports (Pike, 2012; Tulle, 2008a, 2008b, 2008c).

Until recently, older people in many parts of the world were expected to withdraw from everyday work routines due to their frailty and weakness, or as a reward for many years of hard work. During most of the twentieth century, older people were often told to take it easy, preserve their energy and strength, and make sure they had enough rest on a daily basis. Even doctors in North America and much of Europe advised older patients, especially women, to avoid depleting their energy by "doing too much." Therefore, older people have traditionally avoided strenuous physical activity and even feared it as a threat to their health and well-being. For them, playing sports was out of the question because it would put too much strain on their hearts and create shoulder, back, hip, and knee problems. "Acting your age" meant being inactive for people defined as old, although the age at which a person is defined as old varies widely by ethnicity, social class, and gender both within and between societies (Tulle, 2008a).

The legacy of this approach to aging remains influential, even in societies where research has shown that physical exercise will not harm older people unless they have certain chronic conditions or are not physically prepared to engage in activities requiring certain levels of strength and flexibility. But we may still hear an older person say, "I'm too old to do that"—when he really means that he is not physically prepared to do it, or he doesn't want to show that he can't do it as well as he did it in the past.

Aging as a Social and Political Issue

In most societies today, birthrates are declining and people are living longer, due to improved access to health care and rising literacy rates. In 2013, the average life expectancy worldwide was sixty-eight-years-old; for women it was seventy and for men it was sixty-six. Nearly thirty countries had an average life expectancy over eighty years old (WHO, 2013). While many people celebrate longer life expectancy, others are concerned that it will make health care and social services unsustainable at current levels of public funding.

These concerns are intensified by ageist assumptions that older people make no contributions to society and ultimately are a burden that younger people must bear (Pike, 2011). To make matters worse, these assumptions further marginalize older people, encourage them to be physically inactive, separate them from contexts in which they can make contributions, and deny them opportunities to participate in continuing education and professional development needed to maintain their contributions. Also, when ageism and ableist ideology are pervasive in a society, older people often internalize these assumptions and voluntarily withdraw from activities, ceasing to be vital members of their communities and society. As a result, ageism becomes a self-fulfilling prophecy.

Another social and political issue that has emerged in recent years is grounded in the belief that rigorous exercise enables people to stay youthful because it delays and minimizes natural decremental changes that occur with aging. Although we still have much to learn about the effects of various forms and intensity of physical activity on the overall well-being of older people, there are sport scientists and medical practitioners who confidently assert that being physically active is always a good thing—that it will extend and improve the quality of people's lives and help them avoid the illnesses and diseases that older people often experience.[1] But they don't talk about the frequency of sport injuries and the heavy dependence on health care among older athletes who need medical assistance to continue training and competing.

This leads people to believe that if older people do become ill or have a disease, it is due to their life choice not to take care of themselves properly. Evidence shows that this is *not* true (Tulle, 2008c). But if policy makers believe it, they are unlikely to recommend services and medical care for older people, because only "lazy and irresponsible" older people need them. This creates a political situation in which there is little concern about national and community-based programs

for older people. In this way, people who think that physical activity and sports are the answer to numerous social and health problems provide support for a neoliberal political and cultural ideology stressing that when people take personal responsibility for their own lives, most problems will be solved (Collinet and Delalandre, 2015). In connection with aging, this is one way that sports and sport science can influence political decisions that impact people's lives.

Age, Sports, and Ability

Societies in which more than 50 percent of the population live to at least seventy years old are becoming more numerous. Cambridge University historian Peter Laslett (1987, 1996) used the term *Third Age Societies* as he studied what occurs when entire populations become older. One thing that occurs is that the field of gerontology, which involves the study of aging and later life, becomes increasingly important.

Most social gerontologists today point out that while aging is an intrinsically physical process of irreversible decline, the social significance given to this process is important. In particular, their research seeks to address an imbalance in sociological research, which has been dominated by studies of youth as the future producers and consumers of society; at the same time, older people have been overlooked because they've been seen as having few productive and consumptive capacities. The research of social gerontologists also helps those of us in the sociology of sport to develop our own studies of age, sports, and ability, and the meanings given to sport participation at different points during the life span.

There are innumerable studies of the developmental implications of youth sport participation, and we have learned much about age-appropriate physical activity involvement from early childhood through adolescence (Balyi et al., 2013; CS4L, 2013). But studies of the implication and dynamics of sport participation among older people are rare. This is partly because older people are assumed to

---

[1]This is an important and complex issue. It is discussed directly and in detail by Emmanuelle Tulle (2008a, 2008b, 2008c) and less directly by Elizabeth Pike (2011, 2012) and Brad Millington (2012).

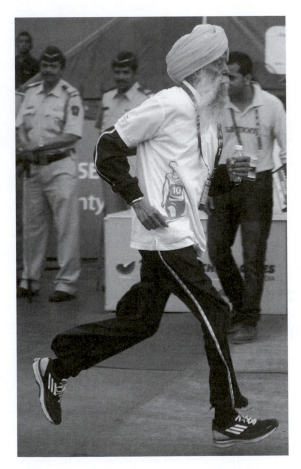

Fauja Singh, a 101-year-old British amateur runner, currently holds the record for the oldest runner to complete a marathon. Here, at the Standard Chartered Mumbai Marathon 2013 in Mumbai, India, he participates in a 4.3-kilometer run for older people. (*Source:* © Divyakant Solanki/epa/Corbis)

be "grown up"—that is, their growth and development are complete, so there is little reason to study physical activities and sports in their lives.

This approach is shortsighted and ignores demographic data indicating that people over the age of sixty are the fastest-growing segment of the population in many societies. Additionally, as the cohorts of people turning fifty years old and older now see themselves as capable of engaging in sports and related vigorous physical activities, there is a need

to understand the full implications of their participation. Historically, public policies and private sector funding has focused on providing young people with opportunities and encouragement to participate in sport activities, but the provision of opportunities and encouragement for older people has largely been ignored (Pike, 2012; Tulle, 2008a).

Unsurprisingly, popular sports worldwide celebrate youth and youthfulness. They often are viewed as stages on which "the future" of societies is exhibited. Sports played by older people are given little attention. Apart from seniors golf tournaments used by corporate sponsors to market products and services to wealthy, influential older men who make product choices for large corporations, there is no consistent coverage of sports involving older athletes. The exception is coverage in which older people make the news as novelties by being the oldest person to run a marathon or the first eighty-year-old to climb a mountain or swim across the local lake.

With this said, many of us have noticed that some elite athletes now play to older ages than in the past (Tulle, 2014). Advances in sport science have improved nutrition and training so that athletes have shorter recovery time as they continue to train intensely. Commentators often refer to the longevity of older players, and sponsors that want to sell products to older consumers are now willing to support older athletes who retain their celebrity personas and their ability to sell products. For example, when David Beckham's contract with the Los Angeles Galaxy in the Major Soccer League ended in 2013, most player personnel directors for elite soccer teams around the world felt that at age thirty-eight he was too old to be of any competitive value. However, several clubs did compete to have Beckham sign a contract with them because of his commercial value. For them, "Brand Beckham" was worth sustaining, even if Beckham himself had passed his prime as a player. But in the end, Beckham decided to retire.

Emerging Ideas About Aging and Sports

The baby-boom generation, born between 1946 and 1964, has until recently been the largest age-based segment of the population in the United States, the United Kingdom, and a few other countries where there was a strong sense of hope and possibility after World War II ended. This positive outlook led couples to have many children over that eighteen-year period, and demographers labeled them the Baby Boom Generation.

Over the years, baby boomers have had a strong influence on everything from the rise of popular culture to the expansion of science and higher education. They also grew up with more access to youth sports, and they attended high school and college at higher rates than previous generations. Now they are in their fifties and sixties and are more physically active than people of that age were in the past. As a result, they are challenging ageist beliefs about older people. Now when active older people receive media attention, commentators are likely to describe them as part of a trend rather than novelties.

On average, baby boomers are healthier than previous generations of older people and they have more resources to continue their physical activities and sport participation. They also have been privileged to live during a period of economic expansion and were children during a time of widespread public support for sport programs. Additionally, the youngest women in this generation were the first in the United States to benefit from the opportunities created by Title IX and similar gender equity laws in other countries. As these factors merged together, many baby boomers made sport participation a total family activity—something that was rare in the past. As a result, they now have more support from family and friends for continuing or initiating sport participation than any previous older generation (Pike, 2012).

This generational shift in ideas and beliefs about age and physical activity does not mean that all older people today are physically active. In fact, the rates of physical inactivity, obesity, and related health problems are disappointingly high. Additionally, some baby boomers accept ableist ideology and deny their own aging, and some others succumb to ageist stereotypes and attempt to hide

their aging with hair dye, diet regimes, cosmetic surgery, drugs, and other enhancement procedures. Some, of course, use sport participation and exercise routines in the hope of looking younger longer—hope fostered through billions of dollars of advertising by the appearance enhancement industry (Pike, 2010).

The point here is that the sheer size of the baby-boom generation, along with its access to resources, has enabled it to have a high degree of cultural clout. And many boomers approach older adulthood with the expectation that if they wish to be active, there should be opportunities for them to do so, or else they will create those opportunities on their own (Brown, 2013). In this sense they are challenging the prevailing ableist ideology and popular ideas about what is natural and normal for older people (Collinet and Delalandre, 2015; Dionigi and O'Flynn, 2007).

At the same time, older people today are challenging the ways in which sports are organized. Many of them combine elements of power and performance with elements of pleasure and participation (see Chapter 3). This provides space for people with differing interests: some focus on results, personal bests, and other aspects of achievement, and others seek social experiences in settings where people are interested in doing physical things for the joy of it.

Older People Only: Age-Segregated Sports

For various reasons, some older people prefer to participate in age-segregated sports. Long-time sport participants may seek events involving peers who share their age-related interests and experiences, whereas new participants often avoid events involving younger people, who may not be sensitive to the concerns of older athletes.

A number of individual sports now sponsor masters or veterans competitions. Cycling, dance, skiing, table tennis, tennis, and triathlon are examples. Swimming and track and field (athletics) have the longest histories of masters-level events. The first

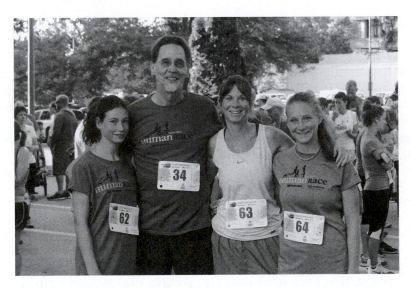

This is one of many three-generation entries into the 5- and 10-Kilometer Human Race in Fort Collins, Colorado, during the summer of 2013. These family members–ages 69, 44, 16, and 14–regularly run races together. (*Source:* © Nancy Coakley)

World Masters Swimming Championships were held in Tokyo in 1986 (Weir et al., 2010), and the same event held in Italy in 2012 attracted nearly 10,000 competitors from seventy-seven affiliated national federations.

The World Masters Games is a multi-sport event held every four years since 1995 for competitors over thirty-five years old. It is recognized by the International Olympic Committee and partners with the International Paralympic Committee to support the Olympic Movement and the sport-for-all philosophy of the Olympic Charter. In 1995, the International Masters Games Association (IMGA) was officially organized with International Federations as its members. More than 8000 athletes participated in the 1983 Games, and the 2013 Games in Torino, Italy, brought together 50,000 athletes representing 100 nations to compete in thirty core sports; athletes at these events were even allowed to form multinational teams. This event attracted less media coverage and fewer spectators than the 2012 Olympic Games, but it had four times as many participants.

The World Masters Games present themselves as inclusive events that focus on the health advantages of lifelong sport participation. They include disability sports events within the regular program, and there are many events designed for athletes of all ages with various impairments. Although these and other veteran events are becoming more popular, they involve only a fraction of the older population worldwide.

Studies of middle-age and older people who participate in masters events are now helping us understand more about the role of sport participation in the aging process (Dionigi, 2006, 2010, 2011; Dionigi and O'Flynn, 2007; Dionigi et al., 2011, 2013; Pike, 2012; Pike and Weinstock, 2014; Tulle, 2007, 2008b). Data from these studies indicate that in most cases, continuing sport participation helps people negotiate the process of getting older. As they move from middle age to later life, they recognize and accept that the level of their performance in sports will decline, although competition remains exciting for them. Some constantly push themselves to excel; others might do so mostly when they enter a new age category and have a chance to place high in their age group in a particular event.

When these athletes talk about sports in their lives, it appears that they use them "to simultaneously resist and accept the aging process" (Dionigi et al., 2013, p. 385). They experience stress, illness, and acute injuries, but staying in sports enables them to maintain their sense of physical competence, experience social and mental stimulation, and feel resilient in the face of advancing age. They don't want age to define them and are pleased when others do not define them in terms of age or think they look younger than they are.

Unfortunately, most of the existing research focuses on white, middle-class people, who often use a particular fitness discourse when they talk about sport participation. At this time we know little about the participation of people of color or people who lack material resources. It is likely that their participation rates are relatively low, but for those who are involved in Masters and other events, it would be useful to know the meanings they give to their experiences and how those meanings change in connection with aging and shifting life circumstances.

There is little doubt that veterans and masters sport programs will increase as a growing population of older people demand them and as people see them as a way to create careers and make money (Brown, 2013; Weir et al., 2010). Economic development officials in cities worldwide now see sport events for older people as a way to increase tourism and bring into the city people who are likely to have money to spend on hotels, restaurants, and other local tourist attractions.

Active older people are also attracted to events in which they can compete without feeling the pressure to constantly improve their performance. Instead of focusing on progressive improvement, they emphasize maintaining their physical abilities so they can remain active as they become older. For this reason, older people often avoid sports with high injury rates. Research in Europe has recently found that the sport participation histories reported by 1739 people over fifty years old

involved progressively less competition and more diversity in terms of how sports were organized (Klostermann and Nagel, 2012).

It is difficult to track changes in how people integrate sport participation into their lives as they age, but from what we know at this time it appears that as people age, they prefer modified versions of competitive activities that are organized to emphasize the pleasure of movement, social experiences, and controlled challenges. Many older people also choose to engage in walking, swimming, strength training, yoga, tai chi, and similar activities that involve no competition or achievement tracking such as times and rankings. They take these activities seriously at the same time that they focus on health, fitness, social experiences, and the overall pleasure of participation. Evidence also indicates that some older people now choose to play physically active video games so they can exercise in the safety and comfort of their homes (Diaz-Orueta et al., 2012).

Overall it is likely that images of older people who are active, fit, healthy, and accomplished athletes will become more visible over time. This might inspire others to be active in ways that challenge the credibility of those who use ageism and ableism to mark older people as incapable and inferior (Pike, 2012). On the other hand, the images could be used by people with a political agenda based on ableist ideology to argue that older people who don't meet exercise expectations should not receive public support because they lack moral worth. This means that as older people become more physically active, the meanings given to age and ability can vary significantly as people promote different social and economic policy agendas.

Age, Ability, and Context

As we grow older, our age intersects with other social factors such as gender, race/ethnicity, and socioeconomic status, and this influences our experiences of sports in later life. For example, older white men's experiences and opportunities are very different from those of older black women; and wealthier people have more choices than people with few material resources. Additionally, the relationship between age and gender has been described as a "double jeopardy," with older women being doubly constrained by age and gender (de Beauvoir, 1972). But this might more accurately be described as "multiple jeopardy" as we also consider the effects of race/ethnicity, socioeconomic status, and other variables (see Pike, 2010, 2012).

Women have longer life expectancies than men in all societies, a social condition described as the "feminization of aging" (Davidson et al., 2011). However, statistics indicate that women are less physically active than men throughout the life span and their activity levels decline significantly in later life (Sport England, 2013; Wilińska, 2010). This is due to their continued domestic responsibilities in later life as they maintain their role as caregivers for grandchildren and their own parents (see Pike, 2010).

Although many sports remain male-dominated, an increasing number of women in some sectors of society see physical activity and sport participation as part of an overall program to maintain their health, strength, and flexibility as they age. The pace and extent of this trend varies greatly from one society and population to another, depending on patterns of gender relations, the popularity and accessibility of personal enhancement technologies, and the experiences and perspectives of older women (Pfister, 2012).

Women sometimes exercise to delay the appearance of aging, which reaffirms ageist ideology at the same time that it may support personal health (Tulle, 2008). Older women, particularly those with high socioeconomic status, can engage in sports activities and belong to leisure clubs as a way to embrace and negotiate the aging process or as a way to fight it (Dionigi et al., 2013). This raises interesting research questions: Do those who use physical activity to fight or "delay" the aging process benefit more or less, and do they drop out more or less often, than those who exercise or play sports for other reasons?

Age and gender also intersect with ethnicity and social class in connection with physical activity and sport participation. Ethnicity issues are complex in the United States and other countries where immigrants come from a wide array of cultures and have immigration patterns that span multiple generations. Patterns for first-generation immigrants from China are likely different than patterns among fifth-generation or later Chinese Americans who have ideas and beliefs about age and ability that are based on their experiences in the United States. Similarly, patterns among first- and later-generation people with Mexican ancestry will differ with their unique experiences. For the most part, research indicates that the longer an immigrant population lives in the United States, the more likely it is that their lifestyles will match those of their status peers in U.S. culture.

As noted in Chapter 9, socioeconomic status is strongly related to patterns of physical activity and sport participation in the United States. Participation is perceived as a personal choice, but choices expand with a person's financial resources. Therefore, older people who are able to maintain their lifestyles will continue with their previous physical activity habits to the extent that their health and general social situation permit.

Most U.S. media images of active older people portray those who are well-off and healthy (Marshall and Rahman, 2015). The images are primarily in commercial ads promoting the "ideal" way to live as retired people, and that life involves cruising and jetting off to attractive tourist destinations and joining friends engaged in never-ending consumption of goods, services and a combination of supplements and prescription drugs. However, more than 90 percent of older people cannot live such a consumption-oriented lifestyle. Their life choices are based on limited financial resources and the accessibility of opportunities to engage in physical activities with friends. Cost, accessibility, and sociability matter the most in their choices about physical activity participation (Pike, 2012). For most older people living primarily on social security and limited savings, choices outside the home are scarce or nonexistent. Research is sorely needed on this topic.

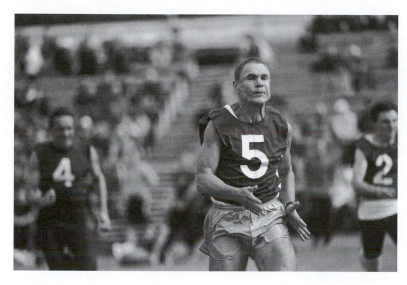

Participants in running and cycling races in Scottish Highland Games have "handicaps" based on past performances. This means that in the 100-meter sprint, the starting line for a sprinter who is sixty-eight years old might be 7 meters closer to the finish line than the starting line for the national Scottish high school champion in the event. This allows men and women of all ages to compete with each other in the same event. (*Source:* © Mark Bryan Makela/In Pictures/Corbis)

CONSTRUCTING THE MEANING OF *ABILITY*

"Ability" is a loaded concept. Different people see various abilities as essential as they view the world from their vantage point. Ask an engineer about ability, and the response will be different from what an artist or auto mechanic might say. On average, men will describe ability in terms that don't match up with what women say, and the same goes for older and younger people, African Americans and Euro-Americans, the wealthy and the poor. Variations also occur from one culture and situation to another (Spencer-Cavaliere and Peers, 2011).

You get the point: Ability is a complex phenomenon, and its meaning shifts depending on the situation and a person's vantage point and experiences. To discuss ability, it is important that we choose our words carefully so we understand each other. In the case of science and research, words must be precisely defined, because they are used to identify the topics we study and the questions we pose. To that end we must also be sensitive to how others define and respond to particular words. Mistakes and oversights interfere with communication and obtaining valid information from others.

The same goes for ability's often misunderstood sibling: *disability*. This point is emphasized by Damon Rose, the editor of the disability website *Ouch!* (http://www.bbc.co.uk/news/blogs/ouch/). Rose is registered as blind and understands how people with disabilities respond to the words used to identify them (Rose, 2004). For example, *handicapped* is an offensive designation. For most people with a disability, **handicapped** means *being held back, weighed down, and marked as inferior due to perceived physical or intellectual impairments.* The word is based on the perspective of non-disabled people who decided that particular impairments should define the identity of those who live with them.

Rose realizes that words have power and may be used to discredit people with certain attributes and perpetuate the barriers that disrupt and influence their lives. This means that as we work to understand the meaning of *dis*ability in sports, it is important that we use terminology that does not unwittingly disadvantage those who already face the challenge of living with and around their physical or intellectual impairments.

The definition of the term "*dis*ability" has been debated for many years by health and medical professionals, government officials, school administrators, physiologists, psychologists, social scientists, and those who live with physical or intellectual impairments (Harpur, 2012). This is because official definitions are used to determine who qualifies for public assistance in schools and government programs, who is protected by antidiscrimination laws, who may park in reserved areas and use designated facilities, who may or may not participate in mainstream or "disability sports," and so on.

According to the World Health Organization, definitions should be taken seriously because disability "is a complex phenomenon, reflecting the interaction between features of a person's body and features of the society in which he or she lives" (WHO, 2011). This is relevant in connection with sports, because disability is nearly a universal aspect of experience. With rare exceptions, each of us will be impaired at some point in time in a way that limits how we function in everyday life—and the likelihood of this being permanent rather than temporary increases with age. The challenges we face when this occurs are many, and often take the form of barriers that are common features of our everyday social and physical environments. This makes it a matter of self-interest to support interventions to remove barriers that limit and restrict activities and participation among people with varying abilities. These barriers are present in (a) physical environments designed solely for people without movement impairments; (b) social norms and organizational structures that ignore, marginalize, or exclude people with certain impairments; and (c) personal attitudes and vocabulary that link disability with inferiority.

None of us is physically or mentally perfect, and we regularly make personal adjustments to reduce the impact of our own lack of ability. If we are lucky, we have access to support systems and assistive devices that make those adjustments more effective and less disruptive. Those of us with corrective lenses, for instance, may take clear vision for granted, but only because an assistive device reduces the impact of our sight impairment in our lives.

It is also important to avoid arbitrary barriers that turn our impairments into disabilities. For example, prior to the late 1990s, if your leg was amputated below the knee, you could not have been a member of your national powerlifting team, because the rules of the International Powerlifting Federation (IPF) stated that to be eligible for official events, a competitor doing a bench press and other compulsory lifts must have two feet in contact with the floor—and a prosthetic foot did not qualify as a foot. This meant that you would have been "*dis*'d" by the IPF—that is, *dis*qualified due to *dis*ability. After a few *dis*'d athletes legally challenged this rule, it was changed so that a prosthetic leg and foot were permitted as replacements for a flesh-and-bones leg and foot.

In this example, the original IPF rule had converted an impairment into disability. The revised rule eliminated disability by removing the barrier that restricted participation. However, the connection between impairments and abilities is often more complex than this. We saw this with Oscar Pistorius, the 100- and 200-meter sprinter from South Africa, who fought a long legal and scientific "classification" battle to qualify for participation in the 2012 Olympics as a runner with two below-the-knee prostheses. The prostheses that Pistorius wore were Flex-Foot Cheetah blades. As he set records in the Paralympics and won a world championship in track and field (athletics), Pistorius was nicknamed "the blade runner" and "the fastest man on no legs." But he was "*dis*'d" when the IOC and the IAAF ruled that he could not participate in the Olympic Games because his prostheses gave him an "unfair advantage" over other Olympic runners in the 100- and 200-meter sprints. After reviewing considerable research evidence and deliberating for nearly a year, the Court of Arbitration for Sport concluded that the carbon-fiber devices used by Pistorius did not give him a net advantage in his events.

The Pistorius case attracted massive media coverage, and it raised many issues about the meaning of ability and disability in sports. These issues are important, but most people with physical impairments are concerned with more basic and practical matters, such as access to sport participation opportunities, adaptive sports equipment, knowledgeable coaches, barrier-free facilities, transportation to and from practice and competitions, and basic support for training.

The Emerging Meaning of *Disability*

The discussion of ability in this chapter is based on the hope that we will gradually replace the current language of disability with a new language of ability that focuses on making sure that no one is denied human rights due to their physical or intellectual abilities (Harpur, 2012). At the same time it also is important to know that the terms *disability* and *disabled* were first used by people who wanted to replace widely used negative terms such as *freak, deformed, invalid, cripple, gimp, lame, spaz, spastic,* and *handicapped* in reference to people with physical impairments, and *imbecile, idiot, lunatic,* *demented, retarded, retard,* and *feebleminded* in reference to people with intellectual impairments.

During most of the twentieth century people believed that impairment and disability were same thing. This belief was consistent with the medical approach used to understand physical and intellectual impairments and how to deal with them. This approach is represented by the medical model as illustrated in Figure 10.1. In this model it is assumed that the goal is to diagnose the origin of the impairment and then use medical strategies to fix, heal, cure, or correct it. If successful, the body or mind would be "normalized" and the person could rejoin mainstream society. If not successful, the next alternative was a rehabilitation program to help the person overcome his or her flawed condition to an extent that would permit at least partial participation in society. As these attempts were made to normalize the body or mind under the guidance of medical experts, people with disabilities were passive recipients of diagnoses and treatments.

The medical model of disability is based on the perspectives of those who are not impaired in ways that lead them to be classified as disabled. But it has remained popular for two reasons. First, many people continue to accept ableist ideology and see disability as an individual condition in need of expert diagnosis and treatment. Second, a massive industry has been built around this approach, and it prospers

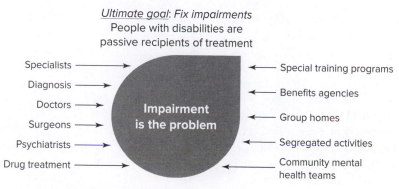

FIGURE 10.1 Medical model of disability.

when the primary goal is to fix or rehabilitate bodies and minds. Both these reasons ignore the possibility that impairments are a normal part of the human condition and that they are converted into disabilities by a combination of negative attitudes, stereotypes, and barrier-filled social arrangements and built environments.

Disability rights activists in the 1960s rejected the passivity prescribed for them by the medical model. An alternative to this model was presented in 1983, when Mike Oliver, a disability studies scholar in England, introduced and advocated the use of a social model to conceptualize and understand disability (see Figure 10.2). Oliver argued that the experience of being disabled was actually a product of social oppression rather than a the result of personal defect requiring a medical "fix" to become "normal" (Oliver, 1983, 1990).

People with disabilities already considered themselves to be normal and resented being seen as flawed and inferior. From their perspective, impairment was a fact of life but their *dis*ability was caused by the social and cultural responses to various physical and intellectual impairments. Therefore, disability became a social issue in need of a political solution rather than a personal trouble in need of medical treatment. The focus on treatment and rehabilitation shifted to a focus on political actions that confronted barriers created by negative attitudes, poorly organized and managed social arrangements, and thoughtlessly designed physical environments. The goal implied by the social model was cultural and environmental transformation instead of medical and pharmacological fixes.

Embracing the social model of disability did not mean that individuals no longer sought medical assistance and treatment to ameliorate the pain or inconvenience caused by impairments. But it did mean that problems caused by disability were most effectively solved through social and cultural change (Couser, 2009; Oliver, 1983, 1990).

The social model identified barriers as the problem and removing them as the goal. For over two decades, this approach unified people in the "disability community" who shared common experiences of oppression and misrepresentation across all disability categories (Beauchamp-Pryor, 2011; Shakespeare and Watson, 2002).

The social model inspired changes worldwide. Locating disability in culture and society rather

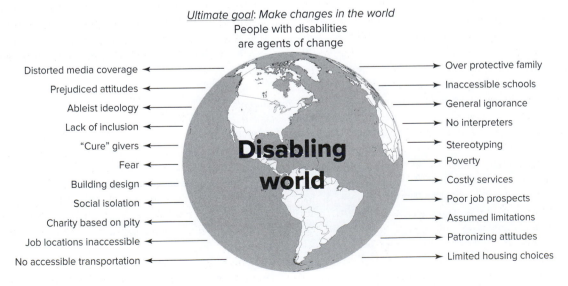

FIGURE 10.2 Social model of disability.

than in the bodies and minds of individuals shifted the focus from rehabilitation to full access, from charity to opportunity, and from risky surgeries to dependable support systems.

As people learned more about disabling barriers built into the structure of everyday life, they called for changes that acknowledged normal variations in human abilities. They realized that they could not eliminate the paralysis caused by a spinal cord injury, but that it was possible to provide wheelchairs to people with those injuries and make sure that the physical environment was designed to accommodate wheelchairs.

The political activism fueled by the social model was liberating and empowering for people with impairments. To focus on social oppression rather than their own bodies as *the problem* served to legitimize previously repressed anger and boost their sense of self-worth. Fighting for rights rather than depending on charity was fulfilling. Most important, their actions led to the passage of new laws mandating accessibility and prohibiting ableism and discrimination. In the United States, the Americans with Disabilities Act (ADA) is a primary example of such a law.

The ADA was passed and signed into law by President George Bush in 1990. It stated that all programs and facilities that are open to everyone must also be open to people with disabilities unless such access creates direct threats to the health and safety of the people involved. When applied to sports this means that people with disabilities must be allowed to participate in programs open to everyone as long as they and the accommodations they require do not threaten the health and safety of other players, cause "undue burden" for the sponsoring organization, or fundamentally change the sport being played (Block, 1995).

Threats to health and safety must be real, based on objective information, and unavoidable, even after reasonable efforts have been made to eliminate them. For example, if a child wears a metal brace to stabilize a leg impaired by cerebral palsy, she must be allowed to play in a youth soccer league if the brace can be covered so it will not hurt anyone

and if the league does not have to make burdensome changes or fundamentally alter its game rules to accommodate her participation. Additionally, if tryouts are required for everyone wanting to play in a program, the girl with the brace may not be prohibited from trying out because of her impairment. However, she may be cut if she does not meet the physical skills standards applied to everyone being assessed. The coach may *not* require that all players on the team must run without a limp, but she may say that being able and willing to run at a reasonable pace is a standard requirement for team membership.

Unfortunately, the fiscal austerity policy approach that has become common in many countries following the global economic crisis has undermined many of the hard-won changes inspired by the social model. This situation and criticisms of the model have fragmented the disability community and enabled people with neoliberal political agendas to revive the medical model and its emphasis on the need for people to be personally responsible for keeping and making themselves well. As a result, programs for people with disabilities have been severely cut or eliminated. Even military veterans with severe impairments caused by injuries sustained in recent wars have seen their programs downsized or eliminated. As this continues there are renewed calls for a revival of political action based on the social model (Oliver, 2013; Oliver and Barnes, 2012).

The Meaning of Ability Differences

Before reading this book, what would have happened if you had been asked to close your eyes and imagine five different sport scenes? Would one or more of those scenes have involved athletes with a disability? Unless you have played disability sports or seen them played by others, it is unlikely that any scene would have included athletes with a disability.

This imagination exercise is *not* meant to evoke guilt. Our views of the world are based on personal experiences; and our experiences are influenced by the meanings given to age, gender, race, ethnicity, social class, sexuality, disability, and other socially significant characteristics in our culture. Neither culture nor society forces us to think or do certain things, but the only way to mute their influence is to critically examine them and learn the ways in which cultural meanings and social organization create constraints *and* opportunities in people's lives, including people with a disability. Once these things are known, strategies for disrupting them can be created.

Consider the case of Danny: At the age of twenty-one he was a popular and highly skilled rugby player. Then came the accident, the amputation of his right arm just below the shoulder, the therapy, and eventually, getting back with friends. But reconnecting with friends after suddenly becoming impaired was not easy. Danny described his experience with these words: "A lot of them found it very difficult . . . to come to terms with it . . . And they found it hard to be around me, friends that I'd had for years" (in Brittain, 2004b, p. 437; see also Smith, 2013).

Chris, an athlete with cerebral palsy and one of Danny's teammates on the British Paralympic Team, explains why his friends felt uncomfortable: "They have very little knowledge of people with a disability, and they think that if they leave me alone, don't come in contact with me, and don't get involved, its not their problem" (in Brittain, 2004b, p. 437).

Chris raises a recurring issue in the history of disability: What happens when people define physical or intellectual impairments as "differences" and use them to create a category of "others" who are distinguished from "us normals" in social worlds?

Throughout history, people with disabilities have been described by words that connote revulsion, resentment, dread, shame, and limitations. In Europe and North America, it took World War II and thousands of returning soldiers impaired by injuries to raise widespread concerns about the words used to describe people with disabilities. Language changed. Today people with intellectual disabilities now have the Special Olympics as a participation option. Elite athletes with physical disabilities may qualify for the Paralympics ("para" meaning *parallel with,* not *paraplegic*). Words like *retard, spaz* (spastic), *cripple, freak, deaf and dumb, handicapped,* and *deformed* have been driven out of favor. But comments such as "She's a quad," "They're amputees," and "What a retard!" can still be heard on occasion.

Improvements have occurred, but when people with a disability are defined as "others," encountering them often forces people to deal with their vulnerability, aging, and mortality. And when it challenges their faulty assumptions about normalcy around which they have constructed their social worlds, it can be very upsetting. Therefore, those identified as physically and intellectually "normal" often ignore, avoid, or patronize people with a disability. This reproduces ableism and undermines the possibility of abandoning ableist ideology.

The fear of "otherness" is powerful, and people in many cultures traditionally restrict and manage their contact with "others" by enlisting the services of experts. These include doctors, mental health workers, psychiatrists, healers, shamans, witch doctors, priests, exorcists, and all professionals whose assumed competence gives them the right to examine, test, classify, and prescribe "normalizing treatments" for "impaired others." Therefore, the history of disability is also the history of giving meaning to difference, creating "others," and using current and limited knowledge to treat "otherness" (Foucault, 1961/1967; Goffman, 1961, 1963).

Disability activist and writer Thomas Couser points out that by defining people with physical and intellectual impairments as others, we marginalize them and create for ourselves the illusion that we live in a normal reality. The implications of this are explored in the Reflect on Sports box "Living in the Empire of the Normal."

Media Constructions of *Dis*Ability

Disability sports receive little media coverage apart from the Paralympic Games, which may be given some coverage in newspapers and television programming, but this occurs only once every two years (Schantz and Gilbert, 2012). World championships and other major events receive little or no mainstream media coverage.

People who make programming decisions for commercial media assume that covering disability sports is a money-losing proposition. Additionally, most media people have never played or even seen disability sports, and they lack the words and experiences that would enable them to provide coverage that might build a media audience.

Research shows that when disability sports have been covered in mainstream media, athletes often are portrayed as "courageous victims" or "heroic supercrips" who engage in *inspiring* athletic performances (Schantz and Gilbert, 2012; Silva and Howe, 2012; Tynedal and Wolbring, 2013). Sociologist Ian Brittain (2004) analyzed this coverage and found that media images and narratives usually fell into one of the following categories:

Patronizing: "Aren't they marvelous!"
Curiosity: "Do you think she can really do that?"
Tragedy: "On that fateful day, his life was changed forever."
Inspiration: "She's a true hero and a model for all of us."
Mystification: "I can't believe he just did that!"
Pity: "Give her a hand for trying so hard."
Surprise: "Stay tuned to see physical feats you've never imagined!"

Images and narratives organized around these themes construct disability in terms of the medical model—focused on personal impairments that must be overcome. This leads people to ignore *why* particular social meanings are given to disabilities and *how* they shape the lives of people with specific impairments (Brittain, 2004; Smith and Thomas, 2005). As a result, media coverage often perpetuates the ableist belief that disabilities are abnormalities and that people with disabilities have identities based on abnormalities.

Media coverage of the 2012 Paralympics in London highlighted certain technologies used by athletes (Wolbring, 2012b). Artificial "running legs" and the athletes who used them were covered as if they were new models of race cars and drivers. But wheelchairs received less coverage and the athletes using them were regularly described as "wheelchair *bound*" rather than wheelchair users. The inference in this coverage was that wheelchairs were confining, whereas the artificial legs were liberating, even transforming. For the commentators viewing these devices from their vantage point in the empire of the normal, this is not surprising. Sleek, efficient legs were for them supernormalizing, whereas through ableist eyes the wheelchair, even a $10,000 racing chair, remained an indicator of disability.

Carla Silva and David Howe at Loughborough University in England were led to similar conclusions by their research (Silva and Howe, 2012). They found that media coverage of Paralympic athletes often represented them as "supercrips" who have overcome astonishing odds to do what they do. This was also true in two promotional media campaigns they analyzed—one in Portugal and one in the United Kingdom. The former focused on Portuguese *Superatleta*—"super athletes"—and used a Superman "S" in the campaign logo. Media ads depicted a person in a wheelchair negotiating his way around an illegally parked car that blocked sidewalk access—as if disability mysteriously infused power into his body. The UK campaign was titled *Freaks of Nature,* and it was launched by a major commercial television company wanting to hype the "staggering ability" of Paralympic athletes at the upcoming 2012 Paralympic Games.

Both campaigns created controversies. Silva and Howe explain that this wasn't surprising, because there is little consensus on how to represent disability in sport events. In the absence of public discourse about the meaning of disability and the experiences of people who face disability in their everyday lives, media people did not know how to talk about it, much less present it to a commercial television audience seeking entertainment.

Silva and Howe fear that the supercrip narratives currently used when covering the Paralympics may reaffirm the neoliberal ableist idea that it is up to people with disabilities to overcome them

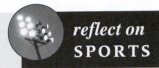

Living in the Empire of the Normal

Mainstream media images of bodies in contemporary cultures highlight healthy, fit, and traditionally attractive models with no visible impairments. Images of impaired bodies are rare, except in notices for fund-raising events to "help the disabled"—usually children shown in vulnerable situations. Only recently have a few people with physical impairments been positively represented in popular media, and most have been skilled athletes. But this is a typical pattern in the "Empire of the Normal," where people with impaired bodies or minds are exiled to the margins of the Empire and controlled by medical experts and "rehab" programs (Couser, 2000, 2009; Goffman, 1961, 1963).

Visible impairments in the Empire of the Normal require polite responses as residents of the Empire repeatedly ask: What happened to you? Why are you this way? Why are you not like me and everyone else in the Empire? Answering these questions is the price of admission into the Empire. Knowing this, people with visible impairments develop "body stories"—narratives that account for their abnormality in a manner that prevents

them from being exiled before they complete their business in the Empire. But completing business often is difficult because the story must be told again and again and again. As a result, their identity comes to be shaped around their impairment rather than their abilities or other traits (Thomson, 2000, 2009).

When people with visible impairments play sports in the Empire, it is usually on the invitation of an established resident, or on the recommendations of a medical expert—physical therapist, doctor, psychiatrist, or psychologist. In fact, the first version of what we now call Paralympic sports was created in a British medical center for war veterans with spinal cord injuries. Ludwig Guttmann, the neurosurgeon who founded the center, felt that playing sports was effective rehabilitation therapy for patients. When he scheduled these events to be played publicly at the same time that the 1948 Olympic Games were being staged in London, he was described as a radical. His action had disrupted the Empire of the Normal and forced its residents to encounter bodies with serious physical impairments. This violated the Empire

on their own so they can live normal lives like "the rest of us." Alternatively, Silva and Howe hope that future coverage will represent Paralympic athletes with a narrative emphasizing that physical difference is a naturally occurring phenomenon that creates for each of us an opportunity to accommodate those differences in ways that make our families, schools, communities, and societies more humane and inclusive.

The Special Olympics for people with intellectual disabilities presents a slightly different challenge to journalists and commentators, because events are organized as competitive at the same time that they emphasize the importance of participation over winning. For example, a study of the television news coverage of the 2009 National Special Olympics in Great Britain found that

commentators used complex and "mixed" messages in their representations of the event (Carter and Williams, 2012). They sustained a relentlessly "positive" tone in their comments, focused on human interest stories, ignored larger social and political issues related to disabilities, and tended to become emotional and use words like *courageous* and *inspirational* when they interviewed family members of the athletes. However, the researchers stated that the commentators did a reasonably good job, given that they had little experience or training preparing them to discuss learning disability issues or to interview people with varying intellectual abilities.

Despite misguided media representations, most athletes with a disability will accept coverage containing misrepresentations over no coverage. Like norm, "Out of sight, out of mind," which had always been respected in the past.

It is rare for people with physical or intellectual impairments to play sports in the Empire because there is a shortage of accessible opportunities, resources for transportation, adapted equipment, knowledgeable coaches, and programs designed to support their achievement and success. Even when opportunities are available, decisions to take them are influenced by responses anticipated from residents of the Empire: How will they define my body? Will they treat me as an athlete or patronize me as a courageous cripple?

Research in the Empire indicates that people identified as disabled define and give meaning to their sport participation as they integrate sport experiences into their lives. When their participation is treated by people from the Empire as trivial or "second class," they can develop self-doubt and a sense of inferiority. Patronizing and artificial praise create anger, disappointment, and loneliness. But when people are genuinely supportive, take players' participation seriously, and appreciate their skills, it builds confidence and confirms a sense of

normalcy, which often is fragile and unstable in the confines of the Empire.

Because power and performance sports are given high priority in the Empire of the Normal, athletes with physical impairments often are discouraged from playing with or alongside athletes residing in the Empire. Instead, they play in "special" programs with others like them, and this influences the meanings they give to their experiences.

In recent years, athletes with physical or intellectual disabilities have seen their sports as sites for challenging dominant body images and expectations in the Empire of the Normal. Developing sport skills, many hope, is a way to break through the walls of the Empire and discredit residents who accept ableist ideology and believe that until impaired bodies are fixed they should not play in the Empire (Thomson, 2002).

At this point in time, it is difficult to say that residents of the Empire will abandon arrangements that privilege them in a manner they've come to expect. So what will it take for the Empire to pull down its walls and work to achieve inclusion?

• •

other athletes, they want to be acknowledged for their physical competence. But they also hope that their visibility and accomplishments will challenge traditional stereotypes and make people aware of issues related to ableism and the need for inclusion in all spheres of society. For this to occur, and to avoid replacing negative stereotypes with a similarly unrealistic supercrip stereotype, people in the media need guidance to provide coverage from vantage points outside the empire of the normal.

Gendering *Dis*Ability

In cultures where femininity is associated with physical attractiveness and sexual desirability, and masculinity is associated with power and strength, gender shapes the ways people negotiate the

meaning of physical disabilities in their lives. This is illustrated in the following stories about Anna, Nick, and Mark, all of whom have participated in research projects on disability.

Anna was born with underdeveloped arms and feet. Despite encouragement and support from a close friend, she resisted going to the gym and becoming involved in sports. She explained her resistance in the following way:

> I really wanted to go—inside, I was dying to be physical, to have a go at "pumping iron". . . But at the time I just couldn't say yes . . . I was too ashamed of my body. . . . It was the same thing with swimming. I just couldn't bear the thought of people looking at me. I felt really vulnerable (in Hargreaves, 2000, p. 187).

Anna's fear of her body being seen and judged is not unique. Negotiating the meanings that we and others give to our bodies is a complex and challenging process. Women who accept dominant gender ideology often make choices that reduce their sport participation. For example, a young woman with an amputated leg might choose a prosthesis that is more natural looking, rather than one that is more functional and better suited to playing sports. As one woman explained, "It's one thing to see a man with a Terminator leg . . . . It may inspire people to say, "Cool." But body image for women in this country is model thin and long sexy legs" (Marriott, 2005).[2]

Nick, a twenty-year-old American college student whose legs had to be amputated after he contracted a rare bacterial disease when he was fourteen, agrees with this explanation. He wears Terminator legs and loves them. He points out that whenever his legs run short on their charge, he doesn't hesitate to plug them into the nearest electrical outlet.

Even though Nick has no problem with people seeing his "Terminator legs," he and other men with a disability face a challenge when negotiating the meaning of masculinity in the face of a disabling physical impairment. This is especially true in the case of men who accept a gender ideology that ties masculinity to physical strength and the ability to outperform or dominate others. An example is provided by Mark.

AS a young man whose legs were paralyzed by an accident, Mark explains that his ideas about masculinity make dealing with his impairment especially difficult. For example, after filling his car with fuel and putting his wheelchair in the back, his car had an ignition problem and Mark could not start the engine. A man waiting for the pump impatiently honked his horn and shouted obscenities out his window. Mark said that before his accident he would have turned around, walked

back, and "laid him out." Not being able to do so led him to say, "Now I'm useless . . . my manhood has been shattered" (in Sparkes and Smith, 2002, p. 269).

Although Mark did not use the same words that Anna used, they each felt vulnerable due to cultural definitions of gender. Some men with a disability who feel vulnerable might, like Anna, avoid participating in sports, whereas others might view sports as sites for asserting or reaffirming their masculinity.

Sociologists Brett Smith and Andrew Sparkes (2002) point out that people create their identities, including gender identities, through narratives—that is, the stories that show and tell others about themselves. Their research indicates that playing power and performance sports is consistent with a narrative in which manhood is constructed through physical accomplishments and dominance over other men.

When traditional gender narratives are not critically assessed, and when alternative or oppositional narratives are not available, both women and men with certain physical impairments will experience challenges related to ability and participation in sports. Women might avoid participation for fear that their bodies will be seen as unfeminine, and men might avoid participation for fear that they will not be able to assert themselves and overpower other men. Therefore, anyone dealing with physical impairment and disability benefits by having access to counter-narratives that construct gender in more inclusive terms.

When there are multiple ways to be a woman or a man, people with visible disabilities have more options for negotiating the meanings that they and others give to their bodies. This was documented in a study of women wheelchair users playing sledge hockey, wheelchair basketball, and table tennis (Apelmo, 2012). The women challenged stereotypical notions of gender in sport by displaying determination, strength, and risk taking, while simultaneously embodying a more traditional femininity in resisting the widespread view of disabled women as non-gendered and asexual. Such an approach might

---

[2]"Terminator leg" is how some people refer to the cyborg-like appearance of hi-tech, battery-powered prosthetic legs that have *not* been disguised to look like flesh and bone, so-called after the cybernetic character played by Arnold Schwarzenegger in the 1984 film *The Terminator* and its many sequels.

SPORT AND ABILITY

Sports are often at the center of inclusion battles involving people with impairments (LeClair, 2012). This is due to three factors:

1. Sports are highly visible and culturally valued activities, and sport participation is seen as self-affirming as well as a way to gain social acceptance.
2. It is widely believed that sport participation is important for personal and health development, because it teaches valuable lessons about hard work, teamwork, and task accomplishment at the same time that it prevents obesity and improves physical function across multiple body systems.
3. Sports are increasingly organized to be exclusive on the basis of ability, and resources for sports are disproportionately allocated to elite training and competition.

Activists have worked at regional, national, and global levels for a number of years to make sport participation a right for all people, including those with a disability. This influenced the passage of the 2006 UN Convention on the Rights of Persons with Disabilities, which clearly placed sport within the usual activities of citizenship and led to calls for accessibility in all sport places and spaces, increased funding, supportive policies, appropriate programs, effective disability organizations, and the involvement of people with a disability in positions of power and influence in sport organizations.

At this point, the primary barriers to regular sport participation faced by people with disabilities include the following:

- Little encouragement and guidance for early physical skills development that is age-appropriate and ability-appropriate
- Few gymnasiums and other facilities that are fully accessible
- Irregular and inconvenient public transportation for people with a disability

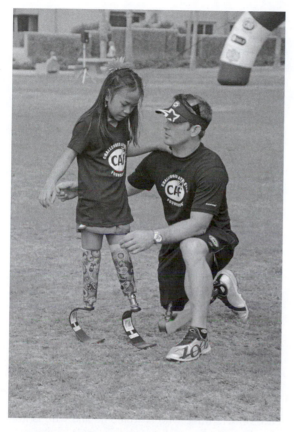

A visible impairment often arouses curiosity and leads others to ask, "What happened [to you to make you different from 'normal' people]?" People with physical impairments answer this question with a story that explains "why my body is different from your body." If this occurs regularly, identity may become linked with impairment and it becomes difficult to be recognized for more meaningful and important dimensions of self. To be known primarily in connection with impairment creates limitations and loneliness–it is *disabling*. Having older role models helps deal with this issue. (*Source:* Photo courtesy of the Challenged Athletes Foundation, http://www.challengedathletes.org)

enable women like Anna to become more physical and have a go at pumping iron, and it might enable Mark to accept help without feeling that he is sacrificing his manhood in the process.

- Too many one-time opportunities and events and too few regularly scheduled programs for participation, training, and competition
- A shortage of expertise in creating participation opportunities that people with a disability perceive as welcoming
- Overprotective family members and a lack of family resources to support regular participation
- Few advocates with the power and influence to mandate the elimination of barriers
- Scarcity of institutionalized sources of year-round information and resources to support participation

These barriers are common worldwide, but they are especially prominent in developing countries where resources are scarce and few people listen to the voices of people with impairments (Bickenbach, 2011; WHO, 2011). As disability rights activists have won incremental success in wealthy, democratic countries, there is a widening gap between the life chances of disabled people in poor versus wealthy countries. Physical education and sport-for-all programs are luxuries that can seldom be afforded in the least developed parts of the world, where access isn't even an issue because sport facilities and programs are non-existent. Additionally, most people with physical or intellectual impairments in poor countries must focus all their personal energy and time on survival.

Religion, culture, language, and the lingering influence of colonialism may also create barriers in many parts of the world. At this point there is limited research investigating the dynamics of disability in parts of the world where poverty, political instability, and wars have undermined possibilities for organized sports, including disability sports. However, in those areas sports may exist sporadically in spaces created by informal collections of people, most often boys or men seeking an opportunity to play (see http://archive.noorimages.com/series/1.34).

Exclusion and Inclusion

Sports are accompanied by mixed messages when it comes to inclusion and exclusion. On the one hand,

popular discourse and beliefs grounded in the great sport myth emphasize that sports are sites at which social barriers disappear as people come together and establish constructive forms of social integration and cooperation. On the other hand, sports usually are organized as exclusive activities in which the majority of hopeful participants are cut or marginalized. Additionally, players often express negative attitudes toward opponents, spectators loudly express their dislike or hatred for opposing teams and fans, and venues hire security forces to try to prevent extreme fan violence that can cause death and destruction.

It is useful to remember this when thinking about inclusion and exclusion in connection with ability and disability: we must seek as much evidence as possible. This is especially important because some people, including some researchers, tend to become emotional and see only positive things when witnessing sport programs that bring together participants.

From a sociological perspective, processes of exclusion and inclusion always involve power relations. The situations in which these processes occur are organized around norms and traditions that influence or determine who is welcome and who is not. Norms and power relations also influence interaction between those who are included, and even regulate the limits of participation for particular people.

Exclusion and inclusion can occur formally or informally. For example, students in wheelchairs in U.S. high schools know that they are excluded from tryouts for the school basketball team just as they have been informally excluded by their peers who play intramurals and pickup games after school. Norms and expectations have been developed by officials in the empire of the normal. For them, sports for students with a disability are an "extra"—something out of the ordinary, that would disrupt existing schedules for "normal" students and require coaches to have specialized knowledge. For these reasons, only a handful of U.S. secondary schools and universities have sports for students using wheelchairs or in need of adaptive equipment. Although the National Federation of

State High School Associations (NFHS) and the National Collegiate Athletic Association (NCAA) may give token recognition to sports for athletes with a disability, the exclusion of disabled students from school sports is systemic, pervasive, and possibly illegal.

Young people with a disability generally have only two options if they wish to play sports: find an organized adapted sports program, or play informal games in which peers are willing and able to develop adaptations. Few communities have adapted youth sport programs, and informal games seldom include young people with the skills needed to make accommodations for a peer with a disability. The dilemma this presents was noted by a ten-year-old boy with cerebral palsy when he said that other kids like him, "but . . . if I'm trying to get in a game without a friend, it's kind of hard" (in Taub and Greer, 2000, p. 406). In other words, without a friend who has enough power with peers and enough experience with disabilities to facilitate a process of adaptation and inclusion, this ten-year-old does not play sports.

Other children with a disability have described their experiences in these ways (in Taub and Greer, 2000, p. 406):

"[Kids] try and shove me off the court, [and] tell me not to play."

"They just don't want me on their team."

"There's a couple of people that won't let me play."

In a study of fifty-three European hearing-impaired athletes, the participants reported that competing with hearing athletes increased their opportunities for competition. Participating in sports with hearing athletes played an important role in the integration of hearing-impaired athletes into mainstream society. If adaptations to communication can be made in these integrated settings, it will greatly increase participation by athletes with certain impairments (Kurková et al., 2011).

Unless these opportunities occur, children with a disability miss opportunities to make friends and participate in activities that have "normalizing" effects in cultures where sports often are contexts for gaining social acceptance and self-validation.

A young person with cerebral palsy expressed the importance of these opportunities with these words (in Taub and Greer, 2000, pp. 406, 408):

> [Playing games] makes me feel good 'cause I get to be with everybody . . . [We can] talk about how our day was in school while we play. Playing basketball is something that I can do with my friends that I never thought I could do [with them], but I can, I can!

Responses to Exclusion When people lack power, they usually respond to systemic and pervasive exclusion with resignation or by seeking contexts in which they feel welcome (Wolbring et al., 2010). Sometimes they find support by aligning themselves with others who have been excluded, or they might accept isolation and the self-doubts that accompany it. Over time, those who are excluded become invisible. In the case of students with a disability, this occurs regularly.

Students with a disability seldom see themselves participating in school sports. For example, when Bob Szyman left his position as secretary general of the International Wheelchair Basketball Federation (IWBF) to teach special education and physical education in Chicago, his goal was to establish a wheelchair basketball league for city high schools. But his biggest challenge was finding students and parents who were excited about such a league. Students with disabilities had no expectations, and there was no wheelchair sport culture in the schools. Additionally, there were no administrators, teachers, or coaches asking why there were no "paravarsity teams" in their district or schools. When Szyman, who now teaches at Chicago State University, organized wheelchair sports camps and competitions, the participants went out of their way to thank him, but they didn't ask why their schools had no sports programs for them. They were so accustomed to exclusion that they had no expectations to be included. Over the past decade, Szyman has had some success in establishing adaptive sport opportunities, but a high school league has not been organized.

Another way of responding to exclusion is illustrated by Tatiana McFadden, who has won ten Paralympic medals in wheelchair racing and won the gold medal in the marathon at the 2012 Olympic Games in London a week after winning the Boston Marathon race. McFadden was born with spina bifida in Russia. Both of her legs were paralyzed, and her mother, who had no means of caring for Tatiana, left her in an orphanage, where she used only her hands to scoot around for the first six years of her life. Near death, Tatiana was noticed by Deborah McFadden, a U.S. Department of Health official who was visiting Russian facilities. McFadden adopted her and used sports to help strengthen her. At eight years old, Tatiana began racing in her wheelchair. But when she went to high school, she was told she could not participate on the track team because her chair gave her an advantage over other runners and was a danger to them as they raced. This left her to race around a track alone in a "special competition," which was meaningless and embarrassing.

Tatiana knew her rights, and she sued the school district and won the right to race on the track with runners, although her time did not count for her team. When she graduated, she went to the University of Illinois at Urbana-Champaign, where she could train in a disability sport program—the best among only a few university programs. Today she is known worldwide as a premier woman wheelchair distance racer as well as an activist who fights for disability rights in sports.

The Emerging Meaning of Inclusion *Inclusion* is the new buzzword in social worlds where various forms of diversity are common. However, people in the empire of the normal often use the term without knowing that it means much more than simply removing boundaries and barriers. They don't understand that hanging up a "Now Open" sign after years of systemic exclusion will not bring about real inclusion.

Social inclusion is a complex process involving the following (Donnelly and Coakley, 2002):

- Investments and strategies that create the conditions for inclusion by closing physical and

social distances and resource gaps that lead people to think in terms of *us* and *them*
- Creating contexts in which previously excluded people can see that they are valued, respected, and contributing members of a group or community
- A proactive, developmental approach to social well-being in which people are supported in connection with their needs
- Recognition of the reality of diversity as well as the commonality of people's lived experiences and shared aspirations

This means that achieving and sustaining inclusion requires sensitivity, knowledge, experience, and hard work. It is an ongoing process rather than a destination, and if people forget to sustain it, backsliding to previous forms of exclusion is likely.

Inclusion of people with disabilities is mandated in the United States by the 1973 Rehabilitation Act. Similar to the mandate for gender equity brought about by Title IX (see Chapter 7), this Act applied to all programs receiving federal aid and stated that people with disabilities could not be denied benefits or opportunities received by other citizens. As with Title IX, it was not fully enforced because people in the empire of the normal claimed that they didn't understand it. This led to the passage in 1990 of the ADA, which mandated access and equity in more specific terms and applied to private as well as public facilities. For example, access was an issue when a building had stairs but no elevator, when streets had curbs that prevented wheelchair mobility, when there were no ramps to doorways and walkways, and when restrooms and toilets were clearly impossible to use by people with a disability. "Access" issues were usually easy to see, but equity was another matter—again, similar to Title IX and gender equity. Those who objected to making changes continued to claim ignorance about the exact meaning of equity.

After the U.S. Government Accountability Office issued a research report showing that students with a disability were generally denied an equal opportunity to participate in school sport programs and therefore denied the health and social benefits of athletic participation, U.S. Education Secretary Arne Duncan issued an equity "guideline" letter in January 2013 (Duncan, 2013; Galanter, 2013; Resmovits, 2013). It told all school officials that because "sports can provide invaluable lessons in discipline, selflessness, passion, and courage," they must make sure that "students with disabilities have an equal opportunity to benefit from the life lessons they can learn on the playing field or on the court" (see Galanter, 2013). Secretary Duncan also provided specific examples of the types of "reasonable modifications" that officials must consider in connection with "existing policies, practices, or procedures for students with intellectual, developmental, physical, or any other type of disability." Examples included the following:

- Using a visual cue in addition to a starter pistol so that students with a hearing impairment who are fast enough to qualify for the track team can compete.
- Waiving a rule requiring a "two-hand-touch" finish in swim events so that a one-armed swimmer with the requisite ability can participate at swim meets

This letter created panic among officials who see nothing but problems in making such accommodations. But it opens the door for students previously excluded from sports to expect that they should be included if they have the requisite skills to make teams. Therefore, a process of inclusion that began in 1973 is taken slightly more seriously today, after more than forty years of resistance to change. Duncan's goal is to push officials to hire teachers and coaches with the sensitivity, experience, and communication skills needed to bring about equity for students with disabilities. His guidelines caught many people off-guard and they will lead some to be overwhelmed, but they are a starting point for producing inclusive school cultures and sport programs.

Education is only one sphere in which inclusion is an issue. Community officials must also consider what inclusion means for their park and recreation programs. Officials in youth sports have seldom thought about these issues. And what does inclusion mean for the relationship between the Paralympic Games and the Olympic Games (Wolbring et al., 2010)? The politics associated with answering these questions are significant. For example, in the case of the Paralympics and Olympics, some people have adjusted to and succeeded in the currently separate programs and want to keep them that way. Others want them merged so that events from each would be held simultaneously instead of scheduling the Paralympics to follow the Olympic Games. Still others think that the technologies allowed in the Paralympics will enable athletes to surpass the records of Olympians and that the Paralympics will eventually become the premier global sport event. However, in the meantime there will continue to be situations in which some athletes with a disability are "too able" for disability-specific sports programs but "not able enough" for mainstream sports programs.

Sport as a Cause of Disability

In Chapter 6, we discussed sports as sites at which disabling injuries occur. Such injuries occur partly because sports involve physical challenges in which risks are inherent. This cannot be avoided, although there are ways to control risks in most sports. But controlling risks is difficult when sports and sport performances are closely linked with issues of masculinity. This inserts physical risk into the identity formation process for males and it influences how they view what happens to their bodies in sports.

The cultural dynamics associated with risk, pain, and injury were outlined in Chapter 5 in the discussion of the sport ethic. To the degree that establishing and maintaining an athlete identity is important in a person's life, overconforming to the norms of the sport ethic becomes an identity strategy that takes priority over risk-control strategies. "Paying the price" by enduring pain and injuries is normalized, even though it increases the chance of sustaining potentially disabling injuries.

Public discourse usually focuses on injuries in collision and heavy-contact sports, such as boxing, football, rugby, and ice hockey. However, as "extreme" sports have become popular and increasingly commercialized, they also have become sites at which disabling injuries occur. Sponsorship money and media coverage have created a context in which athletes in these sports constantly underplay the possibility of serious injuries. Young males in motocross, half-pipe board events, BASE jumping, big air events, and dozens of other extreme sports have constructed narratives that glorify risk taking and confer hero status on those who incur the most gruesome injuries. The women in these events adopt the same narratives to maintain their identities and participation opportunities in these male-dominated sports.

British sociologists Brett Smith and Andrew Sparkes (2002, 2003, 2004; Smith, 2013) have collected data over many years in their interviews with young men who suffered spinal cord injuries in rugby. Among other things, they continue to investigate the process through which these men negotiate the transformation from their former active "able" selves to being a person dealing with a serious physical impairment.

One important aspect of this research is that it can provide data on medical costs, which are assumed to decline with sport participation. For example, we know little about the medical care implications of sport participation among older people, for whom rigorous training and sport injuries often come with high medical costs. It may be that as older people participate in more physically adventurous activities, accidents, and sometimes disabling injuries increase. Does this generate more medical costs than are generated by less-active peers? At this time, we don't know.

DISABILITY SPORTS

When disability is viewed as a weakness or defect that makes the person with an impairment inferior to others, it is important to have a strategy to normalize one's body. During childhood people with an impairment become aware of what makes them different from others. Over time and through their social relationships they develop an understanding of their (dis)ability and how to negotiate its meaning and relevance as they interact with others. In most cases, they also develop strategies that enable them to compartmentalize their impairment so it does not define them, especially in situations when it is irrelevant to what they are doing. This does not mean eliminating the impairment or dismissing it as an irrelevant part of self. Instead, it means presenting one's entire self in a way that does not connote lower status or less character, and it also means that others will see a person as worth knowing despite an attribute that influences ability in certain circumstances. And some people come to transform their impairment into a positive aspect of their lives. Research by Higgins et al. (2002) found that individuals who underwent this transformation process were more likely to accept themselves in ways that enabled them to move ahead with other forms of development. However, not all people with an impairment experience this transformation.

When Ben Quilter was seven years old, he took up judo in order to take part in the same sport as his brother. By the time he was twelve he was competing in regional and national competitions. But then Ben's eyesight began to deteriorate, and at age sixteen he was categorized as a visually impaired competitor. The rules of judo are adapted for visually impaired participants so that they start bouts "gripped up" with their opponent, and there are some changes to the judo ring. However, Ben explains that these changes are sufficiently minor to allow visually impaired and sighted athletes to train and compete with each other. Also, the organization and funding of judo is similar for sighted and visually impaired athletes. In 2008 Ben was selected for the Paralympic Team for the Beijing Games, and the team was announced at the same press launch as the judo team for the Olympic Games. Ben won a bronze medal in the London 2012 Paralympic Games and said that in judo "everything's the same, just train full time with the guys, I'm treated like everyone else really, you wouldn't even know that I had a visual problem."

Ben's experience in judo is an example of how sports can be organized so that people with disabilities are treated on equal terms with other athletes. A related example is the Disability Sports Events (DSE), established in 1961. Based in England, the DSE sponsors competitions in a range of sports for people with any impairment at any age It also hosts a "mini games" multi-sport event for children six to twelve years old. The events include a series of inclusive sports and games to encourage young people with various impairments to become involved in sports. Other young people and volunteers are available to assist athletes if the need arises. One of the sports included is Zonal Tag Rugby, an adapted form of rugby in which participants with various impairments participate and compete in a safe and challenging sporting competition. However, DSE receives no government funding, and relies on fund-raising and sponsorships.

The kind of idealism seen in judo and the DSE is heartening to those who know children who cannot play in existing sports programs that are not organized to be inclusive. It is also heartening to the thousands of veterans returning from battlefields with amputated limbs, sight and hearing impairments, and injuries that impede or prohibit walking. Making sports accessible to them would seem to be a no-brainer, even among those who lack idealism. As veterans return to communities, universities, gyms, parks, and workplaces, idealism is essential if barriers are to be eliminated.

Jayne Craike, who competes on the New Zealand Equestrian Federation national dressage circuit and also represents her country in the Paralympics, encourages people to be idealistic as they envision and work to create the future. She says, "I have to believe that there is still more to come in a world that is continually changing, and that we can make a difference" (Joukowsky and Rothstein, 2002b, p. 55). Craike knows that sports are more than therapeutic tools for people with disabilities. In cultures where sport participation is highly valued, they are normalizing activities; they enable people to

establish important identities; and they are sites for meeting others and forcing everyone who watches to acknowledge that impairments are a normal part of the human condition.

Paralympics: Sports for People with Physical Disabilities

Today's Paralympic Games were first conceived by Ludwig Guttmann, a neurosurgeon and director of Stoke Mandeville, a British medical center for war veterans with spinal cord injuries. When he first came to the center in 1943, he was horrified by the way military veterans were treated. With severe paralysis due to war-related spinal cord injuries, they were merely kept alive without movement or hope. Guttmann came up with the idea that sports could be used as a form of therapy that would enhance the quality of life for his patients.

Guttmann was a strong advocate for his patients and felt that they had been pushed to the periphery of the empire of the normal so that people could avoid facing the reality of their impaired bodies. When the 1948 Olympic Games were scheduled to open in London, Guttmann decided that he could bring recognition to his patients and to the success of his therapeutic approach by scheduling a public display of wheelchair archery and the javelin throw on the same day as the opening of the Olympics. Sixteen people with spinal cord injuries participated.

Guttmann's event received no publicity, but he was energized by its impact on the veterans and he foresaw a time when athletes with disabilities would compete alongside Olympic athletes. He hosted nine "annual" Stoke Mandeville Games, which in 1952 began to attract a few veterans from outside of England. In 1960 during the week after the Olympic Games were held in Rome, Guttmann and others hosted 400 competitors in Rome at the first *Parallel Olympics.* Most of the athletes, who competed in eight different events, were military veterans with spinal cord injuries.

Following the event in Rome, the Parallel Olympics was renamed the *Paralympic Games,* which have been held every four years after 1960, with the first Winter Paralympics held in Sweden in 1976. The Summer and Winter Paralympic Games have grown in scope and popularity, largely due to efforts of people who have worked to nurture and sustain them through significant financial and political challenges.

The mission of the Paralympics is to enable athletes with disabilities to achieve sporting excellence and to inspire and excite the world. Additionally, the hope is to make a better world for all people with physical impairments by challenging the negative attitudes and stereotypes that are significant barriers to the full inclusion of people with disabilities in all spheres of society (Brittain, 2012b; Legg and Gilbert, 2011).

Despite intertwined histories and some shared values, the relationship between the Olympic and Paralympic movements has been complicated and tension-filled. For example, in 1983 IOC president Juan Antonio Samaranch told representatives of Paralympic athletes and disability sport organizations that they could no longer use Olympic images, including the "Olympic rings," at any of their events. The Olympics, explained Samaranch, was a global brand with its own commercial interests and goals, and this meant that the IOC would take legal action against anyone using its logo and other symbols. Even the Olympic flag, he told them, was now a licensed logo, and it could be used only by those who paid for the right to do so (Jennings, 1996a).

Disability sport organizations and their athletes did not want to split from the IOC, so they focused on organizing the Paralympic Games that would follow the 1984 Olympics in Los Angeles. But neither the Los Angeles Olympic Organizing Committee nor the U.S. Olympic Committee (USOC) would support them and their event. So they were forced to hold smaller simultaneous events in New York and Stoke Mandeville, England. At the same time, they formed the International Coordinating Committee of World Organizations for the Disabled (ICC) and made it the governing body for the Paralympic Games.

Dr. Jens Bromann, who had once competed in sports for blind athletes, guided disability sports through this challenging period and was elected president of the new ICC. His efforts, along with support from Korean Olympic officials, made the 1988 Paralympic Games a huge success. Held after the 1988 Olympics in Seoul, Korea, the Paralympics brought together more than 3000 athletes from sixty-one nations. At the opening ceremonies, the Korean organizers presented Bromann a flag they had designed specifically for the Korean Paralympic Games. It was white and had five *tae geuks*, or traditional Korean line symbols, that resembled teardrops in the same positions and colors as the five interlocking rings on the Olympic flag (see image A in Figure 10.3). This design was used to show the connection between the Paralympics and the Olympic movement, and that Paralympic athletes train and compete as Olympic athletes do (Sheil, 2000).

The new Paralympic logo and flag infuriated executives at the IOC because they thought it infringed on their five-rings logo. To appease the IOC, a new logo was launched at the 1994 IPC World Championships (see image B in Figure 10.3). The tae geuks again appeared as teardrops, but officials explained that they now represented the Paralympic motto: "Mind, Body, and Spirit." This flag was used through the 2004 Paralympic Games in Athens. In 2008, after the IPC and IOC resolved many of their differences and agreed to hold events in the same host cities, the IPC adopted a new symbol and flag to represent the unique purpose and identity of the Paralympic Games (see image C in Figure 10.3). It consisted of three elements in red, blue, and green—the colors most often used in national flags. The elements are known as *Agitos* (a Latin word meaning, *I move*), and they appear to be in motion around a central point, representing a dynamic, global "Spirit in Motion"—the new motto of the Paralympics.

The Spirit in Motion flag was first used at the 2008 Paralympics in Beijing, and the IOC did not object. At this point, the "one bid, one city" agreement has been successful, but tensions remain between the two organizations as they compete for sponsors, funding, and media coverage.

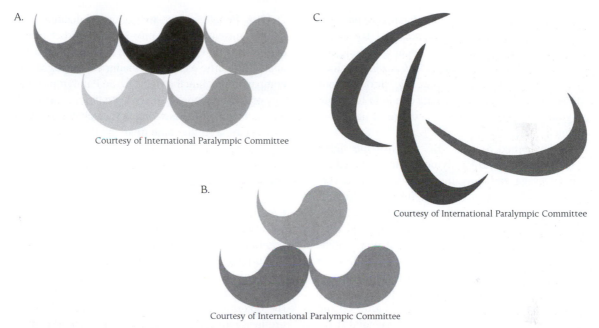

A.

Courtesy of International Paralympic Committee

B.

Courtesy of International Paralympic Committee

C.

Courtesy of International Paralympic Committee

FIGURE 10.3 Logos used on Paralympic flags in 1988 (A), 1994 (B), and today (C).
These three logos have been used by the Paralympics in response to IOC demands that they not use any image that could be compared to the five-rings Olympic logo and flag. The five-teardrops flag and logo (A) was used in Seoul, Korea in 1988; the three-teardrops flag and logo (B) was used from 1994 through 2004, and the Spirit in Motion flag and logo (C) was used at the Beijing Paralympic Games in 2008. (*Source:* Images courtesy of the International Paralympic Committee)

Today the IPC uses a commercial approach similar to the one used by the IOC. Its flag is now a licensed logo—like the IOC flag. But this change raises questions about who will benefit from and be hurt by the commercialization of elite disability sports. Athletes who can attract spectators and sponsors will certainly benefit, but will a focus on these top performers inspire sport participation among people with a disability or will it turn them into spectators? Will people be inclined to donate money to support only elite athletes, or will the Paralympics open doors into the empire of the normal so that people with a disability are seen as deserving the same opportunities received by residents of the empire? Research is needed to answer these questions.

Media Coverage of the Paralympics Now that the IPC has adopted a commercial model, its survival depends heavily on the sale of media rights to events. As we will see in Chapter 11, this shifts the focus from the athletes to spectators and sponsors, and it alters the orientations of those who plan, program, and manage events. Storylines are needed to attract spectators. Individual athletes must be highlighted to keep people interested in who they are and how they perform. The drama and excitement of particular events is crucial, and this must be the focus of marketing.

The Paralympics have never been a highly rated media event and have received little media attention in the past. However, there was a concerted attempt to change this with the 2012 games in London. The media in the United Kingdom covered the Paralympics at an unprecedented level, devoting to it over 150 hours of live television coverage on a primary channel with additional coverage on three cable channels and two major radio channels. The Australian Broadcasting Company provided 100 hours of live coverage, including the opening and closing ceremonies. Media companies in Canada provided nearly 600 hours of live coverage through four online streams along with a daily one-hour highlight program on major English- and French-language channels.

In the United States, NBC paid for the rights to televise the 2012 Paralympics but provided no live coverage and only minimal highlight coverage. This was a great disappointment to officials, athletes, and those spectators in the United States who had followed the progress of athletes and were aware of events that promised interesting match-ups. Critics pointed out that NBC never fails to use uniformed military to market the coverage of NFL games and other professional sports, but they ignored the military veterans participating on the U.S. Paralympic team. This was a financial decision, in that the company executives didn't expect high enough ratings to make money selling advertising time for the events. This is a typical way to do business in the empire of the normal, but it makes NBC stand out as a crude profit seeker at a time when more attention and publicity were given to the Paralympics than ever before in history.

As the IPC goes forward, it will negotiate with the IOC for a share of rights revenues that come in a single amount for both events (Purdue, 2013). In cases where the IPC negotiates exclusive rights for the Paralympics only, its officials will be under pressure to produce large enough audiences to drive the bid amounts up to the levels they need to maintain their organization and present spectator-friendly events. As this occurs, the marketing people at the IPC will present Paralympic events as spectacles. Much attention will be given to popular athletes, high-tech prostheses such as the carbon-fiber legs worn by runners, events where athletes will inspire awe and amazement, and medal counts for countries.

Attempts to market the Paralympics as a spectacle are met with widespread criticism (Brittain, 2004; Darcy and Dowse, 2012; Schantz and Gilbert, 2012; Wolbring, 2012a, 2012b, 2012c, 2012d, 2012e). People object to commercialization and what it means for disability sports. Market forces determine who is funded, which countries win medals, and specific aspects of media coverage. Media companies that buy the rights to the Paralympics and to world championships may hype "bionic athletes" and high-tech prostheses that will catch the attention of spectators. At the same time, the IPC may further complicate an already confusing classification system with new classes of competitors likely to attract spectator attention.

Classification Issues   Creating fair competition has always been a primary challenge for those who organize disability sports. Variations in physical impairments are nearly infinite, and the full impact of impairments is unique to each individual competitor. This means that there are complex rules for determining how athletes are classified and grouped into competition categories. The IPC publishes a twenty-page *Layman's Guide to Paralympic Classification* (IPC, 2007a), another guide for winter sports, and an eighty-two-page classification code book (IPC, 2007b).

The classification code has always created controversy in both its content and implementation (Beckman et al., 2009; Brittain, 2012a; Burkett et al., 2011; van Hilvoorde and Landeweerd, 2008; Wolbring, 2009, 2012d). It requires that each athlete be examined and evaluated, and it allows for protests and appeals when athletes feel they have been misclassified. The code also requires that each federation provide classifier training and certification, because each sport involves different abilities and has its own classification code.

The current categories for the Summer Paralympics include amputees, cerebral palsy, spinal cord injury, and visual impairment. A category for intellectual disability was added in 1996 but then removed when ten of the twelve members of the Spanish basketball team in 2010 were found to have no disabilities. The category was reinstated for a few sports in 2012. In the Winter Paralympics, the categories are visually impaired, seated, and standing. Hearing-impaired athletes don't constitute a major category in the Paralympics because they compete primarily in the Deaflympics, which have taken place since 1924. But this may change in the future.

Ian Brittain (2004), a longtime expert on disability sports, and others have criticized the IPC classification code because it is based solely on medical criteria and it reinforces disability stereotypes (Darcy and Dowse, 2012). Officials at the IPC realize that the code is complex and cumbersome, and they are revising it to accommodate the new commercial realities of disability sports. The new code will be complete by the end of 2016, and it will acknowledge the increased stakes for performing well and winning medals in the Paralympics. The new code also intends to promote the "viewability" of the Paralympics by reducing the number of competitive categories.

Regardless of the changes, athletes in wealthier nations will continue to have a significant advantage over other athletes. Participation in disability sports is especially expensive because it often requires special transportation arrangements, adaptive equipment, and specialized training venues. Therefore, medal counts very closely reflect average per capita income for countries—a pattern even more pronounced in the Paralympics than in the Olympic Games (Buts et al., 2013).

Special Olympics: Sports for People with Intellectual Disabilities

In 1968 the International Olympic Committee granted Eunice Kennedy Shriver permission to use the word "Olympics" for a sporting event that would offer adults and children with an intellectual disability year-round training and competitions in Olympic-type sports (Foote and Collins, 2011). Today the Special Olympics is a multifaceted global organization that sponsors research, builds support communities, and offers health education programs. But its primary purpose is to offer people with an intellectual disability "continuing opportunities to develop physical fitness, demonstrate courage, experience joy and participate in a sharing of gifts, skills and friendship with their families, other Special

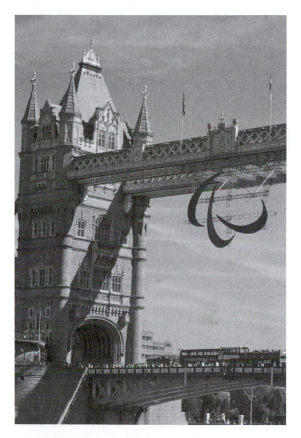

During the London 2012 Olympic Games, the Olympic rings hung from Tower Bridge, London. Immediately following the Games, the rings were removed and replaced with the Paralympic *Agitos* for the duration of the Paralympic Games. (*Source:* © Elizabeth Pike)

Olympics athletes and the community" (http://www.specialolympics.org/mission.aspx).

Some local groups and organizations sponsor and manage sport programs for people with an intellectual disability, but the Special Olympics stands out in terms of its size and influence. It sponsors 50,000 competitions a year—136 each day—around the world. About 6500 athletes from 177 nations participated in the 2015 World Summer Games in Los Angeles, California. The Special Olympics World Games are held every two years, alternating with summer and winter events.

As an organization, the Special Olympics raises funds and organizes events more efficiently than most NGOs in the world. But it has been criticized for organizing its programs in ways that reinforce negative stereotypes and ableist ideology (Hourcade, 1989; Storey, 2004, 2008). Participants in the programs don't learn functional skills that are transferable to their lives in the community, they are treated in paternalistic ways by volunteers and spectators, they are not connected with people who can advocate their interests or be their friends after events are over, and there is no evidence that their lives are changed in any significant ways because of their participation.

In response to these criticisms, people managing the Special Olympics recently developed Unified Sports, a global program in which people with an intellectual disability are paired with teammates from the general community in competitive, developmental, or recreational sports, depending on their interests. The program is designed to facilitate friendships and inclusion in the larger community and enable individuals with impairments to engage with others on the basis of their abilities. The Unified Sports program is based on research and theory, and it is revised as evaluation research identifies weaknesses and strengths (Dowling et al., 2010).

When it was created in 1968, the goal of Special Olympics was to provide dedicated spaces and activities for a population of people who at that time were feared, ridiculed, mistreated, and usually cut off from the empire of the normal. It managed to accomplish this goal, but it had no strategy for systematically engaging participants in the larger community or preparing the community to include people with an intellectual disability into everyday activities so they could live more independently.

Today the organization is actively addressing oversights while retaining its traditional programs for people who need more direct support and assistance. However, most people in the empire of the normal have no experience interacting with intellectually impaired people who have not had opportunities to participate in everyday activities.

To create those opportunities in sports requires a level of awareness and support that remains rare in most social worlds. In the meantime, people with an intellectual disability seek opportunities to play sports in supportive environments that positively connect them with peers and the larger community. One young person who was interviewed in a recent study puts it this way (Darcy and Dowse, 2012, p. 406):

> No one seeks out me or my career to be involved in their program or find out what I'd like to do or provide me with opportunities to try sports on a regular basis like normal kids and if I like it I'll keep doing it but if I don't or it doesn't suit me I want the freedom to choose not to do it again but have another option to try.

Disability Sport Events and Organizations

The range and frequency of physical or intellectual impairments is vastly underestimated in the empire of the normal. People conceal or disguise their physical impairments in public or avoid being seen by others who are likely to stare and then pity or reject them. People with intellectual impairments often are vulnerable to exploitation, so those who care about them often keep them at home or in private, safe settings. Despite these factors, people who share similar characteristics or impairments have created sport organizations to sponsor events. The Dwarf Athletic Association of America (http://www.daaa.org/) sponsors the World Dwarf Games in connection with the annual National Conference for Little People of America (LPA).

The summer and winter Deaflympics are organized by the International Committee of Sports for the Deaf—known in much of the world through its French name, Comité International des Sports des Sourds (CISS). The Deaflympics are run exclusively by the hearing impaired, and only deaf people are eligible to serve on the board and executive bodies. With ninety-six member nations, the International Committee of Sports for the Deaf is organized into four regional confederations: Europe, Asia-Pacific, Pan-America, and Africa (http://www.deaflympics.

com). Hearing-impaired athletes and teams have athletic skills similar to those of the general population, so they do not feel they fit neatly into the Paralympics.

The Cerebral Palsy International Sports and Recreation Association (CPISRA) is the international governing body that coordinates and oversees sports for people with cerebral palsy—that is, those people with disabilities caused by neurological disorders, including stroke and traumatic brain injuries.

The United States Association of Blind Athletes (USABA) supports athletes who are visually impaired. In 2013, it joined with the International Blind Sports Association to sponsor World Youth Championships and the 2013 IBSA Pan American Games in Colorado Springs, Colorado. Skiing and goalball are their most popular sports.

There also are generalist organizations that work with and sponsor events for athletes with a wide range of physical and intellectual impairments. For example, the Challenged Athletes Foundation operates in the United States and works with individuals who want to live active lifestyles by training and participating in one or more sports. The Wounded Warrior Project (WWP) was formed in the United States to assist veterans wounded in the military on or after September 11, 2001. As of early 2014, this included over 51,000 wounded men and women, an estimated 320,000 veterans with traumatic brain injuries, and over 400,000 veterans with post-traumatic stress syndrome. The annual Warrior Games provide competitions and serve as an access point for veterans to become involved in Paralympic sports.

Disability Sport Legacies

The legacy goals of disability sports vary with the organizations that sponsor them. As with sports generally, intended or assumed legacies often differ from reality. As noted above, the Special Olympics may have provided many participants with enjoyable experiences and opportunities to meet people, but the impact was short-lived and did not alter public attitudes about intellectual impairments, foster inclusion, or expand opportunities for people

with an intellectual disability. In this sense, the great sport myth carries over into disability sports and often causes people to overlook what must be done if sports are to have the positive developmental impact they expect them to have.

Until recently people in disability sport organizations had not thought of doing systematic evaluation research that would critically assess whether their goals were being achieved. Of course, different organizations have different goals. In some cases, the primary goal is to give people with particular characteristics or impairments opportunities to play sports with peers under conditions that they control. Having been excluded so completely from sports in the empire of the normal, they have established their own sports and sport events in which they don't have to deal with negative attitudes, curiosity and staring, and feeling like they are oddities. In other cases, the goal is for sport programs and events to empower people with a disability, foster positive public attitudes, and enable people to fully participate in the general community (Brittain, 2012b; Wedgwood, 2013).

Although research on the impact of disability sports is scarce, a few recent studies provide initial assessments of what may or may not be occurring. Interviews with Paralympic stakeholders—people personally associated with the organization—indicated that the athletes were perceived to be personally empowered by their involvement, but other positive outcomes were few (Purdue and Howe, 2012). In fact, the athletes were not perceived as models that inspired people with a disability, because they did not describe themselves as *disabled* and were never shown dealing with everyday issues that others face. Similarly, data collected by Wolbring (2012c) indicated that the physical activity and recreational sport participation rates among people with a disability had not increased with the growing popularity of the Paralympics because structural barriers continued to exist in societies. Being inspired by Paralympic athletes did nothing to eliminate negative attitudes, increase funding for disability sports, improve accessibility to venues, provide convenient transportation, or create

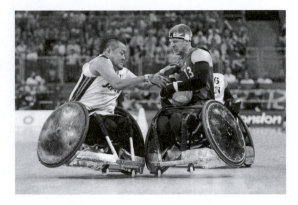

Wheelchair rugby–also known as "quad rugby" and "murderball"–is played in the Paralympics and in national and world championships. Some rugby players use a highly masculinized vocabulary to describe the intimidation and violence that occur in their sport. Although wheelchair rugby challenges stereotypes about people with a disability, it reaffirms a gender ideology in which manhood is defined in terms of the ability to do violence. (*Source:* © Ben Hoskins/Getty Images)

knowledgeable and experienced coaches and support staff (Wilson and Khoob, 2013).

Observations made by disability rights activists support these findings (Ahmed, 2013; Braye et al., 2012). Watching athletes run on $15,000 prostheses or play rugby and race in $6000 wheelchairs did not make disability "cool" or change the reality of dealing with impairments. Also, the dozens of impairment classification categories used to sort competitors seemed irrelevant to many activists, who felt that people could not see themselves in categories created by the IPC. Additionally, individual needs continued to be unmet after the Paralympics. It is true that a few people in the empire of the normal saw athletes perform during the Paralympics, but seeing them did not motivate those people to support local disability programs or vote for legislation to bring about equity. In fact, the activists worried that the opposite was more likely: after seeing the ability of the athletes, people would conclude that disability was not an issue, thereby reproducing

ableist ideology and ableist attitudes (Braye et al., 2012; Rival, 2015).

Finally, males are disproportionately overrepresented among athletes in disability sports. This is partly because more boys and men engage in risky actions that can cause physical impairments, and girls and women with physical or intellectual impairments may be more protected by family members and not encouraged to seek sport participation opportunities. In any case, the culture of disability sports is heavily masculine and this may lead females to feel unwelcome. There may also be subtle sexism in the referral process that moves people from rehabilitation programs into sport programs. If doctors and therapists don't encourage girls and women to move into sports as much as they encourage boys and men, it would reproduce an already male-dominated, male-centered, and male-identified sport culture. The visibility and popularity of wheelchair rugby, or "murderball" as it is known by men in disability sports, reaffirms this point.

TECHNOLOGY AND ABILITY

When athletes use technologies to adapt their bodies to the physical challenges presented by sports, they blur the line between body and machine. Of course, this is neither new nor unique to disability sports. Specialized equipment and technologies (such as climbing shoes or special rowing blades) have long been used in all sports, similar to the wheelchairs, crutches, and prostheses used by people with physical impairments—they help them move more efficiently (Apelmo, 2012).

Various forms of "assistive" performance enhancements are used in most sports. Tennis and baseball players have "assistive" elbow and knee reconstructions using super strong synthetic ligaments or stronger ligaments taken from other parts of their bodies. Endurance athletes sleep in "assistive" hyperbaric chambers to increase endurance by boosting the oxygen-carrying capacity of their red blood cells. Lionel Messi, reputedly the best soccer player in the world today, took growth hormones that added inches to his unusually short stature, and dozens of baseball players and golfers have had Lasik eye surgery to obtain 20/15 vision and the ability to see a baseball or golf ball more distinctly. These athletes don't think of themselves as disabled nor do they see the use of such "assistive" and performance-enhancing procedures as compensation for weakness or cheating, and it is certain that none of them ever thought of participating in the Paralympics.

In the 1980s, biologist Donna Haraway (1985) made the case that many people could be described as cyborgs because they depended on machines and communication technologies to navigate their way through everyday life, and this was well before smartphones appeared as fixed components of human hands. But the most intense and complex example of this cyborg hybridization is probably experienced by severely impaired people who merge technologies with their own bodies to claim and sustain their humanity.

Oscar Pistorius, the South African sprinter, has recently been the most visible sporting cyborg. Identified as "Blade Runner" or "the fastest man on no legs," he was born with no fibula bones in his legs. Oscar's parents decided when he was eleven months old that below-the-knee prosthetic legs and feet would enable him to move more freely, and the surgery was completed in 1987.

As an active, athletic boy, Oscar dreamed of playing elite rugby. Never having experienced a body without prosthetic legs, he did everything his friends did. Through middle school and high school he wrestled and played cricket, rugby, water polo, and tennis. But after he shattered his knee playing rugby in late 2003, his doctor prescribed running as physical therapy. In January 2004 at the age of seventeen he began to train as a sprinter. Two months later he competed in his first 100-meter race,

> The goal for many amputees is no longer to reach a "natural" level of ability but to exceed it, using whatever cutting-edge technology is available. As this new generation sees it, our tools are evolving faster than the human body, so why obey the limits of mere nature?
>
> —Daniel H Wilson, robotics engineer, 2012.

winning a gold medal and setting a world record time of 11.51 seconds in two Paralympic categories: the T44 class for athletes with a "single leg *below knee amputation*" and the T43 class for "double leg *below knee amputation.*"

His success in these races led to his competing in the 2004 Paralympic Games in Athens, Greece, where he won a silver medal in the 100-meter and a gold medal in the 200-meter sprint. Overall, he set four world records at those games, and went on to compete and win in the 2008 and 2012 Paralympic Games.

Team OSSUR has sponsored Pistorius and other record-setting Paralympic sprinters who wear Ossur's carbon-fiber Flex-Foot Cheetah prosthesis. The Flex-Foot replicates the hind leg of a cat, with a small-profile foot that extends and reaches out to contact the ground while the large thigh muscles pull the body forward. These prosthetic legs return about 95 percent of the energy put into them by the runners' upper legs. A human lower leg returns about 200 percent of the energy put into them, which OSSUR researchers have taken as a challenge to duplicate the running power of a human leg, a goal that will take some time to achieve.

In 2007, Pistorius began training like an Olympic sprinter in a quest to qualify for the 2008 Olympics in Beijing. However, his quest was foiled when the IAAF, the global governing body for track and field, disqualified him. After reviewing research they had commissioned, the IAAF executive committee concluded that his prosthetic legs gave him an advantage over Olympic runners (IPC, 2008). In a sense, Pistorius was "*dis*'ed" by the IAAF for being abnormally able.

Pistorius appealed the IAAF decision and asked the International Court of Arbitration for Sport to consider other studies that went beyond the IAAF laboratory tests, which did not assess the carbon-fiber leg in a running situation. He knew from experience that the bladelike legs slowed him at the start of a race, provided poor traction on a wet track, produced rotational forces that were difficult to control, and supplied none of the maneuverability and control supplied by the human leg, ankle, and foot (Longman, 2007a).

After independent researchers conducted further studies, and the international court reviewed the data, the IAAF overturned its ban in May 2008 and ruled that Pistorius was eligible to qualify for the Olympics and participate in other international events. Although he failed to qualify for the 2008 Olympics in Beijing, Pistorius continued training and qualified to compete in the 2012 Olympic Games in London. He was neither the first athlete with a physical impairment to compete in the Olympics, nor the first to use a prosthetic limb, but his story resonated with people as they followed it through globalized media coverage.

Virtual Bodies and Cyborg Identities

The issues raised by Pistorius and his carbon-fiber legs received massive attention. The image of cyborg athletes, as informed by science fiction action films featuring mechanically and genetically engineered bodies, created moral panic among people worried about altering human nature. At the same time, others used the medical model to imagine the liberating possibilities of bionic body parts that could fix physical impairments, make people better than normal, and be improved over time to even negate the effects of aging.

A visible spokesperson for the bionic dreamers has been Hugh Herr, director of the Biomechatronics Research Group at MIT. Herr became a bilateral amputee at seventeen years old, and his dissatisfaction with painful and poorly designed prosthetics inspired him to obtain a PhD in engineering as he developed innovative prostheses, including for his own lower leg, ankle, and foot. Herr predicts

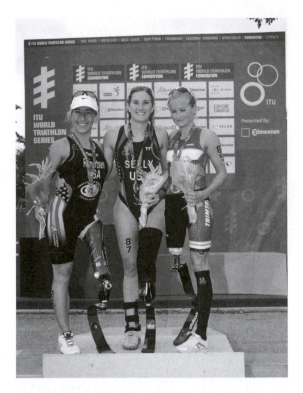

Normal, enhanced, or disabled? The lines between these categories are becoming increasingly blurred. This is creating ethical and practical dilemmas in sport organizations, because it is difficult to preserve a level playing field when engineered enhancements are used. People in Paralympic and related organizations may be ahead of others in dealing with this, because they have already confronted enhancements and developed a classification code that takes them into account. (*Source:* © Rich Cruse/ Photo courtesy of the Challenged Athletes Foundation, http://www.challengedathletes.org)

that there will be "extreme interfaces" between soft and hard materials integrated with skin, bone, muscle, and nerves, making prosthetic body parts move naturally with messages delivered from the brain through synthetic nerves (Moss, 2011; Rago, 2013). This prediction aligns Herr with others described as transhumanists, a collection of dreamers and scientists described in the Reflect on

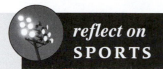

Nobody's Perfect
Does That Mean I'm Impaired?

Ableism leads people in different directions. One of the emerging pathways is being charted by transhumanists, who use the medical model as a lens for imagining the future of human bodies.

Transhumanists believe that all bodies can be improved so that people can achieve goals currently out of reach. They claim that we have not taken full advantage of available enhancement procedures and technologies because we cling to outdated beliefs based on religion and cultural traditions—beliefs no longer in sync with twenty-first-century knowledge.

In the case of sports, transhumanists predict that athletes will seek and use various forms of body- and performance-enhancing technologies that are undetectable without monitoring, scanning, and controlling bodies from birth onward. As athletes demonstrate what is possible by using innovative enhancements, they will expand our sense of what is possible in our relationship with the physical world. This process is already under way with corrective lenses for eyes, joint replacements, ligament transfers and replacements, muscle generation, bone grafts, stem cell therapies, and a wide array of surgeries that enable athletes to return to their sports more quickly than ever before and train themselves back to 100 percent.

The credibility of transhumanists is challenged by critics of ableist ideology, by people panicked about turning humans into cyborgs, and by skeptics who say that transhumanists are opportunists who profit by intensifying people's insecurities about their bodies and then selling them expensive enhancement procedures or technologies.

As you consider the pros and cons of transhumanism, imagine this: You are a top college basketball player looking forward to signing a professional contract, but during your junior year you rupture your ACL during the final minutes of the NCAA finals. Your orthopedic surgeon says she can repair it to provide stability for walking but not for playing competitive basketball, or she can surgically insert a synthetic ligament that is stronger than the original and perfect for playing basketball. Your insurance will cover either surgery. Which one would you choose?

If you choose the synthetic ligament, what would prevent others from having similar surgeries so they could do more intense muscle conditioning to improve their speed and vertical jumping ability? Where and for whom would you draw the line when it comes to such body enhancements? We may find this form of transhumanism to be troubling, but we cannot escape these questions as new technologies are being developed. *What will happen if no lines are drawn?*

• •

Sport box "Nobody's Perfect: Does That Mean I'm Impaired?"

Sport philosophers and others present arguments for banning prosthetics in sports. They say that the precise contribution of prosthetics to performance may never be known, which may put athletes with a disability at an unfair advantage over those who do not or cannot use such technology. Also, the impact of technology on the design of prostheses is likely to affect athletes' abilities and unfairly advantage those with the resources to access the most recent innovations (Burkett et al., 2011; Dyer et al., 2010; Marcellinia et al.,

2012; Normana and Moolab, 2011; Swartz and Watermeyer, 2008; Treviño, 2013).

The proponents of banning prostheses are up against powerful corporations that will showcase and market their new performance-enhancing technologies through the bodies of athletes in the Paralympics and other disability sport events (Wolbring, 2012a, 2012e). In turn, this will be attractive to amputees who see a possibility for exceeding natural limits and "evolving faster than the human body" (Wilson, 2012). Popular culture has already introduced this idea in the form of "iron man" exoskeletons that permit unnatural physical feats.

Access to Technology

We occasionally hear heartening stories about people using assistive devices made of Kevlar, carbon-fiber biologics, and other high-tech materials. For people who compete in the Paralympics, these materials are now used to make light and fast racing wheelchairs, revolutionary running prostheses, racing mono-skis to maneuver down steep mountain slopes, and other assistive devices that extend skills and broaden the experiences through which people can feel joy and accomplishment.

This technology is often seductive when we see it for the first time—so seductive that we may focus on the device and overlook those who might benefit from it. However, as most athletes know, technologies are only as good as the people who use them. And most people with disabilities know that adaptive technologies for sports are prohibitively expensive.

American athlete Diane Cabrera discovered this when cancer took her leg in 2001. A new prosthesis enabled her to walk, but it cost $11,000 and her medical insurance covered only $4000 per year. She spread payments over two years and struggled to find $2200 for additional payments related to diagnostics, fitting, tuning, and maintaining the device. When she needed a new leg socket in 2005 because her original prosthesis no longer fit correctly, she put it off due to cost.

That's what many people do today when they need prostheses. Whereas standard prostheses may be partially covered by insurance, prosthetic limbs and adaptive devices for sports involve additional costs that must be paid by individuals in nearly all cases. Sport prosthetics require replacement every year or two, and other prosthetic limbs should be replaced every four to six years. Racing wheelchairs can cost $5000 or more, and Kevlar wheels push the cost up even higher. When they are customized for rugby, add another $1600. Although Oscar Pistorius does not himself pay for his Flex-Foot Cheetah prostheses, they cost $15,000 to $18,000 for each leg, and they must be replaced or refurbished regularly when training full time. Ossur

can sponsor only a few runners, which means that it would be very costly for an unsponsored athlete to complete against people like Pistorius in the Paralympics.

The cost of adaptive equipment is a significant barrier to sport participation for many people with physical impairments. Adding further to these constraints is the fact that compared to adults in the general population, U.S. adults with disabilities are:[3]

- Twice as likely to have less than a high school degree
- More than twice as likely to be unemployed
- Three times more likely to live in households making less than $15,000 per year
- Twice as likely to live in households with incomes under or just above the poverty line
- Three times more likely to depend on public subsidy programs

People with disabilities also have higher expenses for daily living and required care. These are the realities of social class and disability in the United States. For young elite athletes, there are a handful of sponsorships available from companies that develop and manufacture prostheses and other adaptive technologies. This enables a select few to bypass resource barriers, but others continue to face formidable barriers in terms of accessing and regularly participating in sports at any level.

Federal government assistance for people with disabilities was cut in 2013, even for recent military veterans. States have not made up for these cuts; charity support is unpredictable and declining; and community programs are scarce, even for people with dependable transportation. Such class-based barriers force many people with disabilities to join Diane Cabrera and "make do right now."

---

[3]U.S. Department of Labor, 2011; http://disabilitycompendium .org; http://disabilitystatistics.org/reports/acs.cfm.

TO "*DIS*" OR NOT TO "*DIS*"

Ability is variable, relational, and contextual: it ranges from low to high, and the meaning of that variation depends on the relationships involved, the tasks being done, and the resources available to accomplish them. When people trust and cooperate with each other, they find ways to utilize everyone's abilities so that each person makes contributions to the group. Even when tasks require particular combinations of abilities, abilities are what matter and *dis*abilities are secondary or irrelevant.

Sport teams are perfect examples of this ability complementarity. All team members have different attributes and abilities, and the team's success depends on finding the best ways to combine those abilities during competitions. This approach eliminates *dis*ability, because it does not involve anyone drawing a line between those identified as *able* and *unable* and then assigning them to two mutually exclusive sport participation categories.

The category of "*dis*abled person" or "person with a *dis*ability" has become central to obtaining health care, government insurance coverage, academic support, public subsidies, and the identities of people with particular impairments. Therefore, any attempt to change current categorization methods will meet heavy resistance. Many individuals and families know that they could not survive without the help they currently receive due to a disability classification. But there also are the following problems associated with the current system:

- Classifying a person as disabled is based on political agreements and compromises about the types and degrees of impairments required to be defined as officially *incapable*.
- The category "disabled" has meaning only when distinguished from the category "able-bodied," and this obscures recognition of the abilities of people with impairments and creates a label that is a barrier to participation in mainstream society.

- An official *dis*ability classification system leads many people to assume that an unimpaired body is natural and normal, and that people classified as *dis*abled are subnormal, below average, and less than whole as a human being.
- When people classified as *dis*abled seek equity and full rights of citizenship, people with ableist attitudes see them as wanting "special privileges" and reject their requests.

As long as we use a vocabulary that establishes these contrasting categories, we tend to think, talk, and act in either/or terms, which creates an unequal power relationship and sets into motion social dynamics that undermine inclusion, privilege people in the "able-bodied" category, and marginalize those in the "disabled" category. This fosters social and physical segregation by category, imposes second class citizenship on persons with certain physical and intellectual impairments, encourages their withdrawal from activities, and creates a culture in which everyone spends vast amounts of time and money to eliminate or hide characteristics and impairments that are relatively common among human beings.

As people use the two opposing ability categories as a basis for developing expectations and organizing social relationships, they overlook the complexity of ability, develop distorted views of ability differences, and do not learn to deal with ability variations in constructive and inclusive ways. At the same time, people who are classified as *dis*abled find it difficult to establish and maintain positive self-esteem and to develop and utilize abilities that would enable them to meaningfully participate in mainstream activities (Nario-Redmond et al., 2013).

This is why many people with physical impairments, including athletes at the Paralympic Games, do not describe themselves as *dis*abled. They identify themselves in terms of what they can do, not in terms of what they cannot do. They organize their lives around their abilities, as most other people do. Most people would say this is a normal way to live, and that creating a category that defines people who live normally as subnormal and *dis*abled is likely to interfere with achieving fairness and equity in society.

At this point in time, rejecting the notion of *dis*-ability and defending an "anti-*dis*-ing" position is seen as extreme. However, it also is clear that most people living with an impairment want to be acknowledged for what they can do instead of what they cannot do. If they decide that they do not want to be "*dis*-d," they may challenge others with words similar to these: "My body is normal for me. Your belief that my body is the problem simply hides the fact that the real problem is your fantasy-based definition of a 'normal' body."

This approach implies that to be *dis*'d is counterproductive to development and that achieving a fair and equitable future depends less on knowledge about disability and more on knowledge about whose interests are served by particular ideas and beliefs about age and ability.

Similarly, knowing how people develop ideas and beliefs about what is normal when it comes to bodies, and who benefits from or is disadvantaged by particular conceptions of *normal,* is crucial for transforming society. Therefore, future discussions should focus on how we can eliminate age- and ability-based barriers to sport participation and achieve forms of inclusion that meet everyone's needs.

Summary

ARE AGE AND ABILITY BARRIERS TO PARTICIPATION?

Sports and sport participation are closely tied to culturally based ideas and beliefs about ability and the body. These ideas and beliefs impact each of us, because they serve as a baseline for our own definition of "normal." We experience this impact to different degrees as our abilities and bodies change over time due to aging and impairments caused by injuries, illness, or chronic disease. Because ability and the body are involved in sports and physical activities, these ideas and beliefs affect rates of sport participation and a society's provision of opportunities to participate in sports.

Ableist ideology, ageism, and ableism negatively impact sport and physical activity participation among people whose abilities and bodies do not measure up to prevailing or dominant social conceptions of *normal.* This occurs despite natural physical and intellectual variations among human beings. This is similar to the dynamics of sexism and racism, except that ableist ideology, ageism, and ableism will eventually impact everyone, even those who previously used it to marginalize or disadvantage others.

Ageism accounts for various manifestations of age discrimination. In the case of sports, ageism leads to age-segregated patterns of participation and provision of participation opportunities. This affects older people negatively because of the widespread belief that playing sports is not developmentally important for people who are "grown up."

Ableism accounts for the creation of a *dis*ability category in society and in sports. People are assigned to this category due to visible or functional characteristics and impairments. This locates them outside of the realm of "the normal" and leads them to be seen by many people as flawed and inferior.

Ideas and beliefs about aging vary over time and from one social world to another, but in societies characterized by rapid social and technological change, being younger is valued over being older. This has turned age into a social and political issue in many societies, especially those in which the average age of the population is increasing and older people are becoming increasingly powerful in political terms. This is occurring in the United States and other societies in which numerically large cohorts of people born in the years after World War II are in their fifties and sixties—and soon, seventies and eighties.

Because older people have used a disproportionate share of medical care resources in many societies, sports and physical activities have been identified in neoliberal societies as tools that older people must use to stay healthy and cut medical costs. This new focus raises issues related to gender, ethnicity, and social class, because women, first-generation ethnic immigrants, and people with lower income and education often have very low levels of sport participation. Additionally, the cost of participation in private, for-profit programs puts membership out of reach for nearly all people in these categories.

The meaning of ability varies by situation, but it has been defined in many societies in a way that "*dis*'s"—or classifies as *dis*abled—people perceived as incapable of fully participating in mainstream social and economic life. This turns *disability* into a social and political category that has significant implications for many people.

The meaning of disability differs depending on the assumptions used when defining it. When assumptions are based on the medical model, impairments are the problem, and "fixing" them through treatment and rehabilitation is the solution. When assumptions are based on the social model, problems rest in a world full of physical and social barriers that could be minimized by responsive designs, education, and political change.

Many people with impairments prefer the social model because it provides them with a strategy for challenging the power of the empire of the normal, where they are seen as subnormal outsiders due to their physical or intellectual attributes. The media generally reproduce the norms of the empire as they portray athletes with disabilities as courageous victims or heroic supercrips. Such portrayals are based on misinformation and will change only when media personnel develop the vocabulary that takes them beyond disabilities into the realm of abilities.

Because of their visibility and cultural importance, sports have become sites at which disability issues are confronted and contested. Processes of ability-related exclusion and inclusion in sports have become a focus of many governmental and nongovernmental organizations and officials from international to local levels. Belief in the great sport myth has led to policies that foster inclusion based on the assumption that sport participation will change the lives of people with disabilities. Although this has led to some new programs it has not eliminated the social and structural barriers that interfere with a wide range of participation opportunities.

In the face of exclusion or poorly managed and inconvenient sport programs, people with particular disabilities have created their own sport organizations and events to meet their needs and expectations. In other cases, individuals or groups of people have challenged traditions of exclusion through protests and legal actions. As this occurs, the meaning of inclusion has changed and come closer to involving full equity of opportunities. But there is much left to be done.

Disability sports have traditionally been viewed through the lens of the medical model and seen as forms of physical therapy and rehabilitation. As elite athletes with a disability have attempted to change this approach and be treated like other elite athletes, they have faced resistance from established sport organizations. The IPC, for example, has faced resistance from the IOC, and disability sport events such as the Paralympics receive little support or media coverage compared to other sport events. At the same time, disability sport organizations face their own challenges related to competition classifications based on impairment and potential ability.

The Special Olympics have become a significant global nonprofit organization. With annual revenues approaching $100 million, it provides training and competition opportunities in 170 nations for over 4 million people with an intellectual disability. Because research has indicated that special Olympics programs have not achieved their goal of integrating people with an intellectual disability into mainstream society, the organization has created new programs to emphasize social integration and equity.

The overall legacy of disability sports is now being questioned, because the publicity given to the Paralympics and other elite events has not led to structural changes and new programs benefiting the vast majority of people with disabilities. In fact, much of the attention in elite events focuses on technologies used by athletes with amputations—a classic example being the carbon-fiber Flex-Foot Cheetah prostheses used by Oscar Pistorius and other record-setting runners.

These technologies have led to discussions and heated debates about physically engineered bodies and turning athletes into cyborgs. The influence of ableist ideology and ableism has led some people to promote transhumanism, which assumes that all human bodies can and should be improved with technology—a position that incites moral panic among people who fear that this will eventually dehumanize individuals and disrupt the social order.

These debates cool down once people realize the cost of the technologies being used in the Paralympics today and the estimated costs of future technologies. Due to the practical issue of cost, most people with a disability are not concerned about futuristic prostheses. They don't see themselves buying exoskeletons so they can perform superhuman feats. More realistically, they hope to see restrooms designed so that they can use toilets without performing gymnastics routines and miraculous wheelchair moves.

Finally, the classifications "able-bodied" and "disabled" have been challenged by people with physical impairments who do not consider themselves to be "disabled" and do not want to be *dis*'d. For them, the problem is not disability, but the way people have constructed their conception of "normal" ability.

SUPPLEMENTAL READINGS

Reading 1. We're not handicapped: We just can't hear
Reading 2. How can I wear shoes if I don't have feet?
Reading 3. The hit isn't real unless it bends steel: Men and murderball
Reading 4. Paying the price: The cost of sport prostheses
Reading 5. Tensions in the Olympic family: Siblings with disabilities
Reading 6. "One of God's favorites": Religion and disability

SPORT MANAGEMENT ISSUES

- As the new manager of a community sport center in a region with many middle- and working-class older people, your success depends on programming that attracts older people. Identify the issues you will discuss with your new programming and management staff during a two-day training session with them.
- You are the assistant athletic director in a major urban public school district, and you are responsible for compliance with the new U.S. Department of Education's guidelines on sports for students with disabilities. Outline two different program proposals that you will present to the district school board when they make decisions about how the district will allocate funds to comply with federal guidelines.
- As a sport management student you have been asked by students in special education to work with them in developing a sport and physical activity program for people with disabilities in the surrounding community. The first brainstorming session is soon, and you are preparing the list of issues you will bring to the session. Identify and explain the five most important issues you want the group to consider.

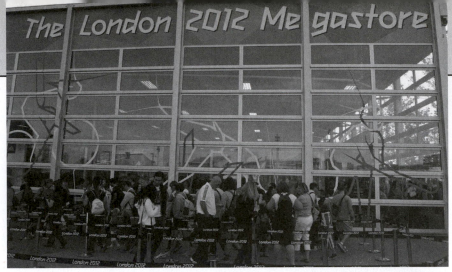

SPORTS AND THE ECONOMY

What Are the Characteristics of Commercial Sports?

Professional sports have become vast global industries, billion-dollar enterprises and powerful cultural forces. Where does this leave their fans?

> —**Jason Kelly, editor, University of Chicago Magazine (2014)**

When sport is regarded solely within economic parameters, . . . there is the risk of reducing athletes to mere merchandise through whom profit may be obtained. The athletes themselves enter into a mechanism that overwhelms them, causing them to lose sight of the true meaning of their activity. . . . Sport is harmony, but if the unrestrained pursuit of profit and success prevails, this harmony is lost.

> —**Pope Francis (2013)**

Having proved [the] effectiveness [of sporting events] in connecting successfully with consumers in existing markets, companies are keen to use sponsorship in order to drive awareness in new, sizeable emerging markets.

> —**Karen Earl, European Sponsorship Association (in Blitz, 2010)**

I see myself as an actor . . . . They tell us who's going to win or be disqualified and we take it from there. . . . Consumers are smarter now, so we admit what we do is entertainment. And we've changed programming. But the bones are the same. Pro wrestling, like action films, is still about good vs evil.

> —**John Cena, WWE wrestler (2009)**

Emergence and Growth of Commercial Sports

Commercialization and Changes in Sports

The Organization of Professional Sports in North America

The Organization of Amateur Sports in North America

Legal Status and Incomes of Athletes in Commercial Sports

Summary: What Are the Characteristics of Commercial Sports?

Learning Objectives

- Identify the conditions under which commercial sports emerge and grow in a society.

- Identify economic and ideological reasons why sports have become so popular in society today.

- Explain how the corporate branding of sports is related to the establishment of ideological outposts around the world today.

- Discuss how commercialization affects the rules, culture, and organization of sports.

- Distinguish differences between aesthetic orientations and heroic orientations, and explain how they are influenced by the commercialization of sports.

- Explain how the owners of the major professional sports have benefited from being allowed to establish cartels, monopolies, and monopsonies.

- Identify the major forms of public assistance received by professional sport franchises and leagues in the United States.

- Identify differences in the legal status of professional and amateur athletes in both individual and team sports.

- Describe the patterns of income received by professional and amateur athletes, and explain why the range of incomes received by athletes is so great today.

Sports have been used as public entertainment through history. However, they've never been so thoroughly commercialized as they are today. Never before have economic factors so totally dominated decisions about sports, and never before have economic organizations and corporate interests had so much power and control over the meaning, purpose, and organization of sports.

The economic stakes for athletes and sponsors have never been higher than they are today. The bottom line has replaced the goal line. Sports are now evaluated by gate receipts, concessions and merchandise sales, licensing fees, media rights contracts, and website hits. Games and events are evaluated using media criteria such as market share, ratings points, and the cost of commercial time. Athletes are evaluated by their entertainment value as well as physical skills. Stadiums, teams, and events are named after corporations and linked to corporate logos instead of people and places that have local historical meaning.

Corporate interests influence team colors, uniform designs, event schedules, media coverage, and the comments of announcers during games and matches. Media companies and other corporations sponsor and plan events, and they own a growing number of sport teams. Many sports are corporate enterprises, tied to marketing concerns and processes of global capitalist expansion. The mergers of major corporate conglomerates that began in the 1990s and now continue in the twenty-first century have connected sport teams and events with media and entertainment companies. The names of transnational corporations are now synonymous with the athletes, events, and sports that bring pleasure to the lives of millions of people.

Because economic factors are so important in sports, this chapter focuses on the following questions:

1. Under what conditions do commercial sports emerge and prosper in a society?
2. What changes occur in the meaning, purpose, and organization of sports when they become commercial activities?
3. Who owns, sponsors, and promotes sports, and what are their interests?
4. What is the legal and financial status of athletes in commercial sports?

EMERGENCE AND GROWTH OF COMMERCIAL SPORTS

Commercial sports are organized and played for profit. Their success depends on gate receipts, concessions, sponsorships, the sale of media broadcasting rights, and other revenue streams associated with sport images and personalities. Therefore, commercial sports grow and prosper best under five social and economic conditions.

First, they are most prevalent in market economies where material rewards are highly valued by athletes, team owners, event sponsors, and spectators.

Second, they usually exist in societies that have large, densely populated cities with high concentrations of potential spectators. Although some forms of commercial sports can be maintained in rural, agricultural societies, their revenues would not support full-time professional athletes or sport promoters.

Third, commercial sports are a luxury, and they prosper only when the standard of living is high enough that people have time and resources to play and watch events that have no tangible products required for survival. Transportation and communications technologies must exist for sponsors to make money. Therefore, commercial sports are common in wealthy, urban, and industrial or post-industrial societies; they seldom exist in labor-intensive, poor societies where people must use all their resources to survive.

Fourth, commercial sports require large amounts of capital (money or credit) to build and maintain stadiums and arenas in which events can be played and watched. Capital can be accumulated in the public or private sector, but in either case, the willingness to invest in sports depends on anticipated payoffs in the form of publicity, profits, or power.

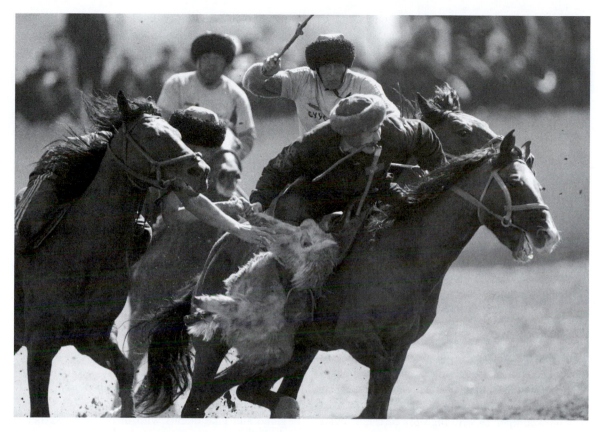

Sports are played in nearly all cultures, but professional sports seldom exist in labor-intensive, poor nations. The Afghan horsemen here are playing buzkashi, a popular sport in their country, but Afghanistan lacks the general conditions needed to sustain buzkashi as a professional sport with fulltime paid athletes and paying fans. (*Source:* © IGOR KOVALENKO/epa/Corbis)

Private investment in sports occurs when investors expect financial profits; *public* investment occurs when political leaders believe that commercial sports serve their interests, the interests of "the public," or a combination of both.

Fifth, commercial sports flourish in cultures where lifestyles emphasize consumption and material status symbols. This enables everything associated with sports to be marketed and sold: athletes (including their names, autographs, and images), merchandise, team names, and logos. When people express their identities through clothing, other possessions, and their associations with status symbols and celebrities, they will spend money on sports that have meaning in their social world. The success of commercial sports depends on selling symbols and emotional experiences to audiences, and then selling audiences to sponsors and the media.

Class Relations and Commercial Sports

Sports most likely to be commercialized are those watched, played, or used for profit by people who control economic resources in society. For example, golf is a major commercial sport in the United States, even though it does not lend itself to commercial presentation. It's inconvenient to stage a golf event for a live audience or to televise it. Camera placement and media commentary are difficult to arrange, and live spectators see only a small portion of the action. Golf does not involve vigorous action or head-to-head competition, except in rare cases of match play. Usually, if you don't play golf, you have little or no reason to watch it.

But golf is popular among wealthy and powerful men, who are important to sponsors and advertisers because they make consumption decisions for themselves, their families, their businesses, and thousands of employees who work under their supervision. They buy luxury cars and other high-end products for themselves, but more important to advertisers is that they buy thousands of company cars and computers for employees and make large investment decisions related to pensions and company capital.

This collection of golf supporters has economic clout that goes far beyond personal and family lives. This makes golf an attractive sport for corporations that have images and products that appeal to consumers with money and influence. This is why auto companies with high-priced cars sponsor and advertise on the PGA, LPGA, and Champions (Senior) PGA tours. This also is why major television networks cover golf tournaments: They can sell commercial time at a high rate per minute because those watching golf have money to spend—their money *and* the money of the companies they control. The converse of this is also true: Sports attracting low- and middle-income audiences often are ignored by television or covered only under special circumstances. If wealthy executives bowled, we would see more bowling on commercial television and more bowling facilities on prime real estate in cities; but wealthy people seldom bowl, and bowling receives little coverage.

Market economies always privilege the interests of those who have the power and resources to select sports for promotion and coverage. Unless those people want to play, sponsor, or watch a sport, it won't be commercialized on a large scale,

nor will it be given cultural significance in society. A sport won't become a "national pastime" or be associated with "character," community spirit, civic unity, and political loyalty unless it's favored by people with resources.

This is why football is now known as "America's game"—it celebrates and privileges the values and experiences of the men who control and benefit from corporate wealth and power in North America. This is why men pay thousands of dollars to buy expensive season tickets to college and professional football games, why male executives use corporation money to buy expensive blocks of "company tickets" to football games, and why corporation presidents write hundred-thousand-dollar checks to pay for luxury boxes and club seats for themselves, friends, and clients. They enjoy football, but most important, it reproduces an ideology that fosters their interests.

Women who want to be a part of the power structure in the United States often find that they must learn to "talk football" so they can communicate with the men who have created organizational cultures and control women's careers. If female executives don't go to the next big football game and take clients with them, they risk being excluded from the "masculinity loop" that is central to corporate culture and communication (Gregory, 2009). When they go to work every Monday during the fall, they know that their ability to "talk football" can keep them in touch with male co-workers.

The Creation of Spectator Interest

Sport spectators are likely to be plentiful in societies where there's a general quest for excitement, an ideological emphasis on material success, childhood experiences with sports, and easy access to sports through the media.

The Quest for Excitement   When social life is highly controlled and organized, everyday routines often cause people to feel emotionally constrained. This fosters a search for activities that offer tension-excitement and emotional arousal.

According to sociologists Eric Dunning and Norbert Elias, historical evidence suggests that this is common in modern societies. Sports, they contend, provide activities in which rules and norms can be shaped to foster emotional arousal and exciting actions, thereby eliminating boredom without disrupting social order in society (Dunning, 1999; Elias and Dunning, 1986).

Sports generally involve a tension between order and disruption. To manage this tension, norms and rules in sports must be loose enough to allow exciting action, but not so loose that they permit uncontrolled violence or other forms of destructive actions. When norms and rules are too constraining, sports are boring and people lose interest; when they are too loose, sports become sites for reckless and dangerous actions that jeopardize health and social order. The challenge is to find and maintain a balance.

This explanation of spectator interest raises the question, "Why do so many people give priority to sports over other activities in their quest for excitement?" Cultural theorists suggest that answers can be found by looking at the connection between ideology and cultural practices. This leads us to consider the following factors.

Class Ideology and Spectator Interest   Spectator interest in sports is highest among those who believe in a meritocratic ideal: the idea that success is always based on skill and hard work, and skill and hard work always lead to success. This belief supports a widely held class ideology in societies with capitalist economies. Those who hold it often use sports as a model for how the social world should operate. When sports promote the idea that success is achieved through hard work and skill, their ideology is reaffirmed, and they become more secure in their beliefs. This is why sport media commentators emphasize that athletes and teams succeed when they work hard and have talent. This also is why corporations use the bodies of elite athletes to represent their public relations and marketing images—the finely tuned bodies of athletes are concrete examples of skill, power, and

success as well as the use of science and technology (Hoberman, 1994). When high-profile athletes can deliver this message for corporations, lucrative endorsements come their way.

Youth Sport Programs and Spectator Interest   Spectator interest often is initiated during childhood sport experiences. When organized youth sport programs emphasize skills, competition, and success, participants are likely to grow up wanting to watch elite athletes. For young people who continue to play sports, watching elite athletes provides them with models for playing and improving skills; for those who discontinue active participation, watching elite athletes provides continuous connections with the images and experiences of success that they learned while playing organized youth sports.

NFL executives understand the importance of this connection between youth sports and spectator interest. For example, as parents learn more about the dangers of brain injuries in football, the NFL has joined with USA Football to conduct a major public relations campaign to convince parents that football is being made safer and that they should encourage their sons to play the game. If youth football programs decline, so does the number of future players, season ticket purchasers, and media consumers of football.

Media Coverage and Spectator Interest   Media promote the commercialization of sports by publicizing and covering events in ways that sustain spectator interest (Cooky et al., 2013). Television increases spectator access to events and athletes worldwide and provides unique representations of sports. Camera coverage enables viewers to focus on the action and view replays in slow motion as they listen to the "insider" comments of announcers—all of which further immerses spectators into vicarious and potentially exciting sport experiences.

On-air commentators serve the media audience as fellow spectators who embellish the action and heighten identification with athletes and teams.

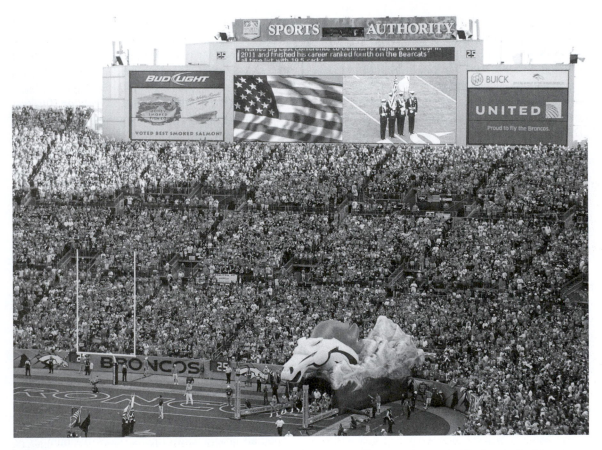

Football is the most widely watched sport in the United States. It offers excitement in the form of rule-governed violence, and it reaffirms the notion that success is achieved through competition and dominating opponents. Youth football teams are very popular, and more young men play high school football than any other high school sport. Football lends itself to media coverage during which replays, slow motion, and expert commentary are used to dissect plays and game plans. (*Source:* © Jay Coakley)

Commentators provide inside stories, analyze strategies, describe athletes as personalities, and magnify the importance of events.

Television recruits new spectators by teaching newcomers the rules and strategies of a sport at home with family and friends without purchasing expensive tickets. This is a painless way to be socialized into a spectator role, and it increases the number of people who will eventually buy tickets, watch televised games, pay for cable and satellite sports programming, and even become pay-per-view customers in the future.

Economic Factors and the Globalization of Commercial Sports

Commercial sports are now global in scope. Globalization has occurred because (1) those who control, sponsor, and promote sports seek new ways to expand markets and maximize profits, and (2) transnational corporations use sports as vehicles for introducing their products and services around the world. This makes sports a form of global cultural trade that is exported and imported in a manner similar to other products.

Sport Organizations Look for Global Markets

Commercial sport organizations are businesses, and their goal is to expand into as many markets as possible. In fact, future profits for major professional sports depend on selling media rights and consumer merchandise. Most leagues now market themselves outside their home countries and use various strategies to develop identification with their sport, teams, and players. In this way, sport organizations become exporters of culture as well as products to be consumed.

The desire for global expansion was the main reason why the NBA allowed its players to compose the so-called Dream Team that played in the 1992 Olympics. The global media attention received by Michael Jordan, Magic Johnson, and other players provided the NBA with publicity worth many millions of dollars. This exposure helped market NBA broadcasting rights and official NBA products worldwide. Today, the NBA finals and the NBA All-Star games are televised annually in over 200 countries and there are 76 international players from 31 countries now playing in the league. Outside the United States, China constitutes the largest NBA market and player development focus. More than 50,000 stores in China sell NBA merchandise, and about 30 percent of all visitors to NBA.com enter through the Mandarin language portal at the site.

The desire for global expansion has led NFL, NBA, NHL, and MLB teams to play exhibition and regular season games in Mexico, China, Japan, England, France, Germany, and Australia and to subsidize leagues and outreach programs for marketing purposes. This spirit of globalization is neither new nor limited to North American sport organizations. The International Olympic Committee (IOC) has incorporated national Olympic committees from every nation worldwide and has turned the Olympic Games into the most successful and financially lucrative media sport events in history. Furthermore, the IOC, like some other sport organizations, has turned itself and the Olympics into a global brand.

The sport with the longest history of global expansion is soccer, which is governed by FIFA—the Fédération Internationale de Football Association. The top soccer clubs in Europe have used multiple strategies to expand their global marketing reach. The best current example is Real Madrid Football Club (FC) in the Liga Nacional de Fútbol Profesional, or La Liga, the premier twenty-team league in Spain. It is valued at $3.3 billion and is owned by about 60,000 club members. It has 50 million social media followers and is rated as one of the twenty most recognizable brands in the world.

Two other sport teams with similar global recognition and value are Manchester United FC in England's Premier League and Barcelona FC in La Liga with Real Madrid. Barcelona, long known as a football club of the working class, has 101 million social media followers worldwide and may be the most recognizable sport brand in the world because of its working-class identification.

As a point of comparison, the New York Yankees and the Dallas Cowboys are valued at $3.2 billion each, but they have fewer than 20 million social media followers between them. Barcelona FC has ten times more followers than the Dallas Cowboys, and about the same number of followers as all thirty-two NFL teams combined. The only U.S. team with a strong global profile is the Los Angeles Lakers, with 26 million social media followers and high brand recognition. These data have attracted the attention of the leaders of U.S. sport leagues because they indicate that there is much room for global expansion.

Corporations Use Sports as Vehicles for Global Expansion

Because certain sports capture the attention, emotions, and allegiance of so many people worldwide, corporations are eager to sponsor them. Corporations need symbols of success and productivity that they can use as "marketing hooks" for products and as representations of their images. For example, people around the world still associate Michael Jordan with the "Air Jordan" trademark copyrighted by Nike; and many people now assume a connection between the Olympics and both McDonald's and Coca-Cola.

In the United States, the "gold medal" achievement for a corporation is to convert the company into a brand that can be associated with various forms of status and identity. Sports serve as effective sites for doing this as sport images and products can be used to represent people's identities at the same time that they can represent other things that give them status in particular social worlds. This dynamic drives consumption and corporate profits. As a result, most people inadvertently boost brand power by wearing clothes that prominently display logos. But corporations have convinced them that this is part of personal identity construction rather than free advertising for a company that cares nothing about them personally.

Companies whose profits depend on selling alcohol, tobacco, fossil fuels, fast food, soft drinks, and candy are especially eager to have their products associated with sports. This enables them to defuse negative publicity about unhealthy and negative aspects of their products and production processes. They want people to think that "if the sports we love are brought to us by beer, cigarettes, liquor, soft drinks, beef burgers, deep-fried foods, candy bars, and fossil fuels, these things must have some redeeming qualities."

We now live in an era of transnational corporations (TNCs) that influence economic activity worldwide, affecting who has jobs, the kinds of work people do, salaries and working conditions, the products that people can buy, where they can buy them, and what they cost. When these corporations sponsor sports, they negotiate deals that promote their interests, increase their power, and create positive images of themselves as "global citizens and leaders." This is worth an investment of billions of dollars each year. For example, eleven global corporations, including Coca-Cola, McDonald's, and Dow (Chemical), each paid $100 million just for the rights to advertise in connection with the 2010 and 2012 Olympic Games in Vancouver and London; and Anheuser-Busch

By unrolling the red carpet to the advertising and marketing of junk-food giants, the IOC is setting a toxic trap to hundreds of millions of parents and kids. —Monika Kosinska, European Public Health alliance (in Jack, 2012)

(Budweiser) spent over $370 million for commercial time during Super Bowls between 2003 and 2016. Like other multinational corporations, these companies buy commercial time during sport events to promote the belief that pleasure and excitement in people's everyday lives depend on them. They use this belief as an ideological outpost in the minds of people worldwide, and as information is filtered through these outposts, corporate executives hope to defuse opposition to the products and operational practices of their companies. When successful, this strategy boosts their legitimacy and contributes to corporate hegemony worldwide.

The success of this strategy led a Coca-Cola executive to tell IOC officials that they owed loyalty to Coke. He explained that

> Just as sponsors have the responsibility to preserve the integrity of the sport, enhance its image, help grow its prestige and its attendance, so too, do you [in sports] have responsibility and accountability to the sponsor (cited in Reid, 1996, p. 4BB).

IOC officials know that drinking cola does not meet the nutritional needs of elite athletes or the health goals of the Olympic movement, but they respond supportively to this executive's message. Coca-Cola has worked for nearly a century to colonize their minds and establish the outposts through which this message has been transmitted. This is why the official program brochure for the Olympics contains these words:

> Without sponsors, there would be no Olympic Games. Without the Olympic Games, there would be no dreams. Without dreams, there would be nothing (cited in Horne, 2007).

Of course, the sponsors themselves could not have written a statement better suited to their purposes. They want people to focus on dreams rather than the realities related to consumption and global corporate expansion; the Olympic Games continue to be awash in Coca-Cola imagery as outposts continue to be established in the minds of billions of potential consumers of soft drinks.

Outposts in Action: Branding Sports When ranchers want to show ownership of animals, they burn their logos into the animals' hides. The brand is their mark of ownership. And in the realm of sports, nearly all major stadiums and arenas in North America now display the brands of airlines, banks, brewers, and a gang of companies selling cars, oil, auto parts, energy, soft drinks, and communications services and products. For the venues in which NFL, NBA, and MLB teams play, these branding or naming rights sell for $3 million to $20 million per year. Deals usually are for ten to thirty years and often include signage in and around the venue, the use of luxury boxes and club seats, promotional rights for events, and exclusive concession rights (for example, the four Pepsi Centers in the United States sell only Pepsi products to fans). This benefits corporations, especially in major cities where four large billboards can cost up to $100,000 a month ($1.2 million per year). Having multiple billboard-like surfaces inside and outside a stadium is viewed as a good investment by corporate executives, especially when the name of their company is used in everyday conversations and they receive "sport perks" for themselves, customers, and friends.

The branding of sports also is apparent inside stadiums, where nearly every available surface is sold for corporate displays. Surfaces without corporate messages are now defined as wasted space, even in publicly owned facilities. This occurs at all levels of sports. For instance, many corporations desperately want to establish outposts in the minds of high school students who are in the process of forming lifelong preferences for products such as soft drinks. David Carter from the Sports Marketing Company in California knows that high school sports need revenues, so he predicts that "commercialism is coming to a school near you: the high school cheerleaders will be brought to you by Gatorade, and the football team will be

presented by Outback [Steakhouse]" (in Pennington, 2004, p. 1).

As corporations brand public spaces, community identities often come to be linked with brands, thereby converting the physical embodiments of local traditions and histories into highly visible signs that promote consumption and identify corporations as providers of pleasure and excitement. In the process, the public good is replaced by the corporate good, even in spaces paid for and owned by citizen-taxpayers.

Sport events also are branded. College football fans in the United States watch everything from the Capital One Orange Bowl to the Chick-fil-A Peach Bowl during December and early January. College football is clearly branded, as are the athletes who wear corporate logos on their shirts, shoes, helmets, and warm-up clothing.

NASCAR auto and truck racing has always been heavily branded. Although they have changed their branding strategies recently, they still have branded races such as Coca Cola 600, Coke Zero 400, Cheez-It 355, Hollywood Casino 400, and Goody's Headache Relief Shot 500. Additionally, racecars are billboards with surface spaces purchased by companies selling products that often cannot be advertised on network television, such as hard liquor and tobacco. This is why it was so important for NASCAR to be nationally televised—the liquor and tobacco companies wanted their brand names in front of a national audience for 250 to 600 laps during races.

Professional events in golf, tennis, beach volleyball, skiing, ice skating, and most other sports are now named after global corporations that want their names and products to be recognized worldwide. Corporations also brand teams in cycling, soccer, rugby, and many other sports. Professional baseball teams in Japan are named after corporations, not cities. Players and even referees in most sports wear the corporate logos of sponsors on their uniforms. Because European soccer was televised for many years by public TV stations that had no commercials, corporations put their logos on the players themselves and around the walls of the

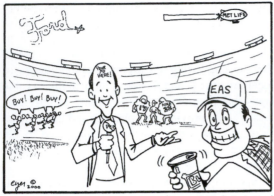

(*Source:* © Frederic A. Eyer)

"This is Pepsi McDonald at Mad Max Fury Road Park where the Microsoft Raiders will battle the Wal-Mart Titans. Team captains, Nike Jones and Budweiser Williams, prepare for the Franklin Mint Coin Toss, right after this message from our sponsor, Ford trucks—giving you power on demand!"

Televised versions of commercial sports have become inseparable from the logos and products of corporate sponsors.

playing fields so that spectators would see them constantly. This tradition continues even though commercial media now own the rights to televise most sport events worldwide.

Corporate branders now give priority to sports that appeal to young males, a demographic category defined as "hard to reach." So there are the X Games, Dew Tour, numerous events sponsored by Red Bull Energy Drink, Van's Triple Crown (surfing, skateboarding, snowboarding), McDonald's All-American High School Basketball Games, the Sprite Slam Dunk Contest, and the Nike Hoop Summit.

Sports agents today tell athletes that they can be brands and their goal should be to merge with other commercial entities rather than simply endorse a company's products. Michael Jordan was the first to do this. He initially endorsed Nike products but gradually became a brand in his own right. Today he has his own line of products in addition to "Air Jordan." Tony Hawk has done this with his own line

of skateboards and other products. However, this strategy is possible only for athletes whose celebrity is great enough to be converted into a brand.

In all other cases, it is corporations who choose who and what they wish to brand. For example, some athletes as young as twelve years old may be known as Nike, Adidas, or Under Armour athletes. Corporate executives now try to brand athletes as early as possible so that they can socialize the athletes to develop marketable personas that can be used to effectively promote corporate interests.

The Super Bowl, far too expensive for any single corporation to brand on its own, is known as much for its ads as for the game itself. Corporate sponsors of the 2016 Super Bowl paid about $5 million for thirty-second commercial spots during the telecast of the game—that's $166,000 per second! Corporate sponsors pay this rate because their ads are seen by live viewers who can't "fast forward" through commercials and they receive exposure beyond the game itself—in terms of previews, summaries, highlights, evaluations, and rankings in other media coverage—and they will be available for years on the Internet where people can see every ad starting with the 1969 Super Bowl. Corporations have branded the Super Bowl to such an extent that it has been described as a program where the commercials are the entertainment, and the game may or may not be entertaining.

Future forms of corporate branding are difficult to predict because it's hard to say where people will draw the line and prevent corporations from colonizing their lives. Ads during television coverage are now inserted digitally on the field, court, and other surfaces of arenas and stadiums so that viewers cannot escape them even when they record events and delete commercials. Corporations spend more of their advertising money today to purchase brand-placement rights, so their names, logos, and products appear directly in the content of sports. This maximizes the branding of playing fields/spaces, uniforms, and athletes' bodies.

The Limits of Corporate Branding   Can corporations go too far in their branding of sports? People

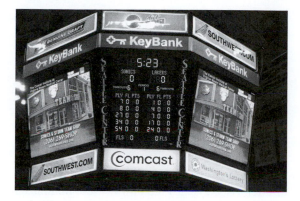

The goal of branding is to establish outposts in people's heads by connecting personal pleasure and excitement with corporations and their products. This is why "sport spaces" are filled with corporate logos and messages. (*Source:* © Jay Coakley)

in New Jersey didn't resist when a local elementary school sold naming rights for its gym to Shop-Rite, a supermarket chain. Most high school and college sport programs have not resisted. Football fans don't object when McDonald's is touted as the NFL's Official Fast-Food Sponsor, and Olympic officials, who claim to be dedicated to health and fitness, have long accepted McDonald's as the Official Restaurant of the Olympic Games. Despite a handful of cases where people objected to ads located on the actual field of play, sports are for sale, and corporations are willing buyers when deals boost their power and profits and promote consumption as a lifestyle.

In less than a generation, sports have been so thoroughly branded that many people, especially those younger than thirty years old, see this situation as "normal"—as the way it is and should be. Does this mean that corporations have established ideological outposts in their heads to the point that they accept corporate power as inevitable and even desirable? If so, corporate hegemony is deeply entrenched, even if some people resist and argue that the control of sports should not rest in the hands of corporate entities accountable only to market forces. If so, commercial sports are a site where people with political and financial resources can package their values and

ideas and present them in a form that most people see as normal, acceptable, and even entertaining.

COMMERCIALIZATION AND CHANGES IN SPORTS

What happens to sports as they shift from being activities organized for players to activities organized for paying spectators and sponsors? Do they change? If so, in what ways?

When a sport is converted into commercial entertainment, its success depends solely on spectator appeal. Although spectators watch sports for many reasons, their interest is tied to a combination of four factors:

- Attachment to those involved ("Do I know, like, or strongly identify with players and/or teams?")
- The uncertainty of an event's outcome ("Will it be a close contest?" and "Who might win?")
- The stakes associated with an event ("How much money, status, or danger is involved in the contest?")
- The anticipated display of excellence, heroics, or dramatic expression by the athletes ("Are the players and/or teams skilled and entertaining?" and "Might they set a record?" or "be the best team ever?")

When spectators say they saw "a good game," they usually mean that it was one in which (1) they were attached personally or emotionally to an athlete or a team; (2) the outcome was in doubt until the last minutes or seconds; (3) the stakes were so high that players were totally committed to and engrossed in the action; or (4) there were skilled and dramatic performances. Events containing all four of these factors are remembered and discussed for many years.

Because attachment, uncertainty, high stakes, and performance attract spectators, successful commercial sports are organized to maximize the probability that all four factors will exist in an event. To understand how this affects sports, we will consider the impact of commercialization on the following three aspects of sports:

1. The internal structure and goals of sports
2. The orientations of athletes, coaches, and sponsors
3. The people and organizations that control sports

Internal Structure and Goals of Sports

Commercialization influences the internal structure and goals of newly developed sports, but it has less influence on long-established sports. New sports developed explicitly for commercial purposes are organized to maximize whatever a target audience will find entertaining. This is not the only factor that influences the internal structure and goals of new sports, but it is the *primary* one. It is apparent in indoor soccer, indoor lacrosse, arena football, beach volleyball, roller hockey, and commercial action sports. Therefore, rules in the X Games are designed to maximize "big air," dangerous and spectacular moves, and the technical aspects of equipment, often manufactured by event sponsors. And when mixed martial arts was commercialized in the form of the Ultimate Fighting Championship (UFC), holding the fights in a cage was clearly an entertainment strategy—and it has worked!

Commercialization also forces more established sports to make action more exciting and understandable for spectators, but the changes seldom alter the basic internal organization and goals of the sports. For example, rules in the NFL have been changed to protect quarterbacks, increase passing as an offensive strategy, discourage field goals, protect players from career-ending injuries, establish "television/commercial time-outs," and set game schedules to fit the interests of commercial sponsors. But the basic organization and goals of the game have remained the same.

Changes in commercialized spectator sports usually do a combination of these six things: (1) speed up the action; (2) increase scoring; (3) balance competition; (4) maximize drama; (5) heighten attachment to players and teams; and (6)

provide "commercial time-outs." A review of rule changes in many sports shows the importance of these factors. For example, the designated hitter position in baseball's American League was added to increase scoring opportunities and heighten dramatic action. Soccer rules were changed to prevent matches from ending in ties. Tennis scoring was changed to meet the time requirements of television networks. Golf tournaments now involve total stroke counts rather than match play, so that big-name players aren't eliminated in an early round of a televised event. Free throws were minimized in basketball to speed up action. A 3-on-3 players sudden-death overtime period followed by a player versus goalie shootout (if needed) is now used by the National Hockey League to eliminate tie games and provide spectators with exciting action.

Although these changes are grounded in commercialization, they haven't altered the internal structure and goals of long-established sports. Teams remain the same size with similar positions, and outscoring opponents remains the primary goal. But games and matches are presented as *total entertainment experiences*. There's loud music, rapidly changing video displays, light displays, cheerleaders and mascots that present entertaining performances, and announcers that heighten drama with excited and colorful descriptions of the action. This entertainment package represents a change, but it affects the context surrounding a game or match rather than the structure and goals of the sport itself.

Orientations of Athletes, Coaches, and Sponsors

Commercial sports occur within a promotional culture created to sell athletic performances to audiences and sell audiences to sponsors. These sports are promoted through marketing hype based on stories, myths, and images created around players, teams, and even stadiums or arenas. Athletes become entertainers, and the orientations of nearly everyone in sports shift toward an emphasis on heroic action and away from aesthetic action. As

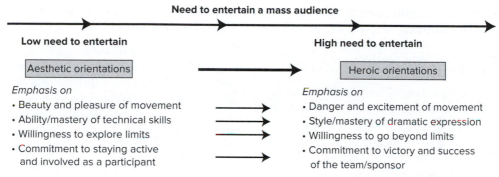

Note: The orientations associated with commercial spectator sports involve a shift from aesthetics to heroics–from skills to spectacle. Spectators need technical knowledge about a sport to be entertained by aesthetic action; when spectators lack this knowledge, they seek and focus on heroic action. Therefore, athletes and others associated with the game emphasize heroic orientations in their performances. "Heroic," as used here, refers to those who "play to the crowd" with entertaining forms of dramatic expression. The extreme version of this occurs in professional wrestling where stereotypical heroes and villains engage in heroic, dramatic, spectacular, and dangerous performances in the ring. Concerns about beauty, mastery, reasoned engagement, and athlete well-being are not the stuff of mass entertainment sports.

FIGURE 11.1 Shifting orientations: What happens when there is a need to entertain a mass audience.

illustrated in Figure 11.1, this shift is designed to attract a mass audience.

Because many people in a *mass* audience lack technical knowledge about the sport they watch, they are entertained mostly by intense action, danger, the dramatic expressions of athletes and coaches, and manifestations of commitment to victory. These things are easily understood by spectators who don't know enough about the sport to be captivated by precise physical skills and subtle strategies.

When spectators lack technical knowledge about football, for example, they are entertained more by a running back's end-zone antics after a touchdown than by the lineman's block that enabled the running back to score the touchdown. Those who know little about the technical aspects of ice skating are entertained more by triple and quadruple jumps than routines that are carefully choreographed and flawlessly executed. Without dangerous jumps, naïve spectators become bored because they don't recognize subtle differences in the skills and routines of skaters. Those who lack

technical knowledge about basketball are more impressed by slam dunks than a well-coordinated defensive strategy that wins a game.

Players realize what a mass audience wants and often "play to the crowd" with heroic displays and exciting or controversial personas. They may even refer to games as "showtime." In commercial terms, a player's style and persona often are as valuable as technical skills. This is why announcers and journalists focus on athletes who can make the big plays and are willing to talk in dramatic terms about their performances. A mass audience is thrilled by long touchdown passes, home runs, and athletes who collapse as they surpass their physical limits.

Overall, commercialization involves a shift in orientations so that the danger of movement becomes important *in addition to* the beauty of movement; style and dramatic expression become important *in addition to* skills; pushing beyond personal limits becomes important *in addition to* exploring limits; and commitment to victory for the team and sponsor becomes important *in addition to* the personal joy of participation. Aesthetic orientations don't disappear in commercial sports, but they are combined with heroic orientations to produce changes in what constitutes a memorable sport event.

Because there are dangers associated with heroic orientations, some athletes try to limit an emphasis on heroic actions in their sports. This has occurred in figure skating as some athletes favor restrictions on the number of triple jumps required in skating programs. They worry that the quest for commercial success jeopardizes their bodies. Other skaters, however, adopt heroic orientations to please audiences and conform to shifts in the orientations of judges, coaches, and other skaters. As a result, they train to successfully land a succession of triple jumps along with quad jumps without breaking bones or destroying the continuity of their skating programs. Aesthetic orientations still exist, but heroic orientations have been woven into popular definitions of "quality" in skating performances.

As heroic orientations become more important, so do concerns about athletes becoming entertainers and sports turning into circus spectacles. For example, as accidents in NASCAR races have been linked to issues of revenge between drivers and strategies to prevent certain drivers from winning series championships, some people wonder if the sport is turning into a weekly circus act (Gluck, 2015). The challenge facing NASCAR executives is to decide whether the races are a form of honest competition or spectacles that pit drivers against each other in demolition derbies.

This issue is not limited to NASCAR. Those who control commercial sports must eventually deal with similar questions. For example, what happens to a sport when heroic orientations are pushed to extremes? Are spectators willing to have aesthetic orientations abandoned in favor of the heroic? What would events be like if this happened? One way to answer this question is to study professional wrestling—a sport turned into heroic spectacle in a quest to be entertaining. This topic is discussed in the Reflect on Sports box "Extreme Heroic Action."

The People and Organizations That Control Sports

When sports depend on the revenues they generate, control in sport organizations shifts away from the athletes and toward those with the resources to produce and promote sports. Athletes in heavily commercialized sports generally lose effective control over the conditions of their own sport participation. These conditions are controlled by a combination of general managers, team owners, corporate sponsors, advertisers, media personnel, marketing and publicity staff, professional management staff, accountants, and agents.

The organizations that control commercial sports are designed to maximize profits. Decision making promotes economic interests and deals with athletes as commodities to be managed. Therefore, athletes in commercial sports usually are cut out of decision-making processes, even when the decisions affect their health and the rewards they receive for playing. This leads them to develop strategies to represent their interests relative to the interests of team owners, agents, advertising executives, media people, and corporate sponsors. For example, athletes in ESPN's X Games constantly struggle to maintain the spirit and norms of their sport cultures as they participate under conditions controlled by ESPN and corporate sponsors.

Like many athletes before them, the athletes in action sports find it difficult to oppose the power of the media and corporate sponsors. If they want the rewards offered in commercial sports, they answer first to the sponsors. This isn't new; sponsors traditionally define the conditions of sport participation. But some people view the power shifts that come with commercialization in critical terms, assessing carefully the pros and cons of a commercial model in which corporations set the terms and conditions of playing sports. Commercialization may not significantly change the structure and goals of some sports, but it does come with major changes in power relations and the organizational contexts in which sports are played.

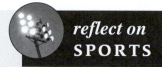

reflect on
SPORTS

Extreme Heroic Action:
Professional Wrestling as "Sportainment"

Professional wrestling is commercialization pushed to an extreme. It isolates elements of commercial sports and dramatizes them through parody and caricature (Sammond, 2005; Schiesel, 2007a; Smith, 2008). In the process, it abandons aesthetic orientations and highlights the heroic.

Starting in the late 1990s, professional wrestling captured widespread spectator interest and was a smashing commercial success. It bodyslammed its way into popular culture worldwide. Its featured events in sold out stadiums nearly every night in North American cities.

Raw Is War and *Smackdown!* were top-ranked programs on ad-supported cable television. Pay-per-view events often subscribed over half a million viewers at $30 per month and up to $50 for special events. Matches were televised in nine languages in 120 countries, wrestling videos were the best-selling "sports videos" in the world, and wrestling action figures outsold all other characters in popular culture.

Branded as World Wrestling Entertainment, professional wrestling events have been among the highest-rated programs on major cable channels. For many

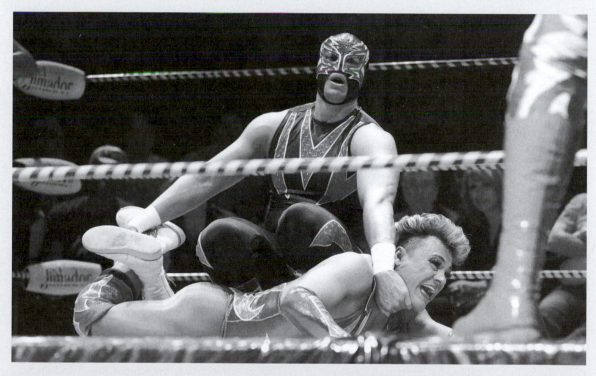

Professional wrestling turns sport into spectacle. Popular worldwide, it is organized around heroic orientations. In Spanish-speaking countries, pro wrestling is known as Lucha Libre–open wrestling in which masks are worn, with the exception of Cassandro, "Queen of the Ring" and the first openly gay celebrity wrestler. Most matches are representations of battles between what fans perceive as good and evil. This well-attended match occurred at the Mayan Theater in Los Angeles. (*Source:* © Splash News//Splash News/Corbis)

Continued

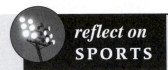

Extreme Heroic Action (*continued*)

years, popular *Monday Night Nitro* and *Monday Night Raw* have cut into the audience for Monday Night Football and the finals of the NCAA men's basketball tournament. Most wrestling programs have had viewer ratings consistently higher than NBA games and always higher than NHL games.

The popularity of professional wrestling is grounded in the heroic actions of performers combined with story lines and personas that engage spectators' concerns with issues related to social class, gender, ethnicity, job security, and national identity. In most cases, story lines and personas are performed by hypermasculine, heterosexual, and homophobic strong men who are arbitrarily victimized or privileged by greedy, underhanded corporate bosses or random, unpredictable events. The men are either supported or undermined by women, represented as alluring and vulnerable sex objects or exotic and heavily muscled sadomasochists. Overall, events are staged to represent male fantasies and fears about sex and power, and their concerns about work in a world where men feel they are losing control.

Sociologist Brendan Maguire uses structural theory to hypothesize that pro wrestling is popular because it "addresses the anxiety and angst associated with community breakdown, social disenchantment, and political correctness" (2005, p. 174). He explains that when community ties are strong and social satisfaction is high and social control is not overly constraining, people have little anxiety and little need to be entertained by dramatic parodies of heroic wrestling action.

Cultural theories, on the other hand, lead to other hypotheses based on past evidence that the popularity of any cultural practice, including professional wrestling, depends on the extent to which it reaffirms the ideologies that people use to make sense of their lives and the world around them. Therefore, the goal of those who produce sport entertainment is to provide people with pleasure and excitement without fostering opposition to the power structure that sustains commercial entertainment. In this way, professional wrestling and most commercial sports reproduce the status quo and existing forms of power relations by presenting actions, story lines, and characters that constitute soap operas for men of all ages and for the women who identify with the orientations and perspectives of men (Schiesel, 2007a).

THE ORGANIZATION OF PROFESSIONAL SPORTS IN NORTH AMERICA

Professional sports in North America are privately owned by individuals, partnerships, or corporations. The wealth and power of owners is greatest at the top levels of professional sports and less so in minor leagues and sports with relatively small audiences. Similarly, sponsors and event promoters range from individuals to large transnational corporations, depending on the size of events.

The Owners of Sport Teams

Most of the individuals or companies that own minor-league teams in North America don't make much money. Many are happy to break even and avoid the losses that are commonplace at this level of sports ownership. Also, many teams, leagues, and events have been financial disasters over the past fifty years. Four football leagues, a hockey league, a few soccer leagues, a volleyball league, four men's and five women's basketball leagues, a team tennis league, and a number of basketball and soccer teams have gone out of business, leaving many owners, sponsors, and promoters in debt. This list covers only the United States and doesn't include all those who have lost money on tournaments and special events.

The owners of major men's professional sport franchises in North America are very different from owners at other levels of commercial sports. Teams or franchises in the NFL, NBA, NHL, and MLB in

2015 were valued from about $186 million (Florida Panthers in the NHL) to about $3.2 billion (Dallas Cowboys in the NFL). Therefore, the owners of teams in these leagues are large corporations and a few very wealthy individuals with assets ranging from hundreds of millions to many billions of dollars. Each of these four major men's leagues is organized as a monopoly, most teams in these leagues play in publicly subsidized facilities, owners make good to excellent returns on their investments, and support from media companies and corporate sponsors almost guarantees continued financial success at this level of ownership.

Similarly, the large corporations that sponsor particular events, from major golf and tennis tournaments to NASCAR and Grand Prix races, know the costs and benefits involved. Their association with top events provides them with advertising platforms and connects them with clearly identified categories of consumers. Media companies also sponsor events so they can control their own programming, as in the case of ESPN's X Games, Red Bull sports, and others.

Major sport sponsorships enable companies that sell tobacco, alcohol, and junk food to link their products and logos to popular activities. Executives at these companies know that people associate sports with strong, healthy bodies instead of cancer, heart disease, diabetes, obesity, tooth decay, and other forms of poor health associated with their products. Their hope is to use sports to increase their legitimacy as "corporate citizens" and defuse resistance to their policies and products.

Investments in sports and sport events are motivated by many factors. In some cases, investors are wealthy fans looking to satisfy lifelong fantasies, build their egos, or socialize with celebrity athletes. Buying a team or sponsoring major events gives them more enjoyment and prestige than other business ventures, often making them instant celebrities.

Those who invest in sports enjoy their status, but they don't allow fun and fantasy to interfere with business and the growth of their capital. They don't enjoy losing money or sharing power. They may look at their athletes as heroes, but they want to control them and maximize investment returns. They may be civic boosters and supporters of public projects, but they define the "public good" in terms that emphasize capitalist expansion and their own business interests, usually to the exclusion of other definitions. They may not agree with fellow owners and sponsors on all issues, but they do agree that their investments must be protected and their profits maximized.

Team Owners and Sport Leagues as Cartels

The tendency to think alike has been especially strong among the owners of teams in the major North American sport leagues. Unity among owners has led to the formation of effective cartels. A **cartel** is *a centralized group that coordinates the actions of a selected collection of people or businesses.* Therefore, even though each sport franchise in each league is usually a separate business, the team owners in each sport come together to form a cartel representing their collective interests. The cartel is used to control inter-team competition for players, fans, media revenues, and sales of licensed merchandise. Additionally, it's used to eliminate competition from others who might form teams and leagues in the same sports. When a cartel succeeds, as it has in each of the major men's professional team sports, it becomes a **monopoly**—*the one and only provider of a particular product or service.*

Each league—the NBA, NFL, NHL, and MLB—is also a **monopsony,** or *a single buyer of a product or service*—in this case, elite athletic labor in a particular sport. This means that if a college football player wants to play professional football in the United States, he has one choice: the NFL. And the NFL, like other monopsony leagues, has developed a system to force new players to negotiate contracts only with the team that drafts them. This enables owners to sign new players to contracts without bidding against other teams, which might be willing to pay particular players more money.

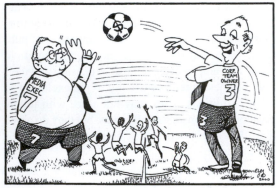

(*Source:* © Frederic A. Eyer)

"Winning is easy when you form a cartel, prevent others from playing, and maintain exclusive control over a highly desired product."

The growth and profitability of commercial sports worldwide have little to do with athletes. Owners, sponsors, and media executives control sports today, and they make money when governments allow them to operate as cartels and keep competitors out of the game.

As a cartel, the owners prevent new leagues from being established and competing with them for players, and they also prevent new teams from entering their league without their permission. When permission is given, it involves conditions set by the cartel. For example, the new team owner is charged an entry fee to become a part of the league and must give back to the cartel some of the team's profits for a certain number of years. Furthermore, a new owner can locate only in a city approved by the cartel, and no current owner can move a team to another city without cartel approval.

Acting as a cartel, the owners in each sport league collectively sell national broadcasting rights to their games and then share the revenues from the media contracts. This maintains the cartel's control over the conditions under which fans can view televised games. This is why games are not televised in the home team's region when they're not sold out, and why cable and satellite fees are so high when fans wish to purchase access to more than the primary games telecast by the major networks. Such a strategy enables team owners to make huge sums of money in their media contracts while forcing people to buy tickets to games and pay high monthly cable or satellite service bills.

Being part of a legal cartel enables most team owners to make impressive sums of money. During the mid-1960s, NFL teams were bought and sold for about $10 million; in 2015 the average franchise value was $2 billion. That's an average per-team capital gain of $1.9 billion, which amounts to an average annual return of $38 million on an original investment of $10 million. This is what a cartel does: it limits the supply of teams and drives up the value of existing teams. Of course, team owners do not include capital gains when they announce that annual profits are low and they must raise ticket prices and have a new stadium so they can be "competitive" with other teams. When you are in a cartel, you can get away with this deception and blackmail without going to jail. Of course, team owners have also used their power to influence the rule makers who set the rules that govern them.

Each league also has unique internal agreements regulating how teams can negotiate the sale of local broadcasting rights to their games. The NFL does not allow teams to sign independent television or radio contracts for local broadcasts of their games, but MLB does. This creates significant disparities in the incomes of baseball teams, because the New York Yankees can negotiate a local media rights deal that may be a hundred times higher than what the Kansas City Royals can negotiate in a much smaller media market.

The biggest differences between the major men's sport leagues are related to their contractual agreements with the players' association in each league. Although each league gives players as few rights and as little money as possible, athletes have struggled over the last five decades to gain control over their careers, regulate the conditions of their sport participation, and increase their salaries. This topic is discussed in the section below titled "Legal Status and Incomes of Athletes in Commercial Sports."

Team Owners and Public Assistance

The belief that cities cannot have "major league status" unless they have professional sports teams and sports megaevents has enabled sports team owners and promoters to receive public money (Delaney and Eckstein, 2003; deMause and Cagan, 2008; Friedman and Andrews, 2011; Scherer and Davidson, 2010; Silk, 2004). Most common is the use of public funds to build arenas and stadiums. As noted in Chapter 9 (pp. 266–267), this "stadium socialism" enables wealthy and powerful capitalists to use public money for personal gain, but when the media discuss this transfer of funds, it is usually described as "economic development" rather than "welfare for the rich."

Team owners and their supporters justify stadium subsidies and other forms of public assistance with a five-point argument (Lavoie, 2000):

1. A stadium and pro team creates jobs; those who hold the jobs spend money and pay taxes in the city so that everyone benefits.
2. Stadium construction infuses money into the local economy; this money is spent over and over as it circulates, generating tax revenues in the process.
3. The team attracts businesses to the city, and this increases local revenues.
4. The team attracts regional and national media attention, which boosts tourism and contributes to overall economic development.
5. The team creates positive psychic and social benefits, boosting social unity and feelings of pride and well-being in the local population.

These arguments often are supported by the economic impact studies commissioned by team owners. However, impact studies done by *independent* researchers generally reach the following conclusions:[1]

1. Teams and stadiums create jobs, but apart from highly paid athletes and team executives, these jobs are low paid, part-time, and seasonal. Additionally, many athletes on the team don't live in the city or spend their money there.
2. The companies that design and build stadiums are seldom local, and construction materials and workers on major projects often come from outside the region or even from outside the country. Therefore, much of the money spent on a stadium or arena does not circulate as stadium boosters predict.
3. Stadiums attract other businesses, but most are restaurant and entertainment franchises headquartered in other cities. These franchises often have enough cash to undercut and drive out locally owned businesses. Some out-of-town people come to the city to attend games, but most people who buy tickets live close enough to make day trips to games, and their purchases inside the stadium don't benefit businesses outside the stadium gates.
4. Stadiums and teams generate public relations for the city, but this has mixed results for tourism because some people stay away from cities on game days. Most important, *regional* economic development often is limited by a new facility because fans who spend money in and around the stadium have fewer dollars to spend in their own neighborhoods. A stadium often helps nearby businesses, but it often hurts outlying businesses. For example, when a family of four spends about $10,000 for average NBA season tickets, and another $4000 for meals

---

[1]Studies of this issue are numerous; the most recent include: see Bandow (2003); Brown et al., (2004); Curry et al., (2004); Delaney and Eckstein (2003); deMause and Cagan (2008); Friedman and Andrews, 2011; Friedman et al., (2004); Lewis (2010); Silk (2004); Smith and Ingham (2003); Spirou and Bennett (2003); Troutman (2004).

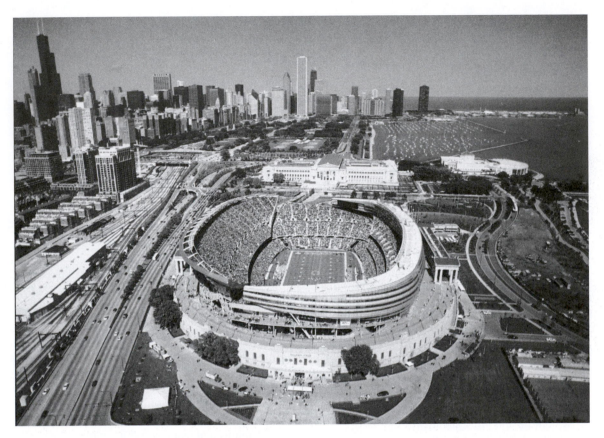

New Soldier Field, home of the Chicago Bears, was remodeled in 2002 with private funds and $432 million of public money—a large government subsidy for a private, family-owned business. Used only ten times a year by the Bears, it is maintained and managed year-round by the city of Chicago. This arrangement made the McCaskey family and other team owners happy because it helped to increase the franchise value of the Chicago Bears from $362 million prior to opening of the new stadium to $1.06 billion six years later. Chicago residents built the stadium and pay maintenance bills, and the team owners enjoy a $702-million increase in team value. (*Source:* © Mike Smith of Aerial Views Publishing, October 5, 2003)

and parking for 41 home games, it will spend less money on dinners and entertainment close to home—if they have any money left!

5. A pro sport team can make some people feel good and may enhance general perceptions of a city, but this is difficult to measure and little is known about its consequences for the city as a whole. Additionally, the feelings of fans often vary with the success of a team, and the feelings of those who are not fans may not be improved by a men's sport team that reaffirms traditional masculinity and values related to domination and conquest.

Independent researchers explain that positive effects are bound to occur when a city spends $500 million to a billion dollars of public money on a project. However, they also point out that the public good might be better served if tax money were spent on things other than a stadium. For example, during the mid-1990s, the city of Cleveland spent nearly a billion dollars of public money to build three sport facilities and related infrastructure. Inner-city residents during the same years pleaded with the city to install a drinking fountain in a park in a working-class neighborhood, and teachers held classes in renovated shower rooms in local public schools because there was no money to fund new educational facilities for inner-city students. At the same time, the owners of the three sport teams received a fifty-year exemption on taxes related to their teams and facilities, and $120 million in tax abatements on other real estate development in the area around the stadiums. This means that the city annually forfeited about $50 million in city and county tax revenues. In the meantime, the franchise values for the NFL, NBA, and MLB teams in Cleveland increased dramatically, giving multi-million-dollar capital gains to each of the wealthy owners.

Sociologists Kevin Delaney and Rick Eckstein (2003) studied the Cleveland case along with eight other cities where public money was used to build stadiums for private use. They concluded that the results in Cleveland were better than in the other cities. However, they found no evidence that the three stadiums fostered a downtown rejuvenation, as stadium proponents had predicted. Neither the number of businesses nor job creation rates increased, and in the three years following the construction, the cost for each new job created was $231,000, nearly twenty times higher than the cost to develop jobs with public programs. The new sport facilities failed to lower poverty rates, improve schools, or increase the availability of safe, low-cost housing (deMause and Cagan, 2008), but they did force poor people to move to other areas of town which gave developers cheap access to land on which they could build.

During the years since these facilities were built, the teams using them have had losing records, and the people of Cleveland see them as confirming their status as losers (Lewis, 2010). But the revenues for the team owners have been more predictable (Rascher et al., 2012), and their franchise values have

increased considerably as the league has negotiated large media rights contracts. The schools remain in poor condition, but the owners have saved considerable money on the sweetheart tax deals they struck with the city and county, so the public subsidies have paid off nicely and made them financial winners.

The people who object to stadium subsidies seldom have resources to oppose the well-financed, professionally packaged proposals developed by the consultants hired by team owners. The social activists who might lead the opposition already deal full time with problems related to unemployment, underfunded schools, homelessness, poor health, and the lack of needed social services in cities. They cannot abandon these tasks to lobby against using public money to benefit billionaire team owners and millionaire celebrity athletes. At the same time, local people are persuaded to think that team owners will abandon their city if they don't pony up public money to build a new facility with the requisite number of luxury suites and club seats.

When thinking about public subsidies to sport teams, it's helpful to consider alternative uses of public funds. For example, my former hometown of Colorado Springs used $6 million of public money in 2000 to construct a youth sport complex consisting of twelve baseball, softball, and T-ball fields of various sizes with bleacher seating; ten soccer/football fields; six volleyball courts; an in-line skating rink; a batting cage (for baseball hitting practice); and multiple basketball courts. At the same time, $300 million of tax money from six Denver metro counties was used to build a new stadium for Pat Bowlen, the wealthy owner of the Denver Broncos. Instead of doing this, the counties could have done what Colorado Springs did and used the $300 million to build 600 baseball, softball, and T-ball fields; 500 soccer/football fields; 300 volleyball courts; 50 in-line skating rinks; 50 batting cages; and 250 basketball courts around the metro area.

Which of these two alternatives would have had the most positive impact on the overall quality of life in the Denver metro area? If the money had been spent on local recreation facilities, individuals and families in the region would now have easy access to one or more of them seven days a week for a nominal cost. Maybe people in the region would be more physically active and healthier. Instead, the region has a 72,000-seat stadium used by the Denver Broncos ten times a year, or thirteen times if they make the playoffs with home-field advantage and win all games leading up to the Super Bowl. Since the stadium was built, the team has played fewer than eleven home games per season except in 2015, and spectators have paid an average of over $85 a seat for 162 games from 2001 through 2015. This amounts to about $820 million; with parking and concessions expenditures, people have paid about $1.4 billion to attend games in a stadium subsidized by their taxes.

Most of this money has gone into the pockets of team owners, executives, and players, who spend part of it in Denver but much of it elsewhere. Also, the owners keep half of the stadium naming-rights money and the other half goes into the public fund to pay maintenance costs for the stadium, which is the responsibility of the taxpayers. Many of the stay-at-home fans of the team pay larger cable and satellite costs to see games and spend at least fifty hours a year sitting down watching Bronco games and consuming food and drinks at home or in bars. They become emotionally invested in the team, players, and outcomes of games and seasons, and they have fun with family and friends when watching and talking about things related to "their" team.

Some people prefer the NFL stadium, but many others might prefer an abundance of local recreation facilities, if they had a choice. Among those preferring the stadium are people with the power and resources to obtain what they want. And they want new stadiums and access to the revenue streams that a stadium generates. They have memberships in athletic and fitness clubs and don't care about building public recreation centers. Even their children play sports in private clubs and on teams that use private facilities. Additionally, they have mini fitness centers in their homes.

This is how power and social class shape local cultures, access to particular kinds of sport facilities, and priorities for spending public money related to sports.

Sources of Income for Team Owners

The owners of top pro teams in the major men's sports make money from (1) gate receipts; (2) media revenues; (3) stadium revenue; (4) licensing fees; and (5) merchandise sales. The amounts and proportions of each of these revenue sources vary from league to league and team to team.

The recent and continuing wave of new stadium construction and renovation is the result of owners demanding venues that can generate new revenue streams. This is why these stadiums resemble shopping malls built around playing fields. Sociologist George Ritzer (2005) describes them as "cathedrals of consumption" designed so that consumption is seamlessly included in spectator experiences. Owners see this as important because it enables them to capture a greater share of the entertainment dollar in a highly competitive urban entertainment market. According to a report in *Forbes* magazine, team owners use the following formula:

> Build new facilities with fewer seats and more luxury boxes, charge higher prices, earn more revenue, hire better players, and reap more wins. Then turn around and raise ticket prices (Van Riper, 2008).

The rest of the formula is to build the stadium mostly with public money so if things go wrong, the local taxpayers are stuck with the losses.

When a new stadium is built, the value of the team that plays there increases at least 25 percent. This means that if a city builds a $700 million stadium for an NFL team that is valued at $2 billion, the franchise value will increase about $500 million to $2.5 billion. This increase goes directly to the owners as part of the assets of the franchise.

To prevent people from realizing how public money is used to subsidize their wealth, the owners make sure that announcers describe *their* teams as *your* New York Giants, Cleveland Cavaliers, Detroit Red Wings, or Colorado Rockies. The owners are happy to support the illusion that their teams belong to the community, as long as they collect the revenues and capital gains while taxpayers take the risks and receive little benefit apart from the emotional perks that come from living in a region that has a professional men's sport team located there.

THE ORGANIZATION OF AMATEUR SPORTS IN NORTH AMERICA

So-called amateur sports don't have owners, but they do have commercial sponsors and governing bodies that control events and athletes. Generally, the sponsors in the United States are corporations interested in using amateur sports for publicity and advertising purposes. The governing bodies of amateur sports operate on a nonprofit basis, although they use revenues from events to maintain their organizations and exert control over amateur sports. They generally hire for-profit companies to organize, publicize, and administer the events for them.

Centralized state-sponsored sport authorities administer amateur sports in nearly all countries except the United States. They work with the national governing bodies (NGBs) of individual sports, and together they control events, athletes, and revenues. Sport Canada and the Canadian Olympic Association are examples of such centralized authorities; they develop the policies that govern the various national sport organizations in Canada, from youth sports to national teams.

In the United States, the organization and control of amateur sports is much less centralized. Policies, rules, fund-raising strategies, and methods of operating all vary from one organization to the next. For example, the major governing body in intercollegiate sports is the National Collegiate Athletic Association (NCAA). For amateur sports not connected with universities, the major controlling organization is the United States Olympic Committee (USOC). However, within the USOC, each of more than fifty separate NGBs regulate and control a particular amateur sport. NGBs raise most of their own funds through corporate

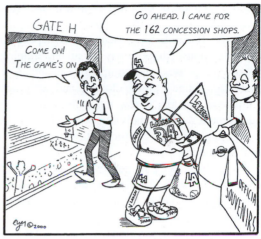

(*Source:* © Frederic A. Eyer)

Recently built stadiums resemble shopping malls, and some fans see attendance as a shopping opportunity. They're a captive audience, and team owners want to capture as many of their entertainment dollars as possible. This fan has taken the consumption bait and is less interested in the game than buying products to prove he was there.

and individual sponsors, and each one sets its own policies to supplement the rules and policies of the USOC and IOC. The USOC has long tried to establish continuity in American amateur sports, but the NGBs and other organizations are very protective of their own turf, and they seldom give up power; instead, they fight to maintain exclusive control over rules, revenues, and athletes. This has caused many political battles in and among organizations.

All amateur sport organizations share an interest in two things: (1) controlling the athletes in their sports and (2) controlling the money generated from sponsorships and competitive events. Sponsorship patterns in amateur sports take many forms. Universities, for example, "sell" their athletic departments, allowing corporations to brand their athletic teams and the bodies of athletes in exchange for money, scholarships, equipment, and apparel. Corporations and universities usually enter these agreements outside of any democratic processes involving votes by students, athletes, or the citizens whose taxes fund the universities.

The NGBs of U.S. amateur sports depend on corporate sponsorships to pay for athlete training, operating expenses, and competitive events. Corporate logos appear on the clothing and equipment of amateur athletes. A few top athletes may sign endorsement deals as individuals, but they cannot do so when the deals conflict with the interests of NGB sponsors.

When this model of corporate sponsorship is used, the economics of sports are linked to the fluctuations of market economies and the profits of large corporations. Corporations sponsor only those sports that foster their interests, and economic conditions influence their ability and willingness to maintain sponsorships. For example, when the Women's United Soccer Association (WUSA) and its 180 professional athletes needed $20 million in 2003 to survive another year, Nike could have reduced the $450-million deal they made with Manchester United, a men's soccer team in England, so it could support WUSA, but it didn't because corporations are about profits, and women's soccer didn't fit into their business plans.

LEGAL STATUS AND INCOMES OF ATHLETES IN COMMERCIAL SPORTS

When sports are commercialized, athletes are entertainers. This is obvious at the professional level, but it's also true in other commercial sports such as big-time college football and basketball. Professional athletes are paid for their efforts, whereas amateur athletes receive rewards within limits set by the organizations that govern their lives. This raises these two questions:

1. What is the legal status of the athlete-entertainers in sports?
2. How are athlete-entertainers rewarded for their work?

Many people don't think of athletes as workers, and they overlook owner–player relations in

professional sports as a form of labor relations. Most people associate sports with play, and they see athletes as having fun rather than working. However, when sports are businesses, players are workers, even though they may have fun on the job. This isn't unique; many workers enjoy their jobs. But regardless of enjoyment, issues of legal status and fair rewards for work are important.

This section focuses on the United States and does not consider all the sports that collect gate receipts but never make enough money to pay for anything but basic expenses, if that. Therefore, we don't discuss high school sports, non-revenue-producing college sports, or other nonprofit local sports in which teams sell tickets to events.

Professional Athletes

The legal status of athletes has always been the most controversial issue in professional team sports.

Legal Status: Team Sports   Until the mid-1970s, professional athletes in the major sport leagues had little or no legal power to control their careers. They could play only for the team that drafted and owned them. They could not control when and to whom they might be traded during their careers, even when their contracts expired. Furthermore, they were obliged to sign standard contracts saying that they agreed to forfeit to their owners all rights over their careers. Basically, they were bought and sold like property and seldom consulted about their wishes. They were at the mercy of team owners, managers, and coaches.

In all sports, this form of employee restriction was called the **reserve system** because it was *a set of practices that enabled team owners to reserve the labor of athletes for themselves and control the movement of athletes from team to team in their sport.*

As long as the reserve system was legal, owners could maintain low salaries and near-total control over the conditions under which athletes played their sports. Parts of the reserve system continue to exist in professional sports, but players' associations (that is, unions) in each of the major professional leagues for men have challenged the system in court and forced significant changes that increased their rights as workers so they could negotiate with owners to control conditions of their work and establish guidelines for their salaries.

In any other business, a reserve system of the type used in sports would violate antitrust laws. Companies cannot control employee movement from firm to firm, and they certainly cannot draft employees so that no other company can hire them, nor can they trade them at will to another company. But this type of reserve system, with modifications since the 1970s, has been defined by the U.S. Congress as legal in sports, and owners use it with minimal interference from any government agency.

Team owners justify the reserve system by saying that it's needed to maintain competitive balance between teams in their leagues. They argue that, if athletes could play with any team, the wealthiest owners in the biggest cities and TV markets would buy all the good athletes and prevent teams in smaller cities and TV markets from being winners. The irony of this argument is that team owners are free-market capitalists who argue that free-market processes would destroy their business! They embrace regulation and "sport socialism" because it protects their power and wealth; they form cartels to restrict athletes' rights and salaries, *but* they advocate deregulation in the economy as a whole. Their positions are ideologically inconsistent, but profitable for them.

Professional athletes always have objected to the reserve system, but it wasn't until 1976 that court rulings gave professional athletes the right to become *free agents* under certain conditions. The meaning of free agency varies, but in all leagues it allows some players whose contracts have expired to seek contracts with other teams that bid for their

> **The NFL is a machine. The operators of the machine pull its levers more frantically every season, pushing it past its breaking point. So the league has stockpiled interchangeable spare parts. The broken ones are seamlessly replaced and the machine keeps rolling.** —Nate Jackson, former NFL player (2011)

services. This change has had a dramatic effect on the salaries of top professional athletes from the late 1970s to the present. Table 11.1 lists average salaries in major sport leagues from 1950 to 2015, and the data show the dramatic increases that occurred after the mid-1970s.

Prior to the mid-1970s pro athletes made from two to four times the median family income in the United States. After free agency was allowed in the 1970s, salaries skyrocketed. With rising revenues from gate receipts and media rights, salaries increased rapidly as teams competed for players and negotiated new Collective Bargaining Agreements (CBAs) with players' unions. In 2015, the ratio of average salaries relative to median family income was 76:1 for the NBA; 64:1 for MLB; 39:1 for the NHL; 32:1 for the NFL; 4.2:1 for the MLS, and 1.1:1 for the WNBA.

Owner–athlete relations change every time a new CBA is negotiated and signed. Although team owners, league officials, and some fans dislike the players' unions, these organizations have enabled players to gain more control over their salaries and working conditions. Labor negotiations and players' strikes in professional team sports have focused primarily on issues of freedom and control over careers, rather than money, although money has certainly been an issue. As a result, free agency now exists for all players after they've been under contract for a certain number of years, and owners no longer have absolute control over players' careers.

Although it's been a struggle for professional team athletes to maintain their unions, they realize that crucial labor issues must be negotiated every time they renew their CBA with the owners' cartel. At this time, the main issues negotiated in CBAs include the following:

1. The definition of league revenues, "and the percentage of those revenues that must be allocated to players' salaries and benefits"

Table 11.1   Average salaries in major U.S. professional leagues, compared with median family income, 1950–2015*

| Year | SPORT LEAGUE | | | | | | Median U.S. Family Income† |
	NFL	NBA	WNBA	NHL	MLB	MLS	
1950	15,000	5,100	NA	5,000	13,300	NA	4,000
1960	17,100	13,000	NA	14,100	19,000	NA	5,620
1970	23,000	40,000	NA	25,000	29,300	NA	9,867
1980	79,000	190,000	NA	110,000	143,000	NA	21,023
1990	395,400	824,000	NA	247,000	598,000	NA	35,353
2000	1,116,100	3,600,000	60,000‡	1,050,000	1,988,034	100,000	50,732
2010	1,900,000	5,150,000	52,000‡	2,400,000	3,298,000	140,000	60,236
2015	2,100,000	5,100,000	72,000‡	2,620,000	4,250,000	283,000	66,632

*Data on players' salaries come from many sources, but I try to be accurate. Average salaries before 1971 are estimates because players' associations did not exist and teams had notoriously inconsistent payroll data.

†This is median annual income for families—that is, households consisting of parents and children. Half of all families fall above the median, and half fall below it. Data are from the U.S. Census; figures for 1950 and 2015 are estimates based on trends (http://www.census.gov/hhes/www/income/data/historical/families/).

‡Estimate based on the salary cap and stated salaries based on years in the league and the round in which players were drafted.

2. The extent to which teams can share revenues with one another
3. Salary limits for rookies signing their first pro contract, salary restrictions for veteran players, and minimum salary levels for all players
4. The conditions under which players can become free agents and the rights of those who are free agents
5. A salary cap that sets the maximum player payroll for teams and a formula determining the fines that an owner must pay if the team's payroll exceeds the cap
6. A total team salary floor that sets the minimum payroll for each team in a league
7. The conditions under which players or teams can request an outside arbitrator to determine the fairness of an existing or proposed contract
8. Changes in the rules of the game

Each of these issues can be contentious in CBA negotiations, or even before a CBA is up for renewal.

If owners don't like the terms of a current CBA and the players' association refuses to talk with them about changes, the owners may use a **lockout**, or *an employer-imposed work stoppage* that, in the case of professional sports, suspends all games and practices until the dispute is resolved and the CBA is revised to the owners' satisfaction. If players don't like the terms of a current CBA and the owners refuse to talk with them, the players may call a **strike**, which is *a work stoppage in which employees refuse to work until a labor dispute is resolved,* and in the case of sports, players agree to sign a new CBA.

Strikes or lockouts occur in either of two situations: (a) when business conditions change to the point that owners or players decide that the existing CBA is no longer fair or reasonable, and (b) when a CBA has expired and the owners and players cannot come to an agreement. Back when players had low salaries and little control over working conditions in their sport, strikes were more likely than lockouts. But now that players have legal leverage as they negotiate their salaries and have been able to control important aspects of their working conditions through CBAs, strikes have become very rare.

At the same time, as corporations and outside investors have become team owners, they seek high investment returns and predictability in their financial projections and feel that they must have more control over players' salaries and benefits. Additionally, they generally detest players' associations because they are much like labor unions. One of owners' strategies has been to request that certain parts of an existing CBA be renegotiated because there are new issues that they face. But if players are happy with the existing CBA, they are not interested in talking about anything with owners.

The result of this situation is that owners have imposed lockouts on players, which means that there are no more games or practices, and players receive no paychecks. NHL owners locked out players in 2004–2005 and 2012–2013; NBA owners locked out players in 2011, as did NFL owners. The owners know that they can outlast the players through a work stoppage. They are independently wealthy and will take short-term losses for long-term gains. The players, on the other hand, have short careers and must take advantage of their youth while they have it. A season-long lockout would mean a 15 to 33 percent loss of sport career lifetime income for each player; for the owners, it's a minor blip in their investment portfolios. Additionally, the owners know that younger, lower-paid players have different contract concerns than highly paid stars, and this will eventually erode unity among the players. Then the owners can make a deal that favors themselves.

The issues in each of the owner-imposed lockouts over the recent past have been different, but in each case the owners wanted to keep a larger share of revenues and give players less. They also wanted lower "caps," or payroll limits for each team so they could pay players less and give teams in the smaller markets a better chance to compete more successfully with wealthier teams in larger markets. The owners also wanted to limit when and how players become free agents, because free agency forces them

to compete with each other when trying to sign good players to contracts. Unregulated free agency gives leverage to the players, and owners don't like that kind of "free-market" situation. Finally, the owners usually want the CBA to contain limits on what they pay top players on their teams. This makes it easier for them to negotiate deals without paying what the players might receive from other teams. In general, the owners don't want to spend more than 40 to 50 percent of total revenues on players' salaries and benefits. Ideally, they'd like to keep 60 percent or more of all revenues so there would be plenty of money left over after they pay all the bills. At this point, most players in the big spectator sports think they should be entitled to 50 cents of every dollar of revenue that is collected by the league and teams. Through the recent lockouts the owners have succeeded in pushing the players' percentage lower. Future lockouts will indicate how low they can force the share of revenues going to players.

As opposed to athletes in high-revenue sports, athletes in most minor leagues and lower-revenue sports have few rights and little control over their careers. The players at this level far outnumber players in the top levels of professional sports, and they often work for low pay under uncertain conditions, and with few rights. Owners almost always have the last word in these sports, although the owners don't usually make large amounts of money.

Legal Status: Individual Sports   The legal status of professional athletes in individual sports varies greatly from sport to sport and even from one athlete to another. Although there are important differences between boxing, bowling, golf, tennis, auto racing, rodeo, horse racing, track-and-field, skiing, biking, and a number of recently professionalized alternative and action sports, a few generalizations can be made.

The legal status of athletes in individual sports largely depends on what athletes must do to train and qualify for competitions. For example, few athletes can afford to pay for all the training needed to develop professional-level skills in a sport. Furthermore, they don't have the knowledge or connections to meet the formal requirements to become an official competitor in their sport, which may include having a recognized agent or manager (as in boxing), being formally accepted by other participants (as in most auto racing), obtaining membership in a professional organization (as in most bowling, golf, and tennis tournaments), or gaining a special invitation through an official selection group (as in pro track-and-field meets).

Whenever athletes need sponsors to pay for training or agents to help them meet participation requirements, their legal status is shaped by the contracts they sign with these people and then with the organizations that regulate participation. This is why the legal status of athletes in individual sports varies so widely.

Let's use boxing as an example. Because many boxers come from low-income backgrounds, they lack the resources to develop high-level boxing skills and arrange official bouts with other boxers. They must have trainers, managers, and sponsors, and the support of these people always comes with conditions that are written in formal contracts or based on informal agreements. In either case, boxers must forfeit control over much of their lives and a portion of the rewards they may earn in future bouts. This means that few boxers have much control over their careers, even when they win large amounts of prize money. They are forced to trade control over their bodies and careers for the opportunity to continue boxing. This is an example of how class relations operate in sports: when people lack resources, they are limited in the ways they can negotiate the conditions under which their sport careers occur.

The legal status of athletes in certain individual sports is defined in the bylaws of professional organizations such as the Professional Golf Association (PGA), the Ladies' Professional Golf Association (LPGA), the Association of Tennis Professionals (ATP), and the Professional Rodeo Cowboys Association (PRCA). When athletes play a role in controlling these organizations, the policies support athletes' rights and enable them to manage the conditions under which they compete. Without such

SIDELINES

(*Source:* By permission of William Whitehead)

Help me, Doc! I make $20 million a year, and I don't feel guilty."

Most athletes generate revenues that match their salaries or prize money. Like other entertainers, a few of them benefit from national and international media exposure. Sport events are now marketed in connection with the celebrity status and lifestyles of high-profile athlete-entertainers.

organizations, athletes in these sports would have few rights as workers.

Income: Team Sports   Despite publicity given to the supercontracts of some athletes in the top professional leagues, salaries vary widely across the levels and divisions of professional team sports. For example, in 2013, there were about 3500 minor league baseball players on 176 teams in North America, and they made from $150 a game at the lowest levels to a high of about $75,000 per year at the top minor league level. The same was true in minor league hockey, where there were at least 2000 players in 2013. The average salary in the nine-team Canadian Football League was about $100,000 but the median salary was half that amount.

Major League Soccer in the United States had an average salary of $115,000 in 2013, but 30 percent of the players made less than $18,000 per year. In the Major Lacrosse League (outdoor) and National League Lacrosse (indoor), average salaries were about $13,000 and $15,400, respectively; and the *most* an NLL player could make was $27,948. The average salary in the Arena Football League was increased to $85,000 in 2013. WNBA players averaged about $52,000 per season, with a $34,500 minimum for rookies and $95,000 maximum for veterans. In most cases, being a professional athlete in team sports continues to be a seasonal job with few benefits and little or no career security.

To understand the range of incomes in pro sports, consider that in recent seasons the total salaries of 15 percent of MLB players have been about the same as the total salaries of the other 85 percent of players. This is why the average—or *mean*—salary in Major League Baseball was about $4.2 million per year, whereas the median salary is less than one-third that amount at $1.2 million per year. The big salaries for a few players drive up the average for the entire league.

Mega-salaries in men's professional team sports did not exist before the 1980s. The data in Table 11.1 show that players' average salaries have grown far beyond median family income in the United States. For example, players in 1950 had salaries not much higher than median family income at that time. In 2012–2013, the average NBA salary was nearly eighty times greater than the median family income!

The dramatic increase in salaries at the top level of pro sports since 1980 can be attributed to two factors: (1) changes in the legal status and rights of players, which have led to free agency and the use of a salary arbitration process, and (2) increased revenues, especially through the sale of media rights, flowing to leagues and owners (see Chapter 12). Data in Table 11.1 show that the increases in player salaries correspond closely with court decisions and labor agreements that changed the legal status of athletes and gave them bargaining power in contract negotiations with team owners.

Income: Individual Sports   As with team sports, publicity is given to the highest-paid athletes in individual sports. However, the reality is that many players in these sports don't make enough money from tournament winnings to pay all their expenses

and support themselves comfortably. Many golfers, tennis players, bowlers, track-and-field athletes, auto and motorcycle racers, rodeo riders, figure skaters, and others must carefully manage their money so that they don't spend more than they win as they travel from event to event. When tournament winnings are listed in the newspaper, nothing is said about the expenses for hotels, food, and transportation or about other expenses for coaches, agents, managers, and various support people. The top money winners don't worry about these expenses, but most athletes in individual sports are not big money winners.

The majority of men and women playing professional tennis, golf, and other individual sports do not make enough prize money to pay their training and travel expenses each year, although many have sponsors that subsidize them. Some athletes with sponsors may be under contract to share their winnings with them. The sponsors/investors cover expenses during the lean years but then take a percentage of prize money if and when the athletes win matches or tournaments.

Sponsorship agreements cause problems for professional athletes in many individual sports. Being contractually tied, for example, to an equipment manufacturer or another sponsor often puts athletes in a state of dependency. They may not have the freedom to choose when or how often they will compete, and sponsors may require them to attend social functions, at which they talk with fan-consumers, sign autographs, and promote products.

Overall, a few athletes in individual sports have large incomes, whereas most others struggle to cover expenses. Only when sport events are broadcast on television can athletes compete for major prize money and earn large incomes, unless they are amateurs or have not bargained for their rights as workers.

Amateur Athletes in Commercial Sports

The term, **amateur**, can mean many things, but it is used here to refer to *athletes whose eligibility requires that they make no money from their athletic*

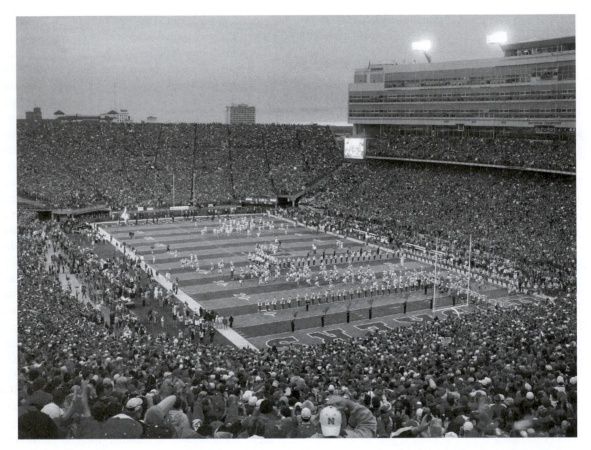

The NCAA strictly limits rewards received by college athletes, even those who generate millions of dollars of income for their universities and the NCAA. A ticket to this University of Nebraska football game costs the same as a ticket to an NFL game, but players receive only "in-kind" rewards for tuition and basic living expenses. When universities profit from big-time football and men's basketball, it's only because they have access to cheap athletic labor. (*Source:* © Bobak Ha'Eri)

performances or in connection with their status as an athlete. In the past, the IOC and the NGBs of many sports required all competitors to be amateurs. But this became increasingly impractical as national and international athletes trained full time. Keeping the amateur requirement would exclude anyone who didn't come from a wealthy background. So the IOC and other sport organizations changed their rules.

The only amateur athletes in the Olympics today are boxers and wrestlers. Allowing professionals to compete in these two sports is seen as a safety issue, so the amateur requirement has been

retained. All other Olympic athletes may compete for prize money and work in sports, which had been prohibited for most of the twentieth century.

Apart from sport governing bodies like the U.S. Golf Association and the U.S. Tennis Association that continue to sponsor official tournaments for amateurs, the only sport governing bodies that use an amateur status eligibility requirement are the Amateur Athletic Association (AAU) and the National Collegiate Athletic Association (NCAA).

The AAU has a long history of sport sponsorship, but today it focuses mostly on youth sports.

It continues to exist only because it signed in 1994 a thirty-year cooperative deal with Walt Disney World Resort. The deal specified that the AAU would hold most of its national championships in over 25 different youth sports at the Wide World of Sports facilities in Lake Buena Vista, Florida. These facilities are located next to Disney World, which meant that as tens of thousands of young athletes came to national AAU tournaments, they would be escorted by families that would turn the trip into a vacation and spend extra days and much money at Disney World. When Disney merged with Capital Cities/ABC in 1995 and acquired the upstart ESPN in the deal, the AAU had another new partner.

This symbiotic relationship between the non-profit AAU and the for-profit Walt Disney Company (and ESPN) was a major marketing triumph for both organizations. The AAU relocated its headquarters to Lake Buena Vista and now holds over 40 national tournaments at the ESPN Wide World of Sports complex. This gave new programming opportunities the young ESPN; it also enabled them to track young athletes and develop storylines for those who might be successful in the future, and it gave them a golden opportunity to recruit new ESPN viewers/subscribers at a young age. Disney World benefitted from the tourism generated by the tournaments and the AAU leaders had new headquarters, an attractive marketing position, and financial security. As they have recruited young athletes and youth sport teams into their organization, families have spent untold millions of dollars as their children have played in what are hyped as national championships year after year after year. This, of course, is a new monetized version of amateurism in which people can generate massive revenues under the cover of non-profit organizations that operate with and like businesses.

This pattern also exists in the NCAA although most NCAA Division III institutions and many Division II institutions are truly amateur. Eligibility for all NCAA sports requires amateur status. This generally means that athletes cannot have played any sport in which they received cash or

in-kind rewards and they cannot have worked in a job where they were hired for their sport skills. However, the NCAA has changed the meaning of amateur many times in its history, especially as it applies to athletes in the Division I revenue-producing sports of football, men's basketball (Schneider, 2011; Zimbalist and Sack, 2013). These changes have been justified in various and sometimes contradictory terms, but they have been made primarily to retain control over athletes while avoiding the charge that big-time college sport programs are using a professional business model and, therefore, should pay players cash salaries and pay taxes on the income made by profit-generating teams (Huma and Staurowsky, 2011, 2012). In fact, it takes 40 bylaws to define "amateur status" in the NCAA rule book, because it is difficult to make sense of amateurism in connection with teams and athletic programs operated as businesses but described as non-profit educational activities.

A recent study by Ramogi Huma and Ellen Staurowsky (2011) found that if football and men's basketball players at 121 universities in the Football Bowl Subdivision (FBS) of the NCAA in 2010 were compensated according to their fair market value (that is, relative to the money they generate), they would "be worth approximately $121,048 and $265,027 respectively for each year they played (not counting individual commercial endorsement deals). This means that collectively those players are annually denied about $1.5 billion of their "fair market value," according to the computations of Huma and Staurowsy (2012)—or about $6 billion over four years. Instead, they received scholarships providing living expenses that, on average, left them living about $3000 or more below the federal poverty line" (Huma and Staurowski, 2011, p. 4). At the same time, their head coaches were making $3.5 million annually, not counting bonuses.

As amateurs, college athletes lack power to negotiate the conditions of their sport participation. Even in revenue-producing college sports, they have few rights and no formal means of filing complaints when they've been treated unfairly or denied the right to play their sports. The athletes are not allowed to share the revenues that they may generate and have had no control over how their skills, names, and images can be used by the university or the NCAA.

Many college athletes recognize that they lack rights, but it has been difficult for them to lobby for changes. Challenging universities or the NCAA in court is expensive and would take years of a young person's life. Forming an athletes' organization might make it possible to bargain for rights, but bringing together athletes from many campuses and sports would require resources that athletes don't have. As a result many college athletes are in a dependent status and under the control of their coaches and athletic departments.

Although the NCAA now allows its Division I member institutions to award multiple year scholarships and adjust scholarship amounts to cover the full cost of attending a particular university, it continues to require that athletes remain amateurs. The NCAA resists defining college athletes as employees, which would change the entire landscape of college sports in the United States.

summary

WHAT ARE THE CHARACTERISTICS OF COMMERCIAL SPORTS?

Commercial sports are visible parts of many societies today. They grow and prosper best in urban, industrial, and post-industrial nations with relatively efficient transportation and communications systems, a standard of living that allows people the time and money to play and watch sports, and a culture that emphasizes consumption and material status symbols.

Spectator interest in commercial sports is based on a combination of a quest for excitement, ideologies emphasizing success, the existence of youth sport programs, and media coverage that introduces people to the rules of sports and the athletes who play them.

The recent worldwide growth of commercial sports has been fueled by sport organizations seeking global markets and corporations using sports as vehicles for global capitalist expansion. This growth will continue as long as it serves the interests of multinational corporations. As it does, sports, sport facilities, sport events, and athletes are branded with corporate logos and ideological messages promoting consumption and dependence on corporations for excitement and pleasure.

Commercialization leads to changes in the internal structure and goals of certain sports, the orientations of people involved in sports, and the people and organizations that control sports. Rules are changed to make events more fan-friendly. People in sports, especially athletes, emphasize heroic orientations over aesthetic orientations and use style and dramatic expression to impress mass audiences. Overall, commercial sports are packaged as total entertainment experiences for spectators, mostly for the benefit of spectators who lack technical knowledge about the games or events they're watching.

Commercial sports are unique businesses. At the minor league level, they generate modest revenues for owners and sponsors. However, team owners at the top levels of professional sports have formed cartels to generate significant revenues. Like event sponsors and promoters, team owners are involved with commercial sports to make money while having fun and establishing good public images for themselves or their corporations and corporate products and policies. Their cartels enable them to control costs, stifle competition, and increase revenues, especially those coming from the sale of broadcasting rights to media companies. Profits also are enhanced by public support and subsidies, often associated with tax breaks and the construction and operation of stadiums and arenas.

It is ironic that North American professional sports often are used as models of democracy and free enterprise when, in fact, their success has been built on carefully planned autocratic control and monopolistic business practices. In practical terms, these team owners have effectively eliminated free-market competition in their sport businesses and used public money and facilities to increase their wealth and power.

The administration and control of amateur commercial sports rest in the hands of numerous sport organizations. Although these organizations exist to support the training and competition of amateur athletes, their primary goal is to control both athletes and revenues generated through membership fees, tournaments, sponsorships, and donations. Those with the most money and influence usually win the power struggles in amateur sports, and athletes seldom have the resources to promote their interests in these struggles. Corporate sponsors are now a major force in amateur sports, and their goals strongly influence what happens in them.

Commercialization transforms athletes into entertainers. Because athletes generate revenues through their performances, issues related to players' rights and their fair share of revenues generated by their performances are very important. As rights and revenues have increased, so have players' incomes. Media coverage and the rights fees paid by media companies have been key in this process.

Most athletes in professional sports do not make vast sums of money. Players outside the top men's sports and golf and tennis for women have incomes that are surprisingly low. Income among amateur athletes is limited by the rules of governing bodies in particular sports.

Intercollegiate athletes in the United States have what amounts to a regulated maximum wage in the form of athletic scholarships, which many people see as unfair when some athletes generate millions of dollars of revenue for their universities. In other amateur sports, athletes may receive direct cash payments for performances and endorsements, and some receive support from the organizations to which they belong, but relatively few make large amounts of money.

The structure and dynamics of commercial sports vary from nation to nation. Commercial sports in most of the world have not generated the massive revenues associated with a few high-profile, heavily televised sports in North America, Australia, Western Europe, and parts of Latin America and eastern Asia. Profits for owners and promoters around the world depend on supportive relationships with the media, large corporations, and governments. These relationships have shaped the character of all commercial sports, professional and amateur.

The commercial model of sports is not the only one that might provide athletes and spectators with enjoyable and satisfying experiences. However, because most people are unaware of alternative models, they continue to express a desire for what they get, even when it is largely determined by the interests of people with wealth and power. Therefore, changes will occur only when spectators and people in sports develop visions for what sports could and should look like if they were not shaped so much by the economic interests of wealthy and powerful people and people hoping to become wealthy and powerful.

SUPPLEMENTAL READINGS

Reading 1. Women's professional team sports can't get traction
Reading 2. Turning spectacle into sport: Mixed martial arts
Reading 3. Red Bull and high-energy sports
Reading 4. Why business and political leaders love new stadiums
Reading 5. Franchise values and making money in professional sports
Reading 6. A tale of two hockey lockouts

SPORT MANAGEMENT ISSUES

• You are in a sport studies course that has students from multiple countries. They ask you what is needed to develop successful commercial sports in a country. Outline the major points that you will make when talking with them, and explain those points in a way that will make sense to people from social and cultural backgrounds that are different than your background.
• Powerful and wealthy people in a country undergoing economic expansion want to create a high level of spectator interest in sports throughout their society. They hire you to

survey the sociology of sport to discover how to create spectator interests. Using material in this chapter, what do you tell them?

- You live in a large city that has been undergoing a steady process of social and economic decline. The state has made $300 million available to build a new arena for the professional hockey team in the city. You have been asked to discuss whether this is a good use of public money. City leaders say that a new arena and a successful hockey team will revitalize the city and create a supportive context for development. You are asked to agree or disagree and to explain your answer.

- You are the athletic director for a large private high school in your community. The school is facing a budget crisis that affects your sport programs. The local soft-drink distributor tells you that his company will give you $50,000 a year if he can put his drink logo on the scoreboard and in a dozen other places in the sport facilities and put soft-drink machines in the locker rooms. He also wants you and the coaches to do a local commercial for his company. The principal and parent board say it is your decision. Now you must explain to them what you've decided. Outline the points you will make to them.

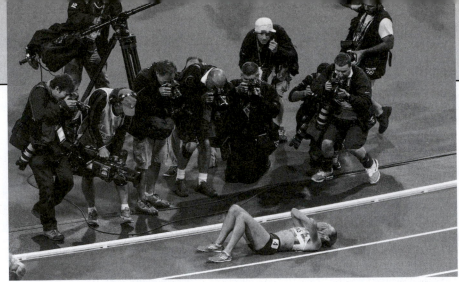

(*Source*: © PCN/Corbis)

SPORTS AND THE MEDIA

Could They Survive Without Each Other?

. . . we're in other businesses besides the business of winning baseball games. . . . We're a media and entertainment company, not just a sports team.

—**Larry Baer, San Francisco Giants president & CEO (in Costa, 2015)**

We are entering a time of commercial and policy confusion for sports broadcast and advertising. . . . The supplementation, augmentation, or replacement of broadcast sports is a generational time bomb.

—**Brett Hutchins, 2015 (in McHugh et al., 2015)**

The NFL and the networks don't want us to experience football as a game, but as a hyper-real production of a game, in the way war movies are hyper-real versions of war.

—**David Zweig, writer and musician (2012)**

Sports is a stealth definer of social values, particularly among young people, and ESPN, the self-described World Wide Leader, is sports's 24/7 purveyor on countless radio stations, TV channels and websites.

—**Robert Lipsyte, sports journalist (2015)**

Learning Objectives

- Identify the major forms of media, what they provide to people, and the influence of commercial forces on media content.

- Discuss whether and how new media, including the Internet, change sport spectator experiences.

- Identify factors that influence the images and narratives presented in the media.

- Discuss how sports and the media depend on each other for commercial success.

- Identify major trends in televised sports and media rights fees.

- Identify economic and ideological factors that influence relationships between sports and the media.

- Explain why corporations that sell alcohol, tobacco, soft drinks, confectionery products (candy), and fast foods are likely to sponsor sports in the media.

- Identify ideological themes around which the media coverage of sports is constructed.

- Describe the major differences in the ways that men and women and blacks and whites are represented in media images and narratives.

- Discuss research findings on audience experiences and the media impact on sport-related behaviors, such as active participation, game attendance, and gambling.

- Identify the factors that influence relationships between sports journalists and athletes.

Mass media, local media, and social media pervade our cultures and our lives. Although each of us incorporates media into our lives in different ways, the things we read, hear, and see in the media are increasingly crucial parts of our experience. They frame and influence many of our thoughts, conversations, decisions, and actions.

We use media images and narratives as we evaluate ourselves, give meaning to other people and events, form ideas, and envision the future. This does *not* mean that we are slaves to the media or passive dupes of those who produce and present media content to us. The media don't tell us *what* to think, but they greatly influence what we *think about* and, therefore what we discuss in everyday conversations. Additionally, our experiences are clearly informed by media content, and if the media didn't exist, our lives would be different.

The Internet and social media have added a new layer to our media experiences. They enable us to go beyond consumption and create images and narratives that we incorporate into our thoughts and actions. But this doesn't occur automatically, nor does it empower us unless we use new media in strategic and informed ways to build relationships and change the world around us.

Sports and the media are interconnected parts of our lives. Sports provide content for all forms of media, and many sports depend on the media for publicity and revenues. To better understand these interconnections, five questions are considered in this chapter:

1. What are the characteristics of the media?
2. How are sports and media interconnected?
3. What images and messages are emphasized in media coverage of sports in the United States?
4. How are media involved in our sport participation and consumption?
5. What are the implications of new media for sport journalism and sportscasting?

CHARACTERISTICS OF THE MEDIA

Revolutionary changes are occurring in the media. The media landscape is changing rapidly and dramatically. Personal computers, the Internet, wireless technology, and mobile communication devices have propelled us into a transition from an era of sponsored and programmed mass media into an era of multifaceted, on-demand, interactive, and personalized media content and experiences; in fact, the time spent each day watching traditional TV is now surpassed by digital media consumption (Hu, 2013). The pace and implications of this transition are influencing our personal and social lives.

Although it's important to discuss new trends and explain what may occur in the future, it is important to understand traditional media and their connections with sports.

Media research in the past often distinguished between print and electronic media. **Print media** included *newspapers, magazines, fanzines, books, catalogues, event programs,* and even *trading cards*—words and images on paper. **Electronic media** included *radio, television, and film.* But video games, the Internet, smartphones, tablets, and online publications have nearly eliminated the dividing line between these media forms.

Today, media provide *information, interpretation, entertainment,* and *opportunities for interactivity and content production.* When media content is provided for commercial purposes, entertainment is emphasized more than information, interpretation, or opportunities for interactivity and content production. In the process, media consumers become commodities sold to advertisers with the primary goal of promoting lifestyles based on consumption.

The media also put us in touch with information, experiences, people, images, and ideas outside the realm of our everyday, real-time lives. But most media content is edited and "re-presented" to us by others—producers, editors, program directors, programmers, camerapersons, writers, journalists, commentators, sponsors, bloggers, and website providers. These people select for us information, interpretation, entertainment, and even opportunities for interactivity to achieve one or more of five goals: (1) make financial profits; (2) influence cultural values and social organization; (3) provide a public service; (4) enhance personal status and reputation; and (5) express themselves creatively or politically.

Commercial forms of sports and traditional media have always had a close relationship. Long before television, newspapers provided sports information, interpretation, and entertainment. Radio did the same. When television began to show people video images of the action, newspapers and radio, including sportswriters and announcers, were forced to change their approach to maintain sales and ratings. There are similar challenges for traditional media today as they compete with on-demand, interactive digital programming as well as privately produced content.

Power and Control in Sports Media

In nations where mass media are privately owned, the dominant goals are to make profits and to distribute content that promotes the ideas and beliefs of people in positions of power and influence. These aren't the only goals, but they are the most influential. Years ago, media expert Michael Real explained that there was no greater force in the construction of media sport reality than "commercial television and its institutionalized value system [emphasizing] profit making, sponsorship, expanded markets, commodification, and competition" (1998, p. 17).

Of course, as the Internet and wireless technology extend content and access, media sport reality is now being constructed in diverse ways. This can be a contentious process as corporations and powerful interest groups attempt to control online access and content. The resulting struggle is a crucial feature of contemporary social worlds.

In nations where mass media are controlled primarily by the state, the primary goals are to influence cultural values and social organization and provide a public service (Lund, 2007). However, state control has steadily declined as media companies have been privatized and deregulated, and as more individuals obtain online access to information, interpretation, entertainment, and opportunities for interactivity and content production.

Power relations in a society influence the priority given to the five goals that drive media content. Those who make content decisions for mass media programming act as filters as they select and create the images and messages to present. In the filtering and presentation process, these people usually emphasize images and narratives consistent with ideologies that support their interests in addition to attracting large audiences. As deregulation and private ownership have increased, the media have become hypercommercialized and media content focuses more on consumption, individualism, competition, and class inequality as natural and necessary in society. Seldom included in the content of commercial media is an emphasis on civic values, conservation, anticommercial activities, and progressive political action. In fact, when groups with anticommercial messages want to buy commercial time on television, media corporations and networks have refused to sell it to them.

There are exceptions to this pattern, but when people use mass media to challenge dominant ideologies, they often encounter difficulties. This discourages transformational programming and leads people to censor media content in ways that defer to the interests of the powerful.

We saw this in 2013 when ESPN withdrew from a partnership with PBS (the Public Broadcasting System) on a *Frontline* program investigating the NFL's handling of head injuries (Miller and Belson, 2013; Sandomir, 2013a). The two-part program, "League of Denial: The NFL's Concussion Crisis," had just been completed when the NFL commissioner met the president of ESPN for lunch. Soon after, ESPN announced it was no longer associated with the *Frontline* program, even though two of its top reporters continued work on the project. Both organizations denied that the $15.2 billion media rights contract between the NFL and ESPN had been the reason ESPN disassociated itself from the PBS program. However, ESPN reporters received a clear message: censor yourself, or others will do it for you when your news reporting could jeopardize income from entertainment programming (Zirin, 2013e).

This does not mean that those who control the media ignore the truth and "force" media audiences to read, hear, and see things unrelated to reality or their interests. But it does mean that, apart from content that individuals create online, average people influence the media only through consumption and program ratings. Therefore, the public receives edited information, interpretation, entertainment, and interactive experiences that are constructed primarily to boost

> Ten years ago, if you wanted to connect with fans, you had to go through a newspaper. Now we connect with them directly and immediately.
>
> —Patrick Smyth, director of media relations, Denver Broncos (in Klemko, 2011)

profits and maintain a business and political climate in which commercial media can thrive. In the process, people who control media are concerned with what attracts readers, listeners, and viewers within the legal limits set by government agencies and the preference parameters of individuals and corporations that buy advertising time. As they make programming decisions, they see audiences as collections of consumers that can be sold to advertisers.

In the case of sports, those who control media decide not only which sports and events to cover but also the images and commentary presented in the coverage. When they do this, they play an important role in constructing the overall frameworks that people in media audiences use to define and incorporate sports in their lives (Albergotti, 2011; Boyle, 2014; Bruce, 2013; Dart, 2012; Rowe, 2009, 2013; Wenner, 2013; Zweig, 2012).

(Source: © Frederic A. Eyer)

"Quick! Bring the camera—the viewers will love this crash!"

Commercial media representations of sports are carefully selected and edited. Commentary and images highlight dramatic action, even when it's a minor part of an event.

Media Representations of Sports

Most people don't think critically about media content (Bruce, 2013). For example, when we watch sports on television, we don't often notice that the images and commentary we see and hear have been carefully presented to create engaging narratives, heighten the dramatic content of the event, and emphasize prevailing ideologies in American society, especially those that reaffirm the interests of sponsors as well as the media companies. The pregame analysis, the camera coverage, the camera angles, the close-ups, the slow-motion shots, the attention given to particular athletes, the announcers' play-by-play descriptions, the color commentary, the quotes from athletes, the postgame summary and analysis, and all associated website content are presented to entertain media audiences and keep sponsors happy. In some cases, sport leagues and their governing bodies hire their own writers and commentators to produce media content, or they deny press credentials to journalists who present content that sport officials don't like (Jennings, 2010).

Sport media commentaries and images in the United States highlight action, competition, aggression, hard work, individual heroism and achievement, playing despite pain, teamwork, and competitive outcomes. Television coverage has become so seamless in its representations of sports that we often define televised games as "real" games—more real than what is seen in person at the stadium. Longtime magazine editor Kerry Temple explains:

> It's not just games you're watching. It's soap operas, complete with story lines and plots and plot twists. And good guys and villains, heroes and underdogs. And all this gets scripted into cliffhanger morality plays. . . . And you get all caught up in this until you begin to believe it really matters (1992, p. 29).

Temple's point is especially relevant today. The focus on profits has increased soap opera storytelling as a means of developing and maintaining audience interest in commercial media sports coverage. Sports programming is now "a never-ending series of episodes—the results of one game create implications for the next one (or next week's) to be broadcast" (Wittebols, 2004, p. 4). Sports rivalries are hyped and used to serialize stories through and across seasons; conflict and chaos are highlighted with a predictable cast of "good guys," "bad guys," and "redemption" or "comeback" stories; and the story lines are designed to reproduce ideologies favored by upper-middle-class media consumers—the ones that corporate sponsors want to reach with their ads. This was apparent in NBC's regular references to athletes' mothers during the 2008 and 2012 Olympic Games. This narrative was planned to fit nicely with Proctor and Gamble's "Thank you, Mom" ad campaign that the company created after it became a $100-million sponsor of the Olympics and paid NBC many millions of dollars for commercial time during the games. It is likely that people at NBC have positive attitudes about mothers, but they had other reasons for making them a centerpiece in the Olympic coverage.

Even though media coverage of sports is carefully edited and represented in total entertainment packages, most of us believe that when we see a sport event on television, we are seeing it "the way it is." We don't usually think that what we see, hear, and read is a series of narratives and images selected for particular reasons and grounded in the social worlds and interests of those producing the event and controlling the broadcast. Television coverage provides only one of many possible sets of images and narratives related to an event, and there are many images and messages that audiences do *not* receive (Galily, 2014). If we went to an event in person, we would see something quite different from the images selected and presented on television, and we would develop our own descriptions and interpretations, which would be different from those carefully presented by media commentators.

New York Times writer Robert Lipsyte (1996) described televised sports as "–sportainment"—the equivalent of a TV movie that purports to be based on a true story but actually provides fictionalized history. In other words, television constructs sports and viewer experiences. But the process occurs so smoothly that most television viewers believe they experience sports in a "true and natural" form. This, of course, is the goal of the directors, editors, and on-camera announcers who select images and narratives, frame them with the stories they wish to tell, and make sure they please sponsors in the process.

To illustrate this point, think about this question: What if all televised sports were sponsored by environmental groups, women's organizations, and labor unions? Would program content be different from what it is now? Would the political biases built into the images and commentary be the same as they are now? It is unlikely that they would be the same, and we would be quick to identify all the ways that the interests and political agendas of the environmentalists, feminists, or labor leaders influenced images, narratives, and overall program content.

Now think about this: Capitalist corporations sponsor nearly 100 percent of all sports programming in commercial media, and their goals are to create compulsive consumers loyal to capitalism and generate profits for themselves and their shareholders. Says media scholar Lawrence Wenner (2013): "The economic influences of media have changed sport, changed our associations with it, and have affected the stories that are told through sport, both in everyday communication and in the service of commerce." For those who are "tuned in" to the commercial media, their experiences as spectators are heavily influenced—that is, "mediated"—by the decisions of those who control programming and media representations.

New Media and Sports

New media, including all digital and social media, radically alter relationships in the production and consumption of accessible content related to sports worldwide. They make possible individually created and selected information, interpretation, and entertainment. Additionally, online interactivity enables people to bypass the gatekeepers of content in the "old" media—that is, journalists, editors, and commentators—as they construct their own interpretations of events, athletes, and the overall organization of sports (McHugh et al., 2015).

In the case of sports, the recent proliferation of mobile devices and growing connectivity change the way many of us access and respond to sport media content. Additionally, many people now have the ability to produce and distribute sport content and commentary. We can interact with fellow fans, ask questions of players and coaches, follow them on twitter, identify scores and statistics, and play online games that either simulate sports or are associated with real-time sport events around the world. This transforms media experiences and mediated realities in dramatic ways (Antunovic and Hardin, 2013a, 2013b; Clavio, 2010; Gantz and Lewis, 2014; Hutchins and Rowe, 2009; Liu and Berkowitz, 2013; MacKay and Dallaire, 2013; McCarthy, 2012; Norman, 2012, 2014).

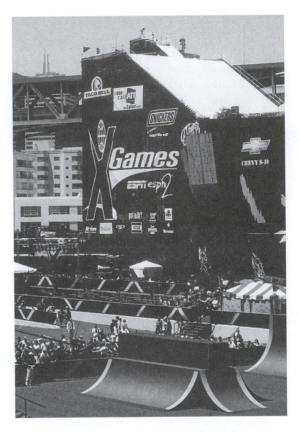

The X Games were created by ESPN. ESPN is owned by ABC. ABC is owned by the Walt Disney Company. The power behind the X Games makes it difficult for the athletes to maintain the culture of their sports on their terms. (*Source:* © Becky Beal)

New Media Consumption   Although people often access online sport content to complement content they consume in traditional media, there is a growing number of others who use new media to replace traditional content (McHugh et al., 2015). This shift in consumption patterns concerns people in media companies that broadcast live sports worldwide, because their revenues in the past have depended on controlling this content and maintaining large audiences to sell to advertisers.

At the same time, sport organizations such as MLB, the NFL, the English Premier Football (Soccer) Division, and others have become more active in managing media representations of their sports so they can directly control information, analysis, and entertainment to promote themselves on their terms. For example, MLB.com offers a $130 per year subscription to access real-time coverage of all regular season games on multiple devices. The site also provides game previews, highlights, statistics, and general commentary, among dozens of other video, audio, and text materials on baseball. This enables MLB and other professional sports to provide media content *and* control the ways that their brands are represented.

Overall, new media allow people to control *when* and *how* they consume sports content, but this changes little from the days of traditional media when content was created by a limited number of powerful sources (Dart, 2014). The real transformational potential of new media rests in how people use them to produce content that offers alternatives to traditional media sources.

New Media Production   At the same time that corporations try to maximize control over online representations of sports, YouTube and other sites provide people opportunities to upload their own information and interpretation of sports as well as representations of sports events and performances. For example, for more than three decades now, young people in alternative and action sports have found creative ways to photograph, film, and distribute images of their activities. Photos and VCR tapes were mailed and passed person-to-person, but distribution today occurs online with images accessible worldwide. Although these images represent what may be described as "performance sports," they're central to the media experiences of many young people who find highly structured, overtly competitive sports such as baseball or football to be constraining and uncreative.

In some cases, young people use new media to represent sports involving transgressive actions such as skating in empty private swimming pools at night or doing **parkour** ("PK"), *an activity in which young men and a few young women use their bodies to move rapidly and efficiently through existing landscapes,* especially in urban areas where walls, buildings, and other obstacles normally impede movement (http://en.wikipedia.org/wiki/Parkour; www.americanparkour.com/). Research on new media representations of these activities is sorely needed. Such representations of parkour have made it a global phenomenon as young men (for the most part) have become aware of the possibility of using the physical environments around them as "sport spaces" in which they can develop skills, express themselves, and even gain widespread recognition by doing things and posting videos that catch the attention of other parkour athletes.

Researchers in many disciplines are now exploring these possibilities as the media landscape is changing in character and scope at a rate unprecedented in human history. Most of this research deals with how people use new media to complement or create informational and interpretive content related to sports already covered in mainstream media.[1] However, there also are a few studies of people using new media to report on sports ignored by mainstream media (Antunovic and Hardin, 2012, 2013, 2015; MacKay and Dallaire, 2012, 2014).

This research highlights and describes exciting possibilities, but it also identifies factors that may undermine those possibilities. Powerful corporations have a high stakes financial interest in controlling new media and using it to add to their bottom line. This includes massive, monopoly-like companies that provide connectivity; mainstream

---

[1]The major sources I've used to explore this issue are these: Boyle, 2014; Browning and Sanderson, 2012; Burroughs and Burroughs, 2011; Connolly and Dolan, 2012; Dart, 2014; Ferriter, 2009; Frederick et al., 2012; Galily, 2014; Gantz and Lewis, 2014; Hutchins, 2014; Hutchins and Rowe, 2009; Kassing and Sanderson, 2013; Kruse, 2011; Lebel and Danylchuk, 2012; Leonard, 2009; Liang, 2013; Liu and Berkowitz, 2013; Madianou and Miller, 2013; McCarthy, 2012; Merrill et al., 2012; Millington and Darnell, 2012; Norman, 2012a, 2012b; Oates and Furness, 2015; Ross, 2011; Sanderson, 2011; Sanderson and Kassing, 2011; Schultz and Sheffer, 2010; Sheffer and Schultz, 2010; Smith and Brenner, 2012; Wenner, 2014; Whannel, 2014; Zimmerman, 2012.

media companies built around newspapers, maga-zines, radio, television, and film; and sport orga-nizations that survive or prosper because of their financial relationships with mainstream media companies. Leaders in this industry are using their resources to enter the new media market, and retain and extend their control over how new media are used, who benefits from their use, and how con-tent is regulated. Therefore, they continue to lobby federal legislators on copyright law, definitions of intellectual property, public domain parameters, lia-bility laws, and a host of other issues that they can use to prevent anyone from threatening their finan-cial interests. At the same time, they extend their control by using new media in strategic ways. Fan-tasy sports and video games are examples of how they enlist people as allies to sustain their power.

The major sociological question related to new media is this: Will they democratize social life by enabling people to freely share information and ideas, or will they become tools controlled by corporations to expand their capital, increase con-sumption, reproduce ideologies that drive market economies, and maintain the illusion that we need them to provide pleasure and excitement in our lives? The answer to this question will emerge as the struggle for control over the media unfolds. At this point the struggle does not involve a fair fight, because people who will benefit from the potential democratizing effects of new media are not even aware of the fight—and the leaders of corporate media are doing all they can to keep it that way.

Fantasy Sports   Consuming sports through the media is a passive activity. People may talk with friends, respond to commentary, even yell at play-ers, coaches, and referees, but these are simply reactions to what is presented by ESPN, NBC, or other media companies. This lack of control can be frustrating to those who follow sports closely and have a deep knowledge of players, game strate-gies, and the decisions made by coaches and upper management. For people accustomed to being in positions of power and control, it can even be alienating. How can these people use what they

know about sport and feel like they are in control as they consume mediated sports? "Fantasy leagues" have become the current answer to this question.

Although the first fantasy sport league, invented in 1979 by a baseball fan, didn't require online access, most fantasy sports today are played online on platforms licensed or controlled by media and sport organizations, such as ESPN and the NFL. For example, playing fantasy football makes every participant a "team owner" who creates a team roster by taking turns with other "owners" to draft current NFL players for their fantasy teams. The weekly performance statistics of the players on an "owner's" team roster are converted into points so that each fantasy team player competes against other team "owners." Usually, all participants pay fees to one of the online services that compile players' sta-tistics, compute scores, and track team records.

Over 40 million people in the United States and Canada play fantasy sports. Players are mostly col-lege-educated white men (over 85 percent) between eighteen and fifty years old with higher-than-average incomes. Collectively, they spend over $5 billion annually to obtain data about players and compete in organized fantasy leagues. Owners typically devote six to ten hours per week consuming media sports and another three hours managing their teams dur-ing the season (FSTA, 2013; Ruihley and Billings, 2013). They also spend close to $500 per year for fees to enter a league, draft and trade players, pay the website host, collect information about players, buy prizes for the owner who wins the season, and play challenge matches with other individual team owners (like side bets during a season).

Fantasy football, baseball, NASCAR, basket-ball, hockey, and other sports transform the rela-tionship between sport media consumers and media content (Schirato, 2012). To "own" players, man-age a team, and compete against others in an offi-cial league gives consumers a sense of control over the sport they enjoy watching and the media content they consume. Media interactivity provides contact with other dedicated fans, reaffirms fan identities, and provides a forum in which status can be gained and the status of others can be challenged.

The outcomes of real games often matter little to fantasy players who focus on the performance statistics of their players, who are on many different teams. Although they often subscribe to expensive cable and satellite television "sport packages" that enable them to watch their players, they focus primarily on the performances of individuals rather than teams. While they watch, they also scout other players and take note of injuries because during the season they can cut, trade, and acquire new players on their fantasy rosters.

Fantasy sports reposition fans relative to players. For example, they can provide the white men who play them with a sense of power and control over players who are unlike them at the same time that they are connected with fellow "owners" who share their interests and backgrounds.

Fantasy league players feel empowered by their "ownership" of teams and players—but the NFL, Major League Baseball, and other sport leagues, as well as mainstream media companies, now use fantasy sports to generate new revenues and to "re-enchant" the spectator experience for those who may become bored as they passively watch games week after week, season after season.

When media executives, team owners, and players discovered in 2002 that fantasy sports increased media sport consumption and fan loyalty in addition to generating $1.5 billion annually, they decided they should control the fantasy business and merge it with their own. Over the next ten years they did just that and began to use their own fantasy league to boost loyalty and encourage consumers to buy expensive cable and satellite packages (at $60 to $100 per month depending on service providers) in which all games in the league are available to consumers.

The NFL, which now provides information for fantasy participants on its NFL Network channel, has also created an NFL RedZone channel to provide game-day *only* coverage of every NFL team whenever it is inside the opponent's 20-yard line. At a subscription cost of $5 to $10 per month, this enables fantasy league players to see every touchdown scored by every team each Sunday afternoon. Even the regular NFL announcers have changed their commentary to call attention to "the red zone," and alert viewers of impending scores so they can learn the fate of their fantasy teams.

The power to control the content of media sport and who may access it under what conditions is a crucial issue in the business plans of sport leagues and media companies, including ESPN/ABC Sports, FOX Sports Media Group (Fox Sports, and Fox Sports 1, launched in August 2013), NBC Sports, CBS Sports, and others. Sports today are global phenomena, which means that sport leagues and media companies think in terms of global power and control. The sponsors that buy commercial time on television and ad space in newspapers and websites are not interested in making deals with media companies or sport organizations unless there are guarantees that media sport programming is dedicated to supporting their products and supporting consumption as a lifestyle. This is especially true in the United States, where all sports are broadcast on commercial television. This means that the feelings of empowerment enjoyed by fantasy league participants are an illusion that is actively reproduced by the sport leagues and media companies that use fan fantasies to increase their power and profits.

Video Games as Simulated Sports   John Madden, known to football fans over the age of forty as a former NFL coach and longtime NFL commentator, is known to the under-forty-year-old game player as a video game brand. *Madden NFL* games are among the most popular video products on the market. When Madden was asked to comment on the video game craze, he said that designers have made video games that look so much like the games on television that television producers are now using special lenses and filters to make televised NFL games appear more like video games.

Game developers work with athletes so that video game situations and players' movements are lifelike. Leagues and players cooperate because they receive rights fees for the use of players' images and the NFL name and logo, but players also want to be portrayed accurately in video games. Even unique mannerisms related to their dramatic on-field personas are included in the game action.

Professional team coaches now worry that video games distract players from live games. Some NFL and NBA players prefer to play video game sports over watching live games. NASCAR, Formula One, and Indy Car video games are so realistic that some racecar drivers use the games to familiarize themselves with the tracks and prepare for the split-second responses required during actual races.

The financial stakes associated with creating realistic and entertaining games are significant. This constantly pushes designers to refine graphics, action, and game possibilities. It also leads them to talk with potential sponsors about product placements and advertisements built into the storylines and actions in the games. As more young people play these video games, corporations see them as vehicles for developing outposts in the heads of game players, fostering a commitment to consumption, and generating revenues for game producers.

A major issue for game developers is obtaining the rights to use the names and images of athletes and sport leagues in their games. *Madden NFL 13,* for example, is produced by EA Sports with permission from the NFL and the NFL Players Association, which receive rights fees from sales of the games. But this also means that everything in the game is subject to NFL approval. Midway Games, on the other hand, developed *Blitz: The League,* a video game modeled after pro football, without buying rights from the NFL. Therefore, they could not use references to the NFL or NFL players' names and images, but they could include images and actions that would not have been approved by the NFL. To heighten the dimension of spectacle in *Blitz,* they incorporated images of blood and gory injuries, near-naked cheerleaders, dirty hits, in-your-face celebrations after big plays, drug use (for energy and strength), and off-field controversies that might boost sales. But Midway Games went out of business just before its 2008 version of the game was released.

Meanwhile, a small but growing number of children are now introduced to sports through video games. For example, children who play games on Nintendo's Wii platform learn rules and game strategies as they play. They see the moves involved in a sport as they manipulate images in the games, and their initial emotional experiences in certain sports are felt in front of computer monitors or televisions rather than on playing fields.

This raises many research questions. After playing interactive video sports, will six-year-olds want to listen to whistle-blowing coaches when they're accustomed to being in complete control of players, game strategies, and game conditions? Will these children bring new forms of game knowledge to situations in which they play informal and formally organized games? How will that knowledge influence the games they play? Will some children simply stay home with their video devices and control their own games without worrying about coaches, playing time, or parental pressure?

Adult game players outnumber children who play, and the majority of players are males between the ages of twelve and thirty. Many male college students are regular game players to the point that status in certain groups reflects prowess in video gaming. Playing games also provides regular social occasions similar to those provided by live sport events, although the players set schedules for video games and can play them when they wish.

At this point, studies of simulated sports and video games indicate the following:

- Gamers often commit many hours to play (Niman, 2013).
- When they play sport-themed video games, the gamers often create their own narratives or stories that fit their interests and perceptions of sports (Crawford and Gosling, 2009).
- Social relationships are formed and nurtured in connection with video games (Hutchins et al., 2009).
- Digital gaming involves a wide range of experiences, feelings, and understandings

because it occurs on the terms desired by the gamers themselves (Crawford, 2015; Witkowski, 2012).

• Sport-themed video games involve embodied experiences different from those associated with the consumption of televised sports (Crawford, 2015).

Future research will try to answer questions such as these: Does playing video games influence how people play sports or what they expect when they play them? If children are introduced to sports through video games, will this influence their expectations and the meanings they give to experiences in live, real-time games? As new media become increasingly integrated into our everyday lives, they will influence sport participation and consumption experiences? Predicting the future is risky, but it is likely that video game experiences will carry over into real-time sports in some way.

SPORTS AND MEDIA: A TWO-WAY RELATIONSHIP

The media and commercialization are related topics in the sociology of sport. The media intensify and extend the process and consequences of commercialization. For this reason, much attention has been given to the interdependence between the media and commercialized forms of sports (Galily and Tamir, 2014). Each of these spheres influences the other, and each depends on the other for part of its popularity and commercial success.

Sports Depend on Media

People played sports long before media coverage of their events. When sports exist for participants only, there's no need to advertise games, report the action, publish results, and interpret what happened. The players already know these things, and they're the only ones who matter. It is only when sports become commercial entertainment that they depend on the media.

Commercial sports require media to provide a combination of coverage, publicity, and news. Sports promoters and team owners know the value of coverage, and they provide free access to reporters, commentators, and photographers. For example, the London Organizing Committee of the Olympic Games and Paralympic Games (LOCOG) accredited 21,000 journalists, media technicians, producers, and camera operators to cover nearly 15,000 athletes during the Olympics and Paralympics; another 6000 to 8000 were credentialed to cover nonsport aspects of the events. NBC sent 2700 people. The BBC deployed 756 staff, and the Associated Press (AP) had 200 journalists and photographers working full time during the games. This made the 2012 Olympic and Paralympic Games the most comprehensively covered event in history. Credentialed media personnel often are given comfortable seats in press boxes, access to the playing field and locker rooms, and summaries of statistics and player information. In return, promoters and owners expect and usually receive supportive media coverage.

Although commercial spectator sports depend on media, most have a special dependence on television because television companies pay for the rights to broadcast games and other events. Table 12.1 and Figure 12.1 indicate that "rights fees" provide sports with predictable, significant, and increasing sources of income. Once "rights contracts" are signed, revenues are guaranteed regardless of bad weather, injuries to key players, and the other factors that interfere with ticket sales and on-site revenue streams. Without these media rights contracts, spectator sports seldom generate much profit.

Television revenues also have greater growth potential than revenues from gate receipts. The number of seats in a stadium limits ticket sales, and ticket costs are limited by demand. But television audiences can include literally billions of viewers now that satellite technology transmits signals to most locations worldwide. For example, the IOC and sponsors of other sport megaevents seek to package the entire world into an audience that can be sold to sponsors.

Table 12.1   Escalating annual media rights fees for major commercial sports in the United States (in millions of dollars)*

Sport	1986	1991	1996	2001	2008	2015
NFL	400	900	1100	2200	3750	4950
MLB†	183	365	420	417	670	1550
NBA	30	219	275	660	765	925
NHL‡	22	38	77	120	70	200
NASCAR	3	NA	NA	412	560	683
NCAA Men's Basketball Tournament	31	143	216	216	560§	771
NCAA (all championships)	NA	NA	NA	NA	18.5	35.7**
WNBA	0	0	0	¶	¶	12

*These amounts have not been adjusted for inflation. Data come from multiple sources, and amounts change whenever new contracts are negotiated.

†Amounts for baseball do not include local television and radio rights fees negotiated by individual teams, national radio rights fees negotiated by the league, or Internet revenues received by the league from individual subscriptions paid to receive games on MLB.com.

‡Includes U.S. rights only for 2001 and 2006; there also are Canadian rights and European rights.

§Includes rights to broadcast on television, radio, and the Internet the men's basketball tournament and other championship events, excluding football.

¶Information has never been disclosed; the new contract that began in 2016 will pay $12 million annually.

**This includes the women's basketball tournament and all NCAA championships in twenty-four Division I sports each year, excluding football.

Additional reasons for increased rights fees include the following:

- The deregulation of the television industry
- A growing demand to watch certain spectator sports
- Increased connectivity with satellite and cable worldwide
- Sponsors willing to pay top prices for access to live sport audiences because commercials are seen by people rather than being skipped over in recorded programs
- The growth of ESPN and other cable channels that collect money from cable and satellite companies as well as commercial sponsors, which gives them two sources of income

These reasons have driven the increases in rights fees as shown Figure 12.1 and Table 12.1. In 1986 the NFL received $400 million in television rights fees, and in 2013 it received over $4.9 billion. Similarly, the rights fees paid to televise the 1984 Olympic Games in Los Angeles amounted to $287 million—ten times *more* than was paid to televise the 1976 Olympic Games in Montreal, and five times *less* than the $1.42 billion that will be paid to televise the 2020 Olympic Games.

This growth in television rights fees makes commercial sports more profitable for promoters and team owners and increases the attractiveness of sports as sites for national and global advertising. Increased attention allows athletes to demand higher salaries and turns a few of them into national and international celebrities, who then use their status to endorse products sold worldwide. For example, the global celebrity and endorsement value of athletes such as David Beckham, Lionel Messi, Maria Sharapova, Usain

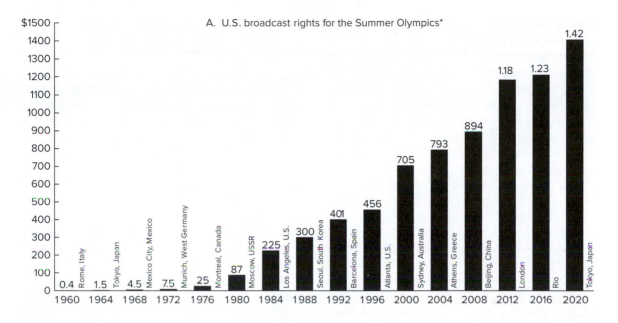

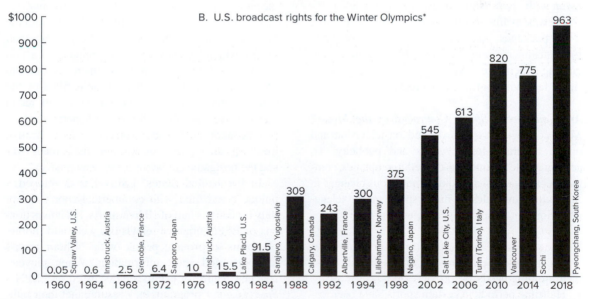

FIGURE 12.1 Escalating media rights fees paid by U.S. media companies to televise the Olympics (in millions of dollars).

*The local organizing committee for the Olympic Games also receives rights fees from other television companies around the world. Europe, Japan, and continental Asia are paying increasingly higher fees. For U.S. rights for Vancouver 2010 through the Summer Games in 2020, NBC Universal has paid the IOC $6.39 billion.

Bolt, Ronda Rousey, and Tiger Woods is primarily due to the invention of satellite television.

The rights fees in Table 12.1 do not include certain streaming rights. For example, in late 2013 the NFL signed a four-year $1 billion deal allowing games to be live-streamed on Verizon phones. But this deal did not include streaming on tablets, which will bring even more money to the NFL, and will force them to define the difference between tablets and smartphones!

The global reach of the web creates new possibilities for large corporations wanting to "teach the world" to consume. However, it also creates challenges because new corporations will compete with traditional media companies for the video rights to sports. This is why NBC developed NBCOlympics.com in 2008, a portal enabling consumers to view events in the 2008, 2010, 2012, and 2014 Olympic Games in Beijing, Vancouver, London, and Sochi, along with on-demand replays and highlights. Coverage was available on mobile devices and cable VOD packages, and other features were available for consumers interested in athlete profiles and gaming experiences. As this approach is expanded, rights fees will continue to increase.

Are Commercial Sports Controlled by the Media?

Most commercial sports depend on television and online coverage for revenues and publicity. To accommodate the interests of media companies, commercial television has required numerous changes in scheduling and rules to make sports more "telegenic." Some of these changes include the following:

- The schedules and starting times for many sport events have been altered to fit television's programming needs.
- Halftime periods in certain sports have been shortened to keep television viewers tuned to events.
- Prearranged schedules of time-outs have been added to games and matches to make time for as many commercials as possible.
- Teams, leagues, and tournaments have been formed or realigned to take advantage of

regional media markets and build national and international fan support for sports, leagues, and teams.

Other efforts to make sports entertaining for media audiences often go unnoticed. For example, the number of words used by announcers and commentators during games has nearly doubled over the past half century (Biderman, 2010a, 2010b). A former director of media relations for an NFL team notes, "Watching sports is mostly boring. Talking and speculating about sports is riveting" (Pearlman, 2011). He realizes that a typical 200-minute NFL game contains an average of 11 minutes of action and 3 minutes of video replays. That leaves 184 minutes to be filled with entertainment that keeps the audience interested. About 60 of those minutes are used by commercials, and commentators fill the rest with observations, analysis, stories, and anything that hypes the meaning and significance of the game for players, teams, owners, coaches, the city, the league, and the fans. The same is true for Major League Baseball games, which typically involve 14 minutes of action during a 150-minute game. Commercials take up 45 minutes, and the rest of the time is filled by the commentators who have studied what will retain viewers' interest. As in all mediated sports, the best commentators are the ones who can create a narrative that keeps the viewers engaged until the game is over and the postgame comments have been made.

In the United States, ESPN has developed a unique connection with commercial sports. It not only broadcasts half of all live sports, but it uses dozens of ESPN-branded television, web, and mobile platforms to provide people with 24-hour access to sports and sport information. When players, coaches, teams, or events are discussed on ESPN's *Sports Center* program, they assume that their public profiles will be enhanced. *Business Week* magazine reporter Karl Greenfield notes that 25 percent of all cable channel revenues in the United States go into ESPN, and it uses its power to shape "the ways in which leagues, teams, and athletes are packaged, promoted, marketed, and consumed by the public." He adds, "In a real sense, ESPN no longer covers

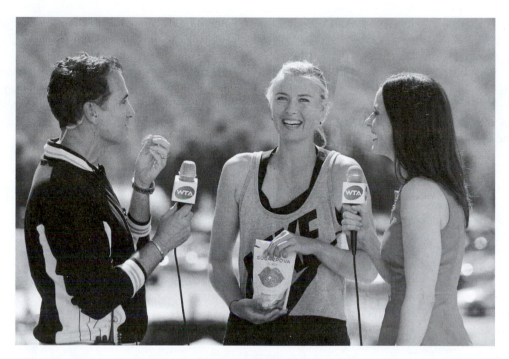

The media enable some athletes to become global celebrities and benefit from windfall income related to their popularity. They know that their celebrity depends on using and maintaining close connections with the media. Tennis player Maria Sharapova, like many top athletes today, is adept at dealing with the media in ways that work to her advantage. (*Source:* © DANNY MOLOSHOK/Reuters/Corbis)

sports. It controls sports" (Greenfield, 2012). This conclusion is put in historical context in a book on ESPN by *New York Times* journalists James Andrews and Tom Shales, who point out that television depended on sports in the past, but today this relationship is reversed, so that now sports depend on television and the new media that keep fans connected to sport "infotainment" 24/7.

Media Depend on Sports

Apart from newspapers and magazines devoted to specific sports, the print media do not depend on sports; nor do films, radio, and the video game industry as a whole. The urgency and uncertainty that are so compelling in sports are not captured and represented in any of these media as they are in visual broadcast media. Overall, the media most dependent on sports for commercial success are newspapers and television.

Newspapers   Newspapers at the beginning of the twentieth century had a sports page, which consisted of a few notices about upcoming activities, a short story or two about races or college games, and possibly some scores of local games. Today, there are daily and weekly newspapers devoted exclusively to sports, and nearly all daily newspapers have sports sections often making up about 25 percent of their news content.

Major North American newspapers give more daily coverage to sports than any other single topic of interest, including business or politics. The sports section is the most widely read section

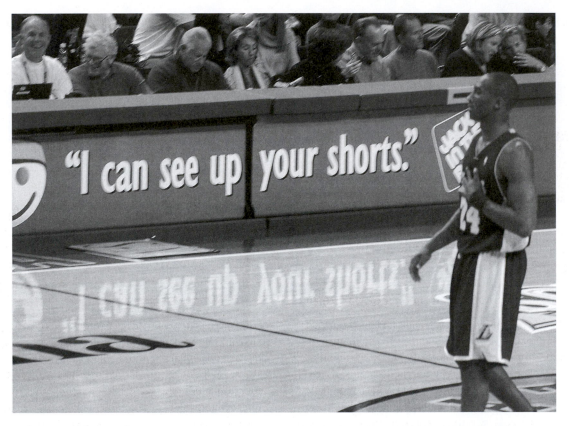

Digital media are especially invasive technologies. Everyone with a smartphone can create media content. Privacy is difficult to maintain, especially among celebrity athletes. They can be represented from multiple and surprising vantage points. This exposes them to scrutiny that athletes prior to this century seldom experienced. (*Source:* © Jay Coakley)

of the paper. It accounts for at least one-third of the total circulation and a significant amount of the advertising revenues for big-city newspapers. It attracts advertisers who want to reach middle-aged males with ads for tires, automobile supplies, new cars, car leases, airline tickets for business travelers, alcoholic beverages, power tools, building supplies, sporting goods, hair-growth products, enhancing sexual performance, testosterone, and hormone therapies. Ads for these products and services are unique to the (men's) sports section, and they generate needed revenues for newspapers.

As the Internet has become a primary source of information about big-time sports nationally and worldwide, many local, small-market newspapers have established online sites for breaking news, regular columns, and blogs. Their print editions may contain this content, but they focus more on local sports, including high school varsity teams, small college teams, and even youth sports.

Television   "Broadcasting right now . . . is about event television, live television, sports events. . . . That's what's really attracting . . . the real eyeballs and the real advertising dollars." This observation by Jeff Zucker (in Gelles and Edgecliffe-Johnson, 2011, p. 9), the former CEO of NBC Universal, explains why media companies in the United States have collectively signed deals paying sport organizations $72 billion for the rights to broadcast their games, matches, and events now and over the next decade.

Such high payouts for sports are a recent development. For example, the NFL's first television contract with CBS in 1962 amounted to $4.65 million, or $330,000 per team. In 2015 the NFL received $4.95 billion—a windfall of $155 million per team. Other sports don't have such lucrative deals, but they have also seen significant increases in their rights fees. For sports that don't share in this media bounty, it is difficult to survive at a professional or elite level.

At a time when television audiences are fragmented and new media capture the interests of many younger viewers, there is a collective urgency associated with certain men's sports and the Olympic Games that creates unified audiences that watch for long stretches without prerecording and editing out commercials. As a bonus for media companies, sports also attract eighteen- to thirty-five-year-old males, a highly sought-after demographic that sponsors cannot reach through other television programming.

Sports now account for a growing proportion of media company income. Half of the operating income of the massive Disney Company is generated by ESPN, as it collects over $6 billion from fees paid by about 100 million cable and satellite subscribers and it sells commercial time to its programming sponsors. Other channels feature sports programming, but ESPN in 2012 produced 35,000 hours of programming and accounted for half of the live sport events televised in the United States (Sandomir et al., 2013).

In an effort to break ESPN's monopoly-like control of premium sports programming, Fox Sports launched Fox Sports 1 in 2013 as a new 24-hour sports programming channel. However, generating the revenues and viewer loyalty possessed by ESPN will be a formidable challenge. NBC Universal (owned by Comcast) has been successful in retaining its hold on the Olympic Games through 2020. Using its cable channels, CNBC, MSNBC, Bravo, and USA Network, it presented over 5500

hours of the 2012 Olympic Games, although it ignored the Paralympics.

An attractive feature of sport programming for the major U.S. networks (ABC, CBS, Fox, and NBC) is that events often are scheduled on Saturdays and Sundays—the slowest days of the week for television viewing. Sport events are the most popular weekend programs, especially among male viewers who don't watch much television at other times. For example, NFL games have consistently accounted for 80 percent of the most-viewed television programs during recent years, and they provide sponsors access to young and middle-age males. Nearly all sport programming is ideal for promoting sales of beer, life insurance, trucks and cars, computers, investment services, credit cards, air travel and erectile dysfunction products. Sponsors realize that sports attract men who make purchasing decisions for hundreds, if not thousands, of employees, as well as for family members when it comes to buying beer, cars, computers, investments, and life insurance.

Golf and tennis are special cases for television programming. They attract few viewers and the ratings are exceptionally low, but the audience for these sports is very attractive to certain advertisers. It comprises people from upper-income groups, including many professionals and business executives. This is why television coverage of golf and tennis is sponsored by companies selling luxury cars and high-priced sports cars, business and personal computers, imported beers, investment opportunities with brokers and consultants, and trips to exclusive vacation areas. This is also why the networks continue to carry these programs despite low ratings. Advertisers will pay high fees to reach high-income consumers and corporate executives who make decisions to buy thousands of "company cars" and computers at the same time that they invest millions of dollars for employee pension plans or 401k plans. With such valued viewers, golf and tennis don't need high ratings to sell their television rights for high fees.

Women's sports also attract television coverage although the amount pales in comparison with coverage of men's sports. Women's events don't receive more coverage partly because female viewers of women's games have not been identified as a target demographic by advertisers who reach women through other means. Furthermore, men make up over half the viewing audience for most women's sports, but they also watch men's sports where sponsors already reach them.

Some cable and satellite television companies attract advertising money by covering sports that appeal to clearly identified segments of consumers. The X Games, for example, attract young males between twelve and thirty years old, which in turn attracts corporate sponsors selling soft drinks, beer, telecommunications products, and sports equipment such as helmets, shoes, skateboards, and dozens of other sport-specific products.

Over the past two decades, television companies have paid rapidly increasing amounts of money for the rights to televise certain sports, as indicated in Table 12.1. This includes nearly $5 billion annually for NFL games and $1.23 billion for the 2016 Olympic and Paralympic Games in Rio de Janeiro, Brazil. This is because NFL games, especially playoff games and the Super Bowl, are the top-10 most watched programs on U.S. television each year; and the Olympics captures high ratings for 16 consecutive days during summer months when ratings are usually low.

Television companies occasionally lose money on sports programming, but potential profits and other benefits are usually worth any risks. Furthermore, regular sports programming is a platform to promote other programs and boost ratings during the rest of the week; and it enhances the image and legitimacy of television among people who watch little other than sports.

As choices for sports television viewing have increased, audiences have fragmented and ratings for many sports have declined, especially during prime-time hours, even as the total number of people watching television sports has remained relatively steady. This means that rights fees for the very large events will remain high, but fees for other events, including "special-interest" events such as bowling, in-line skating championships, and international skiing

races will be limited. When interest in special events is especially strong among particular viewers, pay-per-view (PPV) sports programming can push rights fees to high levels; this continues to occur for championship boxing, professional wrestling, and mixed martial arts. PPV can generate massive revenues, but events must be chosen selectively because most people are not willing to pay upfront for a single event on television. In the meantime, pay TV has become part of people's lives in the form of subscription fees for cable and satellite connections and special sports channels and packages.

Sports and the Media: A Relationship Based on Economics and Ideology

Global economic factors have intensified the interdependence between commercial sports and the media. Major transnational corporations need ways to develop global name recognition, cultural legitimacy, and product familiarity. They also want to promote ideologies that support a way of life based on consumption, competition, and individual achievement.

Media sports offer global corporations a means of meeting these needs. Certain sport events attract worldwide attention; satellite technology transmits television signals around the world; sport images are associated with recognizable symbols and pleasurable experiences by billions of people; sports and athletes usually can be presented in politically safe ways by linking them with local identities and then using them to market products, values, and lifestyles related to local cultures or popular forms of global culture. Therefore, powerful transnational corporations spend billions of dollars annually to sponsor the media coverage of sports. This in turn gives global media companies significant power over sports worldwide.

Finally, many male executives of large media corporations are dedicated sports fans, and they like to be associated with sports as sponsors. Masculine culture is deeply embedded in most of the corporations they control, and they use their sponsorship money to receive VIP treatment at sport events and reaffirm the legitimacy of the masculinized

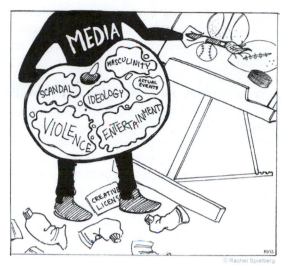

(Source: By permission of Rachel Spielberg)

A few powerful global media companies control most of the media representations of sports worldwide. This monopoly has serious implications for what sports we see or don't see.

corporate cultures in their companies. They also use sport events to entertain clients, fellow executives, and friends as they pay with company credit cards. This combination of masculine ideology and government-supported tax deductions for sport entertainment in the United States is a key factor in the media dependence on sports.

The long-time marriage of sports and media is clearly held together and strengthened by vast amounts of money from corporations whose executives use sports to increase profits and promote ideologies consistent with personal and corporate interests. Ideology is a key factor in the sport–media marriage. This is not a marriage based solely on money, but the goal of the sport–media partnership is to create a global family of eager consumers.

IMAGES AND NARRATIVES IN MEDIA SPORTS

To say that sports are "mediated" is to say that they consist of selected images and narratives.

Much research in the sociology of sport has deconstructed these images and narratives and analyzed the ideas or themes on which they are based. The scholars who have done these studies assume that media sports are symbolic constructions, much like Hollywood action films, television soap operas, and Disney cartoons.

To say that a telecast of an American football game is a symbolic construction means that it presents the ideas that certain people have about football, values, social life, and the characteristics of the viewing audience. Although each of us interprets media images and narratives differently, many of us use mediated sports as reference points as we form, revise, and extend our ideas about sports, social life, and social relations (Bruce, 2013; Crawford and Gosling, 2009; Wenner, 2013).

Because media sports are part of everyday experience today, it's important to consider the following:

1. Media production and representation of sports
2. Ideological themes underlying media coverage
3. Media consumers and the ways they integrate media content into their lives

Media Production and Representation of Sports

When media are privately owned and organized to make financial profits, sports are selected for coverage on the basis of their entertainment and revenue-generating potential. Media images and narratives are selected to represent the event so it meets the perceived interests of the audience and sponsors. Sports that are difficult to cover profitably usually are ignored by the media or covered only with selected highlights.

Sports coverage generally consists of images and narratives that exaggerate the spectacular, such as heroic injuries or achievements. Images and narratives also invent and highlight rivalries and explain why events are important. Furthermore, they create and maintain the celebrity status of athletes and teams. Cultural studies scholar Garry Crawford explains:

The mass-media construction of celebrity often lacks depth of character, as figures are frequently painted in one-dimensional terms. . . . Much of the language used to describe sport stars . . . draws on the narrative of melodrama. Heroes rise and fall, villains are defeated, and women play out their roles as supporting cast members to men's central dramatic roles (2004, p. 133).

Narratives even redeem villains who demonstrate that they can be heroic warriors, with commentators describing them as "loyal blue-collar players"—"willing to take figurative bullets for their teammates"—and "always being there when the chips are down," even if they sometimes have broken rules in the past.

The major media also emphasize elite sport competition. For example, U.S. newspapers and television networks increased their coverage of professional sports through the twentieth century and decreased coverage of amateur sports with the exception of college football and men's basketball. This shift was accompanied by a growing emphasis on the importance of winning and heroic actions and the desire to attract corporate sponsors and a mass audience. It's important to understand this process and the ways that particular images and narratives in media coverage inform popular ideas about sports and about social relations and social life in general.

Ideological Themes in Media Images and Narratives

Sports are represented in the media through images and narratives that are selected from a vast array of possibilities. The traditional media resemble windows through which we view what others choose to put in our range of sight and hear what others choose to say. Therefore, the only way to avoid being duped is to become a critical media consumer or work with others to produce grassroots media representations of sports.

To become a critical media consumer involves learning to identify the ideologies that guide others as they construct media representations for us. In the case of sports, the most central ideologies that influence what we see and hear are those related to success, consumption, gender, race, ethnicity, and nationality.

Success Themes in Media Narratives Media coverage of sports in the United States emphasizes success through individual effort, self-control, competition, teamwork, aggression, adherence to rules, and effective game plans. Also important are big individual plays such as home runs, long touchdown passes, and single-handed goals. The idea that success can be based on empathy, support for others, sharing resources, autonomy, intrinsic satisfaction, personal growth, compromise, incremental changes, or the achievement of equality is seldom included in media narratives, even though these elements exist in sports.

Media representations exaggerate the importance of competitive rivalries as well as winning and losing in athletes' lives. For example, ESPN has organized its coverage of the X Games around the competitive quest for medals when, in fact, many of the athletes and the spectators aren't very concerned about competition or medals (Honea, 2004). Athletes in the X Games and similar events enjoy the external rewards that come with winning, and they certainly want to demonstrate their competence, but they often emphasize self-expression and creativity more than the final scores determined by official judges. Furthermore, friendships with others in the event are more important than media-hyped rivalries and competitive outcomes. However, media narratives highlight rivalries and the desire to win because this reaffirms widely accepted cultural values and can be used to attract sponsors and consumers who may not understand the culture and skills possessed by athletes in action sports.

The success ideology regularly emphasized in U.S. media coverage is less apparent in the coverage that occurs in other nations. Narratives in the United States focus on winners, records, and final scores. Even silver and bronze Olympic medals are often viewed as consolation prizes, and games for third place are seldom played or covered by the media.

The "We're number 1" conceptualization of success that is so common among Americans is seldom used as a media focus in other nations where tie scores are acceptable competitive outcomes and aren't seen as the equivalent of "kissing your sister."

Sportswriters and announcers in the United States focus on "shootouts," sudden-death playoffs, dominating others, and big plays or big hits. Rare are references to learning, enjoyment, and competing *with* others, even though many players see their participation in these terms. Thus, the media don't "tell it like it is" as much as they tell it to reaffirm a discourse of competitive success that closely matches the interests of sponsors and advertisers. This ideological bias does not undermine the enjoyment of sports for most people, but it ignores that there are many ways to enjoy sports, even when they are organized to promote corporate interests.

Consumption Themes in Media Representations of Sports   The emphasis on consumption is clear in most media coverage of sports (Gee et al., 2014; Scherer, 2007; Scherer and Jackson, 2008). About 20 percent of televised sports in the United States consists of commercial time. Ads fill newspapers and magazines, and Internet sites use multiple strategies to present ads mixed with content. "TV time-outs" are now standard in football, basketball, and hockey games. And announcers remind media spectators that "This game is being brought to you by [corporate name]."

Commercials are so central in the telecast of the Super Bowl that the media audience is polled to rate them. Audiences for media sports are encouraged to express their connections to teams and athletes by purchasing thousands of branded objects.

Gender Themes in Media Representations of Sports   Masculinity rules in media sports (Bruce, 2013; Cooky et al., 2013; Cooky et al., 2015; Godoy-Pressland, 2014; O'Brien, 2015; Keats and Keats-Osborn, 2013; Weber and Carini, 2013). Men's sports receive about 95 percent of sports coverage in the media, and both images and narratives tend to reproduce traditional ideas and beliefs about gender. However, recent media coverage of concussions,

serious injuries, permanent sport-related physical and cognitive impairments, athletes in major men's sports coming out as gay, and athletes supporting gay marriage has led to a more multifaceted media narrative about masculinity in sport (Anderson and Kian, 2012). References to men as warriors doing battle and sacrificing their bodies for victories are now accompanied by discussions of safer sports, athlete health, and acceptance of difference. Of course, one reason for this is to create a more positive media image of sports and preserve lucrative revenue flows for media companies. Research is needed to track media narratives to see if this apparent shift is more than superficial, if it exists across sports, and if it persists over time.

Media coverage of women's sports has never been a media priority, and research suggests that this has not changed over the past two decades. In fact, longitudinal research done by Cheryl Cooky, Mike Messner, and their colleagues at the Center for Feminist Research at the University of Southern California shows that sports news and highlights about women's sports have declined since data were first collected in 1989 (Cooky et al., 2013). Tracking coverage on the three major network evening sports news programs in Los Angeles and coverage on ESPN's Sports Center, the data showed that LA sports news devoted 1.6 percent of airtime to women's sports and Sports Center devoted only 1.3 percent.

When Messner and his colleagues issued the first *Gender and Televised Sports* report in 1990, they found that 5 percent of sport news and highlights were devoted to women's sports, but they predicted that this percentage would increase as more girls and women played sports (Duncan et al., 2005). Significant participation increases occurred over the next twenty years, but the airtime given to women's sports has actually declined. The only positive change is that when women's sports have been covered in recent years, the quality of coverage has improved: it is more likely to be serious, and less likely to involve sexist jokes or comments that trivialize and sexualize women athletes. The most recent data for local sports news programs indicated that men appeared as anchors 100 percent of the time, and 99.5 percent of all anchors and ancillary announcers were men. Only one woman appeared as an announcer in any of the programs. Women accounted for 11 percent of the news anchors and ancillary announcers on Sports Center in 2009, down from 12 percent in 2004.

These findings indicate that progressive change in the media coverage of women's sports is neither inevitable nor permanent. This conclusion is supported by a recent review of published research on media coverage of women's sports by sociologist Toni Bruce (2013). Bruce notes that the mainstream media message on women appears to be this: "Go ahead and play but don't expect us to pay attention to your activities." Bruce also explains that media workers don't "actively or consciously try to marginalize women's sport"; however, the standard discourses they use to construct knowledge about sports and create narratives revolve around men and men's sports. Therefore, when news is produced, women's sports are not even on their radar. This means that changes will occur only if those discourses can be disrupted and revised to bring women's sports into the field of vision used by sports media personnel at all levels of news production.

When women's sports events are televised, the narratives constructed by commentators today are more sensitive to the physical skills of women athletes. Over time, and with the help of research by sociologists and communications scholars, announcers and commentators have developed a vocabulary and an approach to telling stories that are less likely to involve the following (Bruce, 2013):

Gender marking—that is, referring to men's events as *the* events and to women's events as *women's* events.
Compulsory heterosexuality—that is, mentioning that women athletes are "normal" because they have a boyfriend, husband, or child, and ignoring the reality that some women athletes are lesbians and that sexuality has nothing to do with athletic ability.

Appropriate femininity—that is, highlighting personal characteristics that distinguish women from men in terms of stature, strength, power, speed, emotional control, and vulnerability.
Infantilization—that is, referring to women athletes as *girls* and calling them by their first names in a way that reduces them to a status subordinate to men, who are referred to by last names and never called *boys.*
Nonsport issues—that is, calling attention to a woman athlete's personality, personal appearance, and personal or family life in a way that makes her athlete identity seem secondary to these important "female matters."
Sexualization—that is, representing women athletes with images that highlight physical attractiveness to the exclusion of sport-related physical attributes, and giving special attention to women athletes who have "redeemed their femininity" by posing for such representations in videos or photo shoots.
Ambivalence—that is, using narratives that recognize and praise sporting skills but also include comments that trivialize or undermine a woman's identity and prowess as a serious athlete.

Toni Bruce notes that coverage today is less likely to involve these things than coverage in the past. But that does *not* mean that they have disappeared or that coverage no longer belittles elite women's sports as deserving less media attention. For example, coverage during the 2012 Olympic Games gave much more attention to Gabby Douglas's hairstyles and her diminutive stature than to her physical strength and fortitude. But the coverage of men's events made no mention of the men's hairstyles or short stature. This is only one example among hundreds of similar cases of media coverage containing stories organized around one or more of the seven factors listed above.

These patterns of media coverage exist worldwide. In an impressive multinational study of 17,777 articles about sports in eighty newspapers from twenty-two countries, it was found that

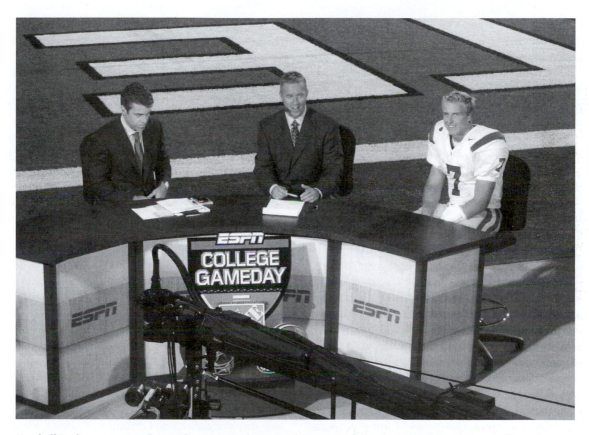

Football is the most popular media sport in the United States, and the demographics of the media audience for college football are attractive for commercial sponsors wanting to reach young people with higher levels of education and higher than average incomes. The coverage reproduces traditional gender ideology. (*Source:* © Bobak Ha'Eri)

85 percent of the articles were about men and men's sports, with female athletes or women's sports being the central focus in only 9 percent of the articles (Horky and Nieland, 2011; Toft, 2011). Further analysis showed that only 8 percent of the articles were written by women, and this percentage had not changed during the past decade.

Men's sport events often are promoted or described as if they had special historical importance, whereas women's sports events usually are promoted in a less dramatic manner (Kian et al., 2008). Men's events usually are unmarked by references to gender, whereas women's events almost always are referred to as women's events.

For instance, there has always been "The World Cup" and "The Women's World Cup" in soccer coverage. This terminology reflects the male-identified and male-centered orientation used by people in the media.

Traditional gender patterns in media coverage have been slow to change partly because sports media organizations worldwide have cultures and structures that are deeply gendered. They've been organized and scheduled around men's sports, just like the work routines and assignments of sport reporters. Therefore, the coverage of women's events often requires changes in institutionalized patterns of sports media work. Furthermore, the vast majority of sports media personnel are men, and the highest-status assignments in sports media are those that deal with men's sports.

Female reporters and announcers today understand that their upward mobility in the sports media industry demands that they cover men's events in much the same ways that men cover them. If they insist on covering only women's events or if they are assigned only to women's events, they won't move up the corporate ladder in media organizations (Bruce, 2013). Advancement also may be limited if they insist on covering men's sports in new ways that don't reaffirm the "correctness" of the coverage patterns and styles developed by men. Although women in the print media regularly cover men's sports, very few women have done regular commentary for men's sports in the electronic media apart from occasional "sideline reporters" who often are expected to look cute and talk to the guys as if they were at a "frat house" with no other women around (White, 2005). One of the exceptions to this pattern occurred in 2008 when Doris Burke was a color commentator for NBA playoff games. Online comments, nearly all from men, were generally supportive of Burke and praised her competence. But a few men were upset. One stated, "I just don't want to hear a woman caller announce *my* game" (emphasis added), and another wrote, "I watched the entire 2nd half on mute because everytime I hear her talk it ruins the game for me." The negative comments were influential, because Burke was removed and neither she nor any other woman has done color commentary on men's games since then.

Race, Ethnicity, and Nationality Themes in Media Representations of Sports

Just as gender ideology influences media coverage, so do racial and ethnic ideology and the stereotypes associated with it (Coogan, 2015; Farrington et al., 2012; Ličen and Billings, 2013; Love and Hughey, 2015; Price et al., 2012; Rowe, 2013; Van Sterkenburg et al., 2012).

Research in the 1970s and 1980s discredited the assumed factual basis of racial and ethnic stereotypes at the same time that media studies identified the ways that ideology influenced sport stories and commentaries, particularly in reference to black athletes. This made white journalists and commentators increasingly aware that the quality of their work depended on avoiding words and inferences based on discredited racial stereotypes. As a result, most of them became more critical about what they wrote and said, and they chose their words more carefully.

But making these changes was difficult for whites who accepted dominant racial ideology and had never viewed it critically or from the perspectives of blacks, Latinos, Asians, and Native Americans. Some media personnel made careless or naïve mistakes, and a few were suspended or fired for them.

Avoiding stereotypes and covering racial and ethnic relations in an informed way are two different things. Sports coverage today pretends that race and ethnicity don't exist; it assumes that sports is a racially and ethnically level playing field and that everyone in sports faces the same challenges and odds for success. But race and ethnicity are influential to such an extent that people cannot talk about them without discovering real, meaningful, and socially important racial and ethnic differences in what they think and feel. Ignoring this story about real differences allows whites in the media and media audiences to be comfortably color blind and deny the legacy and continuing relevance of skin color and cultural heritage in society and sports.

At the same time, blacks, Latinos, Asian Americans, and Native Americans are reminded that mainstream sport cultures have been shaped by the values and experiences of white men, and sport organizations and media companies are controlled by white men. This is simply a fact, and it is not meant to be an indictment of white men. But it does create tension for ethnic minority athletes and unique social dynamics in sports where players are racially and ethnically mixed. This in itself is a newsworthy story, but it would make many people, especially powerful white men, uncomfortable, and it would be difficult for most journalists to tell without being censored. But as long as it remains untold, white privilege in sports will persist without being recognized. Finally, if ethnic minority players or coaches try to tell the story, they're quickly accused of "playing the race card," being arrogant and ungrateful, promoting political correctness, or being bitter because of "imagined abuse."

Media coverage unwittingly reaffirms dominant racial ideology when whiteness is overlooked. For example, when journalists ignore the dynamics of living in a white-dominated, white-identified, and white-centered society, they unwittingly reproduce racial and ethnic stereotypes at the same time that they claim to be color blind.

Pretending to be color blind in a culture where a skin color–based racial ideology has existed for over three centuries ensures that white privilege is seamlessly incorporated into the media coverage of sports. It allows people in sports media to avoid asking why nearly all sports at the high school, college, and professional level are exclusively white or becoming so. It allows the editors at *Sports Illustrated* to never even think of publishing an article about the underrepresentation of African Americans and Latinos in most sports, even when they live in communities where hundreds of high school and college teams in swimming, volleyball, softball, tennis, golf, soccer, lacrosse, rowing, gymnastics, wrestling, and other sports are *all* white.

It also allows journalists to avoid asking critical questions about new patterns of residential and school segregation and growing income and wealth disparity that deeply influences who plays what sports in the United States today. They can put aside questions about why there are fewer African/Asian/Native American and Latino professional golfers today than there were in 1981—fifteen years before Tiger Woods won his first PGA tournament as a professional in 1996. Most important, pretending to be color blind allows media people to ignore whiteness and all racial issues, thereby maintaining a high racial comfort level among white media consumers and advertisers. In this way, ignoring reality becomes an effective strategy for boosting profits.

Scholars in ethnic studies explain that this self-declared colorblindness denies the real history and relevance of skin color and ethnicity in societies where previously unquestioned racism has shaped the distribution of income and wealth and the everyday living conditions of nearly all people. When a color-blind approach governs the coverage of sports, media stories miss significant sport realities and reproduce the racial and ethnic status quo. This allows people in dominant racial and ethnic populations to see and use sports as forms of social escapism—as whitewashed worlds devoid of the complex, messy issues that characterize everyday life.

At the same time, a color-blind approach constantly reminds people in racial and ethnic minority populations that their histories, heritages, and experiences are unrecognized in sports. As a result, some ethnic minority people avoid some or all sports, or they use sports as sites for seeking recognition and respect in the dominant culture. When we view media critically, it becomes increasingly clear that they don't "tell it like it is" as much as they tell it as their target demographics and advertisers want it told.

Ethnicity and Nationality in a Global Context

Themes related to ethnicity and nationality also exist in sports media coverage worldwide (Malcolm et al., 2010; Rowe, 2009, 2013). Although some sports reporters and broadcasters are careful to avoid using ethnic and national stereotypes in their representations of athletes and teams, evidence suggests that subtle stereotypes regularly influence sports coverage (Coogan, 2015; Kelly, 2011; Price et al., 2013; Van Sterkenburg et al., 2010). For example, some media coverage has portrayed Asian athletes as methodical, mechanical, machinelike, mysterious, industrious, self-disciplined, and intelligent. Their achievements are more often attributed to cognitive than to physical abilities, and stereotypes about height and other physiological characteristics are sometimes used to explain success or failure in sports. Latinos, on the other hand, have been described as flamboyant, exotic, emotional, passionate, moody, and hot-blooded.

The sports journalists most likely to avoid such stereotypes are those who have worked to learn about national and ethnic histories and those parts of the world in which teams and athletes live. This is what all good journalists do when they cover events and people. For example, when 28 percent of MLB players are Latino and more players are coming from certain Asian countries, it is reasonable to expect the journalists covering baseball to do their homework and learn about the cultures and baseball histories in those countries, and about the experiences of the athletes who have grown up there.

It also would be professionally responsible for media companies to hire sports reporters and broadcasters who are bilingual and culturally informed so that they could talk meaningfully with players whose lives on and off the field are not understood by most baseball fans. These are important stories as all sports become increasingly globalized. For the media to ignore them is to ignore the reality of sports today.

The most effective way to reduce subtle forms of racial, ethnic, and national bias in the media is to hire reporters, editors, photographers, writers, producers, directors, camerapersons, commentators, and statisticians from diverse racial, ethnic, and national backgrounds. Lip service is paid to this goal, and progress has been made in certain media, but members of racial and ethnic minorities are clearly underrepresented in nearly all sports newsrooms and media executive offices where over 85 percent of the full time reporters and editors are white (Lapchick, 2013).

This skewed pattern is unfortunate because ethnic diversity among media people would enrich stories and provide multiple perspectives for understanding sports and the people who play and coach them. Of course, neither skin color nor gender precludes knowledge about sports or the people involved in them, but knowledge is based on a combination of experience and the richness of the perspectives one uses to make sense of the ethnically and racially diverse social worlds that constitute sports today.

EXPERIENCES AND CONSEQUENCES OF CONSUMING MEDIA SPORTS

Media sports provide topics of conversation, occasions for social interaction, a sense of belonging and identity, opportunities to express emotions, and an exciting distraction for those who are passing time alone. However, few studies have investigated audience experiences to see how people give meaning to media sports coverage and integrate it into their lives. Similarly, we know that media images and narratives influence what people feel, think, and do, but few studies have investigated the consequences of media sport consumption at the individual or collective level.

Audience Experiences

Studies of audience experiences suggest that people interpret media content and integrate media sport consumption into their lives in diverse ways (Bruce, 2013; Gantz, 2013; Wenner, 2013). More men than women are strongly committed to consuming media sports, and strongly committed consumers constitute a relatively small segment of the overall population in most societies, including the United States and Canada (Adams, 2006). However, these studies don't tell us much about the ways that people give meaning to and include the consumption of media sports in their lives.

One exception is a creative study of twenty white men and a few women who had grown up in various towns in western Pennsylvania but had moved to Fort Worth, Texas (Kraszewski, 2008). By various means each person joined with others who had started a tradition of meeting in a sports bar where they watched Pittsburgh Steelers games from August through December. As they met each week their interaction focused on rekindling and nurturing their sense of western Pennsylvania as "home" and their identities associated with their geographical origins. In the process they created a place-image of western Pennsylvania that matched the blue-collar, white European-American, steelworker image of the Steelers. They wore Steelers jerseys, drank Iron City (Pittsburgh) beer in aluminum bottles, and were identified as Steelers fans by the Dallas Cowboys fans in the bar. They avoided talking about social class, race, and jobs and focused on "where they were from"—talking

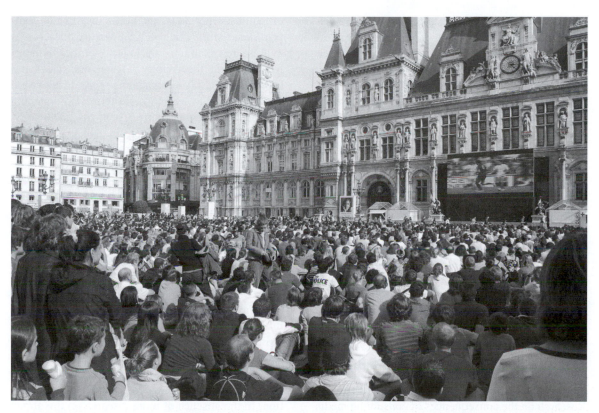

As outdoor screens are used to televise major sport events, such as the Rugby World Cup in Paris (2007), there are new social dynamics associated with media consumption. This crowd was predominantly French, but it also included groups of fans from at least ten other nations. Access to this plaza was open, and spectators were orderly despite a packed crowd and no reserved seats. No sociological research has been done on this phenomenon. (*Source:* © Jay Coakley)

about roads, towns, and other features of the landscape of western Pennsylvania. For them, watching the Steelers on television was a social occasion for interacting with others who reaffirmed their sense of home and their regional identities, despite living over 1200 miles away from where they grew up.

When media scholar Walter Gantz (2013) studied male-female married couples in the United States, he found that they often watched televised sports together and that this usually was a positive activity in their relationships. Men watched sports more than women did and were more likely to be committed sports fans, but when women were

committed fans, their patterns of watching and responding to sports on television were similar to men's patterns. Gantz did find that some couples experienced conflicts related to viewing sports, but most resolved them successfully. Partners usually learned to adjust to each other's viewing habits over time, and when they didn't, it usually meant that they had general relationship problems unrelated to watching sports.

In another study of viewing habits, Whiteside and Hardin (2011) found that even though women participate in sports more often today than in the past, they don't regularly watch women's sports as media spectators. Data indicated that women's leisure time is often spent doing things that fit the interests of other family members rather than using their leisure time for their own interests. They watched men's sports because they watched with the men in their lives. Under these conditions, watching women's sports seldom became a high priority for them.

Future studies will tell us more about the ways that people integrate media sport experiences into their lives and when media sports become important sites at which social relationships occur. For example, we know that social media magnify the voices of sport spectators and provide opportunities to raise their own issues in connection with sports (Millington and Darnell, 2014; Norman, 2012, 2014), but we don't know what that means in terms of their relationships and everyday lives at home, work, school, and in their own sport participation. It will be important to include the use of the Internet and video games in future studies.

Consequences of Consuming Media Sports

Research on the consequences of consuming media sports has focused on a wide variety of issues. Here we'll focus on three: active participation in sports, attendance at sport events, and betting on sport events.

Active Participation in Sports   Does consuming media sports lead people to be more active sport participants or turn them into couch potatoes? This is an important issue, given the health problems associated with physical inactivity in many societies today.

When children watch sports on television, some copy what they see *if* they have or can make opportunities to do so. Children are great imitators with active imaginations, so when they see and identify with athletes, they may create informal activities or seek to join youth sport programs to pursue television-inspired dreams. However, participation grounded in these dreams usually fades quickly, especially after children discover that it takes years

of tedious, repetitive, and boring practice to compete successfully and reach the victory podium.

Research examining the legacies of the Olympics for people in the country hosting the games has shown consistently that watching sports on television is more likely to lead to more television watching than actively playing sports (Conn, 2012; Donnelly, 2008; Green, 2012; Kortekaas, 2012; Thornton, 2013). In light of this evidence it appears that a positive link between watching and doing sports may exist only when parents, teachers, or physical educators strategically connect media representations with everyday sport participation. Research is needed to explore this possibility. In the meantime, an ad for TV coverage of the Olympics on Fox television in late 2012 told viewers that the network had so much sports programming that "there is no need to leave your couch all month long."

Many adults don't play the sports they consume in the media, but some do. Research suggests that those who are not regular participants use media sports as entertainment, whereas those who are avid participants are the ones who use media sports as a source of inspiration for their own participation. In the absence of more research on this topic, we can say only that consuming sports through the media may be connected with activity or inactivity in different situations and with different people.

Attendance at Sport Events   Game attendance is related to many factors, including the consumption of media sports. On the one hand, many people say that they would rather watch certain sport events on television than attend them in person. On the other hand, the media publicize sports, promote interest, and provide information that helps people to identify with athletes and teams and become potential ticket purchasers for events.

Although consuming media sports has generally been positively related to attending live events, this may be changing with widespread use of new media and the existence of large HD televisions. Whereas media companies in the past tried to duplicate the live-event experience on television, now stadium managers try to duplicate the home-viewing experience for those who attend live events. Spectators now want broadband Wi-Fi and high-speed mobile phone connections in stadiums, large HD replay screens, and video screens by concessions and in restrooms so they don't miss the action they paid to see. These stadium upgrades are costly, but without them, more people may choose to stay at home, where they have access to everything they want during a game.

Additionally, there may be circumstances when people who normally pay for their ticket at the gate will stay home to watch a televised game rather than go to the stadium. This might occur when they expect that there will be a large crowd at the game, violent or uncivil behavior on the part of other fans, or bad weather.

Gambling on Sports   Consuming media sports is clearly connected with gambling, but there is no evidence that it causes gambling.

Formal gambling on sports dates back centuries and continues today at horse and dog tracks, in limited terms in Delaware, and in Nevada where people may bet legally on nearly every possible outcome in sport events—such as number of points, who scores first, points in first half or second half, who beats the point spread, and so on.

It has been estimated that sports wagering in the United States amounts to as much as $380 billion annually with over $2 billion bet legally in Nevada during 2014. Sport gambling is most popular among younger men who have above-average income and at least some college education. Male college students have higher rates of gambling than other categories of people, mostly because they think they know more about sports than others.

A 2012 NCAA study (Paskus and Derevensky, 2013) of more than 23,000 students across all three NCAA divisions showed that nearly 60 percent of male students reported gambling for money and 26 percent of the male athletes had bet money on sports, which is a violation of NCAA rules. About one in twenty athletes reported being contacted by outside gamblers looking for inside information they could use to guide their bets on college games. About 60 percent of male athletes and 40 percent of female athletes approved of betting on sports, excluding their own games, and most thought that people could consistently make money by betting on sports.

Sport gambling debts can have destructive consequences, but betting on sports is not generally seen as an important moral or legal issue. Many people today are accustomed to buying state lottery tickets and going to casinos, and they don't favor new restrictions that would limit or ban betting on sports, nor are they seduced by online betting opportunities. However, gambling constitutes a threat to sports because it elevates the stakes associated with competitive outcomes and may lead people to seek an edge by convincing one or more athletes to control the scores of games and matches so that bets can be won when point spreads are not covered by favored teams or athletes. Even a rumor of game or match fixing or point shaving seriously threatens the integrity of competitive outcomes and destroys the foundation for much sport spectatorship. In this sense, consuming media sports does not influence gambling as much as gambling could influence media sport consumption.

SPORT JOURNALISM

Some people trivialize sport journalism by saying that it provides information about people and events that is entertaining but unrelated to important issues in everyday life. However, sports do matter—not because they produce a tangible product or make essential contributions to our survival, but because they represent ideas about how the world works and what is important in life.

Sports are not merely reflections of social worlds; they also are constitutive of those worlds—that is, they're sites at which social worlds are produced, reproduced, and changed. Sport journalists are key players in these constitutive processes, because their representations of sports can influence the ideas and beliefs that people use to define and give meaning to themselves, their experiences, and the organization of social worlds.

Sport Journalists Are Not All the Same

Entertainment is a focus for nearly everyone working in commercial media. Sportswriters generally provide specific information and in-depth analysis, whereas the announcers and commentators for visual electronic media usually focus on providing images and narratives that create anticipation and a sense of urgency among their audience. Exceptions sometimes occur in sport talk radio when analysis and "call-in" interactivity are structured into program format. Additionally, television also includes some sport programming that provides in-depth analysis, but this is relatively rare in its overall programming format.

As athletes, agents, team publicity directors, bloggers, and others contribute online content, traditional sport journalism is changing. Independent investigative journalism has nearly disappeared in favor of entertainment journalism that focuses on personalities and "celebrity chasing" rather than social and political issues in sports. Flashy

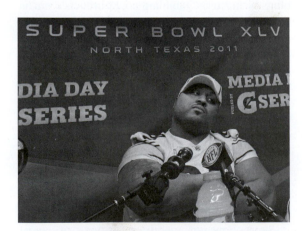

There have always been tensions between elite athletes and journalists, but athletes tolerated journalists because they needed them to communicate with fans. Today that is no longer the case. Social media puts athletes in direct contact with fans, so some of them, like this Super Bowl player, have little patience when forced to deal with journalists and their "inane" questions.
(*Source:* © AP Photo/Eric Gay)

infotainment now takes the place of hard news, media personalities present opinions rather than fact-based stories, and stories holding the powerful accountable for their actions are killed, censored, or never produced.

There are capable investigative journalists working at *Sports Illustrated* and ESPN, but the entertainment side of these media companies limits independent reporting or fosters self-censorship by reporters (Miller and Belson, 2013; Sandomir et al., 2013; Zirin, 2013e). Independent journalists produce stories for blog sites such as *Deadspin* and *SB Nation,* but they are paid as contract workers and rarely have resources for sustained investigative work.

Investigative journalism does not provide a good return on investment for media companies. ESPN is owned by the Walt Disney Company, the largest media conglomerate in the world, and they can make more money providing entertainment than presenting detailed investigations of concussions, tax-avoidance scams, media influence on sports, institutionalized forms of corruption, and other important issues that require critical analysis. They now make more money than ever before, but they are cutting or shortening contracts for their investigative reporters. The same is true for CNN/Sports Illustrated, owned by Time Warner, the second-largest media conglomerate in the world.

As big media exert more control over sports worldwide, those of us who participate in and consume sport can expect fewer media stories about the meaning, purpose, and organization of sports apart from how they are represented by those who control and profit from them.

Sport Journalists on the Job: Relationships with Athletes

As the amount of video coverage of sports has increased, sportswriters have had to create stories that go beyond describing action and reporting scores. This leads them to seek increasingly intimate information about the personal lives of athletes, and this creates tension in athlete–journalist relationships. Athletes today realize that they cannot trust journalists to hold information in confidence, even if the disclosure took place in the privacy of the locker room. Furthermore, the stakes associated with "bad press" are so great for athletes and teams that everyone in sport organizations limits what they say when talking with journalists. As a result, sport stories tend to contain similar and meaningless quotes from athletes game after game, week after week, and season after season.

Salary and background differences between journalists and athletes increase tensions in their relationships. Highly paid black and Latino athletes without college degrees have little in common with middle-class, college-educated, white, Euro-American journalists. As a result, some journalists don't refrain from disclosing personal information about athletes to enhance stories, and athletes define journalists as "outsiders" who can impact their lives without fully understanding who they are and what their identity as an athlete means to them.

Team owners and university athletic departments are so conscious of tensions between athletes and media personnel that they now provide players with training on how to handle interviews without saying things that might sound bad or be misinterpreted.

These tensions also call attention to ethical issues in sport journalism. Many, but not all journalists are aware that they should not jeopardize athletes' reputations simply for the sake of entertainment, and they should not hurt them unintentionally or without good reason. Latino journalist Dan Le Batard, who works for ESPN and the Miami Herald, explains that he tries to be "nonjudgmental" when he covers athletes because all people have flaws and exposing the flaws of athletes who disappoint you with their actions smacks of self-righteousness and raises the ethical issue of invasion of privacy (2005, p. 14). However, journalists constantly face gray areas in which ethical guidelines are not clear, and the need to present attractive stories often encourages them to push ethical limits. As a result, tensions will remain in athlete–journalist relationships.

summary

COULD SPORTS AND THE MEDIA SURVIVE WITHOUT EACH OTHER?

Media and media experiences have become ever-present in the lives of people living in many parts of the world today. This is why we study the relationship between sports and the media.

Media sports, like other aspects of culture, are social constructions. They're created, organized, and controlled by human beings whose motives and ideas are grounded in their social worlds, experiences, and ideologies. The media represent sports to us through selected images and narratives that usually reaffirm dominant ideologies and promote the interests of wealthy and powerful people who own media companies.

New media have altered the way people receive news, consume media content, interact with others who share their interests in sports, connect with athletes and teams, and even express their feelings about everything from on-the-field action to off-the-field management decisions. Therefore, new media extend the boundaries of what we study in the sociology of sport.

People now have access to sports content 24/7 on television, smartphones, tablets, and any Internet-connected device. This means that a person's identity as a fan can be reaffirmed at anytime, anywhere. Fans can also follow athletes on digital sites like Twitter, Instagram, Facebook, Tumblr, and blogs. This eliminates the mainstream media filter and provides them with information that comes directly from athletes.

Fantasy sports and video games are an important component of new media. At this time, they complement existing media, but they're beginning to provide unique sport-related experiences unlike those occasioned by traditional media.

Sports and the media have become increasingly interdependent as both have become more important parts of social worlds. They could survive without each other, but they would be different from the way they are now. Commercial sports have grown and prospered because of media coverage and the rights fees paid by media companies. Without the publicity and money provided by media, commercial sports would be reduced to local business operations with much less scope than they have today, and less emphasis would be placed on elite, competitive sports in people's lives.

Media could survive without sports, but newspapers and television would be different from their current format if they did not have sports content and programming to attract young male audiences and the sponsors who wish to buy access to those audiences. Without sports, newspaper circulation would decrease, and television programming on weekends and holidays would be different and less profitable for television broadcasters.

The symbiotic relationship between sports and the media in most societies today exists because certain sports can be used to attract audiences that sponsors want to convert into consumers of their products and services. The dynamics of this relationship are also influenced by the interaction that occurs among athletes, agents, coaches, administrators, sport team owners, sponsors, advertisers, media representatives, and a diverse collection of spectators. Power relations are a crucial feature of this interaction process, and it is important to understand them when studying the sports–media relationship.

Research indicates that media coverage of sports in the United States emphasizes images and narratives reproducing dominant ideologies related to success, consumption, gender, race, ethnicity, and nationality. As a result, current patterns of power and privilege are portrayed as normal and natural and remain taken-for-granted.

Future research utilizing cultural, interactionist, and structural theories combined with a critical approach will tell us more about the various ways that people make sense of the media representations they consume. This is especially important in connection with the Internet and video games. Patterns of media sport consumption are changing rapidly, and it is important to study them in ways that promote critical media literacy rather than the uncritical celebration of media technology and the promotional culture of most sports coverage.

Few studies have investigated the experiences and consequences of consuming media sports. We know that people make sense of sports media images and narratives on their own terms and that this interpretive process of sense-making is influenced by the social, cultural, and historical conditions under which it occurs. People also integrate media sport experiences into their lives in diverse ways, but we know little about the patterns and consequences of this integration process. For example, research is needed to help us identify the conditions under which the consumption of media sports influences active participation in sports, attendance at live sport events, and gambling on sports.

To understand sports and the media, it helps to become familiar with basic features of sports journalism today. Journalists are key players in the overall process of representing sports to large audiences. In the process they influence ideas and beliefs about sports and social worlds. The interactivity made possible by new media makes journalists more accessible to their audiences while bringing members of the audience into the process of creating media content. Additionally, the need to create stories that capture the attention of media consumers has led journalists to seek stories that disclose private and personal information about athletes. This creates tensions between journalists and athletes, which then influence media representations of sports and the people who play them.

Sports and the media need each other, especially when making profits is a primary goal for each. The sports–media relationship changes as it is negotiated by athletes, facility directors, sport team owners, event promoters, media representatives, sponsors, advertisers, agents, and spectators. Studying the dynamics of this relationship helps expand our understanding of sports in society.

SUPPLEMENTAL READINGS

Reading 1. New media: Consuming sports 24/7
Reading 2. Putting media to use: The NFL as a marketing machine

Reading 3. Live by the tweet, die by the tweet: Learning to use new media

Reading 4. Virtual sports: Play safe, stay home

Reading 5. Media rights deals: What sport has the best deal?

Reading 6. The stronger women get, the more men watch football: A prediction from 1990

Reading 7. People who don't watch sports on TV subsidize those who do.

SPORT MANAGEMENT ISSUES

- Athletes at your university have gotten into trouble using social media. You have been hired to create a social media policy for the athletic department. Identify the three main components of the policy, and describe how you would explain to the athletes why you created each of them.

- You're a new editor at *Sports Illustrated.* At your first editorial meeting the major item on the agenda is the February swimsuit issue. It is decided that it is economically unwise to drop the swimsuit issue, but it is also decided that if the swimsuit issue is continued, there must be other changes in the magazine to present a fair image of women in sports. As a new editor, you are called on to make some suggestions for changes. How would you respond?

- You are called in as an advisor to the President's Council on Fitness and Sports. The two topics being discussed are (1) whether television sports are turning people in the United States into couch potatoes, and (2) whether the television coverage of professional sports is destroying people's interests in local high school, college, and amateur sports. The Council wants advice from you. What do you tell them?

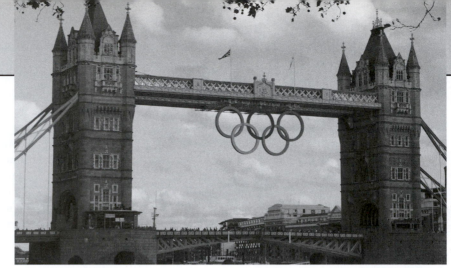

SPORTS AND POLITICS

How Do Governments and Global Political Processes Influence Sports?

Sport has the power to change the world. It has the power to inspire, it has the power to unite people in a way that little else does. It speaks to youth in a language they understand. Sport can create hope, where once there was only despair. It is more powerful than governments in breaking down racial barriers.

> —**Nelson Mandela, former president, South Africa (2000)**

. . . the language of sports is universal; it extends across borders, language, race, religion and ideology; it possesses the capacity to unite people, together, by fostering dialogue and acceptance. This is a very valuable resource!

> —**POPE FRANCIS (2013)**

Many more people in the world are concerned with sports than with human rights.

> —**Samuel Huntington, political scientist (1997)**

Just as athletes and athletic associations sell products, politicians try to associate with sport to help sell themselves and their agendas to a sport-loving public.

> —**Kyle Green and Doug Hartmann, sociologists, University of Minnesota (2012)**

Chapter Outline

The Sports-Government Connection
Sports and Global Political Processes
Politics in Sports
Summary: How Do Governments and Global Political Processes Influence Sports?

Learning Objectives

- Know the differences between politics and government and between power and authority.
- Identify at least five major reasons for governments to be involved in sports.
- Provide examples of how government intervention in sports protects the rights and safety of athletes and nonathletes alike.
- Identify examples of how government intervention in sports may benefit some people more than others.
- Identify the traditional ideals associated with international sports, and discuss those ideals in terms of the realities of international sports.

- Discuss why the Olympic Games are a socially valuable event, and what can be done to make them more socially sustainable.
- Explain the connections between cultural ideology and the sponsorship of sports by nation-states and transnational corporations.
- Discuss the political issues associated with the globalization of sports.
- Give examples of politics in sports, and explain why politics will always be a part of sports.

Organized competitive sports have long been connected with politics, governments, and global political processes. When people say that politics has no place in sports, they usually mean that there is no place in sports for politics that differ from their own.

Politics refers to the *processes of organizing social power and making decisions that affect people's lives in a social world.* Politics occur at all levels of social life, from the politics of friendship and family relationships to national, international, and global affairs (Volpi, 2006). In the sociology of sport we study political processes in communities, local and national sport organizations, societies, and large nongovernment organizations (NGOs) such as the International Olympic Committee (IOC) and the Fédération Internationale de Football Association (FIFA), the international federation that governs world soccer.

Governments are *formal organizations with the power to make and enforce rules in a particular territory or collection of people.* Because governments make decisions affecting people's lives, they are political organizations by definition. Governments operate on various levels from local parks and recreation departments to nation-states, and they influence sports whether they occur in a public park or a privately owned stadium that hosts international competitions. In the sociology of sport we often refer to "**the state**" because this concept *includes the formal institution of a national government plus those parts of civil society—such as education, family, media, and churches—that teach values and ideologies that extend the influence and control of the political agencies that make and enforce laws and govern a society.*

Politics often involve the actions and interactions of governments, but rule-making in sports today goes beyond the political boundaries of the state and occurs in connection with global processes. For example, soccer is a global sport because British workers, students, and teachers brought the game to South America and British soldiers and missionaries brought it to Africa, Asia, the West Indies, and other colonized areas of the nineteenth-century British Empire. Soccer grew around the world through the global processes of migration, capitalist expansion, British imperialism, and colonization—all of which involve politics.

Governments usually are involved in political processes, but today's world includes such rapid global movements of people, products, knowledge, ideas, technologies, and money that these processes transcend particular states and involve transnational corporations and nongovernmental organizations such as Greenpeace, the Red Cross, and sport organizations such as the IOC and FIFA.

This chapter focuses on the relationships between sports and politics. The goal is to explain the ways in which sports are connected with governments, the state, and global political processes. Chapter content focuses on four major questions:

1. Why do governments often sponsor and control sports?
2. How are sports connected with global politics that involve nation-states, transnational corporations, and nongovernmental organizations?
3. What is the role of the Olympic Games and other sport mega-events in global politics and processes?
4. How are political processes involved in sports and sport organizations?

When reading this chapter, remember that power and authority are the key concepts used when studying politics and political processes. **Power** refers to *an ability to influence people and achieve goals, even in the face of opposition from others* (Weber, 1922a). And **authority** is *a form of power that comes with a recognized and legitimate status or office in a government, an organization, or an established set of relationships.* For example, a large corporation, such as Nike or McDonald's, has power if it can influence how people think about and play sports and if it can use sports to achieve its goals. Sport organizations such as the IOC, FIFA, the NCAA, and a local parks and recreation department have the *authority* to administer particular sports as long as the people associated with those sports accept the organizations as legitimate governing bodies. This highlights the fact that *politics* refers to the power to make decisions that affect sports and sport participation.

THE SPORTS-GOVERNMENT CONNECTION

As sports grow in popularity, government involvement usually increases. Many sports require sponsorship, organization, and facilities—all of which depend on resources that few individuals possess on their own. Sport facilities may be so expensive that regional and national governments are the only entities with the power and resources to build and maintain them. Government involvement also occurs when there is a need for a third party to regulate and control sports and sport organizations in ways that promote the public good in a community or society.

The nature and extent of government involvement in sports varies by society, but it generally serves one or more of the following purposes (Houlihan, 2000):

1. Safeguard the public order
2. Ensure fairness and protect human rights
3. Maintain health and fitness among citizens
4. Promote the prestige and power of a group, community, or nation
5. Promote a sense of identity, belonging, and unity among citizens
6. Reproduce dominant values and ideologies in a community or society
7. Increase support for political leaders and government
8. Facilitate economic and social development in a community or society

Safeguard the Public Order

Governments are responsible for maintaining order in public areas, including parks, sidewalks, and streets, among other places. Here are two sections from the Los Angeles Municipal Code, enforced by the city in an effort to safeguard citizens and the public order:

SEC. 56.15. BICYCLE RIDING—SIDEWALKS. No person shall ride, operate or use a bicycle, unicycle, skateboard, cart, wagon, wheelchair, roller skates, or any other device moved exclusively by human power, on a sidewalk, bikeway or boardwalk in a willful or wanton disregard for the safety of persons or property. (Los Angeles Municipal Code, 2013a)

SEC. 56.16. STREETS—SIDEWALKS—PLAYING BALL OR GAMES OF SPORT. No person shall play ball or any game of sport with a ball or football or throw, cast, shoot or discharge any stone, pellet, bullet, arrow or any other missile, in, over, across, along or upon any street or sidewalk or in any public park, except on those portions of said park set apart for such purposes. (Los Angeles Municipal Code, 2013b)

Laws similar to these, full of bureaucratic language, exist in nearly all cities and towns. They set boundaries for where, when, and under what circumstances sports may be played.

Ideally, these laws promote safety and reduce conflict between multiple users of public spaces. For example, state and local governments in many countries ban bare-fisted boxing, bungee jumping off public bridges, and basketball playing on public streets. In the case of commercial sports, governments may also regulate the rights and responsibilities of team owners, sponsors, promoters, and athletes.

Local governments may regulate sport participation by requiring people to obtain permits to use public facilities and playing fields. Likewise, local officials may close streets or parks to the general public so that sport events can be held under controlled and safe conditions. Annual marathons in New York City, London, and other cities worldwide require the involvement of the government and government agencies such as the city and state police.

Safeguarding the public order also involves policing sport events where safety may be threatened by crowds or unruly individuals. During the Olympics, for example, the host city and nation provide thousands of military and law enforcement officials to safeguard the public order. In the face of possible protests and terrorist actions, it is estimated that the Chinese government spent up to $6.5 billion to police and monitor the Beijing area in connection with the 2008 Olympic Games. The Chinese

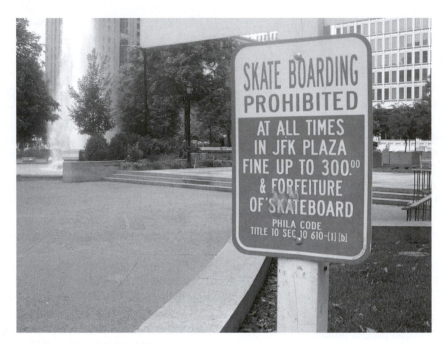

Local governments often regulate where and when certain sports can occur. This is true in Philadelphia's "Love Park," although "street skaters" do break the rules on weekends, holidays, and late at night. (*Source:* © Jay Coakley)

government also employed over 43,000 soldiers, 47 helicopters, 74 airplanes, 33 naval ships, 6000 security guards on 18,000 buses, 30,000 guards at bus stops and terminals, and the personnel to monitor tens of thousands of surveillance cameras in and around Beijing.

Governments also sponsor sports that are used in military and police training. Military academies in the United States sponsor sports for cadets, and the World Police and Fire Games are held every two years because people believe that sport participation keeps prepared soldiers, law enforcement officials, and firefighters to safeguard the public order.

Finally, some governments sponsor sport events and programs for people defined as potential threats to the public order. When public officials believe that sports will keep young people—especially those labeled "at risk"—off the streets and thereby reduce crime rates, vandalism, loneliness, and alienation,

they may provide funding and facilities for sport programs. However, these programs are seldom effective unless they are tied to other efforts to reduce the deprivation, racism, poverty, dislocation, unemployment, community disintegration, and political powerlessness that often create "at-risk youth" and social problems in communities and societies (Coakley, 2002, 2011).

A study by Doug Hartmann and Brooks Depro (2006) suggests that these programs are most likely to be effective in reducing crime rates when they are sponsored in connection with other public efforts that make people in a particular neighborhood aware that the city government and law enforcement is taking them seriously and can be trusted to maintain public order. However, Wheelock and Hartmann (2007) also found that when members of the U.S. Congress debated anti-crime program funding in the 1990s, references to these programs increased their fears of crime by "at-risk" populations (especially black men) and shifted their focus to funding social control programs that emphasized policing and incarceration.

This emphasis on social control raises a critical question about the political interpretation of "safeguarding the public order." For example, it can be used as an excuse to limit the physical and sport activities of people defined by political officials as "undesirable" (Silk and Andrews, 2010). Additionally, when cities host sport mega-events, the goal of "safeguarding public order" is now used to justify the relocation of poor people and the installation of expensive video surveillance systems that effectively eliminate privacy in public areas (Sugden, 2012).

Overall, when safeguarding the public order is the reason for government involvement in sports, the focus of that involvement can influence sports in many ways—sometimes restricting certain forms of sport participation at the same time that other forms are supported.

Ensure Fairness and Protect Human Rights

Governments may intervene in sports by passing laws, establishing policies, or ruling in court cases that protect the rights of citizens to participate in public sport programs. A classic example of this is Title IX in the United States and similar laws that other countries have passed to promote gender equity in sports (Mitchell and Ennis, 2007; Sabo and Snyder, 2013).

Today, many national governments are considering or have already enacted laws mandating the provision of sport participation opportunities for people with a disability. For example, the United States Supreme Court made a ruling in 2001 that ensured fair treatment for Casey Martin, Tiger Woods's former roommate and golf teammate at Stanford University. Martin sued the Professional Golf Association for the right to use a golf cart during competitions because a chronic leg problem impeded his walking.

A federal court in 2008 ruled in favor of the Michigan Paralyzed Veterans of America and forced the University of Michigan to increase its accessible seats for football fans from 88 (in 2007) to 329 in 2010 (out of 107,501 total seats) and to make restrooms accessible even though they were built in previous years not covered by existing ADA law (Lapointe, 2008; Pear, 2008).

In 2013, the U.S. Department of Education's Office for Civil Rights clarified the existing legal obligations of schools "to provide students with disabilities an equal opportunity to participate alongside their peers in after-school athletics and clubs." It also noted that "schools may not exclude students who have an intellectual, developmental, physical, or any other disability from trying out and playing on a team, if they are otherwise qualified" (Duncan, 2013).

In other examples of government actions to guarantee fairness and human rights, the U.S. Congress passed the Amateur Sports Act in 1978 and created the USOC, now the official NGO responsible for coordinating amateur sports in the United States. A major reason for doing this was to protect athletes from being exploited by multiple, unconnected, and self-interested sport-governing bodies that controlled amateur sports through much of the twentieth century. In 1998, the act was revised to require the USOC to support and fund Paralympic athletes because people with a disability were systematically denied opportunities to play elite amateur sports. However, people have differing opinions on how the act should be interpreted and this has led athletes with disabilities to file lawsuits to receive the support and funding that they and many others consider to be fair.

Disputes about fairness and human rights in sports are not always settled by legislative or judicial actions, but as the stakes associated with sports and sport participation increase, government officials are more likely to pass laws and accept sport-related legal cases for judicial rulings. The 2005 and 2012 congressional hearings on steroid use in Major League Baseball were examples of this, even though the hearings accomplished nothing of substance.

Maintain Health and Fitness

Governments often become involved in sports to promote health and fitness among citizens. In nations with state-funded, universal health care programs, governments often sponsor sports and physical activity programs to improve health and reduce expenditures for medical care. Nations without universal health care may also sponsor or promote sports for health reasons, but they have a lower stake in preventive approaches and less incentive to fund them. For example, public schools in the United States have cut physical education programs and communities have defunded recreational sport programs because they are seen as too expensive to maintain.

Although people generally believe that sport participation improves health and reduces medical costs, there's a growing awareness that the relationship between sports participation and health must be qualified because of the following research findings (Bhanoo, 2012; Bloodworth et al., 2012; Gregory, 2012; Leek et al., 2011; Waddington, 2000a, 2007):

- Many illnesses that increase health care costs are caused by environmental factors and living conditions that cannot be changed through sport or fitness programs.
- Some forms of sport participation, including ultra-endurance and heavy-contact sports, do not produce overall health benefits because of the damage they do to the bodies of many participants.
- The culture in certain competitive sports often contributes to injuries and increased health care costs; for example, there are an estimated 300,000 sport-related concussions each year, and more than 62,000 of those are sustained by high school athletes in contact sports alone (Graham et al., 2013). Other injuries, including bone fractures, ligament tears, and tendon damage have increased significantly among high school and college athletes since 2000, and they are costly to treat and rehabilitate (Fawcett, 2012; Healy, 2013; Leet, 2012).
- The demand for health care often increases among competitive athletes because they seek specialized medical care to treat and rehabilitate any injury or physical condition preventing them from meeting their performance expectations.

In light of these factors, some government officials are now cautious and selective when they sponsor sports for health purposes, and they are more likely to support noncompetitive physical activities with clear aerobic benefits than sports with high injury rates.

Promote the Prestige and Power of a Community or Nation

Government involvement in sports frequently is motivated by a quest for recognition and prestige (Hubbert, 2013; Kang et al., 2013; Park et al., 2012; Silk, 2011; Tan and Houlihan, 2012; Yu and Bairner, 2010). This is especially the case for cities and countries that host major sport events such as FIFA World Cups in soccer and the Olympic and Paralympic Games (Booth, 2011; Dorsey, 2013a, 2013b; Schausteck de Almeida et al., 2013; Smale, 2011).

This quest for recognition and prestige also underlies government subsidies for national teams across a wide range of sports, usually those designated as Olympic sports. Government officials use international sports to establish their nation's legitimacy in the international sphere, and they often believe that winning medals enhances their image around the world. This is why many governments provide cash rewards to their athletes who win medals. At the 2012 Olympic Games in London, many governments paid gold medal winners cash bonuses (V. Black, 2012; Caruso-Cabrera, 2012; C. Smith, 2012). In Kazakhstan it was $250,000; in Italy, $182,000; France, $65,000; South Africa, $55,000; Mexico, $37,000. Canada, at $20,000, is among the lowest of international payouts. Russian medal winners received $135,000 for gold, $82,000 for silver, and $54,000 for bronze from the national government but reportedly up to $1 million from local governments in the regions where they resided.

Chinese gold medal winners were paid a reported $55,000, and provincial governments gave houses, luxury cars, or other significant gifts to gold medal winners. Host country Great Britain gave no cash awards to medal winners, although their pictures will go on Royal Mail stamps and they will receive royalties, sometimes reaching five figures, when the stamps are purchased.

U.S. athletes received no money from the government, but the USOC paid medal winners $25,000 for gold, $15,000 for silver, and $10,000 for bronze. But each of the 529 U.S. athletes also received five duffle bags full of items provided by corporations, including a $600 ring (custom sized at registration), an Omega watch worth several thousand dollars, and about 100 other items from Oakley, Nike, Ralph Lauren, and other companies that custom-fit clothes Olympians (Olmsted, 2012). Paralympic athletes also received the rings and additional items.

Attempts to gain recognition and prestige also underlie local governments' involvement in sports. Cities fund sport clubs and teams and then use them to promote themselves as good places to live, work, locate a business, or vacation. Many people in North America feel that if their city does not have one or more major professional sport team franchises, it cannot claim world-class status (Delaney and Eckstein, 2008; deMause, 2011; deMause and Cagan, 2008; Silk and Andrews, 2008).

Even small towns use road signs to announce the success of local high school teams to everyone driving into the town: "You are now entering the home of the state champions" in this or that sport. State governments in the United States subsidize sport programs at colleges and universities for similar reasons: Competitive success is believed to bring prestige to the entire state as well as the school represented by winning athletes and teams; prestige, it is believed, attracts out of state and international students that pay high tuition rates that help support educational programs.

When governments fund sports and sport facilities to boost the profile of a city or nation, they often become caught in a cycle where increased funding is regularly required to compete with other cities and nations doing the same thing with bigger

budgets or newer facilities (Coakley, 2011c; Hall, 2006; Topič and Coakley, 2010). This continuously pushes up the funds and other resources that must be allocated to sports, and it decreases resources for programs having more direct and concrete positive impact on citizens. Government officials often find that using this strategy to boost prestige for a city or nation is costly relative to the public benefits created, especially when most of the direct and tangible benefits go to a relatively small and predominantly wealthy segment of their constituency (Coakley and Souza, 2013).

Promote Identity and Unity

When people identify strongly with a sport, government officials often use public money to support athletes and teams as a representation of a city or nation. The emotional unity created by a sport or team is widely believed to establish or reaffirm an identity that further connects people with the city or nation (Sorek, 2007). For example, when the Brazilian men's soccer team plays in the World Cup, the people of Brazil experience a form of emotional unity and a related sense of attachment to the nation. This attachment means different things to different people, but the expectation is that it will reaffirm national loyalty and highlight everything from the nation's history and traditions to its geography and its place in the global economic or political order.

Research on national identity indicates that it is a much more dynamic social construct than many people have imagined.[1] Its intensity, meaning,

---

[1]Beginning in the mid-1990s, the topic of national identity has received much attention in the sociology of sport. The research done over the last decade has been extensive. The following references are a good starting point for people interested in this topic: Bairner and Hwang, 2011; Bartoluci and Perasović, 2008; Brownell, 2008; Chiang and Chen, 2015; Coakley and Souza, 2013; Darby, 2011; Denham, 2010; Dóczi, 2012; Elling et al., 2014; Gibbons, 2014; Griggs & Gibbons, 2014; Juncà, 2008; Kang, Kim & Wang, 2015; Leng et al., 2014; Licen and Billings, 2013; J. Maguire, 2005; Mehus and Kolstad, 2011; Schausteck de Almeida et al., 2013; Sorek, 2011; Thomas and Anthony, 2015; Topič and Coakley, 2010; Van Hilvoorde et al., 2010; von Scheve et al., 2014.

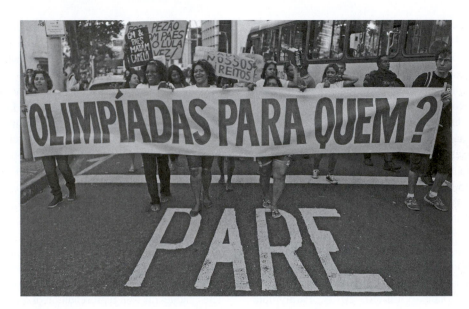

Quantifying and measuring the long-term social impact of sports is difficult. People often assume that sport mega-events such as the Olympic Games and the FIFA World Cup create social integration and national identity. However, this was not the case for the 2014 Men's World Cup or the 2016 Olympic Games in Rio de Janeiro. One year before the Rio Games these protesters carried a sign asking, "Olympics for whom?" They knew that the 2016 Olympic Games would serve the interests of the wealthy and powerful rather than the general population. (*Source:* © Tasso Marcelo/Getty Images)

and the forms through which it is expressed vary widely between and even within nations. Additionally, it changes over time with shifts in national experiences such as those that occur in times of peace or times of war, in the face of positive or negative economic conditions, or when immigration patterns alter a nation's demographic profile.

Consider a recent Olympic qualifying tournament for men's team handball held in Zadar, Croatia. A city of 71,000 people on the coast of the Adriatic Sea, Zadar was repeatedly attacked during the early and mid-1990s by Yugoslav and Serbian forces as Croatia fought a war to break away from Soviet-aligned-Yugoslavia and become an independent nation. Croatia succeeded in gaining its independence, but the people in the Zadar region have only recently felt that the war and its aftermath are behind them. Therefore, when they hosted the handball tournament, the tickets sold out immediately and people from the city

and surrounding area used the team and its matches as opportunities to express deep personal feelings of nationhood shaped by war, economic hardship, recent peace, and hope for future prosperity.

The expressions of national identity in Zadar can be viewed as a sign of resilience and unity with the rest of Croatia, but their intensity, and the ways that they reaffirm a strong sense of separation from people in neighboring Serbia and Bosnia-Herzegovena, cause some people to worry (Bartoluci and Perasović, 2009). They fear that sport-related expressions of national unity, pride, and identity are dangerous under conditions that can turn them into chauvinism and militaristic forms of nationalism (Mehus and Kolstad, 2011; Porat, 2012; Sorek, 2011; Vaczi, 2013).

When government involvement in sport is intended to promote identity and unity, it usually benefits some people more than others. Although emotional unity seldom lasts long, it often serves the interests of people with power and influence because they have the resources to connect it with the images, traditions, and memories that constitute their ideas of nationhood and the importance of loyalty to the status quo. For example, when men's sports are sponsored and women's sports are ignored, the sense of national identity and unity among men may be strong, but women may feel alienated (Adams, 2006). When sports involve participants from only one ethnic group or a particular social class, there are similar divisions in the "imagined community" and the "invented traditions" constructed around sports (Joseph, 2014; Mehus and Kolstad, 2011; Porat, 2012; Shor and Yonay, 2011; Vaczi, 2013, 2015; Wise, 2015).

> The football pitch has become an important tool for integration and a measure of the success of European integration policies. As such, it constitutes a barometer that local, regional, and national policy makers in Europe cannot afford to ignore. —James Dorsey, journalist (2013b)

National and local identities are political in that they can be constructed around many different ideas about who or what the nation or community is. Of course, these ideas can vary widely between particular categories of people. Furthermore, neither the identity nor the emotional unity created by sports changes the social, political, and economic realities of life.

When games end, people go their separate ways. Old social distinctions become relevant again, and the people who were disadvantaged prior to the game or tournament remain disadvantaged after it (Coakley and Souza, 2013; Majumdar and Mehta, 2010). But this raises interesting questions: Do privileged people feel more justified in their privilege, and do people who are systematically disadvantaged in a city or nation feel less justified in making their disadvantage a political issue because everyone, even the rich and powerful, is part of the big "we" that is reaffirmed at sport events? The identity and unity created by sports clearly feels good to many people, and it can inspire a sense of possibility and hope, but it may obscure the need for social transformations that would make social worlds more fair and just.

The recent growth of global labor migration has intensified interest in the relationship between sport and national identity. As globalization has blurred national boundaries and made them less relevant for many people, government officials have used sports and national teams to rekindle the idea of nationhood at the same time that they have used sports and multinational teams to inspire identification with newly created political and economic entities (Tamir, 2014; Topič and Coakley, 2010). For example, as European nations sponsor national sports to reinvigorate old feelings of national identity at a time when immigrant workers bring diverse identities to various nations, representatives of the twenty-eight-nation European Union use golf's Ryder Cup pitting Team Europe against Team USA to promote the formation of a European identity. Satellite and cable companies that serve most European nations have fostered both forms of identification with their sports programming, depending on which one will increase ratings the most.

These developments complicate national identity and make it more difficult to study and understand its connection with sports. Governments continue to use sports to promote identity and unity, but the long-term effectiveness of this strategy is difficult to assess. Many government officials *believe* that sports create more than temporary good feelings of national "we-ness," but nearly all these officials are men, and the sports they support usually have long histories of privileging men.

Research suggests that in well-established nations, the impact of successful national teams on feelings of national pride and identity is minimal (Elling et al., 2012; Van Hilvoorde et al., 2010), and most likely to be boosted among athletes, men, and non-immigrants in the country. Those who are aware of their nation's history and current global status across economic, political, educational, and cultural spheres of life may see sports as important but as only one aspect of national identity. Additionally, people with access to global media may develop attachments to athletes and teams from other countries and pay less attention to the sport profile and accomplishments associated with their own country, except in the case of the Olympics or world championships in certain sports (Topič and Coakley, 2010).

Another identity issue is whether a nation's success in sports makes people in other countries more aware of the nation's existence, attractions, accomplishments, and potential. This has not been studied in detail, but unless a nation receives extensive media coverage in connection with multiple sport events, it isn't likely that winning medals or an occasional championship will lead to more than superficial knowledge about its history and heritage. But research is needed on this issue.

Reproduce Values Consistent with Dominant Political Ideology

Governments also become involved in sports to promote specific political values and ideas among their citizens. This is especially true when there is a need to reaffirm the idea that success is based on discipline, loyalty, determination, and hard work, even in the face of hardship and bad times. Sports are useful platforms to promote these values and foster a particular ideology that contains taken-for-granted assumptions about the way social life is organized and how it does and should operate.

It's difficult to determine the extent to which people are influenced by sports that are represented in specific ideological terms, but we do know that in capitalist societies, such as the United States, sports provide people with a vocabulary and real-life examples that are consistent with dominant political and cultural ideologies.

The images, narratives, and the often-repeated stories that accompany sports in market economies emphasize that competition is clearly the best and most natural way to achieve personal success and allocate rewards to people, whereas alternative approaches to success and allocating rewards—democratic socialism, socialism, communism,

and the like—are ineffective, unnatural, and even immoral.

The Cold War era following World War II was a time when nations, especially the United States, the former Soviet Union (USSR—the Union of Soviet Socialist Republics), and East Germany (GDR—the German Democratic Republic), used the Olympics and other international sport competitions to make claims about the superiority of their political and economic systems and ideologies.

Now that the Cold War is over, powerful global corporations use sports to promote free-market ideology, but governments have not stopped using sports to promote values consistent with ideologies that support their interests. In fact, since the late 1950s the U.S. military has provided "color guard" units to present the American flag at sporting events and has sponsored demonstration "fly-overs" by fighter jet teams to connect the status and place of the military with certain sports, especially NFL football, in the minds of Americans.

Increase Support for Political Leaders and Government

Government authority rests ultimately in legitimacy. If people do not perceive political leaders and the government as legitimate, it is difficult to maintain social order. In the quest to maintain their legitimacy, political officials may use athletes, teams, and particular sports to boost their acceptance in the minds of citizens. They assume, as Italian political theorist Antonio Gramsci predicted, that if they support what people value and enjoy, they can maintain their legitimacy as leaders. This is why so many political leaders present themselves as friends of sport, even as faithful fans. They attend highly publicized sport events and associate themselves with high-profile athletes and teams that win major competitions. U.S. presidents traditionally have associated themselves with successful athletes and teams and have invited champions to the White House for photo opportunities.

Some male former athletes and coaches in the United States have used their celebrity status from

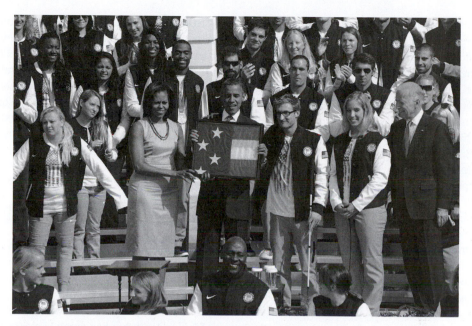

The President and First Lady Michelle Obama welcome 2012 U.S. Olympic and Paralympic teams to the White House lawn, where Navy Lieutenant Brad Snyder, blinded by an IED in Afghanistan, presented the president with a piece of the American flag that was carried during the opening Olympic ceremonies. President Obama has taken many opportunities to be publicly associated with U.S. athletes and sports, because it connects him with what many people see as symbols of U.S. national identity. (*Source:* © Christy Bowe/Corbis)

sports to gain popular support for their political candidacy. In fact, former athletes and coaches have been elected to state legislatures and to the U.S. Congress and Senate by using their status from sports and their sport personas to increase their legitimacy as "tough," "hard-working," and "loyal" candidates who are "decisive under pressure" and "dedicated to being winners."

Facilitate Economic and Social Development

Since the early 1980s, governments have supported or intervened in sports

I am always amazed when I hear people saying that sport creates goodwill between the nations . . . Even if one didn't know from concrete examples . . . that international sporting contests lead to orgies of hatred, one could deduce it from general principles.

—George Orwell, The Sporting Spirit (1945)

to facilitate a particular form of urban economic development (Boykoff, 2014a; Curi et al., 2011; deMause, 2011; Hall, 2006, 2012; Lenskyj, 2008; Schausteck de Almeida et al., 2013; Schimmel, 2013; Silk and Andrews, 2008). National and city governments now spend millions of tax dollars on bids to host the Olympic Games, World Cup tournaments, world or national championships, Super Bowls, College Bowl games, All-Star Games, high-profile auto races, golf tournaments, and track-and-field meets. In many cases, these expenditures of public money are connected with private entrepreneurial projects designed to increase personal and corporate capital and "renew" blighted or declining areas. By using a sport team, a new stadium, or a major sport event to justify spending public money, business-oriented public officials can partner with developers to gentrify declining or deteriorated urban neighborhoods by bringing in upscale businesses, shoppers, and residents, and moving out low-income and homeless people.

Using sports is an effective way to create public support for this type of development project, but many of the projects are risky and controversial as public investments. Most fail to meet the optimistic economic impact projections provided by developers, and benefits are enjoyed by relatively few people (Coakley and Souza, 2013; Cornelissen, 2009, 2010; Darnell, 2010a; Hall, 2012; Kuper, 2010; Majumdar and Mehta, 2010).

Government involvement in sports may also be based on the presumed social effects of sports in a community or society. Many public officials believe the great sport myth and think that sports, in almost any form, bring people together and create social bonds that carry into other spheres of life and increase the social vitality of a city or society. Research generally contradicts this belief, often finding that relationships formed in connection with sports seldom carry over to other spheres, and that some relationships between individuals and groups are characterized by conflicts that can interfere with social development.

Two recent studies have raised additional questions about this issue. Researchers doing an exploratory (or "pilot") study in Canada found that people who worked as volunteers with non-profit sport organizations for longer than one year expanded their network of relationships and were put in touch with valuable resources in the realm of sports. At the same time, however, their involvement in other spheres was limited and nonsport social networks declined in scope (Harvey et al., 2007). Another study done in Canada found that people who had played youth sports were more likely to be involved in community activities through adulthood (Perks, 2007).

Taken together, these studies indicate that sports may be associated with social development under certain conditions and that the social effects of this association may not be immediately observable in people's lives. This doesn't confirm the beliefs of public officials who use sports to promote social development as much as it provides information about how and when government can effectively facilitate social development and what can be expected in terms of social effects.

Additional Examples of Government Involvement in Sports

The previous eight sections did not identify all types of government involvement in sports. Other cases of involvement in the United states include the following:

- Making laws that ban animal sports such as bullfighting or dog and cock fighting and protect the well-being of animals in horse and dog racing, fox hunting, and rodeo
- Making laws that ban, restrict, or regulate gambling on sports, thereby protecting the credibility of competitive sport outcomes and reining in athletes who might be coerced to shave points or fix competitions
- Adjusting the tax code so that the cost of tickets and luxury suites at sport events are partially tax-deductible business expenses
- Interpreting tax law so that highly commercialized college sports are legally defined as nonprofit educational programs
- Interpreting anti-trust and labor law to benefit professional sport team owners, and allowing major sport organizations to claim nonprofit status despite paying executives millions in salaries and bonuses
- Making public funding decisions that influence where public sport facilities are located and what sports they benefit

Even though many people say that politics have no place in sports, governments play a key role in sponsoring and regulating sports. People generally take issue with government involvement only when it does not bring the results they want; otherwise, they seldom notice it.

Critical Issues and Government Involvement in Sports

Advocates of government involvement in sports justify it as serving the "public good." It would be ideal if governments promoted equally the interests of all citizens, but differences between individuals and groups make this impossible. Therefore, public investments in sports often benefit some people more than others. Those who benefit most are the persons or groups who are capable of directly influencing policy makers. This doesn't mean that government policies reflect only the interests of wealthy and powerful people, but it does mean that policy making is often contentious and creates power struggles among various segments of the population in a city or society.

Governments worldwide make decisions about allocating funds between elite sports and sports for all. Elite sports are highly organized, have strong backing from other organized groups, and base their requests for support on visible accomplishments achieved in the name of the entire country or city. Recreational sports serving large numbers of people are less organized, less likely to have powerful supporters, and less able to give precise statements of their goals and the political significance of their programs. This does not mean that government decision makers ignore mass participation, but it does mean that "sport for all" usually has lower priority for funding and support (Conn, 2012; Green, 2006; Green and Houlihan, 2004; Schausteck de Almeida et al., 2012).

Those who believe the myth that there is no connection between sports and government are most likely to be ignored by public officials, whereas those who are aware of government involvement are most likely to benefit when it does occur. Sports are connected with power relations in society as a whole; therefore, sports and politics cannot be separated.

SPORTS AND GLOBAL POLITICAL PROCESSES

Most people have lofty expectations about the impact of sports on global relations. It has long been hoped that sports would serve diplomatic functions by contributing to cultural understanding and world peace. Unfortunately, the realities of sports seldom match ideals. Nation-states and transnational corporations (TNCs) regularly use sports to promote their interests and ideologies, and sports have become much more global today as athletes, teams, events, equipment, and capital investments cross national borders on a daily basis. Issues related to these global processes are often linked with politics, so it is useful to understand them when studying sports in society.

International Sports: Ideals Versus Realities

Achieving peace and friendship among nations was emphasized by Baron Pierre de Coubertin when he founded the modern Olympic Games in 1896. For over a century, his goals have been embraced by many people who assumed or hoped that sports would do the following things:

- Create open communication lines between people and leaders from different nations.
- Highlight shared interests among people from different cultures and nations.
- Demonstrate that friendly international relationships are possible.
- Foster cultural understanding and eliminate the use of national stereotypes.
- Create a global model for cooperative cultural, economic, and political relationships.
- Establish processes that develop effective leaders in emerging nations and close the resource gap between wealthy and poor nations.

Recent history shows that sports can be useful in the realm of **public diplomacy,** which consists of *public expressions of togetherness in the form of cultural exchanges and general communication among officials from various nations.* However, sports have no impact in the realm of **serious diplomacy,** which consists of *discussions and decisions about political issues of vital national interest.* In other words, international sports provide opportunities for political leaders to meet and talk, but they don't influence the content of their discussions or their policy decisions.

Likewise, sports bring together athletes who may learn from and about one another, but athletes have seldom tried to make or influence political decisions, and their relationships with one another have no serious political significance.

Recent history shows that most nations use sports and sport events, especially the Olympic Games, to pursue their own interests rather than international understanding, friendship, and peace (Jennings, 2006). Nationalist themes going beyond respectful expressions of patriotism have been clearly evident in many events, and most nations regularly use sport events to promote their own military, economic, political, and cultural agendas. This was particularly apparent during the Cold War era following World War II and extending into the early 1990s. During these years, the Olympics were extensions of "superpower politics" between the United States and its allies and the former Soviet Union and its allies.

The inherent links between international sports and politics were so clear in the early 1980s that Peter Ueberroth, president of the committee that organized the 1984 Olympic Games in Los Angeles, said that "we now have to face the reality that the Olympics constitute not only an athletic event but a political event" (U.S. News & World Report, 1983). Ueberroth was not being prophetic; he was simply summarizing his observations of events leading up to the 1984 games. He saw that nations were more interested in benefiting themselves than pursuing global friendship and peace. The demonstration of national superiority through sports has long been

> There is simply no sporting event on earth more entangled in politics than [the Men's World Cup]. Anytime you have half the earth tuned in—as colonies play their former colonizers and dictatorships challenge democracies—politics follow like rainbows after rain. —Dave Zirin, independent sport journalist (2010b)

a major focus of world powers, and many nations that seek to extend their political and economic power have used sports to gain international recognition and legitimacy.

For smaller nations, the Olympics, World Cups, and international championships have been stages for showing that their athletes and teams can stand up to and sometimes defeat athletes and teams from wealthy and powerful nations. For example, when the cricket teams from the West Indies or India play teams from England, the athletes and fans from India and the West Indies view the matches as opportunities to show the world that they are now equal to the nation that once colonized their land and controlled their people. When their teams win, it is cause for political affirmation and great celebration.

National and city leaders know that hosting the Olympics is a special opportunity to generate international recognition, display national power and resources to a global audience, and invite investments into their economies. This is why the bid committees from prospective host cities and nations have regularly used gifts, bribes, and financial incentives to encourage IOC members to vote for them in the host city selection process. Illegal and illicit strategies were common during the bidding for the 2002 Winter Olympics, when officials from Salt Lake City offered to IOC members and their families money, jobs, scholarships, lavish gifts, vacations, and the sexual services of "escorts" as they successfully secured the votes needed to host the games (Jennings, 1996a, 1996b; Jennings and Sambrook, 2000). Efforts to influence votes and personally profit from decisions involving billions of dollars still occur, but they are usually done much more carefully and discretely (Booth, 2011; Jennings, 2013a, 2013b).

The link between sports and politics has been clearly exposed by protests and boycotts directed at the Olympics and other international sport events. For example, when Mexican college students used the 1968 Olympic Games hosted by Mexico City as an occasion for protesting police violence and the actions of an oppressive political regime, the police and military massacred hundreds of students and others in a public plaza in the Tlatelolco neighborhood of Mexico City (Poniatowska, 1975). Representatives of governments and National Olympic Committees said little or nothing about the murders because they wanted a "secure" Olympic Games.

In 1980, the United States and sixty-two of its political allies boycotted the Olympic Games in Moscow, the capital of the Soviet Union (USSR), to protest the decision of the Soviets to invade Afghanistan and eliminate Islamic rebels, because the rebels opposed Soviet control of the region. The United States supported the autonomy of Afghanistan, armed the rebels, including Osama bin Laden, and helped to create the terrorist infrastructure that later became Al-Qaeda. In retaliation, the Soviet Union and at least fourteen of its allies boycotted the 1984 Olympic Games in Los Angeles to protest the commercialization of the games and avoid terrorist actions they expected from Americans who had made threats against their teams and athletes.

Each of these Olympic Games was held despite the boycotts, and each host nation unashamedly displayed its power and resources to the world and touted the fact that they topped the medal count for the respective games. Neither boycotting nor hosting the games had any major effects on U.S. or Soviet political policies, although they did intensify Cold War feelings and fears.

Global media coverage of sport mega-events has added new dimensions to the link between sports and politics. Television companies, especially the American networks, have used political controversies to hype the games and increase audience ratings, and they edit programming to highlight the American flag and melodramatic stories about athletes who overcame disadvantage to achieve success and participate in the American Dream (Greider, 2006).

Networks claim that Americans won't watch an Olympics unless the global power and cultural values of the United States are woven into the coverage. Of course, the U.S. media aren't the only ones to do this, but their impact far surpasses the impact of nationalist and ethnocentric coverage in other nations, because the military and economic power and policies of the United States affect the world much more than do the power and policies of other nation-states.

Nationalistic themes in media coverage of international sports are now accompanied and sometimes obscured by images and narratives promoting capitalist expansion and the products and services of transnational corporations. These issues are discussed in the Reflect on Sports box "Olympism and the Olympic Games."

Nation-States, Sports, and Ideological Hegemony

Global politics often revolve around issues of ideological hegemony—that is, whose ideas and beliefs are most widely accepted worldwide and used to guide everything from world trade to who starts wars with whom. In this process, sports usually serve the interests of wealthy and powerful nations. For example, when nations with few resources want to participate in major international sports, they must look to wealthy nations for assistance in the form of coaching, equipment, and training support. As this occurs, people in poorer nations often de-emphasize their traditional folk games and focus on the global sports developed around the values and experiences of nations powerful enough to export their games around the globe and make them the centerpieces of international competitions. If they want to play, those are the sports in which they must excel. To the extent that this makes poorer nations dependent, sports become vehicles for economically powerful nations to extend their control over important forms of popular culture worldwide—and to claim that it is part of the "foreign aid" that they give to poor people and struggling nations (Coakley and

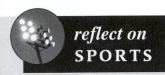

The Olympic and Paralympic Games
Are They Special?

According to the Olympic Charter, the Olympic Games are based on a special philosophy described in these words:

> Olympism is a philosophy of life, exalting and combining in a balanced whole the qualities of body, will, and mind. Blending sport with culture and education, Olympism seeks to create a way of life based on the joy found in effort, the educational value of good example, and respect for universal fundamental ethical principles.

This means that the Olympics should provide opportunities for people worldwide to learn about and connect with one another in ways that lead to respect and peace—a commendable goal given that our future and the future of the earth itself depends on global cooperation.

If the Olympic and Paralympic Games facilitate such an outcome, they are indeed special. But nationalism and commercialism exert so much influence on the coverage of the Games that the goals of global understanding and peace receive only token attention (Lenskyj, 2008).

One factor undermining the philosophy of Olympism is the current method of selling media broadcasting rights for the Olympic and Paralympic Games (Andrews, 2007). Television companies buy media rights so they can re-present selected video images from the Olympics and Paralympics and combine them with their own narratives to attract audiences in their countries. Therefore, instead of bringing the world together around a single unifying experience, the coverage consists of many heavily nationalized and commercialized versions of the Games. Of course, media consumers give their own meanings to this coverage, but they consume images and narratives from only their nation as starting points for making sense of and talking about the Olympics (Buffington, 2012; Licen and Billings, 2013).

Media consumers who want to use the Olympics to visualize a global community constructed around cultural differences and mutual understanding can do so, but current media coverage provides little assistance in this quest. Most coverage highlights the association between human achievement, selected cultural values, and corporate sponsors. In the process, many people come to believe that corporations really do make international sports possible. As they watch television coverage in the United States, about 25 percent of the programming consists of commercial messages from corporations, many of which claim to "bring you the Olympics."

People don't accept media images and narratives in literal terms, but corporate sponsors now bet billions of dollars on the possibility that associating their products and logos with the Olympics and Paralympics will discourage criticism of their products and policies, encourage people to consume those products, and normalize a lifestyle organized around consumption.

The overt commercialism that now pervades the Olympics has led some people to question the meaning of the games themselves (Stockdale, 2012). Bruce Kidd (1996), a former Olympian and a physical and health educator at the University of Toronto, argues that if the Olympic Games are to be special, they must use sports to make people aware of global injustice and promote social responsibility worldwide.

Kidd says that in the spirit of Olympism, athletes should be selected for participation in the games on the basis of their actions as global citizens as well as their athletic accomplishments. There also should be a curriculum enabling athletes to learn about fellow competitors and their cultures. The games should involve formal, televised opportunities for intercultural exchanges, and athletes should be ready to discuss their ideas about world peace and social responsibility during media interviews.

The IOC should sponsor projects enabling citizen–athletes to build on their Olympic and Paralympic experiences through service to others around the world. A proportion of the windfall profits coming from rapidly escalating TV rights fees should fund such projects, thereby giving IOC members opportunities to talk about real examples of social responsibility that they support. The "up close and personal" stories presented in the media could then highlight the socially responsible actions of athletes. Media consumers are increasingly aware that they don't live in isolation from the rest of the world and may find such coverage as entertaining as the current soap opera–like stories of personal tragedies and triumphs.

Additionally, the IOC could control nationalism and commercialism more carefully as it organizes the games and sells broadcasting rights. There is no single best way to do this, but here are six recommendations that would emphasize the spirit of Olympism:

1. *Add to each games "demonstration sports" native to the cultural regions where the games are held.* The IOC should specify that all media companies purchasing broadcasting rights and receiving press credentials must devote 5 percent of their coverage to these native games. Because the media influence the ways that people imagine, create, and play sports, this would provide expanded images of physical activities and facilitate creative approaches to sport participation worldwide. At present, many Olympic sports are simply a legacy of former colonial powers that exported their games as they conquered peoples around the world. But there are thousands of folk games that could inspire new forms of physical activities and sports today, if people knew about them and saw them being played.

2. *Use multiple sites for each Olympic Games.* The cost of hosting the summer Olympic Games was $14.6 billion for Athens in 2004; well over $40 billion for Beijing in 2008; and about $15 billion for London in 2012. Such costs privilege wealthy nations and prevent less wealthy nations from hosting the games and highlighting their cultures. If Olympic events were split into three "event packages," many more nations could host one of the packages and enjoy the benefits of staging the events without accumulating debts that burden local citizens for decades after the event and leave them with a legacy of underused facilities.

3. *Emphasize global responsibility in media coverage.* Television contracts should mandate an emphasis on global social responsibility in the media coverage of the games. Athlete committees, working with scholars from the Olympic Academy, could identify individuals, organizations, and corporations that

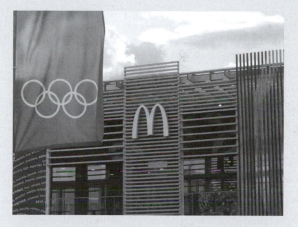

McDonald's and Coke bought the rights to a food and drink monopoly at the 2012 Olympic Games in London. Using marketing logic based on widespread acceptance of the great sport myth, the McDonald's Corporation and the Coca-Cola Company have spent billions of dollars in recent decades to link their logos with the Olympic rings. The hope is that beliefs in the purity and goodness of sports will be associated with their products that are difficult to market as pure and good. (*Source:* © Barbara Schausteck de Almeida)

have engaged in noteworthy forms of social responsibility and assist media companies in producing coverage of these cases. Additionally, a mandated amount of media time should be dedicated to public service announcements from nonprofit human rights groups that work with athletes and sport organizations to promote social justice and sustainable forms of development. This would guarantee that media consumers receive information that is not created or censored by corporations and market forces.

4. *Integrate the Olympics and Paralympics.* Just as the Olympic Movement supports gender equality and opposes racial apartheid in sports, it should include Paralympic athletes in the Olympic Games.

Continued

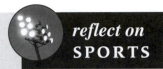

Olympism and the Olympic Games (*continued*)

This would involve common opening and closing ceremonies, awarding the same Olympic medals to athletes in both events, and referring to both as "Olympics." This would send a powerful message to the world saying that the full inclusion of people with a disability is an achievable goal in all spheres of life.

5. *Promote a fair method of calculating medal counts.* National medal counts are contrary to the spirit and official principles of Olympism. They foster chauvinism and hostility, present the achievements of athletes in divisive rather than unifying ways, and privilege large, wealthy nations with resources to train medal-winning athletes. To make medal counts fair, members of the Olympic Academy (scholars who study Olympism) should publish daily during each Olympic Games an "official medal count" in which the size of participating nations is statistically controlled.

Table 13.1 provides an example of how rankings would change if national population size were controlled. The list on the left side of the table ranks nations by the total number of medals won in all the Olympic Games from 1896 through 2013. The list on the right side of the table ranks nations in terms of the number of people in the overall population for each medal won by its athletes: the lower the population number per medal, the more efficient the country is in producing medal-winning athletes.

In this ranking system, Finland is most efficient, because it has had one medal-winning athlete for every 17,904 people in its current population. Great Britain, ranked 21st, has had one medal-winning athlete for every 79,720 people in its population. The United States is 37th with one medal-winning athlete for every 130,521 people in its current population. This could be taken to mean that Finland's system of sport participation and elite athlete training is seven times more efficient than the U.S. system in producing athletes that win Olympic medals, and this does not take into account that the United States has a

much higher Gross Domestic Product (GDP) per capita than Finland has.*

6. *Replace the Olympic motto Citius–Altius–Fortius (Faster–Higher–Stronger) with Health–Unity–Peace.* The current motto creates problems for the Olympic Movement because athletes are reaching the limits of human performance in many sports. Therefore, the only way to go Faster–Higher–Stronger is to use performance-enhancing technologies that are often expensive and not accessible to man athletes worldwide. To ban some of these technologies and spend millions of dollars testing for them seems hypocritical when the current Olympic motto inspires athletes to use them. Therefore, it would be more in keeping with the philosophy of Olympism to adopt a new motto of Health–Unity–Peace.

Of course, people will dismiss these suggestions as idealistic, but the Olympic Movement was founded on idealism and intended to inspire visions of what our world could and should be. Additionally, Olympism, it emphasizes that progress comes only through effort and participation. If the Olympic and Paralympic Games of today are little more than marketing opportunities for transnational corporations and stages for power displays by wealthy nations with medal-winning athletes, now is a good time for those who value Olympic ideals to take action and turn them into reality (Garcia, 2012).

---

*See http://www.indexmundi.com/g/r.aspx?v=67 for information on GDP per capita for all countries. *GDP per capita* is a measure based on purchasing power parity (PPP). *PPP GDP* is gross domestic product converted to international dollars that have the same purchasing power in a particular country as the U.S. dollar has in the United States. This makes it a good statistic to use when comparing the standard of living from one country to another. For our example here, the PPP in the United States is $52,800 and in Finland it is $35,900 (presented in terms of the value of the U.S. dollar in 2014).

Table 13.1   Olympic medal count by total medals (left side) and population per medal (right side), 1896–2013

Rank	Country	Medals	Rank	Country	Medals	Population per Medal
1	United States	2401	1	Finland	302	17,904
2	Soviet Union	1,010	2	Sweden	483	19,649
3	Great Britain	781	3	Hungary	475	20,972
4	France	670	4	Denmark	179	31,176
5	Germany	573	5	Bahamas	11	32,150
6	Italy	550	6	Norway	149	33,595
7	Sweden	483	7	Bulgaria	214	34,413
8	Hungary	475	8	East Germany	409	39,391
9	China	473	9	Estonia	33	39,939
10	Australia	467	10	Jamaica	67	40,385
11	East Germany	409	11	Switzerland	184	42,772
12	Russia	407	12	New Zealand	99	44,773
13	Japan	398	13	Australia	467	48,994
14	Finland	302	14	Cuba	208	54,044
15	Romania	301	15	Netherlands	266	62,901
16	Canada	278	16	Romania	301	63,265
17	Poland	271	17	Bermuda	1	64,237
18	Netherlands	266	18	Czechoslovakia	143	72,153
19	South Korea	243	19	Trinidad & Tobago	18	73,206
20	Bulgaria	214	20	Belgium	142	77,121
21	Cuba	208	21	Great Britain	781	79,720
22	West Germany	204	22	Iceland	4	79,893
23	Switzerland	184	23	France	670	97,537
24	Denmark	179	24	Greece	110	98,069
25	Norway	149	25	Austria	86	98,288

(*Source:* Adapted from http://www.medalspercapita.com/#medals:all-time; and http://www.medalspercapita.com/medals-per-capita:all-time.)

Souza, 2013; Cole, 2012; Darnell, 2012; Forde, 2013).

If people in traditional cultures want to preserve their native games, they must resist dependency status, but this is difficult in international sports when the rules and other structural characteristics of the sports reflect and privilege powerful nations (Topič and Coakley, 2010). For example, when an American sport such as football is introduced to another country, it comes with an emphasis on ideas about individual achievement, competition, winning, hierarchical authority structures, physical power and domination, the body, violence, and the use of technology to shape bodies into efficient performance machines. These ideas may not be accepted by everyone who plays or watches football, but they reaffirm orientations that privilege U.S. interests and obscure the cooperative values that are necessary for the collective survival of most traditional cultures. As an editor at *Newsweek* noted some years ago, "Sports may be America's most successful export to the world. . . . Our most visible symbol has evolved from the Stars and Stripes to Coke and the Nike Swoosh" (Starr, 1999, p. 44).

Ideally, sports facilitate cultural exchanges through which people from different nations share information and develop mutual cultural understanding. But true 50–50 sharing and mutual understanding are rare when nations have unequal power and resources. Therefore, sports often become cultural exports from wealthy nations incorporated into the everyday lives of people worldwide. Local people are free to reject, revise, or redefine these sports, but when "cultural trade routes" are opened through sports, nations that import sports often become increasingly open to importing and consuming additional goods, services, and ideas from the nations that brought them sports (Jackson and Andrews, 2004). To avoid this outcome, the less powerful nations must increase their political power and economic resources; if the imbalance is not corrected it becomes more difficult to resist

Politics runs rampant throughout the sports world, a broad arena in which struggles for racial justice, gender equality, and economic fairness are played out. —The Editors, The Nation (2011)

the political and economic dominance of wealthy and powerful nations.

Political Realities in an Era of Transnational Corporations

Global politics have changed dramatically since the 1970s. Massive corporations are now among the largest economies in the world today, and they share the global political stage with nation-states. This change occurred as nation-states embraced a policy of deregulation, lifted trade restrictions, lowered tariffs, and made it easier for capital, labor, and goods to flow freely around the globe. Although nation-states remain central in global relations, the differences between national and corporate interests have nearly disappeared in connection with sports. This was implied by Phil Knight, CEO of U.S.-based Nike, when he discussed shifts in fan loyalties in the Men's World Cup in soccer:

> We see a natural evolution . . . dividing the world into their athletes and ours. And we glory ours. When the U.S. played Brazil in the World Cup, I rooted for Brazil because it was a Nike team. America was Adidas (in Lipsyte, 1996, p. 9).

For Knight, teams and athletes represented corporations as much or more than nations; and corporate logos were more important than national flags at international events. When Nike paid to sponsor Brazil's national team and used its players to market Nike products, Knight was pushing consumption and brand loyalty over patriotism and public service as global values. For him, sports were outposts in the heads of sport fans and could be used as receptors and transmitters for the messages coming from Nike and other corporate sponsors seeking global capitalist expansion. Like executives from other transnational corporations (TNCs), he believes that sports contribute to the growth of

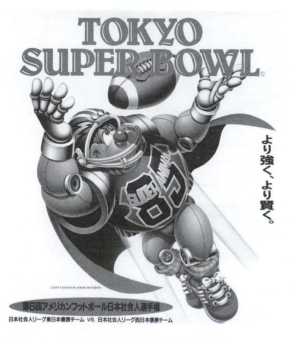

TOKYO SUPER·BOWL

より強く、より賢く。

第6回アメリカンフットボール日本社会人選手権

日本社会人リーグ東日本優勝チーム vs. 日本社会人リーグ西日本優勝チーム

Efforts by the NFL to export football to other nations have failed, largely because it requires expensive equipment and facilities and is tied to meanings and ideologies unique to U.S. history and culture. This advertising poster shows how the NFL was represented by Japanese people as they hosted an NFL preseason game in Tokyo in 1992. The caricature shows a "superanimal" with bionic joints, protective equipment, and a cape.
(*Source:* © Susumu Matsushita)

global well-being when they are used to promote a lifestyle of consumption and the values that support it.

Corporate sponsors now exert significant influence over sport events, at least to the point of directing sport images and narratives toward spectator-consumers rather than spectator-citizens (Brown, 2012). Sports that can't be covered this way—such as those that aren't organized to attract spectators with high purchasing power, or those that don't emphasize competitive outcomes and setting performance/production records—are not sponsored. When spectators and potential media audiences are not valued consumers, and when sports don't represent an ideology of competition and winning, corporations don't become sponsors and commercial media have no reason to cover them.

The global power of transnational corporations is neither unlimited nor uncontested. Individuals and local populations have used their own cultural perspectives to make sense of the images and narratives that come with global sports and give them meanings that fit with their lives (Foer, 2004; J. Maguire, 1999, 2005). However, research that combines cultural theory and a critical approach shows that global media sports and the commercial messages that accompany them often cleverly fuse the global and the local through thoughtfully and carefully edited images that combine local traditions, sport action, and consumer products in seamless and technically brilliant media representations (John and Jackson, 2011; Scherer and Jackson, 2010). The researchers doing this work argue that such fused images "detraditionalize" local cultures by representing local symbols and lifestyles in connection with consumer products that, by themselves, have nothing to do with those cultures.

On a similarly subversive level, Coca-Cola claims that it sponsors the Olympics because it wants the whole world "to move to the beat," to "live Olympic," and experience "unity on the Coke side of life." McDonald's uses a similar approach as the Official Restaurant of the Olympic Games from 1996 through 2016. When asked about the message being sent by having Coca-Cola and McDonald's as sponsors, a spokesperson for the London Organizing Committee explained, "Without our partners such as McDonald's, the games simply wouldn't happen" (Cheng, 2012). A Coca-Cola representative added, "Without the support of sponsors such as Coca-Cola as many as 170 of the 200 National Olympic Committees would be unable to send athletes to compete" (Campbell and Boffey, 2012). A McDonald's spokesperson avoided questions about nutrition and health and stated, "Ultimately it's up to individuals to make the right food, drink, and activity choices for themselves" (O'Reilly, 2012).

The goal of these corporations is to convince people that without them the pleasure and

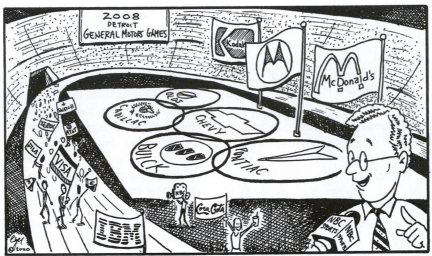

(*Source:* © Frederic A. Eyer)

"NBC Sports has eliminated nationalism in our Olympic coverage and replaced it with global consumer capitalism. Now our commentary will emphasize individualism, competition, and conquest. Enjoy the games—and the commercials that bring the games to you!"

Global politics today involve the interaction of nation-states and transnational corporations. As a result the media coverage of global mega-events is organized around images and messages that link transnational corporations with flags, anthems, and athletes representing nation-states. Patriotic feelings and consumer desires are seamlessly woven together.

excitement of the Olympic Games would no longer exist. This is not true, although there would be less money for IOC expense accounts and the Games might be less glitzy and spectacular, but they could exist without fast-food and soft-drink sponsors. Of course, commercial images and messages do not dictate what people think, but they certainly influence what people think about, and they become a part of the overall discourse that occurs in cultures around the globe.

This description of new global political realities does not mean that sports have fallen victim to a worldwide conspiracy hatched by transnational corporations. It means only that transnational corporations have joined nation-states in the global political context in which sports are defined, organized, promoted, played, presented, and given meaning around the world (Brown, 2012; John and Jackson, 2010; Scherer and Jackson, 2010).

Political Realities in an Era of Globalization

Money, athletic skills, and sports media have all gone global. Even though we pretend that national political boundaries matter for the sake of patriots who track medal counts by country during the Olympics or cheer for their national team in other events, those boundaries have become very porous for many sports. Today, sports are global businesses that transcend and blur political boundaries.

This is not to say that nation-states are unimportant (Rowe, 2013). Most national governments fund sport teams and training centers and present their athletes as representatives of the nation. Additionally, major sport leagues are generally nation-based, and national teams and athletes compete in the Olympic Games, World Cup tournaments, and World Championships. These structures sustain the importance of nations, but as sports become increasingly commercialized, super-rich investors buy sport teams in multiple countries; athletes, coaches, and technical personnel are recruited and seek opportunities and contracts worldwide; spectators follow sports, teams, and athletes outside their own countries; and sports are even transported around the globe as tourists and laborers visit or take up residence in new countries and maintain their connections with the sports of their birth nations. These patterns are not new, but they are more pervasive and growing faster than ever before. As a result, they raise political issues in and out of sports.

Globalization is *a process through which financial capital, products, knowledge, worldviews, and cultural practices flow through political borders and influence people's lives.* Globalization often involves *exchanges* of resources and elements of culture—but those exchanges are seldom equal, because some nations have more power to export and infuse their money and ways of life into other societies. The pace and pervasiveness of globalization increases as transportation and communications infrastructures expand. Globalization is not new, because connections between continents and nations began to grow and encompass nearly all regions of the world in the nineteenth century. But today, the Internet and digital communication have increased the pace of globalization, and this has impacted sports.

Team Ownership and Event Sponsorship Sport team ownership has gone global. Billionaires worldwide see ownership of professional sport teams as investments that bring them worldwide recognition. Oil-rich billionaires from Qatar now own English soccer teams. Russians with billions of windfall dollars made by taking over companies previously owned by the state now own professional teams in top leagues around the world. Asian and North American entrepreneurs and global capitalists now see sport teams anywhere in the world as potential investments that come with publicity perks.

Prior to this century it was unthinkable that a major professional sport team in any country would be owned by someone who was not a citizen of that country. Teams represented cities or well-defined regions, and local owners even hesitated to hire players who were "outsiders." But global media coverage of certain sports has given teams—especially those in the English Premier League, with soccer matches televised in more than 150 nations each week—the visibility needed to become global brands. At the same time the concentration of global wealth has created an international class of multibillionaire investors who see sport teams as investments that will provide good returns if they are marketed worldwide.

As a result, the English Premier League, the highest-profile sport league in the world, has become an investment magnet. During 2003–2013 more than half of the teams were purchased by owners outside the United Kingdom; five of those teams were bought by investors from the United States. Therefore, when the Glazer family, which owns Manchester United, pays a $50 million transfer fee to acquire a player owned by Real Madrid in Spain, NFL fans in Tampa Bay worry. This is because Glazer family also owns the Tampa Bay Buccaneers, and its fans want the Glazers to spend $50 million for a quarterback who would take the team to the Super Bowl. The two teams have separate balance sheets, but the fans of each team wonder if investment decisions for the other team impact decisions for their team.

Professional teams in the United States have also attracted international investors. The Brooklyn (formerly New Jersey) Nets NBA team is owned by Russian billionaire Mikhail Prokhorov, and the Miami Heat NBA team is owned by Micky Arison, an Israeli-born U.S. businessman who co-founded the Carnival [Cruise Line] Corporation. The MLB Seattle Mariners team is owned by Nintendo of America after being purchased by Nintendo's founder, Hiroshi Yamauchi of Japan. The NFL's Jacksonville Jaguars team is owned by Pakistani-born U.S. businessman Shalid Khan, who also owns the Fulham Football Club in the English Premier League.

Major League Soccer has attracted investors from outside the United States, including Austrian Dietrich Mateschitz, owner of Red Bull New York (and NASCAR's Team Red Bull in addition to soccer and Formula 1 teams in Europe). Chivas USA, an MLS team in Los Angeles, is owned by Jorge Vergara, also the owner of Chivas de Guadalajara, a high-profile team in the Mexican soccer league.

The impact of globalization at the level of team ownership is evident worldwide in soccer, basketball, cricket, and rugby. It is also evident in event sponsorship for auto racing, tennis, golf, rodeo, boxing, mixed martial arts, various extreme sports, and professional wrestling. These sports have tours taking athletes to dozens of different countries each year, which makes them ideally suited for global corporations who want to sponsor sports with global appeal among identifiable demographic segments of populations across all countries. The PGA, LPGA, ATP, and WTA now spread their officially sanctioned events in men's and women's golf and tennis in a number of different countries each year to attract spectators, sponsors, and future players worldwide. In fact, the LPGA has so many golfers from Asian countries that it has established a traveling language school to teach English and help native-English speakers learn the basics in other languages so they can communicate with other golfers.

Athletes   Athletes have also gone global. Managers and scouts at soccer and baseball academies see athletes as global commodities that can be trained and then sold around the world to the highest-bidding teams. Professional and U.S. college teams scout for athletic talent worldwide in the hope of finding regions or even towns where genetically gifted and "coachable" (that is, "controllable") athletes can be recruited to come away with them.

Skilled athletes in many sports now also see their job market in global terms and are willing or even desperate to travel to any place in the world where they might be offered a desirable contract (Elliott, 2013).

Most team sports have a hierarchy of "best places to work"—Sweden, Canada, or Russia for men's hockey; the United States or Japan for baseball; the United States or Germany for men's basketball; Germany, the United States, or Australia for women's basketball; England, Germany, or Spain for men's

soccer; France, Spain, or the United States for women's soccer; France or Croatia for men's team handball; Denmark for women's team handball; England, India, or the West Indies for cricket; England, Australia, or New Zealand for netball; and Argentina, Brazil, or the United Kingdom for Formula 1 racing.

In basketball alone, as of late 2013, more than 6700 men and women from the United States had played professionally in other countries during the previous five years (see http://www.usbasket.com/Americans-Overseas.asp). About 850 of those athletes played or are currently playing for teams in Germany; and that's about the same number of U.S. men that played in the NBA over the same period. Additionally, about 230 men and a few women from the United States coach professional or national basketball teams in other countries. These numbers are growing as professional leagues prosper and new leagues are established in China, Russia, Japan, and countries in Eastern Europe and Latin America. For example, former NBA player Stephon Marbury has become one of the most popular athletes in China; he has played on three different Chinese professional teams and in 2015 led the Beijing Ducks to their third Chinese Basketball Association championship in the four years he has played with them.

Athlete migration to U.S.-based professional leagues and the athletic departments of major universities is significant. Athletes born outside the United States make up 80 percent of the players in the NHL, 40 percent of the players in the MLS, 28 percent of players on MLB teams, and 20 percent of NBA players. This has made "translator" a new job category in certain sports. It also creates new challenges for leagues and coaches that have taken on athletes who speak very little English. The English Premier League has players from 100 countries; 62 percent of the players were born outside the United Kingdom, and two of the teams have more than 90 percent of their players from outside the United Kingdom.

Data from the 2008 Olympic Games in Beijing indicated that universities from the Pac-12 Conference had athletes from forty-eight different countries competing in Beijing. Twenty-two universities

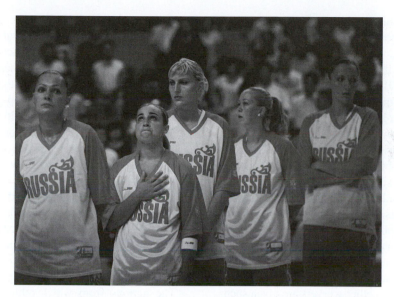

After learning that the U.S. team had no place for her, Becky Hammon (second from left) became a Russian citizen so she could play on the Russian national team in the 2008 and 2012 Olympic Games. When the Russian team played the U.S. team in London, she displayed her feelings for her home country as the U.S. national anthem was played before the game. Hammon is one of many athletes who change their citizenship or take advantage of dual citizenship to play in international events. (*Source:* © AP Photo/Elizabeth Dalziel)

for which data were available had 481 members of their college teams go to the 2008 Olympics, and 258 of those athletes (54 percent) competed for countries other than the United States (Bachman, 2012). When Olympic-level athletes want to attend school and remain amateurs while they train with top coaches and state-of-the-art technology, they seek scholarships in the United States. They know that every Division I university with a full athletic program has training facilities, coaches, and support staff that surpass what is available at the national training centers in most other countries.

Global migration also leads to mixed nationalities and more people with dual or multiple passports. For athletes, this makes country swapping possible. The athlete wants to know: What country shall I represent, or in what country do I have the best chance of making the national team and going to the Olympics? When long-time professional basketball player Becky Hammon was given notice that the U.S. national team had no room for her in 2008, she became a Russian citizen and played for the Russian national basketball team during the 2008 and 2012 Olympic Games. She was widely criticized for doing this, even though she lived part-time in Russia while playing for a professional team there. However, this strategy is used by hundreds of athletes whose mixed ancestry allows them to make choices about which nation to represent (Clarey, 2012). Fortunately for the U.S. team, Missy Franklin, who has dual U.S.-Canadian citizenship because her parents were born in Canada, chose to represent the United States. At least forty other members of U.S. Olympic squads were born in other countries but represented the United States because they had dual citizenship.

Just as some athletes choose to represent one country over another, some countries poach athletes from other countries by promising the athletes rewards and putting them on a very fast track for citizenship (Shachar, 2012). Citizenship can be acquired in less than a day if the country wants the athlete and the athlete agrees to its terms. This form of government involvement in sports is relatively common, and nearly all countries have a "back door" through which athletes can obtain work visas if a professional team wants them to sign to a contract.

It might be difficult for skilled scientists and technology entrepreneurs to obtain U.S. work visas, but the U.S. government waives rules for professional athletes who are granted a special O-1 or P-1 visa, which makes them guest workers with no questions asked and allows them to change teams as many times as they wish. No other workers are given such treatment (Cullen, 2013).

This special exemption from U.S. immigration rules allows the NHL, NBA, and other sport leagues to operate outside normal citizenship and employment restrictions, even if U.S. athletes could be hired instead of athletes from other countries. Members of Congress, even those who are anti-immigration, allowed this to occur because they see sports as special.

When athletes move from one country to another, regardless of their reasons, it raises issues related to (1) personal adjustments by migrating athletes; (2) the rights of athletes as workers; (3) the impact of talent migration on the nations from and to which athletes migrate; and (4) the national identities of athletes and fans (Bradbury, 2011; Carter, 2011; Elliott and Maguire, 2008; Evans and Stead, 2012; Maguire and Falcous, 2010; Roderick, 2012).

The personal experiences of migrating athletes vary from major culture shock and chronic loneliness to minor homesickness and lifestyle adjustments. Some athletes are exploited by teams or clubs, whereas others make much money and receive a hero's welcome when they return home during the off-season. Some encounter prejudice against foreigners or racial and ethnic bigotry, whereas others are socially accepted and form close friendships. Some cling to their national identities and socialize with fellow athletes from their homelands, whereas others develop global identities unrelated to any one national or cultural background. Some teams and clubs expect foreign athletes to adjust on their own; others provide support for those who must learn a new language or become familiar with new cultural norms.

Worker rights vary by nation, and athletes may find that they have more or less protection than they anticipated when it comes to working conditions and how they are treated by management. Much of this depends on their contracts, but state regulations may also apply beyond the contract (Engh and Agergaard, 2015).

The nations from which athletes are recruited usually have less power and resources than the recruiting countries. Over time, there may be such a depletion of talent in a country that the infrastructure for a particular sport is destroyed and local people are forced to follow the sport as it is played in the country that has taken all their best talent (Elliott and Weedon, 2011). This form of "sport talent drain" has a significant impact on countries in Africa and Latin America, where athletes seek contracts in Europe and North America.

At this point little is known about the impact of athlete migration on the identities of the athletes themselves and the feelings of national identity among people in the countries from which they emigrate. Do athletes become citizens of the country to which they are recruited? Does the move to a new country intensify or decrease their sense of national identity? Do people in the country from which athletes are recruited feel resentment about losing their best athletes, or do they see this recruitment as an affirmation of their ability to produce talent in sports? Research is needed to answer these questions.

> Basketball is booming, globally. Almost one in five players last season was not American, and when the U.S. team played China in the 2008 Olympics, 1 billion people watched. Selling 1 percent of them an item of team apparel would mean serious money. —George Will, editorial, *Washington Post* (2011b)

Fans Fans have also gone global. Manchester United in England and the Barcelona Football Club in Spain have fans in nearly every country in the world. Now that many people can receive streamed or televised coverage of games, matches, and events, they often choose to give their sport allegiance to teams and athletes outside their own countries. For example, young soccer fans in Slovenia may pay little attention to club teams in their country because all the top Slovenian soccer players play on professional teams in other countries across Europe. Many Latin American and African fans do the same thing. But in the process they may develop an attachment to one or more teams outside their countries and follow them for much of their lives, even when players from their country are no longer on the rosters.

For this reason the NBA has created a subsidiary, NBA China, with offices in Beijing, Hong Kong, and Shanghai (and Taipei, Taiwan). The opening of these offices was timed to precede the 2008 Olympic Games in Beijing and gave the NBA time to stock stores in China with official NBA products before the opening ceremonies. With 1.4 billion potential sport fans and consumers in China, most sport leagues now cultivate interest there. The NBA was pleased when over 150 million Chinese people watched the national Chinese team play the U.S. team made up of NBA players, or as NBA China would describe them, "shooting and dunking endorsements for NBA media rights and merchandise sales."

Making Sense of Political Realities

It's not easy to explain the relationships between sports and global political processes. Are sports today merely tools of capitalist expansion and new forms of cultural imperialism? Are they being used by wealthy nations to make poor, developing nations dependent on them, or do they enable emerging nations to achieve cultural and economic independence? As globalization occurs, are traditional sports and folk games being replaced by the organized, competitive sports favored by wealthy and powerful nations?

Finding answers to these questions requires research at local *and* global levels. Existing studies suggest that sports favored by wealthy nations are not simply imposed on people worldwide. Even when people play sports that come from powerful nations, they give them meanings grounded in local cultures. Global trends are important, but so are the local expressions of and responses to those trends (Chen, 2012; Cho, 2009; Cho et al., 2012; Dóczi, 2012; Gilmour and Rowe, 2012; Jijon, 2013; John and Jackson, 2011; J. Joseph, 2012a, 2012b; Kobayashi, 2012; Lee and Maguire, 2009; Merkel, 2012; Newman and Beissel, 2009; Poli, 2010; Scherer and Jackson, 2010; Shor and Galily, 2012; Silk and Manley, 2012; Tan and Houlihan, 2012). Power is a process, and it is always exercised through relationships and current forms of social organization. Therefore, research on sports worldwide must examine the processes through which powerful nations exert control over sports in other nations as well as the processes through which people in those nations integrate sports and sport experiences into their lives on their own terms.

POLITICS IN SPORTS

The term *politics* usually is associated with formal government entities in the public sphere. However, politics include all processes of governing people and administering policies at all levels of organization, both public and private. Therefore, politics are an integral part of sports, and local, national, and international sport organizations are generally referred to as "governing bodies."

Most sport organizations provide and regulate sport participation opportunities, establish and enforce policies, control and standardize competitions, and acknowledge the accomplishments of athletes. This sounds like a straightforward set of tasks, but they seldom are accomplished without opposition, debate, and compromise (Green and Hartmann, 2012). Members of sport organizations agree on many things, but conflicts often arise as decisions are made in connection with the following seven questions:

1. *What qualifies as a sport?* There is no universal definition of sport, so each nation, community, and international event, such as the Olympic Games, must develop a definition that makes sense within its circumstances. As a result, official as well as unofficial definitions of "sport" vary widely.

2. *What are the rules of a sport?* The rules in all sports are arbitrary and changeable. The governing bodies of sports often change them to fit their interests or the circumstances in which the sports are played.

3. *Who makes and enforces the rules in sports?* The official rules of every sport are determined by the sport's governing body, but confusion occurs when various organizations representing the interests of different people all claim to be the primary governing body of a sport.

4. *Who organizes and controls sport events?* Until recently, members of the governing body of a sport organized and controlled competitions, but events today may be organized and partially controlled by third parties such as sponsors, media companies, or management groups that specialize in event organization.

5. *Where do sport events take place?* When athletes decide where to play a sport, they choose a place that is convenient for them. When events are staged for commercial purposes, they take place wherever they can generate the most revenue. In the case of international events such as the Olympic and Paralympic Games, various cities make bids to be the host and the members of the organization that owns the event (e.g., the IOC) select the bidding city that provides the most attractive proposal.

6. *Who is eligible to participate in a sport?* Eligibility decisions take into account factors that are defined as relevant by members of a governing body or people managing an event. Age, skill level, academic performance, gender, race/ethnicity, nationality, citizenship, place of residence, and other factors have been used to limit eligibility depending on the concerns and beliefs of the people making eligibility decisions.

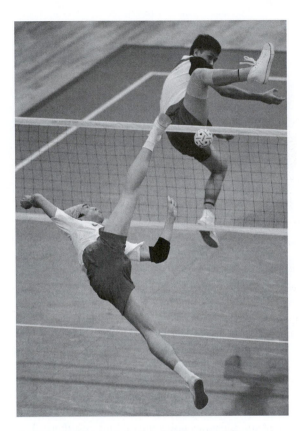

Outside Southeast Asia, Sepak Takraw might be called kick volleyball with no hands or arms allowed; only feet, head, knees, and chest may contact the ball. Based on cuju, an ancient Chinese game, Sepak Takraw has been played in Vietnam, Malaysia, Indonesia, Laos, Thailand, and Myanmar for five centuries. If these nations had conquered and colonized parts of the world and used this game to socialize colonial subjects into their cultures, as did Europeans with their sports, it would exist in enough countries to qualify as an Olympic sport. This is how politics has influenced even the definition of sports. (*Source:* © Chen Yehua/Xinhua Press/Corbis)

7. *How are rewards distributed to athletes and others associated with sports?* When rewards are associated with participating in or staging an event, the question of "Who gets what?" is crucial to everyone involved. Rewards may

include affirmations of status, such as a Most Valuable Player award, or monetary compensation as in the case of revenue-producing sports. The distribution of money often creates friction between the players and the people who organize and manage the team or event.

These questions are inherently political because answers are determined in contexts where there are differences of interest that must be resolved through negotiation (Green and Hartmann, 2012). Most people understand this, but they complain about politics in sports when the outcomes of negotiations are not the ones they favor.

Eliminating politics in sports is not possible. However, it is possible to shape political processes so that the voices of all parties impacted by decisions are heard and taken into account. Many sport organizations are notorious for their lack of transparency and accountability, and this often makes their decisions contentious because people don't know how or why they were made. There will always be differences of interest, but people are more apt to accept political decisions when they have participated in the process of making them and when they can hold accountable those who make them.

summary

HOW DO GOVERNMENTS AND GLOBAL POLITICAL PROCESSES INFLUENCE SPORTS?

Sports and politics are inseparable. Government involvement in sports is generally related to the need for sponsorship, organization, and facilities. The fact that sports are important in people's lives and can be sites for social conflict often leads to government involvement. The forms of involvement vary by society, but their purposes are generally to (1) safeguard the public order; (2) ensure fairness and protect human rights; (3) maintain health and fitness among citizens; (4) promote the prestige and power of a community or nation; (5) promote identity and

unity among citizens; (6) reproduce values consistent with dominant ideology; (7) increase support for political leaders and government; and (8) facilitate economic development.

The rules, policies, and funding priorities set by government officials and agencies reflect political differences and struggles among groups within a society. This doesn't mean that the same people always benefit when government involvement occurs, but involvement seldom results in equal benefits for everyone. For example, funding priorities could favor mass participation instead of elite sports, but this is subject to debate and negotiation. This political process is an inevitable part of organized sports.

History shows government intervention in sports usually favors groups with the most resources and organization, and with goals that support the interests of public officials. The groups least likely to be favored are those that fail to understand the connection between sports and politics or lack resources to effectively influence political decisions. When people believe that sports and politics are unrelated, they're likely to be ignored when officials develop policies and allocate funds.

The connection between sports and global political processes is complex. Ideally, sports bring nations together in contexts supportive of peace and friendship. Although this can and does occur, most nations use sports to satisfy their own interests. Displays of nationalism continue to be common at international events. For example, people who work with, promote, or follow the Olympics often focus on national medal counts and use them to support their claims for national status.

If mega-events such as the Olympics are indeed special events with positive potential, efforts should be made to maximize that potential. Limiting nationalism and commercialism and emphasizing the interdependence of nations would be helpful and could be done many ways.

Powerful transnational corporations have joined nation-states as major participants in global political processes. As a result, sports are used increasingly for economic as well as political purposes.

Nationalism and the promotion of national interests remain part of global sports, but consumerism and the promotion of capitalist expansion have become more important since 1991 and the end of the Cold War.

Within the context of global relations, athletes and teams now are associated with corporate logos as well as nation-states. Global sport events have political and economic implications. They are sites for presenting numerous images and narratives associated with the interests of nation-states *and* corporate sponsors. The dominant discourses associated with sports in the United States are clearly consistent with the interests of corporate sponsors, and they promote an ideology infused with the capitalist values of individualism, competition, achievement, and consumption.

Global political processes also are associated with other aspects of sports, such as the migration patterns of elite athletes and the recruitment patterns of sport organizations. Political issues are raised when athletes cross national borders to play their sports and when leagues and teams bring players from multiple national backgrounds into their countries. The globalization of sports affects the ownership of teams, the movement of athletes around the globe, and the allegiance patterns of sport fans worldwide.

These and other issues associated with global political processes are best understood when studied on both global and local levels. Data in these studies help determine when sports involve reciprocal cultural exchanges leading to mutual understanding among people and when they involve processes through which powerful nations and corporations exercise subtle influence over social life and political events in less powerful nations.

Politics also are part of the structure and organization of sports. Political processes exist because people in sport organizations must answer questions about what qualifies as a sport, the rules of a sport, procedures for enforcing rules, the organization and control of sport events, locations of sport events, eligibility criteria for participants, and distribution of rewards. These political issues are central to sports, and they illustrate why the organizations that make decisions about sports are often described as governing bodies. Overall, sports are inseparable from politics and political processes.

SUPPLEMENTAL READINGS

Reading 1. Politics in organized sports
Reading 2. Protests and boycotts: Politics and the Olympic Games
Reading 3. There's nothing so over as the World Cup
Reading 4. Global politics and the production of sports equipment and apparel
Reading 5. Qatar and Slovenia: Two approaches to using sports as a developmental strategy
Reading 6. The soccer stadium as a political protest site: Looking back at the Arab spring

SPORT MANAGEMENT ISSUES

• You are working for a new office of Sport and Community Development in a midwestern city of 1 million people. As the new director begins to outline a five-year plan, she asks you to list all of the ways that the federal, state, county, and local governments are involved in sports in the city, especially in terms of funding. Identify all the possibilities that you will check out as you begin the project.

• You've been appointed by the International Olympic Committee to a special commission charged with prioritizing possible reforms of the Summer Olympic Games. At the first meeting, each member of the committee must present and justify three suggestions for reform. What are your suggestions, and how do you justify them?

• You work in the personnel office of the Major Soccer League (MSL) in the United States. You must make recommendations about the league's policies related to players who are not U.S. citizens. You must deal with two major questions: (1) Should there be a limit, for each team or the league as a whole on the number of players who are not U.S. citizens? (2) How should the league and its teams provide support for the athletes who come from other countries? Explain your responses and discuss them in the general context of the globalization of sports.

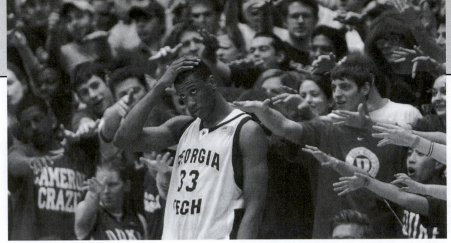

(*Source:* © ELLEN OZIER/Reuters/Corbis)

chapter

14

SPORTS IN HIGH SCHOOL AND COLLEGE

Do Competitive Sports Contribute to Education?

The problem with sports is once you combine it with academics, it starts to take over. So you have to be constantly vigilant to control it and make sure you're sending kids a message about what's going to serve their interests for decades to come.

> —**Amanda Ripley, writer and researcher (in Martin, 2013)**

High school football has never had a higher profile. . . . As players grow bigger, faster, and stronger, there are growing concerns about their health and safety. . . . It all raises a critical question: has the amped-up culture of high school football outrun necessary protections for the boys who play the game?

> —**Rachel Dretzin, Documentary film maker, PBS (2011)**

. . . inequity in college sports has reached such a comical level that it can no longer be justified with a straight face.

> —**Matthew Futterman, journalist, *Wall Street Journal* (2015)**

. . . colleges still send a negative underlying message that black men are only worth educating if they can also play ball. The American university thus remains one of the biggest agents in maintaining stereotypes that say ordinary black men can't think.

> —**Nate Jackson, journalist, *Boston Globe* (2015)**

Learning Objectives

- Identify the arguments for and against interscholastic sports.
- Discuss the research findings about the experiences of athletes in high schools.
- Know the ways that varsity sports influence student culture and the overall social organization of high schools in the United States.
- Explain the conditions under which interscholastic sports may be valuable in high schools and the lives of students who play sports.
- Identify differences between intercollegiate sports in big-time athletic programs and smaller, lower profile programs.

- Explain the research findings on the experiences of college athletes and how participation in sports is related to grades and graduation rates.
- Discus the major reforms that have been made in intercollegiate sports, and explain the purpose and effectiveness of those reforms.
- Assess popular beliefs about the benefits of varsity sports in high schools and colleges.
- Identify the major issues faced by both high school and college sport programs, and explain how they might influence sports in the future.
- Explain why some athletes of color have become socially isolated on predominantly white college campuses.

The emergence of today's organized sports is closely linked with schools in England and North America. However, the United States is the only nation in the world where it is taken for granted that high schools and colleges sponsor and fund interschool varsity sport programs. In most countries, organized sports for school-aged young people are sponsored by community-based athletic clubs funded by members or a combination of public and private sources.

High schools and universities outside the United States may have teams, but they are usually connected with a national sport system and not solely dependent on individual schools or school systems (Brown, 2015; Erturan et al., 2012; Hédi, 2011; Dziubiński, 2011; Pot et al., 2014). Additionally, their meaning and purpose are unlike the meanings given to school teams in the United States, and they are not integral to the culture and social organization of the schools.

Interscholastic sports are an accepted and important part of U.S. high schools and colleges, but when they dominate the cultures and public profiles of schools, many people become concerned about their role in education.

This chapter is organized around four questions about interscholastic sport programs:

1. What claims do people make when they argue for and against the programs?
2. How are sport programs related to education and the experiences of students?
3. What effects do sports programs have on the organization of schools and the achievement of educational goals?
4. What are the major problems associated with high school and college sport programs and how might they be solved?

ARGUMENTS FOR AND AGAINST INTERSCHOLASTIC SPORTS

Most people in the United States don't question the existence of school-sponsored sports. However, budget cutbacks and highly publicized problems in some programs raise questions about the relationship between these sports, the development of young people, and the achievement of educational goals. Responses to these questions vary and almost always are based on strong emotions.

Program supporters claim that interscholastic sports promote the educational mission of schools and the development of young people. Critics claim that they interfere with that mission and distract students from learning and taking seriously their emerging responsibilities as citizens. The main points made on both sides of this debate are summarized in Table 14.1.

When people enter this debate, they often exaggerate the benefits or problems associated with interscholastic sports. Supporters emphasize glowing success stories, and critics emphasize shocking cases of excess and abuse. Research suggests that the most accurate descriptions lie somewhere in between these extreme positions. Nonetheless, supporters and critics call our attention to the relationship between sports and education. This chapter focuses on what we know about that relationship.

INTERSCHOLASTIC SPORTS AND THE EXPERIENCES OF HIGH SCHOOL STUDENTS

Do interscholastic sports affect the educational and developmental experiences of high school students? This question is difficult to answer. Education and development occur in connection with many activities and relationships. Even though interscholastic sports are important in most schools and the lives of many students, they constitute only one of many potentially influential experiences in the lives of young people.

Quantitative research on this issue has seldom been guided by social theories, and it generally consists of comparing the characteristics of athletes and other students. Qualitative research, often based on a critical approach and guided by combinations of cultural, interactionist, and structural theories, has focused on the connections between interscholastic sports, the culture and organization of high schools, and the everyday lives of students.

Table 14.1   Claims that are made in arguments for and against interscholastic sports

Claims For	Claims Against
1. They involve students in school activities and increase interest in academic activities.	1. They distract students from academic activities and distort values in school culture.
2. They build self-esteem, responsibility, achievement orientation, and teamwork skills required for occupational success today.	2. They perpetuate dependence, conformity, and a power and performance orientation that is no longer useful in society.
3. They foster fitness and stimulate interest in physical activities among students.	3. They turn most students into passive spectators and cause too many serious injuries to athletes.
4. They generate spirit and unity and maintain the school as a viable organization.	4. They create a superficial, transitory spirit that is unrelated to educational goals.
5. They promote parental, alumni, and community support for school programs.	5. They deprive educational programs of resources, facilities, staff, and community support.
6. They give students opportunities to develop and display skills in activities valued in society and to be recognized for their competence.	6. They create pressure on athletes and support a hierarchical status system in which athletes are unfairly privileged over other students.

High School Athletes[1]

Studies in the United States consistently show that high school athletes *as a group* generally have higher grade point averages, more positive attitudes toward school, lower rates of absenteeism, more interest in attending college, more years of college completed, greater career success, and better health than students who don't play school-sponsored sports.[2] These differences usually are modest, and it's difficult for researchers to separate the effects of sport participation from the effects of social class, family background, support from friends, identity issues, and other factors related to educational attitudes and achievement.

Membership on a school team is a valued status in many U.S. schools, and for some students it seems to go hand in hand with positive educational experiences, reduced dropout rates, and increased identification with the school. However, research doesn't explain much about why sport participation affects students, and why it affects some differently from others.

Why Are Athletes Different?   The most logical explanation for differences between athletes on school teams and other students is that school-sponsored sports attract students who have good grades and self-confidence, and are socially popular in school.

Most researchers don't have information about the pre-participation characteristics of athletes

---

[1]The term "student-athlete" is not used in this book because *all* members of school teams are students, just like band members and debaters. The NCAA promotes the use of this term as a political strategy to deflect the criticism that big-time college athletic programs are unrelated to the academic mission of universities and to prevent people from defining athletes as employees.

[2]There are hundreds of these studies; the most methodologically respectable of these include the following: Brown, 2015; Carlson et al., (2005); Child Trends (2013); Eitle (2005); Fox et al., 2010; Fullinwider (2006); Guest and Schneider (2003); Hartmann (2008); Hill (2007); Hoffman (2006); Hunt (2005); Kniffin et al., 2015; Leeds et al., (2007); Lipscomb, 2006; Marsh and Kleitman (2002, 2003); Miller et al., (2005); Morris, 2013; Pearson et al., 2009; Pot et al., 2014; Sabo et al., 2013; Schultz, 2015; Shakib et al., 2011; Shifrer et al., 2013, 2015; Troutman and Dufur (2007).

because they collect data at one point in time and simply compare students who play on sport teams with students who don't. These studies are limited because they don't prove that playing school sports changes young people in ways that would not have occurred otherwise.

Fourteen- to eighteen-year-olds grow and develop in many ways whether they play school sports or do other things. This is an important point, because young people who play on varsity sport teams are more likely than other students to come from economically privileged backgrounds and have above-average cognitive abilities, self-esteem, and past academic performance records, including grades and test scores (Child Trends, 2013; Hartmann et al., 2012; Morris, 2013; Shakib et al., 2011; Shifrer et al., 2013). Therefore, students who try out for, make, and stay on school teams are different from other students *before* they play high school sports.

This *selection-in process* is common; students who participate in official, school-sponsored activities tend to be different from other students (Helmrich, 2010). This difference is greatest in activities in which student self-selection is combined with eligibility requirements and formal tryouts in which teachers or coaches select students for participation. Additionally, this combination of self-selection, eligibility, and coach selection, is an extension of a long-term process that begins in youth sports. Over time, students with lower grades and poor disciplinary records decide they don't want to be involved in sports, or they aren't academically eligible to participate, or coaches see them as troublemakers and cut them during tryouts.

Research also shows that students who play varsity sports for three years during high school are different from those who are cut from or quit teams. Those who are cut or quit are more likely to come from less advantaged economic backgrounds and have lower cognitive abilities, lower self-esteem,

> **We let students know: If you participate [in sports], we will control your study life. For kids who really want to play, they've been playing their whole lives and they'll do almost anything to play.** —Jay Sailes, high school principal (in Riede, 2006)

and lower grade point averages than those who remain on teams (Child Trends, 2013; Pearson et al., 2009; Pot et al., 2014; Shifrer et al., 2013; White and Gager, 2007). Furthermore, athletes who receive failing grades are declared ineligible and become "nonathletes" and have low grades when researchers collect data and compare their grades with the grades of eligible athletes!

Another factor that has not been studied is the control that parents, teachers, and coaches have over the lives of athletes on school teams, especially when the athletes are "in season" and their daily activities, especially academic activities, are closely monitored by coaches and parents (Riede, 2006). Homework checks, study halls, grade checks, and class attendance are standard procedures in the lives of athletes when their season is ongoing. Although this probably adds structure to daily schedules, its impact on learning and academic growth is not known.

Overall, school sports have selection-in, filtering-out, and in-season control processes, each of which contributes to differences between athletes and other students. To control for these processes and determine if and when playing sports produces unique, positive educational or developmental outcomes, researchers must collect data at regular intervals over four years from an entire sample of students so they can measure and track changes that are due to sports participation rather than other things.

Studying Athletes in Context Research published over the past half century presents mixed and confusing findings about the effects of playing school sports. This is because most researchers assume that playing on a school team has the same meaning in all contexts for all athletes in all sports and therefore must have the same consequences. But this is not true. Meanings vary widely depending on three factors:

1. The status given to athletes and sports in various contexts
2. The identities young people develop as they play sports
3. The ways that young people integrate sports and an athlete identity into their lives

For example, playing on a junior varsity team or being a mediocre player on the varsity fencing team often involves different implications for the status and identity of a young man in comparison with being an all-state football or basketball player on a state-championship team—even if the young man is on a fencing team at a private school that

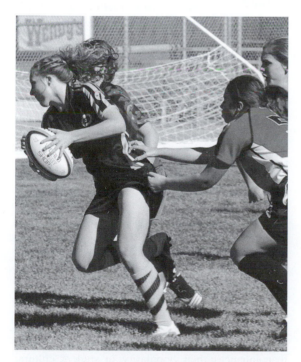

Self-selection, combined with academic eligibility and coach selection, ensures that athletes often have different characteristics from other students before they ever play on school teams. Athletes may learn positive and/or negative things in sports, but it's difficult to separate those things from other forms of learning and development that occur during adolescence. (*Source:* Jay Coakley)

has produced many college and Olympic champions. Similarly, being a young woman ranked the number-one high school tennis player in the state would involve different status and identity implications from being a young woman who is a substitute on the junior varsity softball team.

When researchers at the University of Chicago used data collected over four years from two large samples of high school students, they found that interscholastic athletes at schools located in low-income areas were more likely to be identified as good students than were athletes playing at schools located in upper-middle-income and wealthy areas (Guest and Schneider, 2003). Additionally, having an athlete identity was positively associated with grades in schools located in lower-income areas but negatively associated with grades in wealthier areas where taking sports too seriously was possibly seen as interfering with preparing for college and careers. Therefore, the academic implications of being an interscholastic athlete depended on the different meanings given to playing sports and having an athlete identity in different social class contexts in American society (Morris, 2015; Shakib et al., 2011; Shifrer et al., 2013, 2015).

Research also indicates that the meanings given to playing interscholastic sports vary by gender and have changed since the late 1960s (Fox et al., 2010; Hoffman, 2006; Miller et al., 2005; Miller and Hoffman, 2009; Pearson et al., 2009; Shifrer et al., 2013, 2015; Troutman and Dufur, 2007). For example, young women on school teams have had lower rates of sexual activity (fewer sex partners, lower frequency of intercourse, and later initiation of sexual activity) than their female peers who didn't play sports, whereas young men on school teams had higher rates of sexual activity than other young men in the schools (Miller et al., 1998, 1999). This difference persists because playing on school teams enhances the social status of young people and gives them more power to regulate sexual activity on their own terms (Kreager and Staff, 2009).

During the 1990s, it appears that many young women used this power to resist sexual relationships that they defined as inappropriate or exploitive, whereas young men used their power to gain sexual favors from young women (Risman and Schwartz, 2002). But these patterns could be different today or change in the future as the meanings given to being on school sport teams change and as there are shifts in students' ideas about sex.

Research also suggests that identifying oneself as a "jock" in some U.S. high schools connects a student with peers who are socially gregarious and more likely than other students to engage in risky actions such as heavy and binge drinking (Miller and Hoffman, 2009; Miller et al., 2005; Veliz et al., 2015). This issue needs more study, but it seems that playing on certain school teams provides students with more choices for aligning themselves with various cliques or social groups that have different priorities for what they like to do. The choices made by athletes probably influence how others identify them and where they fit into the overall social organization of the school. In some cases, this "positions" them with others who value academic work, whereas in other cases, it positions them so that they focus on social activities with other jocks who like to party even if it detracts from academic achievement.

Identifying the influence of playing high school sports in a person's adult life is much more difficult than identifying the effects that occur during late adolescence. The meanings people give to sport participation change over time and vary with a wide range of social and cultural factors related to gender, race and ethnicity, and social class. For example, when we hear that many CEOs of large corporations played sports in high school, it tells us nothing about the role of sport participation in the long, complex process of becoming a CEO. The occupational experiences of top CEOs, most of whom are white men, are strongly related to their family backgrounds and social networks, and cannot be separated from the gender, ethnic, and class

> You're only 17 once. I have the rest of my life to worry about pain and stuff like that. I can only play football for so long. I might as well use the time I have and worry about the effects later. —High school football player in the *Frontline* documentary "Football High" (2011)

relations that exist in the United States. This does not mean that these men didn't work hard or that sport participation was unrelated to their development, but the importance of playing varsity sports cannot be understood apart from many other factors that are clearly related to becoming a CEO.

Overall, research in the sociology of sport indicates that the effects of playing school sports depend on the contexts in which sports are played, the organization of sport programs and teams, and the social characteristics of athletes (Crissey and Honea, 2006; Fox et al., 2010; Hartmann, 2008; Hartmann and Massoglia, 2007; Hartmann et al., 2012; Pearson et al., 2009). Therefore, when young, white women from upper-middle-class families play lacrosse in a small, private, elite prep school where grades are all-important, the effects of participation are likely to be different from the effects that occur when young ethnic minority men from working-class families play football in a large public school where they have opportunities to be noticed in positive ways and to connect with adult mentors more than other students have.

Student Culture in High Schools

Sports are usually among the most important activities sponsored by high schools, and being on a school team can bring students prestige among peers, formal rewards in the school, and recognition from teachers, administrators, and people in the local community. Athletes, especially boys in high-profile sports, often are accorded recognition that enhances their popularity in student culture. Pep rallies, homecomings, and other sports events are major social occasions on school calendars. Students often enjoy these events because they provide opportunities for social interaction outside the classroom. Parents favor them because they're associated with the school and crowds are controlled by school authorities; therefore, they will allow their children to attend games and matches even when they forbid them from going other places.

The popularity of school sports has led sociologists to ask questions about their impact on students' values, attitudes, actions, and experiences.

High School Sports and Popularity For many years, student culture was studied simply in terms of the factors that high school students used to determine popularity. Research usually found that male students wished they could be remembered as "athletic stars" in high school, whereas female students wished to be remembered as "brilliant students" or "the most popular." Although these priorities have changed over the last two generations, the link between popularity and being an athlete has remained relatively strong for male students (Shakib et al., 2011). At the same time, the link between popularity and being an athlete has become stronger for female students, although other characteristics, such as physical appearance and social skills, are also important—more important than they are for young men.

Most high school students today are concerned with academic achievement and attending college; furthermore, their parents regularly emphasize these priorities. But students also are concerned with four other things: (1) social acceptance; (2) personal autonomy; (3) sexual identity; and (4) becoming an adult. They want to have friends they can depend on, control their lives, feel comfortable with their sexual identity, and be taken seriously as young adults.

Because males and females in North America are still treated and evaluated differently, adolescents use different strategies for seeking acceptance, autonomy, sexual identity, and recognition. For young men, sports provide opportunities to demonstrate the physical and emotional toughness that is traditionally associated with masculinity, and successfully claiming a masculine identity is

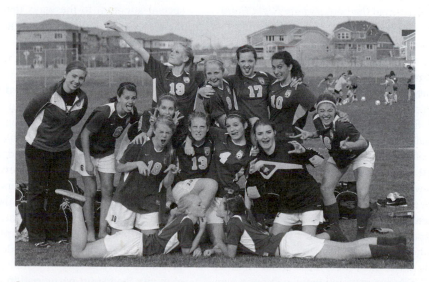

Sport participation often gives young women opportunities to establish personal and social identities based on skills respected by peers and people in the general community. However, even though playing sports often is enjoyable, as for the members of this soccer team, it usually does not bring as much status and popularity to girls as it does to boys in U.S. high schools. (*Source:* © Danielle Hicks)

assumed to bring acceptance, autonomy, and recognition as an adult.

For young women, sports are not used so much to claim a feminine identity that brings acceptance, autonomy, and recognition as an adult, but playing sports is used to achieve and express the personal power that enables young women to achieve these things. My hypothesis is that young women in high school at this point in time are less likely than their male peers to view sports as a self-identification focal point in their lives and more likely to view them as part of a larger project of achievement that involves academic, social, and other personal accomplishments. If this is the case, the visibility and status gained by high school athletes have different implications for young men than for young women in high school student culture and beyond (Shakib et al., 2011).

High School Sports and Ideology   Sport programs do more than simply affect the status structures of high schools. When Pulitzer Prize–winning author H. G. Bissinger wrote the book *Friday Night Lights* about a high school football team in Odessa, Texas, he observed that football "stood at the very core of what the town was about. . . . It had nothing to do with entertainment and everything to do with how people felt about themselves" (1990: 237).

Bissinger noted that football in Odessa and across the United States was important because it celebrated a male cult of toughness and sacrifice and a female cult of nurturance and servitude. Team losses were blamed on coaches who weren't tough enough and players who weren't disciplined and aggressive. Women stayed on the sidelines and faithfully tried to support and please the men who battled on behalf of the school and town.

Attending football games enabled students and townspeople to reaffirm their ideas about "natural differences" between men and women. Young men who did not hit hard, physically intimidate opponents, or play with pain were described as "ladies," and a player's willingness to sacrifice his body for the team was taken as a sign of commitment, character, and manhood. At the same time, women who

didn't stand by and support their men were seen as gender nonconformists.

Bissinger also noted that high school sports were closely linked with a long history of racism in Odessa, and that football was organized and played in ways that reaffirmed traditional racial ideology among whites and produced racial resentment among African Americans. Ideas about race and certain aspects of racial dynamics have changed since 1988 when many whites in the Odessa area referred to blacks as "niggers" and blamed people of color for most of the town's social and economic problems. White people are not as likely today to say that black athletes succeed on the football field because of their "natural physical abilities" or that white athletes succeed due to character, discipline, and intelligence.

Bissinger's book fails to deal with many aspects of high school life, but a study by anthropologist Doug Foley (1990a, 1999a) provides a more complete description and analysis of the place of sports in a high school and the town in which it exists. Foley studied an entire small Texas town but paid special attention to the ways that people incorporated the local high school football team and its games into the overall social life of the school and the community. He also studied the social and academic activities of a wide range of students, including those who ignored or avoided sports.

Foley's findings revealed that student culture in the high school "was varied, changing, and inherently full of contradictions" (1990a, p. 100). Football and other sports provided important social occasions and defused the anxiety associated with tests and overcontrolling teachers, but sports were only one part of the lives of the students. Athletes used their sport-based status as a basis for "identity performances" with other students and certain adults, but for most students, identity was grounded more deeply in gender, social class, and ethnicity than sport participation.

Foley noted that sports were socially important because they presented students with a vocabulary they could use to identify values and interpret their everyday experiences. For example, most sports came with a vocabulary that extolled individualism, competition, and "natural" differences related to sex, skin color, ethnicity, and social class. As students learned and used this vocabulary, they perpetuated the culture and social organization of their school and town. In the process, traditional ideologies related to gender, race, and class continued to influence social relations in the town's culture, even though some people questioned and revised those ideologies and redefined their importance in their lives.

> **High school sports, once viewed as a bastion of wholesomeness, is being transformed into a cutthroat business at the highest levels of play, with teenage athletes the prized assets.** —Benjamin Hochman and Ryan Casey, *Denver Post* journalists (2011)

The point of Foley's study and other research on socialization as a community process is that the most important social consequences of high school sports are not their impact on grades and popularity but their impact on the overall culture of the school and community as well as young people's ideas about social life and social relations. Examples of this are highlighted in the PBS *Frontline* documentary "Football High" (Dretzin, 2011).

High School Sports as Learning Experiences

Early in the twentieth century, educators included physical education and sports in U.S. schools because they believed that learning should encompass body and mind (Hyland, 2008). Physical activities and sports, they thought, could be organized to teach important lessons. But the widespread acceptance of the great sport myth and the related belief that "sports build character" led to the assumption that playing sports automatically transformed young people in positive ways, no matter how the sports were organized. There was no need for research to identify what participants learned or how to teach things beyond tactics and techniques. Individual testimonials about "sport making me what I am today" fueled the mythology that sport was like an automatic car wash: those who enter will be cleansed, dried, and sent off with a shiny new look.

As a result, there are no "learning evaluations" at the end of seasons, coaches aren't held accountable as teachers, and there is an amazing lack of systematically collected evidence documenting the dynamics of teaching and learning in various sports played by over seven million high school students every year. The downside of this lack of knowledge is that we can't prove what young people learn in sports or when and why they learn certain things, either positive or negative. Nor can we rate the effectiveness of various coaching strategies for teaching what we want young people to learn in sports. And what is it that we want young people to learn? If we knew these things, we could present evidence to school boards when they make funding decisions. Too many people simply assume and say the same things: sport teaches discipline, teamwork, and the value of hard work. But they provide only anecdotal evidence about themselves or someone they know. What we need is systematic research identifying the conditions under which school teams provide worthwhile educational experiences for students.

INTERCOLLEGIATE SPORTS AND THE EXPERIENCES OF COLLEGE STUDENTS

Does varsity sport participation affect the educational and developmental experiences of college athletes?[3] This question cannot be answered unless we understand that college sport programs are very diverse. If we assume that all programs are like the ones we see or read about in the media, we are bound to have distorted views of athletes, coaches, and intercollegiate sports.

---

[3]This chapter focuses primarily on four-year institutions in the United States. Although junior colleges and two-year community colleges comprise 25 percent of all higher education institutions with intercollegiate sport programs and have about 10 percent of all intercollegiate athletes, there is little research on them.

Intercollegiate Sports Are *Not* All the Same

The amount of money spent every year on intercollegiate sports varies from less than $500,000 at some small colleges to over $160 million at the University of Texas. Large universities usually sponsor ten to eighteen varsity sports for men and a similar number for women, whereas small colleges may have only a few varsity sports and many club teams. In small colleges, coaches may be responsible for two or more teams and teach courses as well. Larger universities may have twelve or more coaches for football alone and multiple coaches for most sports. Few of these coaches teach courses, and most have no formal connection with academic programs at universities.

Schools with intercollegiate sports are generally affiliated with one of two national associations: the National Collegiate Athletic Association (NCAA) or the National Association of Intercollegiate Athletics (NAIA). The NCAA is the largest and most powerful association, with 1200 member institutions, about 460,000 athletes, and a budget of over $500 million per year. Member institutions are divided into five major categories, reflecting program size, level of competition, and the rules that govern sport programs. Division I includes (in 2015–2016) 351 schools with "big-time" programs. This division contains three subdivisions:[4]

1. Football Bowl Subdivision (FBS) consists of 120 universities that have big-time football teams; each institution is allotted eighty-five full scholarships for football players.
2. Football Championship Subdivision (FCS) consists of 127 universities that have football programs and are allotted only sixty-three scholarships that can be awarded to (or split between) no more than eighty-five students.

3. Non-Football (NF) subdivision consists of 100 universities that do not have football teams but have big-time basketball and/or other big-time sports.

NCAA Divisions II and III contain 300 and 444 schools, respectively. These schools have smaller programs and compete at less than a big-time level, although competition often is intense. Division II schools may award limited scholarships but rarely give a full scholarship to an athlete. Division III schools do not award athletic scholarships.

Some colleges and universities choose to affiliate with the NAIA rather than the NCAA. The NAIA has about 250 member schools, an estimated 60,000 athletes, and a budget that is less than 1 percent of the NCAA budget. NAIA schools have teams in up to twelve sports for men and eleven for women. Athletic scholarships are not common and seldom cover more than 25 percent of college costs Most member institutions are small private schools, many with religious affiliation, and their athletic programs have minimal budgets. The NAIA struggles to maintain members in the face of NCAA power and influence.

Christian colleges and Bible schools also have sport programs. About 115 of these are affiliated with the National Christian College Athletic Association (NCCAA), although many have dual membership in the NCCAA and either the NAIA or NCAA Division III. The National Junior College Athletic Association consists of about 436 junior and community colleges; some of its 50,000 athletes receive scholarships, nearly all of which cover only partial expenses.

Even though the vast majority of intercollegiate sport teams are not big-time, people use what they see and read in the media to make conclusions about all college sports. But this is a mistake because most sports at most schools do not resemble the sports covered by the mainstream media. Tables 14.2 and 14.3 identify the percentage of schools in each category and the percentage of athletes that play in each category. For example, Table 14.2 shows that Division I

---

[4]These numbers continue to change regularly as conferences and universities position themselves to maximize revenue generation for their sport programs.

Table 14.2   Percentage distribution of all colleges and universities with sport programs by athletic organization and division, 2014

Organization	Division	Percent of All Institutions
NCAA	Div. I	16.5
NCAA	Div. II	13.8
NCAA	Div. III	20.9
NAIA		12.4
NJCAA*		24.5
All Others[§]		11.9

Table 14.3   Percentage distribution of all college athletes by athletic organization and division, 2014

Organization	Division	Percent of All Athletes
NCAA	Div. I	29
NCAA	Div. II	18
NCAA	Div. III	30
NAIA		8
NJCAA*		9
All Others[§]		6

Source: Adapted from association data, 2014.
*National Junior College Athletic Association
[§]Includes all colleges and universities having sport programs but not maintaining membership in any of the above organizations.

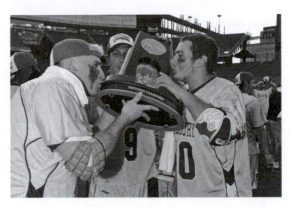

Sports in Divisions II and III receive little attention. Little coverage was given to the 2012 Division III national lacrosse championship in which the Salisbury Sea Gulls defeated SUNY Cortland. The experiences of athletes in these programs differ from the experiences of athletes in big-time programs, but research documenting and analyzing the differences and their educational implications is lacking. (*Source:* © Michael Tureski/Icon SMI/Corbis)

universities comprise 16.5 percent of all institutions of higher education with intercollegiate sports; and Table 14.3 shows that only 29 percent of all intercollegiate athletes play on teams in Division I universities. NCAA Division III has the highest proportion of athletes—30 percent—in 444 schools that award no athletic scholarships.

Although it's important to study all these categories, most research focuses on the Division I universities. Therefore, this chapter, based on the literature in the sociology of sport and other disciplines, provides a limited view of intercollegiate sports. This is important to remember when we discuss issues and problems because they vary widely from one division to the next.

Athletes in Big-Time Programs

Being an athlete in a big-time intercollegiate program is not always compatible with being a student. A recent survey of 21,000 NCAA athletes showed that most of them spend close to forty hours per week doing their sports; football players reported spending forty-five hours a week on their sport (Petr et al., 2011), and most athletes said they spent more time on their sport than on academic work.

Research by sociologists Patricia and Peter Adler (1991, 1999) helps to put these data in context. After five years of observing, interviewing, traveling with, and hanging out with athletes and coaches for a big-time college basketball team, the Adlers concluded that playing on such a team and being seriously involved in academic courses seldom go hand in hand. The young men on the team began their first year of coursework with optimism and idealism because they expected their academic experiences to contribute to their future occupational success. However, after one or two semesters, the demands of playing basketball, the social isolation that goes along with being an athlete, and the powerful influence of the team culture drew them away from academic life.

The men discovered that selecting easier courses and majors was necessary if they were to meet coaches' expectations. Fatigue, the pressures of games, and over forty hours a week devoted to basketball kept them from focusing seriously on academic tasks. Furthermore, nobody ever asked them about their academic lives; attention always focused on basketball, and few people expected these young men to identify themselves as students or give priority to coursework. Racial ideology and stereotypes accentuated this social dynamic as many people assumed that young black men playing basketball had no interests or abilities other than their sport.

When these young men received positive feedback, it was for athletic, not academic, achievement. Difficulties in their courses often led them to view academic life with pragmatic detachment—that is, they didn't become emotionally invested in coursework and they chose classes and arranged course schedules that enabled them to meet the demands of their sport. They knew what they had to do to stay eligible, and coaches would make sure their course schedules kept them eligible. Gradually, most of the players detached themselves from academic life on the campus.

Academic detachment was supported in the team culture. These young men were with one another constantly—in the dorms, at meals, during practices, on trips to games, in the weight room, and on nights when there were no games. During these times, they seldom talked about academic or intellectual topics, unless it was in negative terms. They encouraged cutting classes, and they joked about bad tests and failing papers. They provided each other with support for their identities as athletes, not students.

Academic detachment did not occur for all team members. Those who managed to balance their athletic and academic lives were the ones who entered college with realistic ideas about academic demands, had parents and peers who were familiar with academic demands in college, and entered the university with solid high school preparation and the ability to develop relationships with faculty and other students. These relationships were important because they emphasized academic achievement and provided support for academic identities.

The Adlers also found that the structure of big-time intercollegiate sports worked against maintaining a balance between athletics and academics. For example, as high-profile people on campus, these young men had many social opportunities, and it was difficult for them to focus on coursework instead of their social lives. Road trips to away games and tournaments took them away from classes for extended periods. They missed lectures, study groups, and tests. Their tight connections with fellow athletes isolated them from the academic life of the university.

Unlike other students, these young men generated revenue and publicity for the university, the athletic program, and coaches. Academic detachment was not a problem for the school as long as the young men did not get caught doing something illegal or resist the control of their coach. It became a problem only when it caused them to be ineligible.

The Diversity of Athlete Experiences

Some big-time intercollegiate sport teams are characterized by chronic problems, low graduation rates, and hypocrisy when it comes to education. However, teams in nonrevenue-producing sports are more likely to be organized so that athletes can combine sport participation with academic and social development. This combination is most likely when athletes enter college with positive attitudes about school and the value of a college education and then receive support for academic involvement and the formation of academic identities.

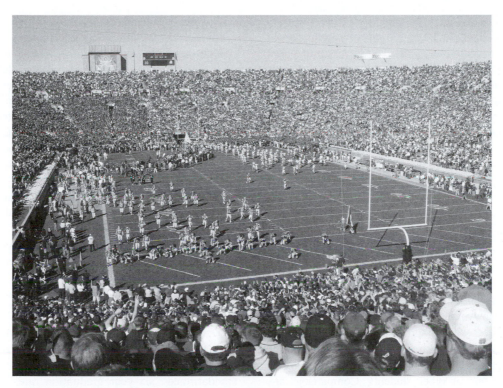

Athletes in big-time college sports face difficult choices when allocating time and energy to academic work, sport participation, and social activities. Studying for tests is difficult when the stakes associated with your games often involve millions of dollars for your school and when your coach wants you to give 110 percent every day to the team. Also, playing in front of 80,000 people in a stadium with millions watching on television distracts eighteen- to twenty-two-year-olds from academic assignments. (*Source:* © Bobak Ha'Eri)

Athletes on teams in which there is strong support for academic success may train hard and define athletic success as important, but most of them take their education seriously and try to maintain a balance between their academic and athletic commitments. The athletes who do this most effectively are those who have the following: (1) past experiences that consistently reaffirm the importance of education; (2) social networks that support academic identities; (3) perceived access to career opportunities following graduation; and (4) social

relationships and experiences that expand confidence and skills apart from sports.

Coaches in programs that actively support academic success may schedule practices and games that do not interfere with coursework. Athletes may miss games and meets to study for or take tests, write papers, or give presentations. Team members may discuss academic issues and support one another when it comes to academic performance. In other words, there are sport programs and teams that do not subvert the academic mission of higher education (Simon, 2008). Usually they're found in

NCAA Division III and some NAIA programs, but they also exist in some low-profile, nonrevenue-producing Division I and II sports and in many women's sports. However, as sport cultures are increasingly organized to emphasize year-round dedication to improvement and competitive success, and as coaches must have winning teams to keep their jobs, it becomes difficult to balance athletics and academics even in low-profile sports (Hyland, 2008; Morgan, 2012).

Grades and Graduation Rates: Athletes in Big-Time College Sports

Unlike athletes in low-profile intercollegiate programs, athletes in big-time, revenue-producing sports often have different backgrounds from other students on campus. They're more likely to be African American, come from lower socioeconomic backgrounds, and be a first generation college student in their families. This makes it difficult to compare their academic achievements with the achievements of other students. Comparisons are also difficult because grade point averages (GPAs) have different meanings from one university to another and from department to department within a single university. Even graduation rates are poor indicators of academic outcomes because academic standards and requirements vary from one university to another and between programs in universities.

Some studies report that college athletes earn higher grades than other students, and some report the exact opposite. Some studies show athletes attending graduate school more often than nonathletes, and others show athletes taking an abundance of courses requiring less than average academic work.

When comparing the grades received by athletes with grades received by other students, it is important to take into account two factors related to the academic careers of athletes:

1. Athletes in certain sports are overrepresented in specific courses and majors. This phenomenon is known as *clustering*. It occurs for various reasons: when athletes lack academic confidence and seek support from teammates in the same courses or major, when black athletes find a department where faculty members are aware of racial issues and treat them with respect, and when coaches assign athletes to classes involving little work or classes taught by faculty members willing to give good grades to athletes regardless of the quality of their coursework.

2. Athletes in football and men's basketball often enter college with lower than average high school GPAs and lower ACT and SAT scores than other students, including most other athletes, at their universities. Their academic goals may differ from the goals of other students, and this influences their academic choices and performance.

Data on academic progress and graduation rates also are confusing because they're computed in many ways. The NCAA now publishes standardized "six-year graduation rates" for all member institutions and for each major division, which has made is possible to do basic comparisons of universities and sports. These rates for Division I universities during 2011–2012 provide the following information about athletes who receive full or partial athletic scholarships (NCAA, 2012):

- Sixty-five percent of the athletes who entered Division I universities in 2005 graduated within six years, whereas 63 percent of the general student body graduated in six years. Therefore, athletes as a group have a graduation rate similar to other college students—even though athletes have a higher proportion of men and African Americans and a lower proportion of Asian Pacific Americans than there are in the general student body.

- Graduation rates are lowest in revenue-producing sports, especially men's basketball (47 percent) and football (59 percent); these

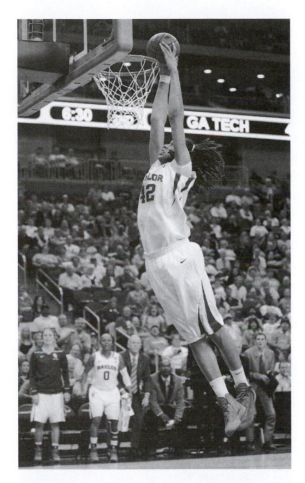

Graduation rates for female athletes are higher than for men who play college sports. However, as women's teams have become entertainment oriented, graduation rates have declined slightly. Research shows that women tend to allocate more time to academic work as they make choices between school, sport, and social life. (*Source:* AP Photo/Charlie Neibergall)

rates are below the rates for all athletes (65 percent) and the general student body (63 percent).

- The graduation rate for African American male athletes (49 percent) is significantly higher than the rate for African American men in the general

student population (39 percent). The rate for black female athletes (64 percent) is higher than the rate for black women generally (48 percent). Graduation rates for black male athletes have increased since 1986 when minimum academic standards for scholarship athletes were established for Division I universities. However, the data on graduation rates among black students continue to indicate that "predominantly white campuses are not places in which students of color feel welcome and supported, whether or not they are athletes" (Edwards, 2011; Hawkins, 2010; Lapchick, 2005, 2010).

What do these patterns mean? With whom should we compare athletes when we assess the academic integrity of big-time sports—with regular full-time students who work full time, who have equivalent scholarships, who enter college with similar grades and test scores, or who come from similar socio-economic backgrounds?

Richard Southall and his colleagues at the College Sport Research Institute (CSRI) at the University of North Carolina have developed an adjusted graduation gap measure that compares athletes with other full-time students. From 2010 through 2016 they found that athletes consistently had lower graduation rates than full-time students, with the differences being dramatic for football and men's and women's basketball (http://csri-sc.org/research/).

Overall, there is no single ideal comparison. Furthermore, even though graduation is an important educational goal, it should not be the only criterion used to judge academic success. College degrees are important, but they don't mean much unless sufficient learning has occurred. It's difficult to measure learning in a survey of athletes, but it is possible to hold athletic departments academically accountable.

The Challenge of Achieving Academic Goals

Graduation rates among athletes have increased as eligibility rules have become stricter. The most recent new rules for athlete eligibility went into effect in August, 2016. They require that first year athletes must have had at least a 2.3 GPA in sixteen specific core high school courses with ten of those courses completed before starting senior year, be a high school graduate, and have an SAT score of 900 or an ACT score of 75. Lower SAT or ACT scores require a higher GPA. For example, an SAT score of 740 or an ACT score of 61 requires a 2.7 high school GPA in core courses to be eligible for competition and to receive a scholarship at a Division I school (NCAA, 2015).

These changes in NCAA eligibility rules were designed to do three things: (1) send messages to high schools and high school athletes that a commitment to academic achievement is required to play college sports; (2) set new guidelines for universities that haven't taken seriously the academic lives of athletes; and (3) encourage universities to provide athletes with the support they need to succeed academically.

Boosting eligibility standards has been somewhat successful, but many intercollegiate programs still fall short of meeting reasonable academic goals. Reforming big-time college sports is difficult because they are tied to many interests unrelated to education. Some young people in those sports are in college only to obtain the coaching and experiences needed to stay competitive in amateur Olympic sports or to enter professional sports as soon as an opportunity presents itself. Coaches, especially those in Division I, view their sports as businesses, and they are hired and fired on the basis of win–loss records and the amount of revenue that they create for the athletic program.

Academic administrators, including college presidents, generally use high-profile sports as public relations and fund-raising tools instead of focusing on them as educational programs. The corporations that sponsor teams and buy advertising on telecasts of college sports are not concerned about athletes' education as long as their teams attract positive attention to the company's products. Similarly, local businesses that make money when the home team attracts fans are not concerned about graduation rates as long as sports fill the town with spectators for every home game.

> We've reached a point where big-time intercollegiate athletics is undermining the integrity of our institutions, diverting presidents and institutions from their main purpose. —William E. Kirwan, chancellor, University of Maryland (in Pappano, 2012)

Because of persisting problems, the NCAA passed new academic rules for institutions in 2005. These rules shifted more responsibility for academic reform to athletic departments in Division I universities. The rules, which now apply to over 6200 Division I teams, establish a minimum academic progress rate (APR) *and* a minimum graduation success rate (GSR).

The APR is calculated at the beginning of each semester by awarding a team 1 point for each of its players who is academically eligible and 1 point for each player who has returned to school for that semester. A formula is used to adjust the calculations for teams of different sizes, but the perfect score for all teams is 1000 points. A team that does not have a score of at least 925 points—which would imply a graduation rate of about 60 percent—is subject to losing one or more of its allotted scholarships in the following year, depending on the difference between the team's score and the minimum 925 points. The APR is based on rolling data from the previous four academic years so that one bad year doesn't affect a team unfairly.

The GSR also is calculated by using four years of rolling data. Therefore, the rate for 2015 was based on the proportion of athletes who entered the university in 2006 through 2009 and graduated within six years after they first registered for courses. The GSR is not reduced when athletes in good academic standing transfer to other universities or enter professional sports.

If the NCAA continues to enforce these rules, coaches and athletic departments have two options: (1) take academic issues more seriously, or (2) find ways to get around the rules without being caught. This makes academic support programs an important part of big-time athletic departments. The

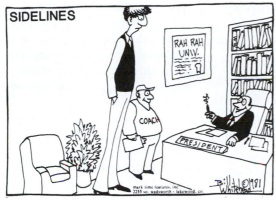

(*Source:* By permission of William Whitehead)

"I like your new recruit, coach; he's an excellent example of higher education!"

In big-time intercollegiate sports, coaches and university presidents have frequently distorted the meaning of higher education.

financial stakes are too high to leave eligibility to chance.

Academic Support Programs   Athletic departments with big-time sport programs now maintain academic support programs. Although the stated role of people working in these programs is to help athletes succeed in their academic work, the fact that they are administered by and located in athletic departments raises questions about their real goals. These questions are asked every time it is reported that paid staff wrote papers and did other assignments for athletes (Benedict and Keteyian, 2013; Dohrmann and Evans, 2013; Smith and Willingham, 2015).

Although these programs have existed at least since the early 1980s, they've attracted little research. A study in the mid-1990s suggested that academic support programs for athletes were useful but they didn't boost graduation rates (Sellers and Keiper, 1998). The first published evaluation of an academic support program was done at the University of Minnesota in 2007 (Kane et al., 2008). The evaluation resulted in the development of a model and recommendations for how to improve academic support for athletes and how to measure improvements through regular program evaluations. This model was well received by others concerned about academic integrity in college sports, but there is no research on how it has been used and whether it is effective.

When journalists at *Sports Illustrated* did an eight-month investigation of alleged improprieties in the football program at Oklahoma State University between 1999 and 2011, they found convincing evidence that football players "routinely had their coursework completed by tutors" working for the athletic department or by other university staff members (Dohrmann and Evans, 2013c). Former players also reported that they would be given answers to upcoming tests and that coaches would register them in courses for which they did little work to receive passing grades.

Academic support programs usually operate under the supervision of the athletic department. When coaches of football and men's basketball—coaches making between $1 million and $9 million per year—receive bonuses of a few hundred thousand dollars when their teams win conference championships and have good GPAs, it creates pressure on the staff in the support programs to do all they can to help athletes stay eligible and receive good grades. We know little about how this occurs, and it is unlikely that athletic departments would give permission for studies to be done.

Future Reforms   For nearly four decades the NCAA has tried to improve the academic experiences and graduation rates of college athletes. But at the same time, research suggests that there is a growing separation between the culture of intercollegiate sports and the general university culture (Bowen and Levine, 2003; Bowen et al., 2005; Lawrence et al., 2007; Smith and Willingham, 2015).

This separation is fueled by historical, commercial, and political factors that currently shape the culture of college sports (Nixon, 2014). These factors are so powerful that a group of college professors formed The Drake Group (TDG, www.thedrakegroup.org/), the goal of which is to reform intercollegiate sports and defend academic integrity in higher education. TDG lobbied the U.S. Congress, asking it to investigate the nonprofit status of college sport teams organized to make profits. When Congress formed an investigative committee, the NCAA acted quickly to highlight academic success stories in college sports and the committee pulled back its investigation. TDG remains active and argues that until intercollegiate sports are monitored by an independent agency, the educational mission of universities will continue to be compromised.

The fact that powerful commercial forces influence big-time college sports leads many of us who have studied college sports to be skeptical about the real impact of reform efforts (Coakley, 2008b; Morgan, 2012; Oriard, 2012; Thelin, 2008; Zimbalist, 2013). But others remain hopeful that meaningful changes will occur if the NCAA makes a serious and sustained commitment to enforcing academic standards and using penalties that have serious financial and reputational consequences for universities and athletic departments (Chelladurai, 2008; Simon, 2008).

DO SCHOOLS BENEFIT FROM VARSITY SPORTS?

High school and college sports affect more than just athletes. In this section, we look at the influence of these programs on high schools and colleges as organizations. In particular, we examine school spirit and budgets.

School Spirit

Anyone who has attended a well-staged student pep rally or watched the student cheering section

> **I'm a UCLA Prostitute. I sell my body to them. They pay me to perform for them. When my teammates and I perform well, the school makes lots of money . . . Regardless of how much money the school makes, we get the same, just our scholarship.**
> —College football player (in Anderson, 2004)

at a well-attended high school or college game or meet realizes that sports can generate impressive displays of energy and spirit. This doesn't happen with all sport teams, nor does it happen in all schools. Teams in low-profile sports usually play games with few, if any, student spectators. Teams with long histories of losing records seldom create a spirited response among more than a few students. Many students don't care about school teams and resent the attention given to some teams and athletes. But there are regular occasions when sports are sites at which students and others associated with a school can come together to express spirited feelings about their teams and schools. These provide the scenes covered in the media and talked about by some people as they reminisce about their time in high school.

Proponents of varsity sports say that displays of school spirit at sport events strengthen student identification with schools and create solidarity among students. In making this case, a high school principal in Texas says, "Look, we don't get 10,000 people showing up to watch a math teacher solve X" (McCallum, 2003, p. 42). Critics say that the spirit created by sports is temporary, superficial, and detrimental to educational goals.

Being a part of any group or organization is more enjoyable when people have opportunities to collectively express their feelings. However, considerable resources in the form of time, energy, and money are devoted to producing this outcome in connection with sports. Students focus time and energy on these occasions by making signs, planning social events in connection with games, and showing support for players. Cheerleaders practice and attend games. Athletes practice, play, and travel ten to twenty hours a week, think about games, and view their "athlete" status as central to who they are in the school. Teachers attend games, mix with and "police" student spectators, serve as score and time keepers, and perform other game-related duties.

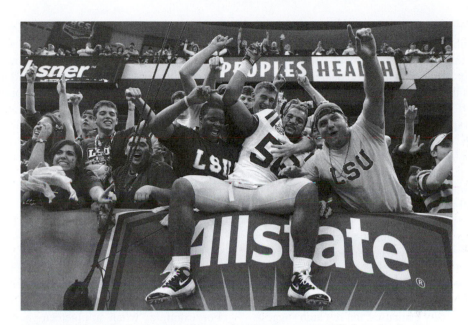

Is this a display of school spirit? If it is, what does it mean? Will these students study harder, graduate at a higher rate, or donate more money to the school than other students? Is this an expression of identification with the school, and what does that mean? Unless we can answer these questions, how do we know if school sports should be supported because they foster school spirit and identification? (*Source:* © Jamie Schwaberow/NCAA Photos)

Administrators devote time and energy to making sure the games, athletes, and students represent their schools in positive ways.

Parents pay participation fees, assist coaches with never-ending fund-raising for teams, run concession stands, and work behind the scenes to support their children who play or watch games. Coaches and school athletic program staff are paid, and they are part of a district and state structure consisting of people who are full-time sport management staff with offices and expense accounts. There also are people hired to do pre- and post-game cleanup of gyms, bleacher areas, and outdoor fields. Others are hired to groom and line the fields, repair damage to equipment and facilities, and set up bleachers and scoring tables. Referees are trained and hired, and the physical facilities of the entire school are managed to host up to three or four events per week smoothly and safely. Finally,

local journalists and other newspeople come to and report on games as the only school activities worth covering in local news.

Now imagine if all this time, energy, and material resources were used to create curricula, engage in well-planned course projects, maintain classrooms and laboratories, train and pay teachers, reward students for academic accomplishments, and present the school as a valuable learning site to the entire community (Ripley, 2013a, 2013b). Would learning be defined as more central to students and in the overall organization of schools? This is what occurs in many other post-industrial countries that are ranked far higher than the United States when it comes to knowledge and test scores in math, reading, and world affairs.

In contrast, in the United States, people, including educators, uncritically assume that sports are so crucial in the organization of schools that no one even thinks of discussing this issue or what U.S. education might be like if sports were community-based rather than school-sponsored activities. Again, the great sport myth is accepted in a way that undermines thinking about how school spirit might be more effectively organized around something other than sport teams and the sport events that increasingly conflict with academics rather than compliment them (Ripley, 2013a, 2013b).

The spirit associated with high-profile intercollegiate sports is exciting for some students, but only a small proportion of the student body attends even highly publicized games. Either the students aren't interested or the athletic department limits student tickets so they can sell seats at a higher price to other fans.

The games of big-time sport teams often are major social occasions that inspire displays of spirit on many university campuses, but research suggests that this spirit has little to do with the educational mission of the university or creating general social integration on a campus (Clopton, 2008, 2009, 2011; Clopton and Finch, 2010; Pappano, 2012). It does create regular occasions for a segment of students, more often white males than women or ethnic minority students, to party, binge drink, avoid the library, and study less, especially when their team is successful and winning games regularly (Clotfelder, 2011; Higgins et al., 2007; Lindo et al., 2012).

Finally, we know that sports can generate impressive displays of school-related spirit in local communities. In fact, games played by teenagers, who often are perceived as "problems" in shopping areas and neighborhoods, become the main source of local entertainment in many towns and smaller cities in the United States. Does this lead to support for the schools and their educational programs, or does it focus attention more on the performance of sport teams rather than the academic performance of local students?

Research is needed on this issue. People assume that support for teams translates into support for schools, but we don't know how or under what conditions this occurs. For example, people regularly watch, talk about, and cheer for high school and

university sport teams at the same time that they vote down bond issues to fund local schools and vote for state legislators who cut billions of dollars from state university funding. How and under what conditions do those cheering fans support funding for the high schools and universities that sponsor the teams they follow? We know little about this, although many people uncritically assume that spirit generated by sports is always good for education.

School Budgets

Public high schools and colleges have different budget issues because of the ways they are funded, although private high school and colleges face similar issues. The financial stakes associated with big-time intercollegiate sports puts about 250 universities in a budget category of their own. For example, when a nineteen-year-old sophomore shoots a crucial free throw during the NCAA tournament, it could be worth $1.5 million for his university—and this does not include the millions of dollars that will be won or lost by gamblers who have bet on the game. This is not the case in high school sports. Therefore, high school and college budget issues are discussed separately.

High Schools   Most interscholastic sport programs are funded through school district appropriations that come from property taxes. In most cases, expenditures for these programs account for less than 1 percent of school operating budgets. When certain sports have large budgets, money also comes from gate receipts and booster clubs.

In the face of recent budget shortfalls, many high schools have used various fund-raising strategies: (1) collecting sport participation fees from the families of students who play on school teams; (2) fostering booster clubs; and (3) seeking corporate sponsorships. But each of these alternatives creates problems.

Participation fees privilege students from well-to-do families, discourage students from low-income families, and create socioeconomic divisions in the student body. But they are widely used and range from a low of $25 to a high of over $1000 for some sports that require big budgets to pay for equipment, travel, and facilities. Some families pay thousands of dollars for their children to play school sports, which creates serious problems for coaches when parents who have just written a check for $500 make it known that they don't want their child sitting on the bench.

Relying on booster club support also creates problems because most community boosters want to fund boys' football or basketball teams rather than the athletic program as a whole, and many parent booster clubs focus only on the sports that their children play (Fry, 2006). This practice intensifies existing gender inequities and has led to Title IX lawsuits, none of which have been decided in favor of boosters who ignore girls' teams. Additionally, some boosters feel that they have the right to give advice to coaches and players, intervene in team decision making, and influence the process of hiring coaches. Community boosters may focus on win–loss records so they can tout their influence when they interact with friends and business associates; for them, educational issues may take a back seat to building a team that will win a state championship and boost their personal status.

Corporate sponsorships connect the future of interscholastic sports to the advertising budgets and revenue streams of businesses. This means that schools can be left empty-handed when advertising budgets are cut or sponsorships are not paying off enough to satisfy company owners, stockholders, and top executives. Other problems occur when the interests of corporate sponsors don't match the educational goals of high schools. For example, promoting candy, soft drinks, and fast-food consumption with ads and logos on gym walls, scoreboards, and team buses contradicts health and nutrition principles taught in high school courses. This subverts education and makes students cynical about the meaningfulness of their curriculum. Additionally, certain corporations want to "brand" students as young as possible so they sponsor sports in the hope of turning students into loyal consumers.

High school budget issues have become increasingly contentious with the rising expectations of parents and athletes seeking athletic programs that match the individualized attention they've received in private club programs (Hochman and Casey, 2011a). As more students come out of club programs, they are focused on obtaining a college scholarship, so they expect coaches, trainers, equipment, and facilities that will help them achieve this goal, even if it is unrealistic.

This issue is not going away, even though budget crises are forcing some schools to drop all sports. The result is emerging inequality with public schools in upper-middle-class areas and private schools with students from wealthy families funding elaborate sport programs and facilities while schools in low-income areas struggle to maintain a few teams using outdated and rundown facilities and equipment.

Colleges and Universities The relationship between sports and school budgets at the college level is complex (Lifschitz et al., 2014). Intercollegiate sports at small colleges are usually low-budget activities funded through student fees and money from the general fund and the college president's office. The budgets at 128 NCAA FBS universities range from about $18 million to $160 million. However, athletic departments use many different accounting methods, making it difficult to compare them. For example, some departments may "hide" profits to maintain their nonprofit status for tax purposes, and others may "hide" losses to avoid criticisms that sport teams are too costly and take money away from academic programs.

There are about 1900 intercollegiate sport programs in the United States. Less than twenty of them consistently make more money than they spend. Table 14.4 shows the amount of debt incurred in 2012 by universities with the biggest and "most successful" sport programs. Among the 128 FBS universities—the ones with top-rated football and basketball programs—annual losses averaged about $12.3 million per university. Among the 125 FCS universities, average losses

Table 14.4   Median university revenues and expenditures by subdivisions in Division I, 2012

	Median Total Revenues*	Median Generated Revenues	Median Total Expenses	Median Net Revenue (or Deficit)**
Football Bowl Subdivision (N = 120)	$55,976,000	$40,581,000	$56,265,000	−$12,272,000
Football Championship Subdivision (N = 127)	$13,761,000	$ 3,750,000	$14,115,000	−$10,219,000
Division I—No Football (N = 100)	$12,756,000	$ 2,206,000	$12,983,000	−$ 9,809,000

Source: NCAA 2004–2012 Division I Intercollegiate Athletics Revenues and Expenses Report (https://www.ncaapublications.com/p-4306-revenues-and-expenses-2004-2012-ncaa-division-i-intercollegiate-athletics-programs-report.aspx).
*This amount includes money from students fees, the general university budget, and donations given to the foundation in addition to generated revenues.
**This is the amount of overspending (that is, generated revenues minus expenses) that must be paid with "external" funds from student fees, the general budget, and donations; during the period 2011–2015, this amounted to over $10.3 billion in subsidies with over half coming from student fees (Wolverton et al., 2015).

were $10.2 million per university, and among the 94 universities in the No Football Subdivision, average losses were $9.8 million (Berkowitz and Upton, 2013; Berkowitz et al., 2013).

The general pattern since 2007 is that athletic department income has increased primarily due to increased television rights money, but spending has increased at a similar rate. Most athletic departments spend more than they take in, and then use student fee money and money from the general university budget to make up the difference. This has occurred during a period when student tuition and fees have soared at a record pace and faculty salaries have been nearly frozen and their workloads have increased.

Two facts that shock most people are these: (a) during the 2011–2012 academic year, the 227 FBS and FCS universities received $2.3 billion in subsidies from student fees, state government money, and the university's general fund. This amounts to about one-third of all the money that these athletic departments spent during the year; and (b) during 2010–2011, FBS universities spent $92,000 per athlete on all their teams, but spent only $13,600 per student—a nearly a 7-to-1 ratio (Berkowitz and Upton, 2013; Desrochers, 2013).

In the Southeastern Conference, where universities pour money into their football teams, $164,000 was spent per athlete and $13,400 was spent per student—more than a 12-to-1 ratio. In FCS universities, $36,700 was spent per athlete and $11,800 was spent per student—more than a 3-to-1 ratio. It is also expected that these athlete-to-student spending gaps have increased since 2010 as athletic departments continue on what is an unsustainable spending spree.

Another troubling issue is that the twenty-three athletic programs that claimed to have made more than they spent during 2011–2012 collectively received about $52.4 million in subsidies from student fees and the universities. For example, Florida State generated $92.3 million in income during 2011–2012 and spent $90.3 million, but received subsidies of $7.8 million—so they reported just over $100 million in so-called "income" and a so-called "profit" of $9.8 million.

"Generated" or real income consists of money from ticket sales, media rights contracts, donations, and some merchandise sales. "Subsidies" consist of student fees and money from the universities' general funds and state appropriations. But subsidies do not include other forms of government support such as the tax deduction taken by the wealthy fans that buy luxury suites and high-priced tickets to football and men's basketball games and deduct up to 100 percent of their costs as either "business expenses" or "charitable contributions," thereby cutting about 40 percent of total costs off their taxes—money that could be used to fund public programs; additionally, tax-free bonds, often held by wealthy individuals and institutions, are used to build new university sport stadiums with luxury suites for wealthy fans and their friends.

Budget information for most colleges and universities shows that sport programs exist because they are funded by student fees and by money from general university funds and the state. Every now and then a wealthy individual or corporation gives a large amount of money to an athletic program so it looks like it is profitable. This has occurred at the University of Oregon, where Phil Knight, CEO of Nike and an Oregon graduate, has donated about $300 million to the athletic department. This has led some people to suggest that it should change its name to Nike University. The athletic program at Oklahoma State University received $265 million from billionaire T. Boone Pickens and used it to help turn its football team from a perennial loser into a consistent winner. Unfortunately, Pickens did not know that this turnaround was allegedly aided by improprieties such as paying football players, maintaining their eligibility through academic fraud, tolerating their drug use, and recruiting skilled players with sexual favors supplied by female students helping out the team.

NCAA data show that the median athletic expenditures at Division II schools with football teams increased from $2.9 million in 2004 to $5.1 million in 2011, and a few schools had expenditures over $15 million, but no school generated more than $9.7 million; the median amount of revenue generated was only $618,000 (Fulks, 2012a).

For schools without football teams, expenditures were $3.6 million in 2011, with median revenues of $297,000. The median loss for men's programs in Division II was $1.9 million and for women's programs it was just under $1.2 million. Football lost the most money of any teams—a median of about

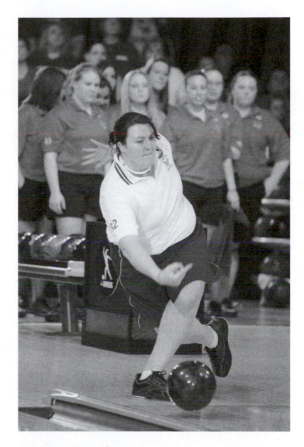

In most NCAA schools, women's sport programs have smaller financial deficits than men's sports. This means that men's sports have a higher net cost than women's sports in most schools. The budget for this 2008 and 2011 Division I championship bowling team at the University of Maryland Eastern Shore is a small fraction of the budgets for most men's sports. (*Source:* © Alyssa Schukar/NCAA Photos)

$1 million, compared with women's basketball, which lost a median of $313,000. Because most Division II revenues come from student fees and there are more female than male students in these schools, men's sports, especially football, are disproportionately subsidized by women. In Division II programs without football, the net cost of men's and women's programs was nearly the same.

A similar pattern exists in Division III. For schools with football, the median expense for the athletic program was $2,858,000 in 2011, an increase of almost 85 percent over expenses in 2004. Schools without a football team spent a median of $1,383,000 in 2011—a 109 percent increase from the median $660,000 spent in 2004. Revenues are negligible in Division III sports, most games and matches have free admission and there is no television coverage for which teams are paid. This means that the expenses per athlete are relatively high—in 2011, about $5600 in schools with football and $5100 for schools without football. Football remains the costliest sport; men's programs cost a median of $985,000 with football but only $380,000 without football. In programs with football, the women's programs average $649,000, but only $423,000 in programs without football. In the latter case, women's sports cost more than men's sports by about $40,000 per year.

Although the cost of sport programs in Divisions II and III pales in comparison to many programs in Division I, schools in each division are sites for increasing tension between core educational values and decisions that favor intercollegiate sports in admissions and resource allocation in campus budgets (Bowen and Levine, 2003; Bowen et al., 2005). This tension has been building since the 1980s, and some faculty members now believe that academic quality suffers when so many campus resources are dedicated to recruiting athletes, financially supporting teams that have ever-growing training and travel expenses, and building facilities for sports that are not systematically organized to be educational. They also ask if it is sensible to provide coaches with money to recruit students with highly specialized sport skills when the head of the sociology department or the faculty advisor for the school newspaper does not have a similar recruiting budget. Sports, they say, can exist without recruiting because many students want to play on school teams for reasons other than athletic scholarships and media coverage.

Current research indicates that sports and sport experiences have a wide range of consequences depending on the meanings that people give to them and the ways they are integrated into people's lives in particular social and cultural contexts. At this point, we've only begun to study those meanings, contexts, and consequences in education, even though U.S. schools have sponsored competitive sport teams for well over a century.

HIGH SCHOOL AND COLLEGE SPORTS FACE UNCERTAINTY

Despite their popularity, interscholastic sports are surrounded by uncertainty today. Some of the issues causing that uncertainty are similar for high schools and colleges, whereas others are unique to each level. In this section we focus first on the similar issues and then deal with issues unique to each level of participation.

Issues Facing High School and College Sport Programs

High school and college sport programs both face issues related to cost containment and growing budget inequality between programs in schools at the same level of competition. The second issue is the changing orientations and rising expectations of parents and athletes, who now make their own sport-related goals a priority when searching for a sport program.

A third issue facing both high school and college programs is how to minimize concussions, repetitive head trauma, and other serious injuries that could significantly reduce participation in certain sports and bring about major structural and cultural changes in athletic departments.

A fourth issue is how to create and maintain sport programs that support the educational mission of the school and promote learning experiences for all students without overshadowing the academic focus of teachers and students. Finally, both high schools and colleges continue to face the issue of gender inequities and the issue of providing participation opportunities for students with disabilities.

Viewed collectively, these five issues are bringing high school and college sport programs to a crossroads. The people running these programs are facing serious decisions on matters that can no longer be pushed aside and ignored. Dealing with these issues requires systemic strategies as well as strategies matched to individual schools and sport programs, regardless of the competitive level at which their teams play. However, these issues are not just matters for sports. They have implications for the quality of education in the United States. Sports have become such a central component of U.S. schools that strategies for dealing with them have implications far beyond the playing field and the lives of individual students.

Cost Containment and Budget Inequality The cost of programs at both high school and college levels has been increasing at a rate that far exceeds inflation and the cost increases for other segments of secondary and higher education. With growing pressure to contain costs and eliminate operational deficits, most sport programs today face serious budget questions. Money is tight across all of education, and those who administer sport programs cannot assume that their desires to spend can be covered by increases in general funding at either the high school or college level.

> In fact, college athletics in general are more the province of the privileged than the poor . . . Beneath the thin layer of sport entertainment that makes its way onto television are the bulk of college athletes: Well-off and white. —Tom Farrey, ESPN, in *Game On* (2008)

As academic and athletic programs deal with funding cuts, both have used special fees and fundraising to preserve what they currently do. Schools in wealthy districts or schools that draw students from relatively wealthy families have usually been able to sustain and even increase spending as other schools face grim or desperate circumstances. In some schools, programs have been trimmed to teams in just a few sports, and in others the entire sport program has been dropped. But across all programs there is growing inequality in funding for sports, even among schools that compete at the same level.

Budget and program inequality among high schools is related primarily to the residential distribution of wealth across neighborhoods, towns, and even regions of the country. At the college level it is related to the distribution of media rights revenues and gate receipts for spectator sports. As a result, a relatively small percentage of programs enjoy the resources needed to build state-of-the-art facilities, attract skilled athletes, and pay qualified coaches and staff. At the same time other programs struggle to meet expenses and they cut corners that sometimes raise safety issues for athletes.

Exacerbating this inequality at the high school level is the emergence of private schools that have the resources to field excellent teams across a number of different sports (Hochman and Casey, 2011b). These schools can recruit students without being limited by the geographical restrictions that exist for public schools, so they can pick the best athletes and offer them tuition assistance or even full scholarships. If they also have an attractive academic program, students from wealthy families will bypass the public school in their area and attend a private school with a well-funded sport program and a collection of highly skilled athletes.

As this occurs around the United States, schools with top teams in football and boys' and girls' basketball seek national ranking and play games out of state as they face off with the other high-budget teams across the country. Some people have suggested that there should be regional or even a national conference for these teams so they could play each other every year and sell broadcast rights to games.

Sport program inequality is gradually becoming a castelike system in which inequality reproduces itself year after year. Adding to this trend is the fact that the best high school athletes are increasingly coming out of youth sport club programs in which participation costs are so high that they exclude well over half the young people in most regions of the country. This means that the socioeconomic haves are the young people with the best opportunities to develop their skills, attend high schools with large budgets, and then receive the majority of athletic scholarships in college—scholarships that, for some of them, have more status value than financial value, because they have enough money to pay college expenses. In this way, inequality in high school programs increases the inequality in college programs.

The sport program inequality at the college level is easy to see in Division I of the NCAA, but it also exists in Divisions II and III. The absolute dollar differences in Division I budgets are staggering, although the proportional differences in all three divisions show massive budget gaps. For example, the University of Texas spent about $161 million on its sport programs in 2013–2014, which is more than the combined athletic expenses of the twenty lowest-budget programs in the FBS and FCS subdivisions of Division I. Big-budget schools don't win all their games, but they continue to have income that increases the budget gap in college sports. This is why, as of 2012–2013, about 92 percent of all NCAA Division I championships in history have been won by fewer than seventy schools—about 20 percent of the Division I membership—a pattern that has become even more apparent in recent years.

Inequality at the college level has become so great that representatives of schools in Division I can no longer agree on rules, rule changes, and rule enforcement procedures (Nixon, 2014). This is because about sixty-six of these athletic departments from the top five out of thirty-four athletic conferences exist in a totally different world than the athletic departments in the other schools. Basically, they are running professional programs while everyone else runs wannabe or amateur programs. The professional programs want rules that fit their situation, although they still want their workers (the athletes) to toil under a strict minimum wage as they receive many millions of dollars from deals with media companies.

Efforts to reduce inequality in the United States always run into massive resistance regardless of the context. The resistance to cost-containment

policies is also strong. Could there be a ceiling on college team budgets and coach salaries? Could television rights money be redistributed across more schools? The chances of doing these things are slim, which means that program inequality will continue to shape the sports landscape at both the college and high school levels.

Changing Orientations and Rising Expectations
As the stakes associated with sport participation have increased, there has been a corresponding increase in the expectations and goals of parents and athletes. Young people today have been raised in a culture emphasizing self-improvement, growth, and achievement, and in no sphere of society is this emphasis stronger than it is in sports. At the high school level, a growing number of athletes seek opportunities to develop the skills and visibility that maximize their chances to receive a college athletic scholarship. They also believe that year-round involvement in a single sport is essential to achieving this goal, and they seek schools and coaches that fit their expectations.

When a local public school does not meet their expectations, parents and athletes seek other schools if they have a choice. If not allowed to switch schools, they might seek a private school or even move into another area where there is a public school program that offers what they want. In either case, they will expect to receive personal attention and coaching. Another alternative that is becoming increasingly popular in soccer, volleyball, lacrosse, and a few other sports is to remain on a high-profile club team that plays year-round and regularly goes to state, regional, and national tournaments scouted by college coaches. But these clubs are expensive, often costing $10,000 or more per year depending on the travel and tournament fees.

The president of Biocats, a multi-state scouting service for young athletes, has observed this change in many high schools:

> . . . parents and kids have never experienced anything beyond "It's all about me" in club sports. We have to re-educate kids and parents when they get to high school: "This isn't a club." (In high school)

it's not about you. It's about team, school, and community. You are serving them. In the club, they are serving you (Hochman and Casey, 2011b).

It is difficult to say how these changing orientations and rising expectations play out at the college level. Certainly there are more prima donna athletes focused on their personal goals. This results in more athletes switching schools to find the attention they expect, and it may lead to more athletes joining collective efforts forcing schools to provide better health care and insurance, compensation for the use of their names and images to boost revenues, and regulations limiting the hours they must spend on their sports each day and week. If this is where changing orientations and rising expectations lead, it will have a dramatic impact on the organization of college sports.

Concussions, Repetitive Head Trauma, and Other Serious Injuries   Concussions and the possibility of incurring permanent brain damage while playing school sports, especially football, is a hot-button issue for high school and college sports. It is also an anxiety-provoking liability issue for coaches, athletic directors, and school administrators. With football being the most popular and heavily promoted sport in high schools and college, the fact that half of all reported concussions in organized school sports occur in football raises this anxiety level even further.

High school administrators know that the vast majority of athletes on interscholastic teams are under the age of informed legal consent, and that the school has a special responsibility to protect them while they are under their supervision. If studies continue to show that sport-related concussions or repetitive sub-concussive head trauma can cause death, permanent brain injuries, or an inability to meet academic expectations, they must drop football and possibly other sports, or find ways to drastically reduce head trauma during practices and games. Some teams now limit practice hours spent doing full contact drills and scrimmages, but they have increased the number of games that football

teams play in a season, including playoffs (Brady and Barnett, 2015). Many coaches now teach tackling moves that limit head involvement, but these moves often are lost in the speed of real game action. New concussion diagnosis and treatment protocols are mandated in high school sports, but these only reduce the likelihood of playing with a head injury rather than preventing head injuries.

As research continues to show that repetitive subconcussive head trauma can cause temporary or permanent brain damage that could affect grades, college admissions, future job prospects, and general health and well-being, lawsuits will be filed. Defendants in those lawsuits are coaches, school athletic directors and principals, district and state athletic directors, and boards of education. Regardless of the possible legal outcomes, the mere threat of personal and school liability raises the cost of insurance and puts school personnel in an uncertain legal position. This means that dealing with head trauma among athletes is no longer a choice. To avoid assertive actions puts your school, school district, and state high school activities association on the line as well as the careers and family assets of personnel associated with sports.

The issue of concussions and other serious injuries plays out in a slightly different way at the college level. Athletes in college have reached the age of (informed) legal consent. But this means that the NCAA, universities, athletic departments, and teams have the responsibility to fully inform athletes of the risks they agree to take in their sport. Until now all these parties have been grossly negligent. There has been no NCAA policy on concussion protocols, even though the stated purpose of the organization is to protect "student-athletes." Universities have not provided in-depth education sessions to inform athletes of the risks they face in certain sport situations, despite having concussion and brain trauma experts on their faculties and in their medical schools, and despite claiming that college sports are important educational experiences.

A concussion lawsuit was filed against the NCAA and other defendants in 2011 by an individual, but he was joined by additional for-mer players with alleged symptoms of brain inju-ries. Therefore, the suit sought approval as a class action claim on behalf of thousands of former col-lege athletes (AP, 2013; Hruby, 2013a, 2013b).

The case was settled in July 2014, with the NCAA agreeing to establish a $70 million fund to pay for exams to assess whether former play-ers have neurological ailments possibly related to previous concussions. The NCAA also agreed to provide an additional $5 million for research on concussions, and to create a protocol on when athlete can return to play after sustaining a con-cussion. No damages would be paid to any play-ers for the treatment of neurological ailments.

Although college athletes suffered over 30,000 reported and diagnosed concussions between 2004 and 2009, they were denied an opportunity to file a class action suit in which all of them would be represented in one case. This enabled the NCAA to escape the payment of significant damages, such as those being paid to former play-ers by the NFL. Former college players may now sue as individuals, but that is very expensive to do, and the chances of winning such a case is remote at best.

Like the NFL, the NCAA avoided an admission of negligence or wrongdoing in failing to inform players what was known about head injuries. There-fore, they will pay no damages to any former play-ers, and their insurance will cover nearly all of the settlement. A few of the former athletes involved in the suit did not accept the settlement because it failed to cover any treatment, but they could do nothing to reopen the case.

Although the settlement in this case did not hurt the NCAA financially, and high schools have not yet paid a major settlement, emerging research on brain injuries continues to make concussions and head trauma a "crossroads issue" for high school and college sports. If scientists don't develop a way to prevent a brain from moving inside a skull when the head comes to a sudden stop or is twisted vio-lently, the people who run school-sponsored sport programs will be forced to turn in a safer direction

as they enter the crossroads. Staying the course will not be an option.

Educational Relevance   As a form of physical activity and exercise, sports can be important in edu-cational terms. However, this depends on how they are organized, the context in which they are played, and the meanings given to them. Unfortunately, when it comes to high school and college sports we have ignored these conditional factors and used the great sport myth to assume that all sports are essen-tially "educational" and that playing sports always involves positive and valuable learning experiences. This has prevented educators, including coaches, from having critical discussions about what they want to happen in school-sponsored sport programs, how they can use teaching and learning theory (ped-agogy) to make those things happen, and how they can determine whether they have been successful.

Much of the reason why sport programs have become increasingly detached from academic pro-grams is that many people simply assume that sport is education and that playing sports is learning. On the basis of these assumptions, which research shows to be faulty, educators in the United States have made a very specialized form of elite, com-petitive sports a central feature of our schools with-out having systematically collected evidence or sound educational theory to justify this decision or guide its implementation.

These assumptions about sport participation are especially problematic when we consider the power of sports in U.S. culture. Once sports are integrated into the culture and structure of schools, there is a tendency for them to dominate the public profile of the school; capture the attention of students, teach-ers, staff, and administrators; and take on a pur-pose and importance of their own—a purpose that is connected with winning records, championship trophies in the entrance of the school, public rela-tions, entertainment, and media coverage. Overall, sports become both the symbolic and the real rep-resentation of the school itself.

When this occurs, sports are likely to collide with and overshadow the academic mission of the school (Nixon, 2014). Then people say that we have to have sports because they are the reason many of our students come to school every day. Or we need to have them because they are the only things that bring us together as a school community. Or we need them because they are the "front porch" of the university. And these statements are accepted without asking why our curriculum is so bad that students tolerate it only because they must do so to play sports, or without asking what other ways we might come together as a community, or create ways to make Nobel Prize winners and cutting-edge knowledge the front porch of the university.

Without asking these critical questions, schools end up spending much more to support athletes than regular students (Marklein, 2013). To question these spending patterns in the United States is to invite widespread criticism grounded in highly charged emotions, defensiveness, and personal attacks (Martin, 2013). The criticism consists mostly of statements about "what sports meant to me" and "what sports mean to my kids." But these responses actually support the relevance of the question, because they clearly show how important sports have become in schools, and how people take this for granted without asking serious questions about their educational relevance.

Such spending patterns would be viewed as strange by students from countries with highly rated educational systems, where the academic context of the school is where they learned about teamwork, how to constructively handle failure and success, how to work hard and complete projects, how to be resilient when learning is difficult, and how to see learning as the reason for the existence of schools and their attendance at school (Ripley, 2013a, 2013b). This is not to say that young people from these countries do not play sports. They do, and sports are important to many of them. But for them, sports are community-based and do not dominate the social, cultural, and physical landscapes of their schools.

It is unrealistic to suggest that schools drop sport programs, although budget cuts are forcing some to do so. But it is not unrealistic to suggest that educators ask critical questions and take seriously the research that explains how and when sports alter the cultures and organization of their schools. Then they can make a decision to keep, change, or abandon sport programs. A good place to start is to ask what they would think about a higher education system in a country where the highest-paid person in all the top universities is either a football or men's basketball coach, the most revered people on campus are football or male basketball players, and the university spends six times more money per capita to support athletes than to support students who are not on college teams.

Gender Inequity A program in which students in the United States play the same sports across multiple generations ignores educational theory and fails to recognize the changing and diverse sport interests that exist in a culture that prizes individuality and innovation. For example, when high schools emphasize the same few power and performance sports for over a century, they discourage participation by some boys and many girls who prefer sports emphasizing pleasure and participation—sports that may not have existed 40 to 100 years ago. The progress that has been made toward achieving gender equity is due to adding new sports, such as soccer and lacrosse, to athletic programs, and further progress toward equity requires similar changes.

Students who do not measure up to their bigger, faster, taller, and stronger classmates require alternatives to or modifications of traditional power and performance sports. Although sports like football and basketball receive much attention and many resources, there could be teams in Ultimate (Frisbee), disc golf, racquetball, flag football, in-line skating, orienteering, slacklining, wall climbing, mountain biking, BMX, water tube polo, roller hockey, skateboarding, and other sports for which there is enough local interest to field teams. With guidance, the students themselves could at least partially administer and coach these teams and coordinate exhibitions or meets and games with teams from other schools. Does there really have to be an official state champion for a sport to be educational?

Girls' sports in high school continue to lack the support that boys' sports enjoy. This problem has a history that goes far beyond high school, but the result, as illustrated in Table 14.5, is that many more boys than girls play high school sports—nearly 1.3 million more in 2015. Additionally, progress toward gender equity stalled in 2000 and there has been some backsliding during recent years (Table 14.5).

Gender inequities at the college level are grounded in similar social and cultural dynamics, but the inequities go deeper and are manifested in many realms, such as operating budgets, recruiting money, and coaches' salaries. These differences in all NCAA programs for 2014 are shown in Figure 14.1. Even though women were 53 percent of the student body, they constituted only 44 percent of the athletes. Additionally, they received 46 percent of the scholarship dollars, 33 percent of recruiting dollars, 35 percent of

Table 14.5   Girls and boys participating in high school sports, 1971–2015 (in millions)

Academic Year	Girls	Boys	Difference
1971–1972	0.29	3.66	3.37
1975–1976	1.65	4.11	2.46
1980–1981	1.85	3.50	1.65
1985–1986	1.81	3.34	1.53
1990–1991	1.89	3.41	1.52
1995–1996	2.47	3.63	1.16
2000–2001	2.78	3.92	1.14
2005–2006	2.95	4.20	1.25
2010–2011	3.17	4.49	1.32
2014–2015	3.29	4.52	1.23

Source: National Federation of High Schools; http://www.nfhs.org/ParticipationStatistics/ParticipationStatistics

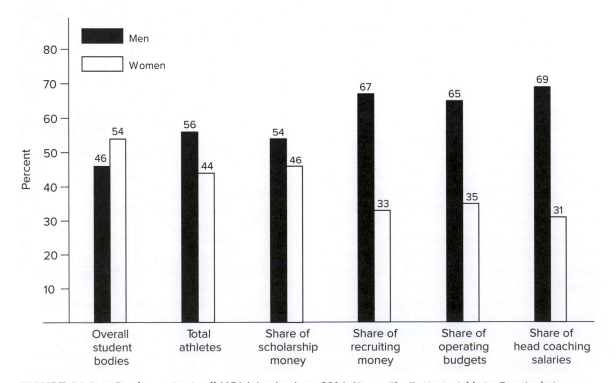

FIGURE 14.1   Gender equity in all NCAA institutions, 2014. (*Source:* The Equity in Athletics Data Analysis Cutting Tool; http://ope.ed.gov/athletics/GetAggregatedData.aspx)

the total athletic department operating expenses, and 31 percent of the salaries for head coaches (although they have more teams than the men do).

Many people justify these gender inequities by noting that men's teams generate more revenues than women's teams. Others say that a portion of the revenues claimed by men come from student fees and state funds plus the potential for men to generate revenues is due to larger gender inequities that lead people to value men's sports more than women's sports. This means that the question for colleges and universities is whether gender inequities in the larger society should shape funding priorities in their sport programs. At this point, it appears that they do.

Gender-related participation inequities in high school and college are due primarily to the size of football teams and the increasing costs associated with fielding football teams. A few universities in the top five intercollegiate conferences (Atlantic Coast, Big Ten, Big 12, Pac-12, and Southeastern) have football and men's basketball teams that generate enough revenues to fund the overall budgets for women's sports, but as the expenses for football and men's basketball increase, there is a need for increased subsidies to sustain women's and most other men's teams.

In terms of gender equity, the supporters of intercollegiate football face a glaring contradiction. On the one hand, they say that football is an educational activity and that they should not have to pay taxes on their increasing revenues or treat players as employees. On the other hand, when gender equity is discussed, they claim that college football is a business affected by objective market forces out of their control and that it should not be treated as an educational activity. This is why Title IX remains controversial—it exposes the contradictions of big-time sport programs and turns football supporters into flip-floppers.

The current organization and operation of high school and college football are the primary causes of persistent gender inequities in participation and funding because teams are large and the sport is expensive.

The other major reason for persistent gender inequities is that athletic programs remain grounded in a culture based on the values and experiences of men. This will not change until more women are hired as coaches of both women's and men's teams and as athletic directors. But the chance of this happening in the near future is remote for at least three reasons. *First*, most people working in school sport programs today are not familiar with the full meaning of gender equity as it is described in Title IX law, and certainly don't know how to implement the law (Staurowsky and Weight, 2011). *Second*, when football is the centerpiece of sport programs at the school and conference levels, women are not likely to be hired in top leadership positions because it is widely believed that they cannot effectively work

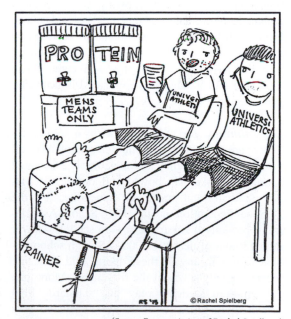

(*Source:* By permission of Rachel Spielberg)

If it weren't for our football team, women's teams would have no funding on this campus.

Many people do not know that major college football teams, with a few exceptions, lose money each year and are supported by student fees and other external funds. Consequently, they perpetuate misleading information year after year.

with a football coach and team (Schull et al., 2013). *Third*, when women who are coaches or lower-level administrators raise questions about gender inequities, they are usually defined as troublemakers and marginalized in the athletic department or in the coaching job market (Fagan and Cyphers, 2012).

Changing the organization and culture of sport programs is a formidable task, and it is nearly impossible when those in charge see no reason to change or see change as a threat to their status and power. However, in the case of programs described and funded as "educational," there's no justification for paying women any less than men or defining women as unqualified for leadership jobs because some people believe that they cannot understand football or work effectively with powerful and highly paid football coaches. Ellen Staurowsky, a former athletic director and a respected scholar in sport management, points out that everyone in athletic departments at the high school and college level should have regular opportunities to receive training in Title IX law and how to effectively implement it in their programs (Staurowsky and Weight, 2011). This would be a valuable step forward in achieving gender equity.

Opportunities for Students with a Disability
Where are disability sports in high schools? For all practical purposes, they are invisible. The "adapted sports" of basketball, bowling, floor hockey, soccer, softball, and track are sanctioned by the National Federation of State High School Associations, but only 0.7 percent of high schools—fewer than 130 out of nearly 18,000 U.S. high schools— have teams in any of these sports, and these are located in only seven of the fifty states. More than 7.71 million students play on "standard" high school sport teams; fewer than 9000 students play on adapted sport teams, and nearly half of these play in three sports—bowling, softball, and soccer (NFHS, 2013).

Some athletes with a disability play on standard teams, but apart from them, there is only one varsity athlete in adapted sports for every 950 athletes on high school teams. Students with a disability are "off the radar" for most high school sport programs

and nearly all college programs. Consequently, students miss opportunities to play with and watch their peers with various (dis)abilities compete and share sport experiences with them. This is a missed educational opportunity for all students.

Competitive sport participation by students with a disability often requires a combination of creatively designed programs. There are sports in which athletes with a disability can be included in standard games, meets, and matches, but when this isn't possible there should be school teams in one or more adapted sports. When there's a shortage of athletes at individual schools, there should be teams from districts or combinations of schools; when practical, another alternative is to have students without disabling impairments play with "handicaps" to provide the required number of team members.

Finally, when students lack school teams and play on community-based teams sponsored by disability organizations, their participation should be publicized, supported, and formally rewarded, as is done for athletes on school teams.

There are many ways to support athletes with a disability. Appropriate strategies will vary from one school to another, but they can be developed if people are creatively inclusive in how they organize sports. However, this seldom occurs unless there are people at the school and district levels who are active and assertive advocates for students with impairments that prevent them from playing on existing school teams. These advocates now have guidelines established by the U.S. Department of Education to increase their legitimacy and political clout within the schools.

Colleges and universities have done little to nothing to provide sports for people with a disability (Wolverton, 2013). Only a dozen programs have recognized programs, and they are funded through student services rather than athletic departments. The programs are at the universities of Alabama, Arizona, Illinois, Missouri, Oklahoma State, Central Oklahoma, Oregon, Edinboro (Pennsylvania), Penn State, Rutgers (new program), Texas at Arlington, and Wisconsin at Whitewater. The sports offered include men's and women's wheelchair basketball, track and road racing, tennis, golf, rowing, and wheelchair rugby (Gerber, 2015).

Although some Paralympians train in these programs, it is difficult to schedule games and meets with other university teams due to the distance between schools and the expenses associated with travel.

At a few of these universities participation occurs totally in-house in the form of training and intramural competitions. Despite recommendations and guidelines provided by the U.S. Department of Education, few people in higher education have done anything beyond mentioning disability sports in passing conversations. Brad Hendrick, the Director of the Division of Disability Resources and Education Services at the University of Illinois at Urbana-Champaign notes that administrators and athletic directors are quick to list reasons that programs can't be developed rather than thinking creatively about how they can be developed (Walker, 2013).

The existence of the Paralympics has not had an impact on program development, even though it would make sense for universities to sponsor Paralympic sports just as they sponsor Olympic sports in their athletic departments. As it is now, college students with a disability must seek opportunities to play sports outside the university, even though they pay student fees and should have access to the same opportunities that other students have.

It is difficult to predict how quickly people in the schools will respond to the Department of Education guidelines and take seriously the sport participation of students with disabilities. It could take decades for measureable progress to be made and at least a generation before sport participation opportunities for students with a disability are a taken-for-granted part of secondary and higher education.

Issues in High School Sport Programs: A Focus on Sports Development

Some high school administrators, athletic directors, and coaches think that educational quality is somehow linked to the development of a sport program that focuses on winning records and being ranked highly among schools in the state or nation. Their goal is to create a sport program that resembles a big-time intercollegiate program. This leads to excessive concerns with building high-profile programs that become the focus of attention in the school and community.

People who focus on sports development often give lip service to keeping sports in proper perspective but fail to acknowledge that emphasizing sports in the school often marginalizes many students with no interest in sports. Additionally, in their zeal to create and maintain high-profile programs, administrators often make decisions that overlook the educational needs of all students in the school.

Sports development today goes hand in hand with informal requirements that athletes specialize in a single sport year-round, even though this may limit their overall social and educational development. This approach turns off students who want to play sports but don't want to make them the center of their lives. At the same time, other students become so dedicated to sports that they see education as secondary in their lives at school.

Adherence to a sports development model often is driven by boosters and booster organizations that raise funds and provide other support to one or more sport teams in a school. However, individual boosters and booster organizations are seldom regulated by schools or school districts, and they exist primarily in wealthier areas, often giving unfair advantage to a single team in a school or an entire athletic program relative to programs in poor areas where resources are scarce and teams struggle to exist. Many boosters who provide resources, sometimes out of their own pockets, feel they have a right to intervene in the process of evaluating and hiring coaches, and they generally focus on coaches' win–loss records rather than their teaching abilities.

Issues in College Sport Programs

This is a challenging time for college sports, especially at the big-time level. They are facing more issues today than at any time in the past century. Scandals and rule violations, lawsuits related to player compensation, and distorted racial and ethnic priorities are discussed in this section.

Scandals and Rule Violations   A steady and sometimes overwhelming number of scandals in college sports capture headlines and much attention. The most publicized and horrific case involved Jerry Sandusky, a retired assistant football coach at Penn State, who used his affiliation with the Penn State football program to lure boys into relationships and sexually abuse them. When an assistant coach observed an incident of Sandusky committing sodomy on a young boy in a Penn State football shower, he reported it to head football coach, Joe Paterno, rather than to state child protection authorities. Paterno took his time reporting it to Penn State officials, who took no action. It wasn't until a former victim came forward that an official state investigation began; this led to Sandusky's conviction on forty-five counts of child abuse and child sexual abuse.

The independent investigation of this case concluded that the university administration's failure to take state-mandated actions and report the incident was due to "a culture of reverence for the football program that is ingrained at all levels of the campus community" (Freeh Sporkin and Sullivan, LLP, 2012, p. 17). As a result, a serial sexual predator operated freely for at least thirteen years alongside the football program. The Penn State president, athletic director, and director of campus security were all fired for their cover-up of Sandusky's actions. It appeared that protecting the football program was a higher priority for them than following state law or protecting children from Sandusky's predatory behavior.

The Penn State scandal, along with other scandals, led many people to conclude that universities have lost institutional control of their sport programs. For example, when Gordon Gee, president of Ohio State University, was asked if he would dismiss the football coach for failing to report multiple NCAA rule violations by members of the football team, he said, "No—are you kidding? Let me be

very clear, I'm just hopeful the coach doesn't dismiss me" (Wickersham, 2011). Gee was the highest-paid university president in the United States, but when he made his comment he was making almost $2 million less than the football coach. He made his comment in a joking manner, but many saw it as an indication that big-time college sport programs had become more powerful than the universities that sponsor them. Under these conditions, it is not difficult to understand that the hubris and the sense of entitlement that come with such power open the door for scandals and rule violations.

Player Rights and Compensation   The increased revenues and stakes in big-time college sports, especially in football and men's basketball, have raised questions about the rights of athletes and the compensation they receive. Furthermore, athletes in these sports now realize that this "system is entirely based on their acceptance of their own powerlessness as the gears of this machine [and if] they choose to exercise their power, the machine not only stops moving, it becomes dramatically reshaped" (Zirin, 2015a).

This realization led Kain Colter, quarterback for Northwestern University's football team, to organize his teammates and petition the National Labor Relations Board (NLRB) to form a union. Their goals were fourfold: (1) to prevent their coach from terminating the scholarships of injured players; (2) to have the university take player safety more seriously, especially related to concussions and head trauma; (3) to have health insurance that cover full treatment for football-related injuries, even after eligibility ends; and (4) to limit the hours that coaches could keep them in practices each week, because they often worked 50-hours or more. Notably, they were not seeking to be paid for their participation.

The response to this move was immediate and dramatic. Their coach, the university president, and people around the country said that the players would destroy college sports. Eventually, the NLRB stated that even though the players fit the definition of employees and had the right to vote on unionization, such an action would impact all of college sports, and the board members didn't think they should make such a momentous decision.

The Northwestern players lost, but their case raised questions about the rights and treatment of college athletes, especially those whose labor generates billions of dollars in revenues. This forced the NCAA to respond and part of that response was to allow the wealthiest and most powerful conferences more autonomy to make their own rules. Subsequently, this has led to series of changes so that universities can now award multiple year scholarships and increase the amount of a scholarship to cover the full cost of attendance at the university. Additionally, meal restrictions were lifted so athletes could have more food without violating NCAA rules, which would also give them the calories needed to meet in-season energy needs.

The Pacific 12 conference went further to guarantee four-year scholarships for athletes receiving full awards. Aid is now available to athletes needing to complete graduation requirements after their eligibility ends. Medical insurance is expanded to cover athletes up to four years after leaving the university. Athletes are now allowed to transfer to another Pac-12 school and receive a scholarship immediately rather than waiting for a year. And the conference now includes athlete representatives in the conference governance structure. Clearly, such changes benefit athletes at the same time that they alter the dynamics of recruiting, coach–athlete relationships, the overall health care received by athletes, and the potential power that athletes have in their sports.

More potentially disruptive challenges to the NCAA and the operation of college sports were initiated in 2009 by former UCLA basketball star, Ed O'Bannon, and Sam Keller, a former Arizona State and Nebraska quarterback. When O'Bannon noticed that his likeness was being used in an EA Sports video game, he along with Keller and other players whose likenesses were also being used filed a class action suit against EA Sports, the Collegiate Licensing Company that negotiates licensing fees

for the NCAA, and the NCAA that receives fees for selling rights to the players' likenesses.

The former athletes won this case and were awarded $40 million. All athletes who had appeared in the video games since 2003 were eligible for compensation. But O'Bannon continued his suit against the NCAA saying that it violates anti-trust laws by preventing athletes from earning money from the sale of their names, images, and likenesses. In practical terms, he wanted athletes to share in the revenues generated by the sale of media rights, jerseys and apparel bearing their names, and other commercial ventures using their names and images.

A judge decided in O'Bannon's favor in a 2014 decision stating that the NCAA was in violation of anti-trust law and that universities could pay athletes up to $5000 per year that would be available to them after their college sport careers ended. The NCAA appealed this decision and a panel of judges disallowed the lower court's ruling on compensation, but also ruled that the NCAA ban on athlete compensating athletes was anti-competitive and in violation of anti-trust law. Therefore, it questioned the NCAA's claim that the integrity of college sports required that athletes remain unpaid amateurs and it requested a full analysis of the NCAA's "amateurism defense" that has been used since 1984 to legally deny payments to athletes.

If the O'Bannon suit is not settled out of court, it is likely to go to the U.S. Supreme court. More important, the case leaves open the door for other lawsuits charging that the NCAA violates anti-trust laws by putting any limits on the amount of an athletic scholarship and prohibiting cash payments to athletes. In fact, Jeffrey Kessler, a high powered attorney representing college football and men's basketball players, is arguing in *Jenkins* v. *NCAA* that there should be a free market for recruiting and compensating athletes in revenue producing sports. In the early 1990s, Kessler represented NFL players in their successful quest for free agency, and now he is representing college players in a similar quest. If there is a ruling in favor of the athletes, universities would be forced to make scholarship and payment offers to high school recruits who would choose the best offer on the table.

The NCAA predicts disaster if it loses this case (or similar cases), but lawyers representing the players note that the NCAA uses a free market argument to justify multi-million dollar contracts for football and men's basketball coaches. They say that if that argument applies to coaches, it also should apply to athletes, and if coaches' salaries have not destroyed college sports, players' salaries won't destroy it either; the free market will set its own limits. But it would also impact the entire system of college sports.

Distorted Racial and Ethnic Priorities In 2015, black students made up about 12 percent of the total student body at Division I universities. Figure 14.2 shows that at the same time, black men and women were 22 percent of the athletes, 53 percent of football players, 66 percent of the men's and 57 percent of the women's basketball players.

Sixty-seven percent of all black male athletes played football or basketball—the only sports that produced revenues and the sports with the lowest graduation rates. This also means that, in some big-time sport programs, black male athletes consistently generate revenues that fund other sport teams on which all or nearly all of the players are white.

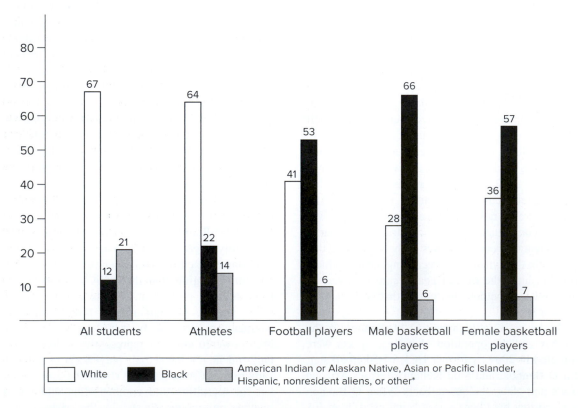

*Racial and ethnic classifications are based on self-identifications.

FIGURE 14.2 Percentages of students and athletes in NCAA Division I universities by race and ethnicity, 2014–2015. (*Source:* Lapchick, 2015; http://web1.ncaa.org/rgdSearch/exec/saSearch; http://www.census.gov/hhes/school/data/cps/2014/tables.html)

Overall, 1 of every 7 black men on Division I campuses is an athlete; this is the case for 1 of every 29 white men, 1 of every 25 black women, and 1 of every 33 white women. This gives many people the impression that black males are super-athletes who attend college only because of their physical skills. At the same time it leads people to overlook the fact that more than 99.5 percent of all black American men between the ages of eighteen and twenty-three do not have athletic scholarships.

Overall, these data suggest that if African Americans excel in revenue-producing sports, universities will actively identify and recruit them, but the same universities do a poor job of recruiting African American students who don't excel at scoring touchdowns or making jump shots. There is no denying that a few African Americans benefit from athletic scholarships. But the problem is that universities have capitalized on the racist myth that blacks can use sports to improve their lives, while ignoring their responsibility to recruit black students and change the social climate on the campus so that black students feel welcome, supported, and respected, even if they don't score touchdowns or score 20 points a game.

A related problem is that many black athletes feel isolated on campuses where there are few black students, faculty, and administrators (Bimper, 2015; Bruening et al., 2005; Comeaux and Fuentes, 2015; Hawkins, 2010; Martin et al., 2010; Singer and Carter-Francique, 2013; Smith, 2009; Torres, 2009). This isolation is intensified by many factors, including these:

1. Racial and athletic stereotypes make it difficult for black athletes to feel welcome on campus and develop relationships that support their academic success.
2. Athletes must devote so much time to their sports that it is difficult for them to become involved in other spheres of campus life.
3. Campus activities often fail to represent the interests and experiences of black students, who consequently often feel like outsiders.
4. When campus life is unrelated to their experiences, black athletes may withdraw from activities that could connect them with other students.
5. White students who lack experience in racially diverse groups might feel uncomfortable interacting with black students from backgrounds unlike their own.
6. When white students think that black athletes have things easy and are unfairly privileged, it creates tension that undermines meaningful interaction.

Feelings of social isolation are especially intense when black athletes come from working-class or low-income backgrounds and white students come from upper-middle-income backgrounds (Torres, 2009). This combination of ethnic and socioeconomic differences can also create tensions, unless the administration, faculty, and professional staff provide regular opportunities for students to interact in ways that increase their knowledge of peers from different backgrounds. Putting athletes in their own dorm wings, creating special academic support programs for them, and giving them athlete centers where they eat and hang out with other athletes might make general campus isolation more tolerable, but it does not foster learning and development (Hawkins, 2010).

Most research on black players in the sociology of sport has focused on black men, so we don't know much about the experiences of black women who play sports in predominantly white institutions. Black women athletes face the dual challenges of complex racial and gender dynamics on campus and in the athletic department (Bernhard, 2014; Bruening, 2004, 2005; Bruening et al., 2005; Carter-Francique, 2014; Carter and Hawkins, 2011; Carter-Francique et al., 2011; Gabay, 2013; Hughes, 2015). They see few women of color in positions of power and authority in their schools and athletic departments, so they might not feel fully included in either sphere.

A key issue for some black women is that Title IX law has benefited white women more than black women. For example, over 75 percent of all black women with scholarships in Division I NCAA schools in 2015 were playing on basketball or track teams, and black women received less than 4 percent of the scholarships in the other sixteen women's sports. This means that nearly 25 percent of all black women with scholarships play on teams where they may be the only black athlete, and it's likely that their experiences are different from the experiences of black women on basketball and track teams.

Title IX has fueled the growth of soccer, crew (rowing), golf, rifle, and lacrosse, but these sports are played primarily by white women in upper-middle-class families. Most black women who play on these teams in college do not have black teammates and their experiences can be socially isolating. For this reason, Tina Sloan Green of the Black Women in Sport Foundation claims that "Title IX was for white women" and that the experiences of black girls and women have been overlooked in the expansion of college sports for women (Suggs, 2001).

Universities must be more aggressive and creative in recruiting and supporting ethnic minority students who aren't athletes and in doing the same for ethnic minority coaches and faculty. It's not fair to recruit black or other ethnic minority athletes to campuses where they have little social support and feel that students and faculty don't know much about their history, heritage, and experiences. If universities effectively included racial and cultural diversity within all spheres of campus life, recruiting black athletes would not indicate a distorted set of campus priorities. When universities present to the world images of physically talented black athletes and intellectually talented white scientists, racism is perpetuated, whether intentionally or not.

summary

DO COMPETITIVE SPORTS CONTRIBUTE TO EDUCATION?

The United States is the only nation in the world where it is taken for granted that high schools and colleges will sponsor and fund interschool sport programs. There are arguments for and against this practice, but most of the claims made on both sides are not based on good research.

Generalizing about high school and college sport programs is difficult because programs and the conditions under which participation occurs are so diverse. However, it's important to study school sports to determine if and when they contribute to positive educational outcomes for athletes, the overall organization of the school, and students in general. At a minimum, if the programs provide no educational benefits for the athletes, they cannot be justified as school-sponsored activities.

Research shows that young people who play on high school teams have better overall academic records than those who don't. But much of this difference is explained by the processes through which students are selected-in and filtered-out of school teams. Young people with characteristics consistent with academic achievement are favored in these processes, so it is not surprising that athletes, on average, have different characteristics from other students.

The most effective way to determine what occurs in connection with school sport participation is to study athletes and teams in context over time. This enables a researcher to identify the factors that influence sport experiences, the meanings that young people give to those experiences, and how young people integrate them into their identities and everyday lives.

Sport experiences vary widely and are given different meanings that tend to be influenced by gender, race and ethnicity, social class, (dis)ability, and the social and cultural context of the family, school, and local community. Although there is reasonably consistent evidence indicating that the social dynamics on certain high school sport teams increase the likelihood of binge drinking among all athletes and higher rates of sexual activity and bullying among certain male athletes, most studies suggest that athletes have higher than average rates of educational achievement and fewer problems than other students.

Research also indicates that some schools, coaches, parents, and athletes lose sight of educational goals in their pursuit of competitive success in sports. Sports can be seductive, and people connected with high school teams usually require guidance to keep their programs in balance with the academic curriculum. Unless sport teams are explicitly organized to achieve positive educational outcomes, the chances of achieving them decrease. When people assume that sport participation automatically builds character and enhances learning, it undermines the planning and evaluation that must be a part of any school activity, especially those that are as costly and popular as school sports.

The possibility that sport participation interferes with the education of athletes is greatest in big-time intercollegiate programs. The status and identity that often comes with membership on highly visible and publicized sport teams makes it difficult for many young people to focus on and give priority to academic work. This is especially the case among young men who see their destinies being shaped by sport achievements, not academic achievements. With this said, data indicate that athletes as a category have higher graduation rates than the general student population. However, graduation rates among athletes vary widely by gender, race, and sport.

High school and college sports usually create spirited feelings among some students, faculty, and staff in schools. But little is known about the characteristics of this spirit or if and when it contributes to the achievement of educational goals—or disrupts the achievement of those goals. Although many different activities can be used to unite students and link them with community and society, sports often are used to do this in the United States. Sports are popular activities, but there is much to be learned about the conditions under which they are most and least likely to produce particular educational and developmental outcomes.

Most high school sport programs don't seriously cut into funds for academic programs. The money they require is well spent if they provide students with opportunities to learn about their physicality, develop physical and interpersonal skills, and display their skills in ways that lead them to be recognized and rewarded by others. However, when budgets are strained, many sport programs depend on participation fees, boosters, and/or corporate sponsors to survive. When this occurs, schools in lower-income areas are at a serious competitive disadvantage. Over time, these strategies to fund school sports lead to and intensify social class and racial/ethnic divisions in schools and school districts.

Funding issues are complex and often confusing in intercollegiate sports. However, it's clear that very few programs are self-supporting and nearly all of them depend on subsidies from student fees, donations, and general campus funds. As intercollegiate programs boost their focus on achieving commercial goals, the likelihood of achieving educational goals usually declines. The allocation of general funds and student fees to intercollegiate sports becomes an increasingly contentious issue when athletic departments and sport teams have become so separate from the rest of campus culture that faculty and students see no reason to support them.

High school and college sport programs now face a number of "crossroads issues." These include cost containment and budget gaps between schools; rising expectations among athletes and their parents; dealing with concussions, repetitive head trauma, and other serious injuries; creating and sustaining programs with explicit educational relevance; eliminating gender inequity; and creating opportunities for students with a disability. Each of these issues creates a serious challenge for athletic directors and coaches.

Issues unique to high school sport programs consist of clarifying the meaning of sport development so that it is compatible with the education mission of schools and making sure that boosters and other community supporters understand that clarification. The unique issues faced in college sport programs are reducing scandals and rule violations, settling the class action likeness lawsuit filed on behalf of Ed O'Bannon, dealing with increasing the cash value of scholarship awards to cover the full cost of attending college, and eliminating the distorted priorities related to race and ethnicity in the university and in athletic departments.

The decisions made on these crossroads issues will have a significant impact on the future direction of high school and college sports.

SUPPLEMENTAL READINGS

Reading 1.   Research faculty are not eager to study intercollegiate sports

Reading 2.   A brief history of NCAA academic reforms

Reading 3.   School–community relations

Reading 4.   Bibliography of research on college sports

Reading 5.   Ethnicity and sport participation among high school girls

Reading 6.   Conformity or leadership in high school sports

Reading 7.   Should intercollegiate athletes be paid?

SPORT MANAGEMENT ISSUES

- You're a reporter for a newspaper in a small midwestern U.S. city. A chronic budget crisis leads the local school board to consider dropping varsity sports. The board has scheduled a meeting to discuss this issue with people in the community. To prepare for the meeting, you review the arguments you expect to hear on both sides of the issue. What are those arguments, and who do you expect to be the most vocal proponents of each?

- You're a member of a school board in an urban school district. The board has just been presented with data showing that varsity athletes in the fifteen high schools in your district receive higher grades than nonathletes. A group of parents is using the data to request more funds for interscholastic sports in the district. What are the questions you would ask about the data, and why would you ask them?

- The academic experiences of athletes in colleges with big-time sport programs are different from the experiences of athletes in colleges with lower-profile programs. If you were talking to a group of high school seniors interested in playing college sports, how would you explain these differences?

- The intercollegiate sport programs at your school are in bad financial shape. Because of large losses, the students have been asked to increase their student fees by $100 per semester to maintain the programs. If the fee increase does not pass, all the intercollegiate sport programs will be dropped and replaced by low-cost, student-run club sports. How would you vote? Use material from this chapter to support your decision.

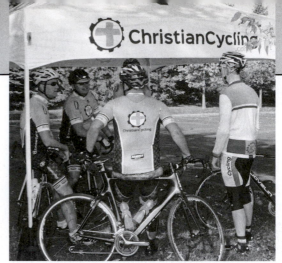

(*Source:* © ChristianCycling.com)

chapter

15

SPORTS AND RELIGIONS

Is It a Promising Combination?

In fandom, as in religious worship, our social connections are brought to life, in the stands as in the pews. It serves as a reminder of our interconnectedness and dependency. . . . In short, if you look hard at sports, you can't help but see contours of religion.

> —**Michael Serazio, Communication Department, Fairfield University (2013)**

. . . [Using mixed martial arts as] outreach is part of a larger and more longstanding effort on the part of some ministers who fear that their churches have become too feminized, promoting kindness and compassion at the expense of strength and responsibility.

> —**R. M. Schneiderman, journalist,**
> ***Newsweek*/The Daily Beast (2010)**

My audience is God. . . . The right way to play is not for others and not for myself, but for God. I still don't fully understand what that means; I struggle with these things every game, every day.

> —**Jeremy Lin, NBA player (in Brooks, 2012)**

I've a wife and two kids to provide for and if it means killing you in the ring, that's what I will have to do. . . . I read the Bible quite a lot. . . . It gives me strength to know that if God is in my corner then no one can beat me . . . . If you put Him first then everything will work out.

> —**Tyson Fury, British and Commonwealth Heavyweight boxing champion (in Gore, 2010)**

Today, all 30 N.B.A. teams have volunteer chaplains, with no guidance or oversight from the league. . . . For some players, attending chapel service has become as much a part of their pregame routine as having an ankle taped.

> —**Andrew Keh, journalist (2015)**

Chapter Outline

How Do Sociologists Define and Study Religion?
Similarities and Differences Between Sports and Religions
Modern Sports and Religious Beliefs and Organizations
The Challenges of Combining Sports and Religious Beliefs
Summary: Is It a Promising Combination?

Learning Objectives

- Understand why sociologists study religion in society.
- Discuss the similarities and differences between sports and religions, and why it may be difficult to make clear distinctions between them.
- Discuss why Christianity in general and Protestant beliefs in particular have become regularly connected with sports.
- Identify forms of world religions other than Christianity, and discuss why they have not become closely connected with sports and sport participation.

- Discuss challenges faced by Muslim women who want to play sports.
- Explain how Christian sport organizations have used sports.
- Identify the ways that Christian athletes and coaches have used religion in sports.
- Identify and discuss the conflicts faced by Christian athletes in violent spectator sports, and explain strategies for dealing with them.
- Discuss what has occurred when sports and Christian beliefs have been combined in recent history.

The relationship between sports and religions varies by time and place. Physical activities and sports in many traditional cultures are included in rituals that are linked to the supernatural. For example, the histories of many Native American cultures show that games and running races often had spiritual significance. The histories of Jews and Christians in Europe and North America indicate that there have been times during which religious authorities approved of physical activities, games, and sports and times during which authorities condemned them as indulgent and sinful. There have been religious approaches to the body—sometimes linking it with weakness and sin, and other times linking it with strength and godliness.

During the last half of the twentieth century, most religious organizations in North America and Europe approved of sports and even sponsored them. Furthermore, some individuals today combine sport participation with their religious beliefs and publicly proclaim the personal importance of this combination. This is especially common among Christian athletes in the United States.

The purpose of this chapter is to examine the connections between religions and sports. This relationship is complex because religious beliefs are combined with sports in diverse ways, depending on the experiences, relationships, and interests of individuals and groups.

The major questions we'll discuss in this chapter are these:

1. How is *religion* defined, and why do sociologists study it?
2. What are the similarities and differences between sports and religions?
3. Why have people combined sports and religious beliefs, and why are Christians more vocal about this combination than are Jews, Muslims, Hindus, Buddhists, Sikhs, and other people whose religious beliefs are not based on Christianity?
4. What are the issues and controversies associated with combining religious beliefs and sport participation?

When discussing the last question, special attention is given to the prospect of using religion as a platform for eliminating racism, sexism, deviance, violence, and other problems in sports and sport organizations.

HOW DO SOCIOLOGISTS DEFINE AND STUDY RELIGION?

A sociological discussion of religion often creates controversy because people tend to use their own religious beliefs and practices as their only point of reference. Tensions are inevitable whenever people are asked to think critically and analytically about the beliefs they use to make sense of their experiences and the world around them.

In sociological terms, **religions** are *socially shared beliefs and rituals that assume the existence of supernatural entities or powers with a moral purpose, and that people accept on faith and use as a source of meaning, guidance, and transcendence* (Bruce, 2011). Religious beliefs and rituals link people's lives with a supernatural realm or a divinity, including God or gods.[1] This link is grounded in faith—the foundation of all religions.

Religions are powerful because people use them as sense-making perspectives and guides for action. For this reason, they share certain characteristics with ideologies. Both are components of culture organized around beliefs accepted on faith or taken for granted, and both are used to explain the meaning of objects, events, and experiences and to guide choices and actions. However, ideologies focus mostly on secular, here-and-now, material world issues, and they're neither automatically nor inevitably linked with the supernatural or a divinity. Religions, on the other hand, always bring a divinity or the supernatural into the sense-making process and connect meaning and understanding to

---

[1]The word *God* refers to the Supreme Being or the Creator in monotheistic religions. The words *god(s)* and *godliness* refer to deities across all religions, including polytheistic religions, in which people believe in multiple deities, or gods.

a sacred realm that transcends the here-and-now material world.

Although ideologies are linked with the secular world and religions are linked with a supernatural realm, they often overlap, making it difficult to clearly differentiate them. For example, if people have a religious belief that God created male and female as two distinct human forms, they could use it to develop and support a gender ideology organized around male-female sex differences and the assumption that it is neither moral nor natural to blur or make light of those differences. When this occurs, secular ideologies take on moral significance and ideologically based actions become moral actions. This is why Islamic jihadist ideology is a powerful force in the world today—it establishes a connection between selected Islamist beliefs and a here-and-now quest for political control. As a result, the actions of jihadists are given moral urgency and legitimacy in their view of the world.

Because religion informs widespread views of the world and influences social relationships and the organization of social life, it also informs ideas and beliefs about the body, movement, physical activities, and even sports. However, as we examine the relationship between religions and sports, it's useful to know that religions are linked with the supernatural and sacred—that is, with things that inspire awe, mystery, and reverence. For example, many Christians define churches as sacred places by connecting them with their God. Therefore, the meaning of a church to Christians can be understood only in terms of its perceived link with the supernatural. On the other hand, sport stadiums are secular places and have no connection with the sacred or supernatural as defined by Christians. They may be important to people, but they are understandable in terms of everyday, secular meanings and experiences.

The importance of distinguishing between the sacred and secular is illustrated by answers to the following questions. First, do you think that people in your town would object to a sport stadium having Pepsi, Budweiser, and McDonald's logos on the scorer's table and on scoreboards placed around the venue? Second, do you think those people would accept the same logos placed on the pulpit and incorporated into its stained-glass windows in their church, temple, or mosque? My guess is that having logos in the stadium is a non-issue, but putting those logos in a place of religious worship is certain to cause controversy, with people saying that they degrade the sacred meaning given to their (God's) house of worship and the sacred objects in it.

The diversity of religions and religious beliefs around the world is extensive. Human beings have dealt with inescapable problems of human existence and ultimate questions about life and death in many ways. In the process, they've developed rich and widely varied religions. When sociologists study religions, they examine the ways that believers use religion as they give meaning to themselves, their experiences, and the world around them. They also focus on the ways that religious beliefs inform people's feelings, thoughts, and actions. When religious beliefs set some people apart from others and connect power, authority, and wisdom in the secular world with a divinity or supernatural forces, religion has significant social consequences.

The social consequences of religion and religious beliefs vary widely, and they can include the following:

- Powerful forms of group unity and social integration, *and* devastating forms of group conflict and violent warfare
- A spirit of love and acceptance *and* forms of moral rejection and condemnation
- Humble conformity with prevailing social norms *and* a righteous rejection of prevailing norms
- A commitment to social equity *and* commitment to policies and practices that produce inequalities between men and women, racial and ethnic groups, social classes, homosexuals and heterosexuals, and people with and without certain physical or intellectual impairments

Of course, none of these consequences is inevitable. Each occurs only in connection with the ways that people interpret religious beliefs and incorporate them into their lives.

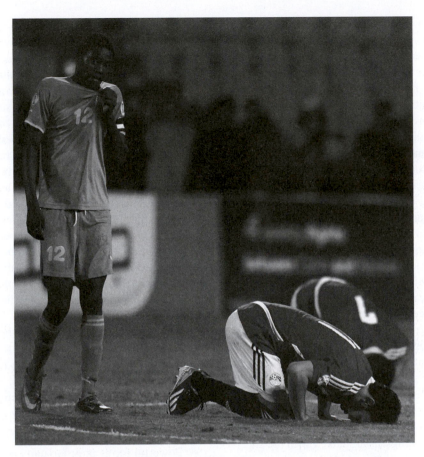

In societies where Christianity is dominant, there usually are reasonably clear distinctions between the secular and sacred. In societies where Islam and Hinduism are dominant, it is very difficult to make this distinction because the secular and sacred are almost seamlessly merged in daily life. After defeating Zimbabwe in a 2014 World Cup qualifying match, these Egyptian Muslim players give thanks to Allah. (*Source:* © AMR ABDALLAH DALSH/Reuters/Corbis)

SIMILARITIES AND DIFFERENCES BETWEEN SPORTS AND RELIGIONS

Discussions about sports and religions often are confusing. Some people view sport as a form of religion, or at least "religion-like," whereas others assume that the "true nature" of religion is essentially different from the "true nature" of sport. Still others view sports and religions as two distinct sets of cultural practices, which may be similar or different

depending on how people create, define, and use them. The purpose of this section is to explain and clarify each of these three positions.

Sports as Religion

Attending an NFL game or a World Cup soccer match and being a part of 75,000 or more people yelling, chanting, and moving in unison reminds some people of a religious experience. Some people go so far as to say that sports *are* religion because they involve passions, dedication, identities, and ritualistic actions and they are played with bodies made in the image of God (Bain-Selbo, 2008, 2009; Bauer, 2011; Thoennes, 2008). Others stop short of this position and say that sports are simply religion-like because they share some characteristics and can produce similar consequences (Baker, 2007; Forney, 2007; Serazio, 2013; Sing, 2013). In both cases, the following similarities between sports and religions have been noted:

- Both have places or buildings for communal gatherings and special events—sports have stadiums and arenas, and religions have churches and temples services.
- Both emerge out of a disciplined quest for perfection in body, mind, and spirit—sports emphasize perfection through disciplined physical performance, and religions emphasize perfection through disciplined moral purity.
- Both are controlled through structured organizations and hierarchical systems of authority—sports have commissioners, athletic directors, and coaches; and religions have bishops, pastors, and priests/ministers/rabbis.
- Both have events that celebrate widely shared values—sports involve contests that celebrate competition, hard work, and achievement; and religions involve ceremonies and rituals that celebrate commitment, community, and redemption.
- Both have rituals before, during, and after major events—sports have initiations, national anthems, halftime pep talks, hand slapping, and band parades; and religions have baptisms, opening hymns, regular sermons, the joining of hands, and ceremonial processions.
- Both have heroes and legends about heroic accomplishments—sports heroes are elected to "halls of fame," and their stories are told repeatedly by journalists, coaches, and fans; and religious heroes are elevated to sainthood, and their stories are told repeatedly by religious writers, ministers, and believers.

- Both evoke intense emotions and give meaning to people's lives—sports inspire players and fans to contemplate human potential, and religions inspire theologians and believers to contemplate the meaning of existence.
- Both can distract attention from important social, political, and economic issues and thereby become "opiates" of the masses—sports focus attention on athlete-celebrities, scores, and championships; and religions focus attention on everlasting life and a personal relationship with the supernatural, rather than here-and-now issues and the material conditions of people's lives.

This list helps us understand why some people describe sport as religion or religion-like.

Sport and Religion Are Essentially Different

Some people argue that religion and sport each have a unique, separate truth, or "essence." The essence of religion, they believe, is grounded in divine inspiration, whereas the essence of sport is grounded in human nature.[2] They argue that religion and sport reveal basic truths that transcend time and space, and people "live out" these truths every day, *but* the truths offered by religion are clearly different from the truths offered by sport.

People who think this way are called **essentialists** because *they assume that the universe is governed by unchanging laws and that meaning and truth are inherent in nature.* When they study religion and sport, they argue that the fundamental character of religion is essentially different from the fundamental character of sport, and they identify the following differences:

- Religious beliefs, meanings, rituals, and events are fundamentally mystical and sacred, whereas

---

[2]These people use the singular rather than the plural form when they refer to *sport* and *religion*. This is because they assume that all forms of sport contain and express the same essence, as do all forms of religion.

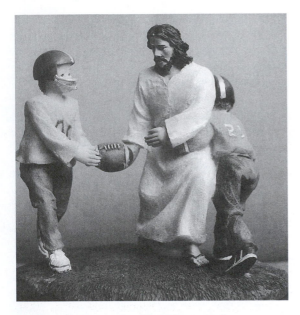

This statue is created and sold by a Christian business. It illustrates that religions, like sports, are socially constructed cultural practices, which change in connection with larger social forces and contexts. To represent Jesus playing a heavy-contact sport that involves brutal body contact and borderline violence is to re-imagine biblical portrayals of him in light of the cultural importance of football in the United States. (*Source:* © Jay Coakley)

sport beliefs, meanings, rituals, and events are fundamentally clear-cut and secular.

- The purpose of religion is to transcend the circumstances and conditions of the material world in the pursuit of eternal life, whereas the purpose of sport is to embrace material reality and seek victories through physical performance.
- Religion involves faith in the primacy of one's beliefs, whereas sport involves competition to establish objective superiority.
- Religion emphasizes humility and love, whereas sport emphasizes personal achievement and conquest.
- Religious services highlight a collective process of acknowledging the sacred and supernatural, whereas sport events highlight a collective

commitment to a here-and-now outcome with secular significance.

Essentialists argue that there are fundamental differences between Super Bowl Sunday and Easter Sunday, even though both are important days in the lives of many people. Similarly, they see fundamental differences between a hockey team's initiation ceremony and a baptism, a seventh-inning stretch and a scheduled prayer, a cathedral and a stadium.

Some essentialists are religious people who believe that religion and sport are fundamentally different because religion is divinely inspired and sport is not. They often claim that the essentially sacred character of religion is corrupted when combined with the essentially secular character of sport (Hoffman, 2010; White, 2008). Nonreligious essentialists don't believe in divine inspiration, but they also argue that the cultural meanings and social consequences of religion and sport are fundamentally different.

Religions and Sports as Cultural Practices

Most sociologists study religions and sports as cultural practices that are created by people over time as they live with each other and give meaning to their experiences and the world around them. This is a *social constructionist approach,* and it is based on evidence showing that religions and sports have diverse forms and meanings that are understandable only in connection with the social and cultural conditions under which people create and maintain them. Furthermore, these forms and meanings change over time as social and cultural conditions change.

Social constructionists generally use cultural and interactionist theories to guide their work. That is, they focus on social relations and issues of power and study the meanings given to the body by people who have different religious beliefs. They also examine the ways that religious beliefs influence movement, physical activity, sport participation, and even the organization of sports. They ask why sports and religions are male-dominated spheres of life and then they study gender ideology in relation to religion, the body, and sports. They also investigate the ways that people combine religious beliefs with sport participation and the social consequences of those combinations in particular social worlds.

Social constructionists realize that the meanings and practices that constitute sports and religions vary by time and place. Religious beliefs and rituals change with new revelations and visions, new prophets and prophecies, new interpretations of sacred writings, and new teachers and teachings. These changes often reproduce the cultural contexts in which they occur, but there are times when they inspire transformations in social relations and social life. Sports are viewed in similar terms—as socially constructed and varying cultural practices that usually reproduce existing meanings and social organization but have the potential to challenge and transform them.

Studying Sports and Religions: An Assessment

The question of whether sports and religions are essentially the same or different does not inspire critical sociological analysis. More important to sociologists are the ways that people participate in the formation and transformation of social and cultural life and how sports and religions are involved in those processes. A constructionist approach guided by cultural, interactionist, and structural theories leads directly to questions about people's experiences and relationships. It also focuses on the different meanings that religions and sports hold for different people and how those meanings are influenced by the social and cultural contexts in which they are formed and changed (Yamane et al., 2010).

Unfortunately, research on sports and religions is scarce. Scholars who study religions are seldom interested in studying sports, and scholars who study sports are seldom interested in studying religions. The studies that do exist focus primarily on Christian belief systems, particularly in North America. Therefore, we know little about sports and major world religions, even though it would be useful to understand how various religious beliefs are related to conceptions of the body, expressions of human movement, the integration of physical activity into everyday life, and participation in sports. Such knowledge could be used to create more culturally inclusive sport programs.

There have been a few recent studies of the influence of Islamic beliefs on the sport participation of Muslim women (Ahmad, 2011; Benn et al., 2010; Dagkasa et al., 2011; Maxwell et al., 2010; Samie, 2013; Samie and Sehlikoglu, 2015; Toffoletti, 2012). For those who study sports and gender, it is helpful to understand that religious beliefs often define, in moral terms, expectations related to gender. This makes religion important to include in their analyses because these expectations regulate bodies and influence sport participation patterns in different cultures (BBC, 2012a; Damon, 2009; Ellin, 2009; Farooq and Parker, 2009; Jobey, 2012; Siemaszko, 2011). Islam has received more attention than other religions in this regard, because it has very specific beliefs about the clothing that must be worn by women, especially when they might be seen by men.

Despite the relative shortage of information about sports and religions other than Christianity, issues related to this topic are discussed in the section, "Sports and World Religions" on pages 516–523. But first, we focus on why certain forms of Christianity have become closely associated with organized competitive sports.

MODERN SPORTS AND RELIGIOUS BELIEFS AND ORGANIZATIONS

Despite important differences between the organization and stated goals of sports and religions, people have combined these two spheres of life in mutually supportive ways (Baker, 2007; Deardorff and White, 2008; Lämmer et al., 2009; Parker and Weir, 2012). In some cases, people with certain religious beliefs have used sports for religious purposes, and in other cases, people in sports have used religion to define and give meaning to their sport participation.

The frequency with which people combine Christian beliefs and sports raises interesting questions. Why have Christian organizations and beliefs, in particular, been combined directly and explicitly with sports? Why haven't other religions been combined with sports and sport participation to the same extent? How have Christian organizations used sports, and how have athletes and sport organizations used Christianity and Christian beliefs? What are the dynamics and social significance of these combinations? These issues are discussed in the following sections of the chapter.

The Protestant Ethic and the Spirit of Sports

Historical evidence helps explain links between modern sports and contemporary Christian beliefs. In the late nineteenth century, German sociologist-economist Max Weber did a classic study titled *The Protestant Ethic and the Spirit of Capitalism* (1904/1958). His research focused on the connection between the ideas embodied in the Protestant Reformation and the values underlying the growth of capitalist economic systems. He concluded that Protestant religious beliefs, especially those promoted by the reformer John Calvin, helped create a social and cultural environment in which capitalism could develop and grow. Weber explained that Protestantism promoted a "code of ethics" and a general value system that created in people deep moral suspicions about erotic pleasure, physical desire, and all forms of idleness. "Idle hands are the devil's workshop" was a popular Protestant slogan.

Weber also used historical data to show that this "Protestant ethic," as he referred to it, emphasized a rationally controlled lifestyle in which emotions and feelings were suppressed in a dual quest for worldly success and eternal salvation. This orientation, developed further in Calvin's notion of predestination, led people to define their occupation as a "calling" from God and to view work as an activity through which one's spiritual worth could be proven and displayed for others to see. This was socially significant because it linked the economy and material success with moral worth: Being rich was a sign of "being saved"—as long as you didn't spend the money on yourself.

The Protestant work ethic has been integrated into different cultures in different ways since the nineteenth century. However, it has always emphasized values that are consistent with the spirit that underlies organized competitive sports as they've been developed in Europe and North America. Sociologist Steven Overman explains this in his book, *The Protestant Work Ethic and the Spirit of Sport: How Calvinism and Capitalism Shaped American games (2011).* Overman shows that the Protestant ethic has emphasized a combination of the following seven key *virtues:*

1. *Worldly asceticism*—the ideas that suffering and the endurance of pain has a spiritual purpose, that godliness is linked with self-denial and a disdain for self-indulgence, and that spiritual redemption is achieved only through self-control and self-discipline.
2. *Rationalization*—the idea that truth can be discovered through human reason, and that virtue is expressed through efficiency and measurable achievements.
3. *Goal directedness*—the idea that spiritual salvation and the moral worth of human action depend on achievement and success.
4. *Individualism*—the ideas that salvation is a matter of individual responsibility, initiative, and choice, and that people control their spiritual destiny by accepting a personal relationship with God/Christ.
5. *Achieved status*—the idea that worldly success is associated with goodness and salvation, whereas failure is associated with sin and damnation.
6. *The work ethic*—the ideas that work is a calling from God and that people honor God by working hard and developing their "God-given potential" through work.
7. *The time ethic*—the ideas that time has a moral quality and that wasting time is sinful and a sign of weak moral character.

Overman theorizes that these seven virtues are closely matched with the orientation and spirit that informs the meaning, purpose, and organization of modern sports, especially power and performance sports in the United States. This theory is only partially supported by evidence because these virtues have been integrated into people's lives in many different ways, depending on historical and cultural factors. Furthermore, some of these virtues are not exclusive to Protestantism—they also exist in forms of Catholicism and other religions, although no religion other than mainstream Protestantism is organized around a set of virtues exactly the same as these seven.

Overman's theory helps to explain some of the ways that people in Europe and North America view the body and sports. Traditional Catholic beliefs,

for example, emphasize that the body is a divine vessel—a "temple of the Holy Spirit" (I Corinthians 6:19). As a result, Catholics living in the nineteenth and early twentieth century were taught to keep the body pure, but purity was achieved through sexual abstinence and restraint, not through playing sports. Most Protestant believers, on the other hand, emphasized that the body was a divine tool to be used in establishing mastery over the physical world (Genesis 1:28; I Corinthians 9:24–27; Philippians 4:13). The perfect body, therefore, was a mark of a righteous soul (Hutchinson, 2008; Overman, 2011).

Protestant beliefs have also supported the idea that individual competitive success is a means of demonstrating a person's moral worth. Overall, organized competitive sports, because they're oriented around work and achievement, are logical

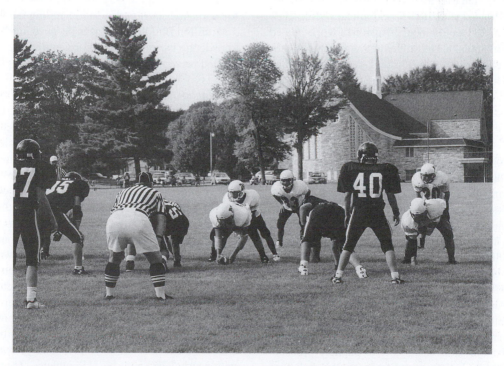

Organized competitive sports emphasize work and achievement. These values are compatible with values underlying Protestant religious beliefs. Therefore, playing football on a church-sponsored team is believed to be consistent with secular and Protestant-Christian values. (*Source:* © Kristie Elbert)

sites for the application of Protestant beliefs. Unlike free and expressive play, sports often are worklike and demand sacrifice and the endurance of pain. Therefore, Protestant/Christian athletes can define sport participation as their calling (from God) and make the claim that God wants them to be the best they can be in sports, even if sports sometimes require the physical domination of others. Furthermore, Christian athletes can define sport participation as a valuable form of religious witness and link their efforts in sports to moral worth and personal salvation.

Evidence supports this aspect of Overman's theory in that athletes from Protestant nations disproportionately outnumber athletes from nations where people are primarily Muslim, Hindu, or Buddhist (Lüschen, 1967; Overman, 2011). Even the international success of athletes from non-Protestant nations is often traceable to the influence of cultures where Protestant beliefs are dominant. However, the recent and rapid global diffusion of work-related achievement values has muted the influence of religious beliefs on athletic success. As a result, many athletes from non-Protestant nations excel in sports and win international competitions today.

Sports and World Religions

Most of what we in North America know about sports and religions focuses on various forms of Christianity, especially evangelical fundamentalism. Little is written about sports and Buddhism, Confucianism, Hinduism, Islam, Judaism, Sikhism, Shinto, Taoism, or the many variations of these and other religions.

The beliefs and meanings associated with each of these religions influence how people perceive their bodies, define and give meaning to physical activities, and relate to each other through human movement. However, few people other than evangelical fundamentalist Christians use sports to publicly proclaim their religious beliefs, or use their religious beliefs to give spiritual meaning to sport participation.

It appears that no religion has an equivalent of the self-proclaimed "Christian athlete," which is visible character in competitive sports in North America, Australia, New Zealand, and parts of Western Europe. This may be due in part to the Christian notion of individual salvation and how certain believers have applied it to everyday life. Additionally, some world religions focus on the transcendence of self, which means that believers seek to merge the self with spiritual forces rather than distinguishing the self by using sport participation to achieve personal growth and spiritual salvation. In fact, the idea of physically competing against others to publicly distinguish the self violates the core beliefs of many religions.

Unfortunately, our knowledge of these issues is limited. We know more about the ways that some North American athletes and coaches convert Zen Buddhist beliefs into strategies for improving golf scores, marathon times, and basketball teamwork than we do about the ways that Buddhism is related to sports and sport participation among the world's 500 million Buddhists. This is because much of our knowledge is grounded in Eurocentric science and limited personal experiences.

Buddhism and Hinduism: Transcending Self
Buddhism and philosophical Hinduism emphasize physical and spiritual discipline, but they do not inspire believers to strive for Olympic medals or physically outperform or dominate other human beings in organized competitive sports. Instead, most of the current expressions of Buddhism and Hinduism focus on transcending the self and the material world. Beliefs emphasize that physical reality is transient and the human condition is inherently fragile—neither of which is consistent with training to be an elite athlete, signing endorsement contracts, or being inducted into a sport hall of fame. For example, 80 percent of the 1.3 billion people in India identify themselves as Hindu, and athletes from India have won only twenty-six medals in Olympic history, compared with nearly 2700 won by U.S. athletes. This is due to many factors, and religion is one of them. China, where Buddhism is practiced by about 300 million people (similar to the size of the U.S. population),

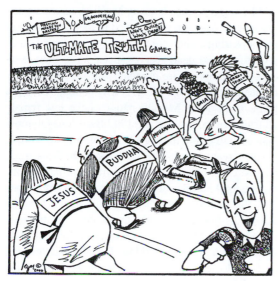

(*Source:* © Frederic A. Eyer)

"Well, fans, this is the race we've waited for. The winner of this one will lead us to Ultimate Truth!"

Scholars who study religions and sports are not concerned with the truth or falsity of religious beliefs as much as they are concerned with the ways that religions influence the meaning, purpose, and organization of sports in society.

sent teams to the Olympics only four times prior to 1984 and until recently was not very successful in the competitions. But during the past three decades, political interests have trumped religious interests and athletes from China are now medal threats in international competitions.

It is primarily elite athletes from Christian, capitalist countries that use the meditation practices and rituals from these religions to improve sport performances and give spiritual meaning to competitive sports. However, a segment of a growing Hindu nationalist movement in India uses exercises, games, and sports combined with yoga and prayers to develop loyalty and affection for Hindu culture and Hindu nationhood (McDonald, 1999). This is consistent with historical evidence showing that sports have long been used as sites for training minds and bodies for military service and "defending culture." However, when this training is tied to religion and

religious practices, it takes on new meaning because the secular and the sacred are combined for political purposes. When this occurs, sports are given a low priority because the focus often turns to identifying secular enemies and morally justifying wars against them.

People revise religious beliefs as changes occur in their cultures and as belief systems travel from one culture to another. This is true for Buddhism and Hinduism as well as other world religions. Of course, there are many variations of Buddhist beliefs and practices, and most of them reflect the orientations of particular teachers or Masters. The island of Taiwan, off the southeast coast of China, is home to a form of "humanistic Buddhism" in which sports have been used to promote health and teach Buddhist principles (Yu, 2011). Competitive success is important, but more important is focusing on good everyday thoughts, words, and deeds.

Traditional Hindu practices in India are heavily gendered and call for women to be secluded and veiled—that is, confined to private, family-based spaces and covered with robes and scarves. These practices were originally linked with a caste system in which religion was used to justify and maintain social inequalities. The caste system consisted of complex norms and beliefs that regulated activities and relationships throughout Indian society. Individuals were born into a particular caste, and their caste position marked their social status in society as a whole.

Officially, the caste system is illegal today, but its cultural legacy continues. This explains why women with a heritage traced back to middle and upper castes have considerable freedom, but women and many men from lower-caste heritage live with persistent poverty, unemployment, and illiteracy. Current patterns of sport participation are influenced by these factors, even though people may embrace "modernized" Hindu beliefs that accommodate increasing secularization in Indian society. Although the caste system was never grounded exclusively in Hindu religious beliefs, Hinduism was organized by upper caste people so that it reproduced the social importance of castes and caste membership.

This topic has yet to be studied in terms of its connection with sports and other physical activities. Additionally, there is a need for research on how Hindus in India and other areas combine religious beliefs with an intense passion for cricket.

Islam: Submission to Allah's Will   Studying Islam and sports is a challenge because Muslims, like many Buddhists and Hindus, make few distinctions between the secular and the sacred. Every action is done to please Allah (God) and is therefore a form of worship. Religious beliefs and cultural norms are merged into a single theology/ideology, with an emphasis on peace through submission to Allah's will.

Muslims have long participated in physical activities and sports, but participation is regulated by their beliefs about what pleases Allah. The connection between sports and the mandate to submit to Allah's will has not been studied until recently (Amara, 2007, 2008, 2010; Benn et al., 2010, 2011; Dagkasa et al., 2011; Farooq and Parker, 2009; Jobey, 2012; Samie, 2013; Samie and Sehlikoglu, 2015; Toffoletti, 2012).

There are noteworthy past and present examples of African American Muslims who excel in sports. However, the traditions of sport participation and the quest for excellence in sports are not as strong in Muslim countries as they are in secularized, Christian-Protestant countries, partly because low per capita income makes full-time training nearly impossible for many Muslims in rural and less developed regions of the world.

Although Muslim nations in many parts of Central and Southeast Asia have no religious restrictions on girls and women playing sports, Islamic beliefs in other parts of the world legitimize patriarchal structures and maintain definitions of male and female bodies that discourage girls and women from playing sports and restrict their everyday access to sport participation opportunities.[3]

---

[3]Patriarchy is a form of gender relations in which men are legally privileged relative to women, especially in regard their access to political power and economic resources.

Physical activities in many Muslim nations are sex segregated. Men are not allowed to look at women in public settings, and women must cover their bodies with robes and head scarves, even when they exercise. These norms are especially strong among fundamentalist Muslims, which is why national Olympic teams from some Muslim nations have few female athletes. For example, at the 1992 Barcelona Olympic Games, half of the thirty-five nations with no women on their teams were Muslim nations. In 2004, only four Muslim nations had no women on their teams, but the total number of women from Muslim nations was the lowest since the 1960 Olympics (Taheri, 2004). The nations with the tightest restrictions include Iran, Afghanistan, Oman, Kuwait, Pakistan, Qatar, Saudi Arabia, the United Arab Emirates, and Sudan. However, an increasing number of women from Islamic countries have participated in recent Asian Games, especially those held in 2006 and 2008 in Doha, Qatar.

Iran regularly holds events exclusively for women, the latest being the Fourth Women Islamic Games in September 2005. But these games are not televised because the women are allowed to dress as they wish, and there is a fear that men may watch them. No men are allowed in or near the event, and armed women guards guarantee that men keep their distance. The connection between gender, sport, and Islam is discussed further in the Reflect on Sports box "Allah's Will."

The popularity of sports among men in Islamic countries is often tied to expressions of political and cultural nationalism rather than to religious beliefs. Similarly, when Muslims migrate from Islamic countries to Europe or North America, they sometimes play sports, but their participation is tied more to learning about life and gaining acceptance in their new cultures than expressing Muslim beliefs through sports (Amara, 2013). Muslim girls and women in non-Islamic countries have very low sport participation rates (Kay, 2006), and Muslim organizations are unlikely to sponsor sports for their members. However, some people, including scholars in the sociology of sport, have organized programs that enable Muslim women to train and

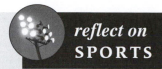

reflect on SPORTS

Allah's Will
Challenges for Muslim Women in Sports

Imagine facing death threats whenever you play sports. Imagine winning an Olympic gold medal, receiving death threats from people in your country who brand you as an immoral and corrupt woman, and then being forced to live in exile. At the same time, imagine that you are a heroine to many young women, who see you as inspirational in their quest for equal rights and opportunities to play sports.

This was the situation faced by Hassiba Boulmerka, the gold medalist in the 1500 meters at the 1992 Olympic Games in Barcelona, Spain. As an Algerian Muslim woman, she believed that being an international athlete did not require her to abandon her faith or her commitment to Islam. But those who condemned Boulmerka said that although it is permissible for women to participate in sports, it was not permissible to do so in shorts or T-shirts, or while men are watching, or when men and women train together, or when facilities do not permit total privacy, or, if you are married, unless your husband gives his permission.

To complicate matters, some Islamic feminists accused Boulmerka of allowing herself to be used by a sport system based on men's values and sponsored by corporations that promote a soulless, consumer culture. To participate in such a system, they said, was to endorse global forces that oppress humankind.

More recently, eighteen-year-old tennis phenomenon Sania Mirza from India was given heavy police security at a tournament in Calcutta, India, after receiving alleged threats from Muslim men saying that she violated Sharia Law stating that any woman in public must cover her entire body except for her hands and face. Mirza's shorts and sleeveless shirts were called "indecent" and "corrupting," and in 2008, the disputes over her tennis clothes

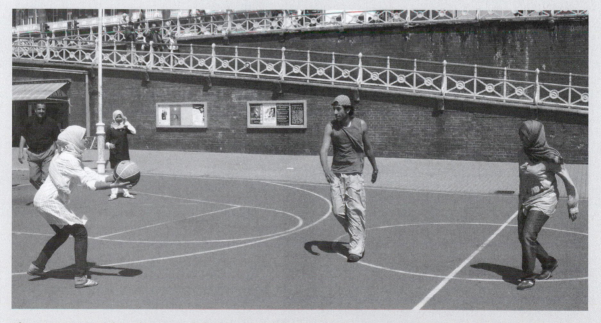

The participation of Muslim women in sports, regardless of their clothing, initiate heated debates about religion and gender. As this Muslim family play on a beachside court in Brighton, England, the daughters wear the hijab and veil. Elite athletes now have clothing designed specifically to allow them to compete and still follow the modesty rules in their religion, although they continue to face sport governing body rules that disallow this clothing. But Muslim women have challenged the rules and won in most cases. (*Source:* © Jay Coakley)

Continued

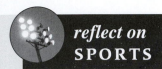

Allah's Will (*continued*)

led her to consider quitting her tennis career. Instead, she decided to boycott tournaments in her home country. At the same time, Indian corporations seek the now twenty-one-year-old Mirza to endorse their products, knowing that many young Indian women look up to her.

The issues facing Mirza were avoided by twenty-five-year-old Bahrain-born sprinter Ruqaya Al Ghasara. Since 2004 she has been winning medals and setting records while wearing her trademark white headscarf and red bodysuit. When Al Ghasara won the 100-meters at the West Asian Games in 2007, she told reporters, "I have no problems with the hijab. I have a great desire to show that there are no problems with wearing these clothes. Wearing a veil proves that Muslim women face no obstacles and encourages them to compete in sport" (Algazeera, 2006). When pressed further, she said, "It's not just a matter of wearing a piece of cloth. There is something very special about wearing the hijab. It gives me strength. I feel lots of support from society because I am wearing the Islamic hijab. There is a relationship between the hijab and the heart" (IAAF, 2007).

These three scenarios illustrate that the bodies of Muslim women are "contested terrain." Today, they remain at the center of deep political, cultural, and religious struggles about what is important, what is right and wrong, and how social life should be organized. Muslim women in sports embody and personify these struggles. On the one hand, these women are active subjects asserting new ideas about what it means to be a Muslim woman. On the other hand, they're passive objects used in debates about morality and social change in the world today.

Of course, there are significant variations in the rights and autonomy of women in different countries where Islam is the dominant religion. But in general, struggles over issues of religion and gender will continue for Muslim women participating publicly in sports (BBC, 2012a; Ghanem, 2012; Jobey, 2012; May, 2012; Sehlikoglu-Karakas, 2012; Siemaszko, 2011; Wilcke et al., 2012). At the same time, Muslim women living in predominantly Christian countries sometimes use sports played in private as a refuge and an opportunity to spend time with peers who share their beliefs (Jiwani and Rail, 2010; Kay, 2006; Walseth, 2006). But coming to terms with "Allah's will" continues to be a challenge for many Muslim women. Their sport participation often depends on the support of people working in sport organizations. For those in sport management it raises an important question: *What strategies are most effective in promoting inclusion and accommodating religious diversity in programs and facilities?*

· ·

play sports under conditions consistent with their modesty norms. So far, these programs have been moderately successful in attracting and providing participation opportunities for girls and young women (Ahmad, 2011; Kay, 2006; Weaver, 2005).

Judaism: Sports and Struggle The link between Judaism and sports is weak, but the link between Jews and sport participation is strong. This apparent contradiction is understandable when we remember that Jews constitute an ethnic population as well as a religion, and that Jews have faced discrimination in nearly every society in which they've lived, except Israel. The following two statements help us understand sport participation among Jews:

Jews are not sportsmen. Whether this is due to their physical lethargy, their dislike of unnecessary physical action or their serious cast of mind—it is nevertheless a fact . . . .

Sport valorized Gentile masculine values like aggression, strength, speed, and combativeness. . . . I loved it. Nothing my [Jewish] father could do or say stopped me from embracing baseball, basketball, or football over religion.

The first statement, based on an anti-Semitic stereotype, was made in 1921 by Henry Ford, possibly the most influential man in the United States at that time. The second statement was made by Alan Klein (2008), a Jew born in Germany just after the gas chambers had been shut down following World War II. Ford invented the assembly line and founded the Ford Motor Company; Klein came to the United States, played sports, earned a Ph.D., and became an anthropologist noted for his excellent research on sports.

Like many Jews, Klein was attracted to sports as a reaction to anti-Semitism (Brenner and Reuveni, 2006). He played typical American sports to assimilate, to fit in at a time when being like everyone else kept him from feeling different in his school and community. Excelling in sports disrupted the stereotype that Jews were "thinkers instead of doers"—smart people with frail bodies. Similar dynamics led Jews to dominate professional basketball in the United States from 1920 through the late 1940s, and boxing from 1910 to 1940 (Klein, 2008a).

Today Jews sponsor the quadrennial Maccabiah Games in the year following the Olympics. These games are cultural rather than religious in origin and purpose; they were founded to foster Jewish identity and traditions and to showcase highly skilled Jewish athletes. The 2013 Maccabiah Games, often described as "the Jewish Olympics," involved more than 9000 athletes from seventy-seven nations, including 1100 athletes from the United States. In addition to thirty-eight competitive sport events, there are cultural and educational programs, all designed to create strong ties with Judaism, Israel, and the global Jewish community (Chabin, 2013).

Shinto: Sumo in Japan   Sumo, or traditional Japanese wrestling, has strong historical ties to Shinto, a traditional Japanese religion (Light and Kinnaird, 2002). Shinto means "the way of the gods," and it consists of a system of rituals and ceremonies designed to worship nature rather than reaffirm an established theology.

Modern sumo is a nonreligious activity, although it remains steeped in Shinto ritual and ceremony. The dohyo (rings) in which the bouts take place are defined as sacred sites. Religious symbols are integrated into their design and construction, and the rings are consecrated through purification ceremonies, during which referees, dressed in priestly garb, ask the gods to bless the scheduled bouts. Only the wrestlers and recognized sumo officials are allowed in the dohyo. Shoes must not be worn, and women are never allowed to stand on or near an officially designated ring.

The wrestlers take great care to preserve the purity of the dohyo. Prior to their bouts, they ritualistically throw salt into the ring to symbolize their respect for its sacredness and purity; they even wipe sweat off their bodies and rinse their mouths with water presented to them by fellow wrestlers. If a wrestler sheds blood during a bout, the stains are cleaned and purified before the bouts continue. Shinto motifs are included in the architecture and decorations on and around the dohyo. However, wrestlers do not personally express their commitment to Shinto, nor do Shinto organizations sponsor or promote sumo or other sports.

In recent years, the popularity of sumo has declined at the same time that the sport has attracted participants from other parts of the world. Not being raised to know or respect Shinto and the traditional sacred rituals associated with the sport, these new wrestlers bring a secular orientation to the ring. This, combined with championships being won by non-Japanese wrestlers and a 2010 gambling scandal, has eroded the religious foundations of the sport (McCurry, 2011; Sanchanta, 2011).

Religion and Life Philosophies in China   Anthropologist Susan Brownell (1995, 2008) has studied physical culture and forms of Taoist, Confucian, and Buddhist ideas and practices in her comprehensive studies of the body and sport in China. She notes that each of these life philosophies is actually a general theory of the nature and principles of the universe. As with Islam, this makes it difficult to separate "religious beliefs" from cultural ideology as a whole. Each of these life philosophies emphasizes the notion that all human beings should strive to live in accord with the energy and forces of nature. The body and physical exercise are seen as important parts of nature, but the goal of movement is to seek harmony with nature rather than to overcome or dominate nature or other human beings.

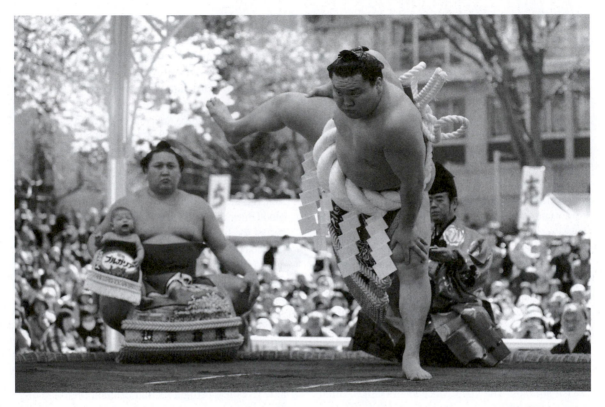

Sumo wrestling in Japan is steeped in centuries-old Shinto rituals of purification. However, as sumo has become a more global sport, there is less awareness of and respect for its connection with religious beliefs and practices. As the Shinto foundations of sumo fade, its meaning in Japanese culture is changing. (*Source:* © Franck Robichon/ epa/Corbis)

Tai chi is a form of exercise based on this cultural approach to life and living. Some versions of the martial arts are practiced in this spirit, but others, including practices outside China, are grounded in secular traditions of self-defense and military training. China's success in recent international competitions, raises other questions about the possible connections between religious beliefs and sport participation. Therefore, future research will examine the implications of Taoism, Confucianism, and Buddhism as they have been integrated into the lives of various segments of the vast and diverse Chinese population.

Native Americans: Merging the Spiritual and Physical   Historically, Native Americans have often included physical games and running races in religious rituals (Nabokov, 1981). However, the purpose of doing this is to reaffirm social connections within specific native cultural groups and gain skills needed for group survival. Outside these rituals, sport participation has had no specific religious meaning.

Making general statements about religious beliefs and sport participation among Native Americans is difficult because beliefs vary from one native culture to another. However, many native cultures maintain animistic religious beliefs emphasizing the spiritual integration of material elements, such as the earth, wind, sun, moon, plants, and animals. Many native games contain features that imply this integration, and, when Native Americans play sports constructed by people from European or other backgrounds, they often use their religious beliefs to give their participation a meaning that reaffirms their ways of viewing the world and their connection with the sacred.

Anthropologist Peter Nabokov has studied running among Native Americans and notes that prior to their contact with Europeans they ran for practical purposes such as hunting, communicating, and fighting; but they also ran to reenact myths and legends and to reaffirm their connection with the forces of nature and the universe. More recently, Native American athletes whose identities are grounded in native cultures often define sport participation in terms of their cultural traditions and beliefs. However, little is known about how they incorporate specific religious beliefs and traditions, which vary across cultures, into sport participation that occurs outside of their cultures or how young Native Americans who play sports connect their participation to religious beliefs.

Sports and World Religions: Waiting for Research

We need more information about the connections between various world religions, ideas about the body, and participation in physical activities and sports. This information would help us understand the lives of billions of people who participate in various forms of physical activities and sports but do not connect them directly with religious organizations or use them as sites for religious witness. This is different from the tendency of some Christians to attach their religion to institutionalized, competitive sports that already exist for nonreligious purposes.

How Have Christians and Christian Organizations Used Sports?

Unlike other religions, Christianity has inspired believers to use sports for many purposes. These include (a) promoting spiritual growth; (b) recruiting new members and promoting religious beliefs and organizations; and (c) promoting fundamentalist beliefs and evangelical orientations.

To Promote Spiritual Growth During the mid-1800s, influential Christian men, described

as "muscular Christians" in England and New England, promoted the idea that the physical condition of a man's body had religious significance. They believed that the male body was an instrument of good works and that meeting the physical demands of godly behavior required good health and physical conditioning. Although most religious people at the time didn't agree with this approach, the idea that there might be a connection between the physical and spiritual dimensions of human beings grew increasingly popular (Baker, 2007; Guttmann, 1978, 1988).

The idea that the body had moral significance and that moral character could be strengthened with physical conditioning encouraged many religious organizations to use sports in their efforts to recruit boys and men. For example, the YMCA grew rapidly between 1880 and 1920 as the organization built athletic facilities in many communities and sponsored sport teams. Canadian James Naismith invented basketball in 1891 while he was a student at the Springfield, Massachusetts, YMCA. William Morgan, the physical activities director at a YMCA in Holyoke, Massachusetts, invented volleyball in 1895.

Religious beliefs about developing and strengthening the body were not applied to girls or women during the nineteenth and early twentieth centuries. For most people, "a female muscular Christian was a contradiction in terms [and] . . . Muscular Christianity represented a reaction against the 'femininization' of American middle-class culture" (Baker, 2007, pp. 44–45). In fact, when activist women opened the first YWCA in Boston in 1866 their focus was on "prayer, Bible study, and Christian witness" devoted to helping women find decent housing and obtain job training so they could work and support themselves; playing sports was not part of the program (Baker, 2007, p. 62).

Although mainline Protestants endorsed sports for boys and men through the end of the nineteenth century, some of them came to wonder about the religious relevance of the highly competitive sports that emerged during the first half of the twentieth century. Scandals, violence, and other problems in sports caused evangelicals, in particular, to question their value. Protestant leaders were also wary of women playing sports because it contradicted their belief that God created men and women to be different and that female athletes would subvert God's plan (Jonas, 2005).

It wasn't until the late 1940s that evangelical Christians again made a direct connection between sports and their religious beliefs (Ladd and Mathisen, 1999). And they were not alone in embracing sports in the years following World War II. Protestant churches and congregations, Catholic dioceses and parishes, Mormon wards, the B'nai B'rith, and some Jewish synagogues also embraced sports as worthwhile activities, especially for young men. These organizations sponsored sports and sport programs because their members and leaders believed that sport participation developed moral character and prepared young men for the military.

During the 1960s and 1970s, athletic-minded evangelical Christians began to focus on sport as a realm in which they could bring their religious beliefs to athletes and then use the visibility and popularity of athletes to spread those beliefs to sport fans and the general public (Krattenmaker, 2010). The widespread acceptance of the great sport myth contributed to their success. People already believed that the essential purity and goodness of sports would be internalized by athletes willing to learn what sport would teach them. When athletes accepted and gave witness to Bible-based values, people saw the connection between sport participation and Christianity as logical and credible.

The connection between Christian values and the perceived purity and goodness of sports was clearly highlighted in 1971 by Billy Graham, the best-known and most highly respected evangelist of the later twentieth century. A long-time outspoken promoter of sports as a builder of moral character, Graham summarized the spirit in which many religious organizations have viewed sports over the last century:

The Bible says leisure and lying around are morally dangerous for us. Sports keep us busy; athletes, you notice, don't take drugs. There

are probably more committed Christians in sports, both collegiate and professional, than in any other occupation in America (in *Newsweek,* 1971, p. 51).

Graham's statement about drugs sounds outdated today, but he accurately noted that many Christians see sports as activities that symbolize and promote moral development. This perception, despite evidence to the contrary, remains strong in North America.

To Recruit New Members and Promote Religious Beliefs and Organizations   Using sports to promote particular religious beliefs was a key strategy of Christian missionaries who accompanied European and North Americans who colonized traditional cultures. Since the mid-1800s, this strategy was used to attract and recruit boys and men to churches and religious organizations, especially in England and the United States (Putney, 2003). This practice became so common in the United States after World War II that sociologist Charles Page referred to it as "the basketballization of American religion" (in Demerath and Hammond, 1969, p. 182).

In the early 1990s, for example, Bill McCartney, the former football coach at the University of Colorado, used sport images and metaphors as he founded a religious organization, The Promise Keepers, and recruited men to join. McCartney and others in the evangelical men's organization preached that a "manly man is a Godly man." Similarly, other Christian fundamentalist organizations have used images of tough athletes to represent ideal "Christian men." This strategy of presenting a "masculinized Christianity" was designed to attract men into churches so they could reclaim their status as moral leaders, honor their commitment to their wives and families, and present a masculinized version of biblical values (Beal, 1997; Randels and Beal, 2002). This approach continued in 2013 with a six-city Promise Keepers men's conference titled "Awakening the Warrior."

Church-affiliated colleges and universities in the United States have also used sports as recruiting and public relations tools. Administrators from these schools know that seventeen-year-olds today are more likely to listen to recruiting advertisements that use terminology, images, and spokespeople from sports. Plus, a winning sport program can provide exposure and publicity for particular religious beliefs (Michaelis, 2011; Zillgitt, 2011).

Even a half century ago, when the famous preacher Oral Roberts founded his university in Tulsa, Oklahoma, he highlighted the importance of its sport program in this way:

> Athletics is part of our Christian witness. . . . Nearly every man in America reads the sports pages, and a Christian school cannot ignore these people. . . . Sports are becoming the No. 1 interest of people in America. For us to be relevant, we had to gain the attention of millions of people in a way that they could understand (in Boyle, 1970, p. 64).

Jerry Falwell, noted television evangelist, introduced intercollegiate athletics at his Liberty University in the 1970s with a similar explanation:

> To me, athletics are a way of making a statement. And I believe you have a better Christian witness to the youth of the world when you competitively, head-to-head, prove yourself their equal on the playing field (in Capouya, 1986, p. 75).

Then, in his opening prayer, Falwell declared, "Father, we don't want to be mediocre, we don't want to fail. We want to honor You by winning" (in Capouya, 1986, p. 72). More recently, university chancellor Jerry Falwell Jr. proudly stated that he was carrying out his father's vision (Pennington, 2012b).

Other church-affiliated colleges and universities have used sports in similar but less overt ways to attract students. Catholic schools—including the University of Notre Dame, Gonzaga, Georgetown, and Boston College—have used football and/or basketball programs to build their prestige as church-affiliated institutions. Brigham Young University, affiliated with the Church of Latter Day Saints (Mormons), also has done this. Smaller Christian colleges around the United States formed the National Christian Collegiate Athletic Association (NCCAA) in the mid-1960s and today they continue to sponsor championships and recruit Christian student-athletes to their schools.

Some religious organizations are developed around sports to attract people to Christian beliefs and provide support for athletes who hold Christian beliefs. Examples include Sports Ambassadors, the Fellowship of Christian Athletes (FCA), Athletes in Action (AIA), Pro Athletes Outreach (PAO), Global Sports Outreach, Baseball Chapel, and dozens of smaller groups associated with particular sports. These organizations have a strong evangelical emphasis, and members are usually eager to share their beliefs in the hope that others will embrace Christianity as they do.

Many Christian organizations and groups also use sports as sites for evangelizing. At the 2012 London Olympics there were 193 approved multifaith chaplains to talk with athletes. Athletes in Action used the 2012 Olympics to reach 2500 Olympic athletes through its events in the Olympic Village. They trained fifty AIA leaders from twenty-five countries to continue their discipleship programs after the games, delivered sport ministry training and materials to 200 churches in six cities in Europe, and planned to expose 200 million people worldwide to their ministry, primarily through the film *Struggle in Triumph,* which was produced in thirty-six languages specifically for the 2012 games. As they interact with athletes, they are guided by the words of Terry Bortz, the global media director for AIA, who says, "You can be one of the top athletes in the world, but if you don't have Christ [in your life], you are really empty" (http://www.youtube.com/watch?v=jOnFviF68WE; see also, Blazer, 2015).

Such efforts to evangelize are not new, but today they are highly organized and coordinated in connection with major events, such as the Super Bowl, the men's World Cup, the Pan American Games, and other sport mega-events.

Apart from major events, RBC Ministries and the FCA, both fundamentalist Christian organizations, publish *SportsSpectrum* and *Sharing the Victory (STV),* widely circulated magazines that use a biblically informed perspective to report on sports and athletes. Articles highlight Christian athletes and their religious testimony. Most athlete profiles emphasize that life "without a commitment to Christ" is superficial and meaningless, even if one wins in sports.

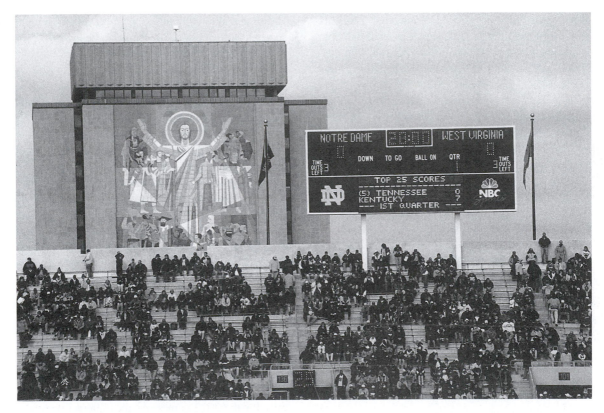

The public profiles of some universities are linked to both sports and religion. This is the football stadium at the University of Notre Dame, with the library in the background. The outside wall of the library presents a mural image of Christ, now known as "Touchdown Jesus" among Notre Dame fans. (*Source:* © Jay Coakley)

This method of using athletes to evangelize is now a key strategy. As one FCA official asked, "If athletes can sell razor blades and soft drinks, why can't they sell the Gospel?" This approach corresponds with the fact that some high-profile media evangelists pair up with celebrity athletes whose statements about their fundamentalist Christian beliefs serve to promote the ministry of the evangelist (Barr, 2009).

A similar strategy has been adopted by top Catholic officials. In 2004, Pope John Paul II established a new Vatican office dedicated to "Church and Sport." Although its primary stated goal is to reform the culture of sport, it is also concerned with making Catholicism relevant in the lives of people, especially men, who are no longer involved in their parishes or using Catholic beliefs to guide their lives.

Today, the office now sponsors a talk radio sport program to attract Italian men who no longer see the Catholic Church as relevant to them; soccer is a central focus of the program on Vatican radio. It has also published three books, each of which summarizes presentations on sports from a Catholic perspective and intends on being a guide for Catholics associated with sports (Pontifical Council for the Laity, 2006, 2008, 2011). Pope Francis has supported the connection between Catholicism and sport through many of his addresses on the topic (http://www .laici.va/content/laici/en/sezioni/chiesa-e-sport /magisterium.html).

To Promote Fundamentalist Beliefs and Evangelical Orientations   Most of the religious groups and organizations previously mentioned promote a specific form of Christianity—one based on a loosely articulated conservative ideology and a fundamentalist orientation toward life.

Religious fundamentalism is based on the belief that the secular foundation of modern societies is inherently corrupt and can be redeemed only if people reorganize their personal lives and the entire social order to manifest the absolute and unchanging Truth contained in a sacred text (Hadden, 2000; Marty and Appleby, 1995; Pace, 2007). Religious fundamentalists emphasize that this reorganization requires people to be personally committed to the supernatural or transcendent source of truth (God, Allah, Christ, Mohammed, "the universe," the spirit world), which provides answers to all questions. These answers are revealed through sacred writings, the verbal teachings of divinely inspired leaders and prophets, and personal revelations.

Fundamentalist movements in all religions arise when people perceive moral threats to a past way of life that was, according to their beliefs, based on moral principles. Therefore, fundamentalists emphasize the "moral decline of society" and the need to return to a time when religious truth was the foundation for culture and social organization. This belief may be so deeply held that it creates a social and political split between fundamentalists and the rest of society.

Ladd and Mathisen (1999) explain that fundamentalist Christians in the United States have used sports, in part, to reduce their separation and gain acceptance from people in the rest of society. The ways that sports have been used by Christian fundamentalist movements in other predominantly Protestant societies suggest that this is seen to be an effective strategy although there certainly are important variations between countries (Butterworth and Senkbeil, 2015).

How Have Athletes, Coaches, and Teams Used Religion?

Athletes, coaches, and teams use religion, religious beliefs, prayers, and rituals in many ways. Research on this topic is scarce, but there is much anecdotal information suggesting that religion is used for one or more of the following purposes:

1. To cope with uncertainty
2. To stay out of trouble
3. To give meaning to sport participation
4. To put sport participation into a balanced perspective
5. To establish team solidarity and unity
6. To reaffirm motivation and social control on teams
7. To achieve personal and competitive success

To Cope with Uncertainty Through history, people have used prayers and rituals based on religion, magic, and/or superstition to cope with uncertainties in their lives (Cherrington, 2012, 2014; Weber, 1922b/1993). Because sport competition involves uncertainty, it is not surprising that many athletes use rituals, some based in religion, to help them feel as if they have some control over what happens to them on the playing field.

A study of Olympic-level wrestlers in Europe found that some of them found reassurance through their prayers before matches. Saying silent meditative prayers, they explained, helped them relax their minds and gain control before stepping onto the mat (Kristiansen and Roberts, 2007). This strategy has been described by a German sport scientist as "Glaubensdoping," or "faith doping" (Güldenpfennig, 2001). This term would not be used in the United States, where prayers and religious rituals are commonly used prior to competition.

Not all religious athletes use prayer and religious rituals in this manner, but many call on their religion to help them face challenges and uncertainty. Therefore, many athletes who pray before or during games seldom pray before or during practices when uncertainty isn't an issue. For example, Catholic athletes who make the sign of the cross when they come up to bat or shoot a free throw during a game don't do the same thing when they bat or shoot free throws during practices. It is the actual competition that produces the uncertainty and then evokes the prayer or religious ritual.

Sometimes it's difficult to separate the use of religion from the use of magic and superstition among athletes. **Magic** consists of *recipe-like rituals designed to produce immediate and practical results in the material world.* **Superstitions** consist of *regularized, ritualistic actions performed to give a person or group a sense of control and predictability in the face of challenges.* Thus, when athletes pray, it may be a form of religion or a form of magic and superstition, but for the person doing it, the purpose is usually to deal with the uncertainty that exists in competitive sports.

To Stay Out of Trouble   Christian athletes often say that religion helps keep them "on track" and avoid the risky lifestyles that often exist in the social worlds that develop around certain sports. For example, an NFL player said, "Before I found the Lord, I drank! I whoremongered! I cussed! I cheated! I manipulated! I deceived!" (in Corsello, 1999, p. 435).

The fact that religious beliefs may separate athletes from risky off-the-field lifestyles and keep them focused on training in their sports has not been lost on coaches who are attracted to the possibility that religion may help athletes control their actions and avoid trouble that could disrupt team focus (Corsello, 1999; Plotz, 2000).

Some team owners also see "born-again athletes" as good long-term investments because they "are less likely to get arrested" (Nightengale, 2006). Religious beliefs also may keep athletes out of trouble by encouraging them to become involved in church-related and community-based service programs. This involvement also separates them from risky off-the-field lifestyles.

The pro-religion position of team owners and coaches must be qualified in connection with Tim Tebow, a former college and professional football player known for his public statements and gestures that expressed his Christian beliefs. As Tebow's persona attracted millions of fans and unprecedented media coverage, his religious celebrity also created so many disruptive issues for his team and teammates that managers were hesitant to add him to their roster (Fleming, 2013).

To Give Meaning to Sport Participation   Sport participation emphasizes personal achievement and self-promotion, and it involves playing games that produce no essential goods or services, even though people create important social occasions around sport events. This makes sport participation a self-centered, self-indulgent activity. Although training often involves personal sacrifices and pain, it focuses on the development and use of personal physical skills, often to the exclusion of other activities and relationships. Realizing this can create a crisis of meaning for athletes who have dedicated their lives to personal achievements in sports (Carter, 2011).

One way to deal with this crisis of meaning is to define sport participation as an act of worship, a platform for giving witness, or a manifestation of God's plan for one's life (Hoffman, 2010; Krattenmaker, 2010). For example, U.S. track-and-field athlete Jesse Williams put it this way at the 2012 London Olympics: "Jesus Christ is the reason why I am able to perform at this level, and I know He has a plan for me. That puts things into perspective before, during and after competition. I know God has put me in this place to represent Him". Many Christian athletes and coaches like to quote Colossians 3:23 in the Bible: "Whatever you do, work at it with all your heart, working for the Lord, not for men." This enables them to define their sport participation as a sacred rather than a secular activity. As a result, their doubts about the worthiness of what they do are eliminated because playing sports is sanctified as a calling from God. Additionally, it is comforting to know that your sport career is part of God's plan.

To Put Sport Participation into a Balanced Perspective   It's easy to lose perspective in sports, to let it define you and foreclose other parts of your life. In the face of this threat, some athletes feel that religious beliefs enable them to transcend sports and bring balance to their lives. Domonique Foxworth, a former NFL player, explains that "there is no better way to calm an eager rookie before a big game than to put the game in perspective by reminding him of his spiritual beliefs" (Foxworth, 2005, 2D). This makes playing sports part of God's plan, and it becomes easier for athletes to face challenges and deal with the inevitable disappointments experienced in sports. In the process, they keep sports in perspective.

Usually, it is close relationships that help athletes maintain perspective. But one player notes, "If you ain't got no family, no loving wife, or other things like that, it's God. . . . He's the only thing that's gonna save you" (Briggs, 2011).

To Establish Team Solidarity and Unity Religious beliefs and rituals can be powerful tools in creating bonds between people. When they're combined with sport participation, they can link athletes together as spiritual teammates, building team solidarity and unity in the process. Many coaches know this, and some have used Christian beliefs as rallying points for their teams (Wolverton, 2013).

This use of religion can backfire when athletes object to expectations to pray or profess agreement with religious statements. This occurred at New Mexico State University when four Muslim football players filed a lawsuit accusing their coach of religious discrimination because he labeled them "troublemakers" after they objected to reciting the Lord's Prayer in a team huddle after each practice and before each game. The university settled the case out of court, suggesting that they agreed that a football coach doesn't have the right to turn his team into a Christian brotherhood (Fleming, 2007).

Objections to pregame prayers in public schools have led some U.S. students and their parents to file lawsuits to ban religious expression in connection with sport events. However, coaches and athletes continue to insist that prayers bring team members together in positive ways and serve a spiritual purpose in players' lives. This controversial issue is discussed in the Reflect on Sports box "Public Prayers at Sport Events."

To Reaffirm Motivation and Social Control on Teams Religions also can sanctify norms and

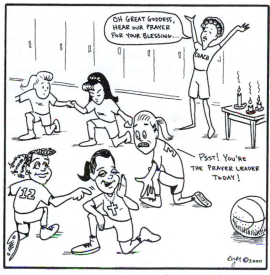

(*Source:* © Frederic A. Eyer)

"She says this prayer is 'voluntary.' Who's she trying to fool?!?"

When coaches use religious beliefs and rituals on sport teams, they may create solidarity or dissent. Coaches say that team prayers are voluntary, but players may feel pressure to pray or not play, regardless of their religious beliefs.

rules by connecting them with divinities. In this way, some Christians connect the moral worth of athletes with the quality of their play and their conformity to team rules and the commands of coaches. This combination of Christianity and sport is very powerful, and coaches have been known to use it as a means of motivating and controlling athletes. Coaches see obedience to their rules as necessary for team success, and religious beliefs can sometimes be used to promote obedience by converting it into a divine mandate.

To Achieve or Explain Competitive Success People often debate whether it is appropriate to pray for victories or other forms of athletic success. Some argue that using prayer this way trivializes religion by turning it into a training strategy. Others say that if prayers bring a sense of harmony and feelings of self-worth to an athlete, praying could enhance performance (Briggs, 2011; Krattenmaker, 2012).

Some Christian athletes believe that God intervenes in sports. For example, Colorado Rockies chairman and CEO Charlie Monfort assembled a Major League Baseball team that in 2007 had many Christians in management, coaching, and on the roster. When the team experienced success, Monfort said, "I think character-wise we're stronger than anyone in baseball. Christians . . . are some of the strongest people in baseball. I believe God sends signs, and we're seeing those." Dan O'Dowd, the team's general manager concurred with his boss, saying, "You look at some of the games we're winning. Those aren't just a coincidence. God has definitely had a hand in this."

Of course, athletes and others connected with sports list many different reasons for praying about their sport participation (Hopsicker, 2009). But it is unlikely that nearly every major professional sport team in the United States would have a chaplain unless owners and managers thought it would improve performance. This also may be why 193 national teams at the 2012 Olympics brought chaplains with them to London. Reid Priddy, who led the U.S. volleyball team to a gold medal in the 2008 Beijing Olympics, explained his success on the court in this way: "Right before the . . . Olympic Games I really felt the freedom from God to be a fierce competitor—not just a really nice and supportive teammate" (FCA, 2012).

THE CHALLENGES OF COMBINING SPORTS AND RELIGIOUS BELIEFS

Organized competitive sports and religions are cultural practices with different histories, traditions, and goals. Each has been socially constructed in different ways, around different issues, and through different types of relationships. This means that combining religious beliefs with sport participation may require adjustments—either in a person's religious beliefs or in the way a person plays sports. Although a growing number of athletes around the world combine Islamic beliefs with their sport lives, this section focuses specifically on the challenges faced by Christian athletes.

Challenges for Christian Athletes

Physical educator Shirl Hoffman (2010) has made the case that there are built-in conflicts between some Christian religious beliefs and the actions required in many power and performance sports. Christianity, he explains, is based on an ethic that emphasizes the importance of means over ends, process over product, quality over quantity, and caring for others over caring for self. But power and performance sports emphasize winning, final scores, season records, personal performance statistics, and self-display.

Do these differences present challenges to Christian athletes? For example, do Christian boxers wonder if pummeling another human being into senseless submission and risking the infliction of a fatal injury is an appropriate spiritual offering? Do Christian football players see problems associated

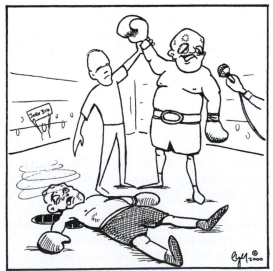

(*Source:* © Frederic A. Eyer)

"I just want to thank my Lord and Savior, who made this knockout possible."

Statements like this are common in post-game interviews. They assume that the "Lord and Savior" is somehow glorified by what occurs in sports. Data suggest that most Christian athletes don't question the logic of this assumption.

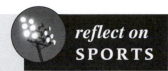

reflect on SPORTS

Public Prayers at Sport Events
What's Legal and What's Not?

Prayers before sport events are common in the United States. They're said silently by individuals, aloud by small groups of players or entire teams in pregame huddles, and occasionally over public address systems by students or local residents.

Public prayers are allowed at private events, and all people in the United States have the right to say silent, private prayers for any purpose at any time. As long as an event is not connected with a public, tax supported organization or as long as people pray privately, prayers are legal in connection with sports.

A 1962 U.S. Supreme Court decision banned organized prayers in public schools when they are said publicly and collectively at sport events sponsored by state organizations, such as public schools. This ruling caused controversy in Texas in 1992, when two families near Houston filed a lawsuit requesting a ban on prayers in public schools. They appealed to the First Amendment of the U.S. Constitution, which says, "Congress shall make no law respecting an establishment of religion." The federal district judge in the case ruled that public prayers are permitted as long as they are nonsectarian and general in content, initiated by students, and not said in connection with attempts to convert anyone to a particular religion. But this decision was qualified during an appeal when the appellate judges ruled that sport events are not serious enough occasions to require the solemnity of public prayer; therefore, the prayers are unconstitutional.

Despite this decision and two similar decisions in 1995 and 1999, people in many U.S. towns, mostly in Southern states, have continued to say public prayers before public school sport events. These prayers often are "local traditions," and people object when federal government judges tell them that they are unconstitutional. They argue that it violates their constitutional right to "freedom of speech."

The issue of prayer related to public school teams continues to be contentious. In 2014, a high school coach in North Carolina was ordered to stop baptizing his players and leading his team in prayers (Stuart, 2014). A similar order was given in 2015 to a high school coach in Georgia when some of his players were baptized before practice. In front of a local news camera, the coach declared,

"We did this right before practice! Take a look and see how God is STILL in our schools!" (Estep, 2015).

Although these and many other cases have not resulted in lawsuits, local authorities have confirmed that they violate the U.S. Constitution—a conclusion reaffirmed whenever cases have gone to court (Willett et al., 2014).

Those who have filed lawsuits argue that the prayers are grounded in Christian beliefs and create informal pressures to give priority to those beliefs over others. They also say that those who don't join in and pray are subject to ridicule, social rejection, or efforts to convert them to Christianity. The people who support public prayers say they don't pressure anyone and that Christianity is the dominant religion in their towns and in the United States. However, they also assume that the public prayers will not be Jewish, Islamic, Hindu, Buddhist, Baha'i, or Sikh prayers and that they will not contradict their Christian beliefs.

When judges rule on these cases they usually consider what would occur if prayers at public school sports events represented beliefs that contradicted Christian beliefs. Would Christians object if public prayers praised Allah, the Goddess, or multiple deities? What would happen if Muslim students said their daily prayers over the public address system in conjunction with a basketball game, if teams were asked to pray to Allah or the Prophet Muhammad, or if all football games were rescheduled to accommodate Muslim customs during their three- to four-week observance of Ramadan in October? These are important questions because over four billion people in the world do not hold Christian beliefs and nearly 1 in 4 Americans have beliefs that are not Christian.

These are the reasons that judges have regularly ruled that public prayers are not allowed at sport events sponsored by state organizations such as public schools. This continues to create management challenges for officials in schools and sport programs, as local populations become increasingly diverse in terms of religious beliefs. *What would you do if you were a coach and half of your team members wanted to read out loud from the Koran/ Qur'an in the lockerroom before games?*

with using intimidation and "taking out" opponents with potentially injurious hits and then saying that such behaviors are "acts of worship"? Do athletes believe that they can use physically injurious actions as expressions of religious commitment simply by saying that they are motivated by Christian love?

For most of the twentieth century these questions were not asked, because it was assumed that sports, especially violent sports, were pagan rather than Christian activities. Athletes were not seen as representatives of Christian ideals. But acceptance of the great sport myth and the belief that sport participation imparts purity and goodness made it possible to claim that being a tough, aggressive athlete was consistent with Christian values.

Research suggests that Christian athletes combine their religious beliefs with sport participation in diverse ways (Baker, 2007). However, in elite power and performance sports most self-described Christian athletes don't think about possible conflicts between their religious beliefs and their actions in sports (Oppenheimer, 2013; Sinden, 2013). At the same time, a few athletes do struggle with the conflict between the moral ethos of sports and the moral ethos of their Christian faith. To be selfless, a primary goal in most religious belief systems, including Christianity, is contrary to what is required to excel in sports (Brooks, 2012). This has recently become an issue among some Christians who wonder if brain damage caused by football interferes with using the sport as a form of witness (Watson and Brock, 2014; Krattenmaker, 2012).

Although there is little research on this topic, Christian athletes in power and performance sports could use one or more of three strategies to reduce doubts about the moral value of what they do in sports.

1. They could focus on the ascetic aspects of sports and see themselves as enduring pain for God's sake.
2. They could strive to be the best they can be as athletes so they can more effectively use sport

as a platform for evangelizing or doing good works off the field.
3. They could drop out of power and performance sports, and seek other sports and activities that fit more closely with their religious beliefs.

Figure 15.1 illustrates the two factors most likely to create conflict and doubts experienced by athletes and the strategies used to reduce them. On the basis of statements made by athletes on the FCA and AIA websites, it appears that Strategy B, options 1 and 2, would be most commonly used.

Challenges for Christian Sport Organizations

The record of Christian organizations indicates that they give primary emphasis to building faith one person at a time. Consequently, they do not devote many resources to eliminating problems in sports other than to condemn overcommercialization and drug use.

> Since the dawn of civilization, we human beings have persistently created God in our own image. —William J. Baker (2000, p. 6)

Noted sports historian William Baker points out that evangelical Christians generally assume that reform occurs only when individual athletes accept Christ into their lives, so their emphasis is on evangelizing over social action and social justice.

Their approach is based on the "primacy of faith"—the idea that faith rather than good works alone is the basis for spiritual salvation. Critics of this approach argue that faith without good works is meaningless, and that people who do good works can be saved even if they haven't given their lives to Christ. But this is a matter of faith rather than the sociology of sport.

Adapting Religious Beliefs to Fit Sports

Religions and sports change as people's values and interests change and as power shifts in society, but it appears that sports change little, if at all, when combined with religion. Instead, it seems

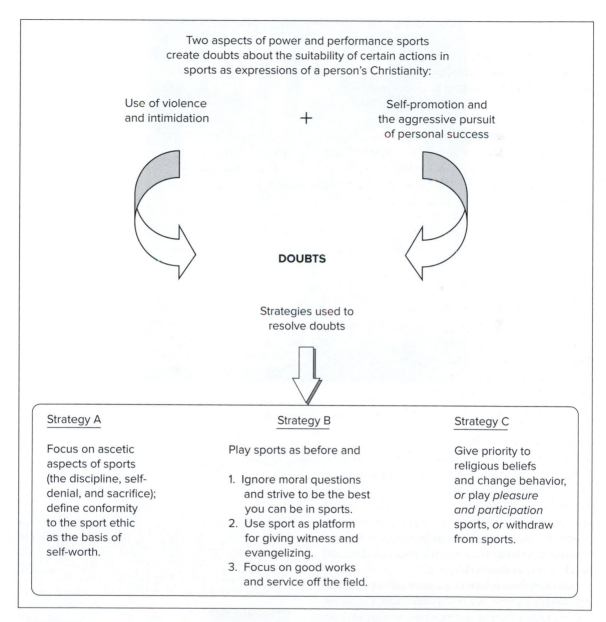

Two aspects of power and performance sports create doubts about the suitability of certain actions in sports as expressions of a person's Christianity:

Use of violence and intimidation

$+$

Self-promotion and the aggressive pursuit of personal success

DOUBTS

Strategies used to resolve doubts

Strategy A

Focus on ascetic aspects of sports (the discipline, self-denial, and sacrifice); define conformity to the sport ethic as the basis of self-worth.

Strategy B

Play sports as before and

1. Ignore moral questions and strive to be the best you can be in sports.
2. Use sport as platform for giving witness and evangelizing.
3. Focus on good works and service off the field.

Strategy C

Give priority to religious beliefs and change behavior, *or* play *pleasure and participation* sports, *or* withdraw from sports.

FIGURE 15.1 Christian religious beliefs and power and performance sports: a model of conflict, doubt, and resolution.

that religious beliefs and rituals are called into the service of sports, or modified to fit the ways that dominant sports are defined, organized, and played in society (Oppenheimer, 2013).

Robert Higgs makes this point in his book *God in the Stadium: Sports and Religion in America* (1995). He explains that the combination of sports and Christian beliefs has led religion to become

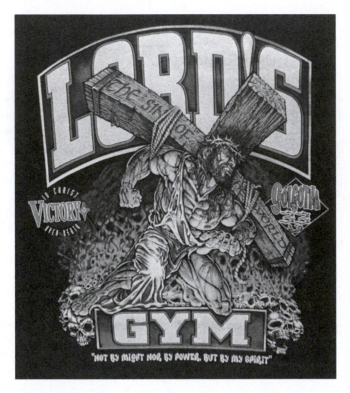

"Not by might nor by power, but by my spirit." History shows that people construct images of deities to fit their values and ideals. This is illustrated in this image of a pumped-up Christ on a T-shirt sold in a Christian gift shop. Christians who value muscles tend to have an image of Christ as muscular. (*Source:* © Jay Coakley)

"muscularized" so that it emphasizes a gospel of discipline, duty, and self-righteousness rather than a gospel of stewardship, social responsibility, and humility. Muscularized religion gives priority to the image of the knight with a sword over the image of the shepherd with a staff. This approach, emphasizing a Christian's role as "the Lord's warrior," fits nicely with the power and performance sports that are popular today.

Although a few Christian athletes have expressed concerns about social justice in sports, most have used Christian religious beliefs to transform winning, obedience to coaches, and a commitment to excellence in sports into moral virtues. Therefore, Christian beliefs generally reproduce sports as they currently exist. At this point, the only exception to this appears to be recreational sports where athletes have agreed upfront to use Christian beliefs to guide their actions during play.

summary

IS IT A PROMISING COMBINATION?

Religion focuses on a connection with the sacred and supernatural, and religious beliefs influence the feelings, thoughts, and actions of believers. This makes religion significant in sociological terms.

Discussions about sports and religions often focus on how these two spheres of cultural life are similar or different. Certainly, they are socially similar because both create strong collective emotions and celebrate collective values through rituals and public events. Furthermore, both have heroes, legends, special buildings for communal gatherings, and institutionalized organizational structures.

On the other hand, those who assume that sport and religion each have essential characteristics that are fixed in nature argue that the inherent differences between these spheres of life are more important than any similarities. Some argue that sports corrupt religious beliefs.

Most scholars in the sociology of sport conceptualize religions and sports as socially constructed cultural practices with meanings that may overlap or differ, depending on social circumstances. This constructionist approach is based on evidence that sports and religions are subject to change as people struggle over what is important and how to organize their collective lives.

Little is known about the relationships between sports and major world religions other than particular forms of Christianity. It seems that certain dimensions of Christian beliefs and meanings have been constructed in ways that fit well with the beliefs and meanings underlying participation and success in organized competitive sports. Organized competitive sports offer a combination of experiences and meanings that are uniquely compatible with the major characteristics of the Protestant ethic.

Sports and certain expressions of Christianity have been combined for a number of reasons. Some Christians promote sports because they believe that sport participation fosters spiritual growth and the development of strong character. Christian groups and organizations have used sports to promote their belief systems and attract new members, especially young males who wish to see themselves as having "manly virtues." They also have used popular athletes as spokespersons for their messages about fundamentalist beliefs.

Athletes and coaches have used religious beliefs and rituals for many reasons: to cope with the uncertainty of competition; to stay out of trouble; to give meaning to sport participation; to put sport participation into a balanced perspective; to establish team solidarity and unity; to reaffirm motivation and social control on teams; and to achieve and explain competitive success.

Although the differences between the dominant ethos of Christianity and the dominant ethos of competitive sports would seem to create problems for Christian athletes and sport organizations, it appears that this rarely occurs. With the exception of sports played at the recreational level and sponsored by Christian organizations, Christian athletes define their religious beliefs in ways that generally reaffirm the ethos of competitive sports.

Neither Christian athletes nor Christian organizations have paid much attention to what might be identified as moral and ethical problems in sports. Instead, they've focused their resources on spreading religious beliefs in connection with sport events and sport involvement. Their emphasis has been on playing sports for the glory of God, using athletic performances as a platform for giving Christian witness, and working in church and community programs.

In conclusion, the combination of sports and religious beliefs offers little promise for changing dominant forms of sport, especially in the United States. Of course, individual athletes may alter their sport-related behaviors when they combine sports and religion in their own lives, but at this time such changes have had no observable effect on what occurs in elite, competitive sports.

SUPPLEMENTAL READINGS

Reading 1. Christian sport organizations
Reading 2. Ramadan as an issue for Muslim athletes
Reading 3. Self-indulgence for the "glory of God": Christian witness in high-performance sports
Reading 4. Skateistan: Skateboarding and gender barriers

SPORT MANAGEMENT ISSUES

- Your university has a growing number of Muslim students. The Muslim women have requested private access to a small gym in an older, secondary recreation center, because some of them are prohibited by their religion or their families from being seen by men while they exercise. Non-Muslim women in campus sororities object, saying that this is a case of granting Muslims special privileges. You have been asked to mediate what has become a potentially volatile campus issue. Describe two possible resolutions to this situation, and explain the rationale for each.
- You are working for USA Track & Field. Both the Fellowship of Christian Athletes (FCA) and Athletes in Action (AIA) have requested office space at your headquarters in Indianapolis. Along with other top staff you've been asked to explain your position on this matter. What issues would you raise in your statement at the upcoming staff meeting?
- You run the youth sport programs in the parks and recreation department of a midsize city, which has a diverse population that includes Muslims, Orthodox Jews, Hindus, and fundamentalist Christians. Each group has requested exclusive programs because they don't want their children to become confused about their religious beliefs as they play sports. The city government emphasizes policies of inclusion and has refused their requests. What management strategies might you use to defuse tensions as these different religious groups of people come together in each of your leagues?

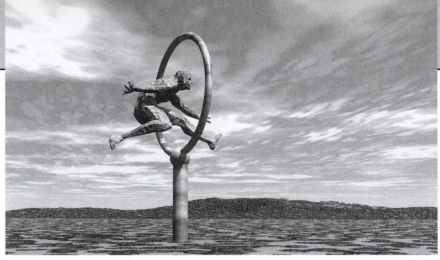

chapter

16

SPORTS IN THE FUTURE

What Do We Want Them to Be?

Our sports belong to us. They came up from the people. They were invented for reasons having nothing to do with money or ego. Our sports weren't created by wealthy sports and entertainment barons like the ones running sports today.

> **—Ken Reed, Sport Policy Director, League of Fans, 2011**

What we have is a crisis of imagination. Albert Einstein said that you cannot solve a problem with the same mind-set that created it. . . . Money should be spent trying out concepts that shatter current structures and systems that have turned much of the world into one vast market.

> **—Peter Buffett, philanthropist (2013)**

Over the next decade . . . (in) the highest echelons of sports, merely "able-bodied" athletes may no longer be able to compete effectively. . . . Will professional sports teams let superabled people play, or is that cheating?

> **—Daniel Wilson, author and robotics engineer (2012)**

. . . a public sociology of sport must account for and intervene into the barriers within sport. . . . It should go beyond critical sociological research and try to find resolutions to social problems in sport at local, national, and international levels.

> **—Peter Donnelly et al., Centre for Sport Policy, University of Toronto (2011)**

Learning Objectives

- Discuss how the power and performance model and the pleasure and participation model can be used to envision possibilities for what sports might be in the future.

- Explain why both power and performance sports and pleasure and participation sports will grow in the future.

- Identify and give examples of the five general societal trends that will influence sports in the near future.

- Distinguish between conservative, reformist, and radical goals for changing sports.

- Identify the pros and cons of the four different vantage points for making changes in sports.

- Discuss how cultural, interactionist, and structural theories can be used in the process of making changes in sports.

- Understand why athletes are hesitant to become change agents in sports and society.

People often describe the future in science-fiction terms that arouse extreme hopes or fears. This sparks interest, but such images are rarely helpful because the future seldom unfolds as rapidly or dramatically as some forecasters would have us believe.

The future emerges in connection with social change, and social change is driven by the actions of people who create a reality that fits their visions of what life should be like. Some people have more power and resources to turn their visions into reality, but they seldom want revolutionary changes because their privileged positions depend on stability and controlled change. This often impedes progressive changes in favor of increasing the efficiency and profitability of existing ways of life.

Although power relations cannot be ignored, people do have different ideas about what sports should and could be in the future. Accordingly, the goal of this chapter is to respond to the following questions:

1. What models of sports might we use to envision possibilities for the future?
2. What current trends must be acknowledged as we consider the future of sports?
3. What factors shape current trends, and how will they influence the future of sports?
4. How can we become effective agents in creating the future of sports?

ENVISIONING POSSIBILITIES FOR THE FUTURE

Sports are social constructions. This means that the sports that are funded and publicized the most at any particular place and time are likely to be consistent with the values, ideas, interests, and experiences of those who have power in a social world. However, sport forms are not accepted by everyone, and people often modify them or develop alternatives in the process of resisting or challenging them.

Dominant sports in most societies have been and continue to be organized around a **power and performance model.** However, people may reject all or part of power and performance sports

as they seek experiences grounded in alternative values and interests. Many of these people create sports organized around one of more elements of a **pleasure and participation model.**

These two models do not encompass all possibilities for envisioning sports in the future, and there are many sports that combine features of both. But we can use them here as starting points for thinking about what we'd like sports to be in the future.

Power and Performance Sports

Power and performance sports will continue to be highly visible and publicized in the near future. They're based on key aspects of dominant ideologies in most post-industrial societies, as demonstrated by their emphasis on strength, power, speed, competition, and competitive outcomes.

Although power and performance sports take many forms, they're all built upon the idea that excellence is achieved through dedication, hard work, and a willingness to take risks and competitive success proves excellence. They involve setting records, pushing human limits, using the body as a machine, and employing science and technology in the process. According to many athletes in power and performance sports, the body is to be disciplined and monitored so as to meet the demands of sports.

Power and performance sports are exclusive in that participants are selected for their abilities to achieve competitive success. Those who lack such abilities are cut or relegated to lower-status programs. Organizations and teams have hierarchical authority structures in which athletes are subordinate to coaches and coaches are subordinate to owners and administrators. It is widely accepted that coaches can exceed standard normative limits when motivating and training athletes to outperform others. Athletes are expected to obey coaches and show that they are willing to make sacrifices in their quest for success.

The sponsors of power and performance sports stress the value of winning. Being endorsed by winning athletes and teams is important when selling products and promoting the sponsor's brand.

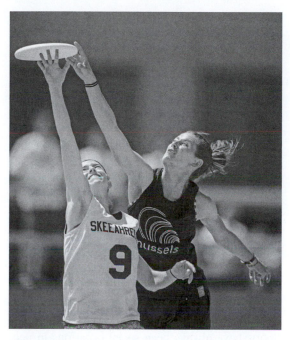

Club sports and intramurals often include elements of both power and performance and pleasure and participation sports. Ultimate is a good example of such a hybrid sport. (*Source:* © Kevin Leclaire/Courtesy of UltiPhotos)

Sponsors assume that their association with winning athletes and teams enhances their status and makes them special in the eyes of people they wish to influence. As long as current sponsors desire this connection, power and performance sports will remain dominant for the foreseeable future in most societies.

Pleasure and Participation Sports

Although power and performance sports are highly visible, many people realize that there are other ways to organize and play sports that more closely match their values and interests. This realization has led to the creation of numerous sport forms organized around *pleasure and participation* and emphasizing freedom, authenticity, self-expression, enjoyment, holistic health, support for others, and respect for the environment. They focus on personal engagement and the notion that the body

is to be nurtured and enjoyed in a quest for challenging experiences rather than trained and subordinated in a quest for competitive success.

Pleasure and participation sports tend to be inclusive, and skill differences among participants often are accommodated by using "handicaps" that allow everyone to experience challenges in organized physical activities. Sport organizations and teams based on this model have democratic decision-making structures characterized by cooperation, power sharing, and give-and-take relationships between coaches and athletes. Humiliation, shame, and derogation are inconsistent with the spirit underlying these sports.

Pleasure and participation sports are characteristically sponsored by public and nonprofit organizations and by corporations seeking exposure to a defined collection of consumers. Additionally, some corporations may sponsor these sports as part of an overall emphasis on social responsibility and a commitment to health promotion, among other commendable goals.

CURRENT TRENDS RELATED TO SPORTS IN SOCIETY

Becoming aware of current trends and the factors that influence them is the starting point for being effective agents in creating the futures we want to see. The complexity of social worlds complicates the identification of trends, so it's useful to think of the factors that support the growth of power and performance sports on the one hand, and pleasure and participation sports on the other. Making this distinction helps us clarify our goals and use social theories more effectively as we participate in the process of influencing the culture and organization of sports.

Factors Supporting the Growth of Power and Performance Sports

There are strong vested interests in power and performance sports among those who control resources in wealthy post-industrial societies. For example, when the goal is to use strength, power, and speed to outperform others, sports reaffirm gender differences and a form of gender ideology that privileges men. As long as men control corporate resources there will be an emphasis on sponsoring power and performance sports. Currently, this helps to explain why American football, the classic embodiment of these sports, has become the most popular spectator sport in the United States and continues to attract billions of dollars in television rights fees and other revenues. Athletes in the NFL and other power and performance sports are portrayed in the media as heroic figures, as warriors who embody a corporate emphasis on productivity, efficiency, and dedication to achieving goals in the face of all barriers. Spectators are encouraged to identify with these athletes and express their identification through the consumption of licensed merchandise and other products.

Because power and performance sports often involve pushing human and normative limits, they are relatively easy to market and sell when combined with storylines that resonate with consumers. This is why the media focus on individual athletes and their personal stories, often turning athletes into celebrities apart from the sports they play. Dedicated long-time fans may be satisfied with coverage focused on the action and competitive strategies in matches and games, but less-knowledgeable fans are more likely to be entertained by narratives about players' lives.

Sportainment coverage is common in commercial power and performance sports, because it feeds and extends storylines that maintain audience interest even when action in the event is boring for many viewers. It also sustains interest in a sport between events and in the off-season and builds to a climax as the next event or new season begins. This boosts ratings and provides an opportunity to initiate and extend engaging narratives that foster consistent media sport consumption.

Factors Supporting the Growth of Pleasure and Participation Sports

Sports have always been social occasions in people's lives, and people incorporate into them the things that give them pleasure or reaffirm their

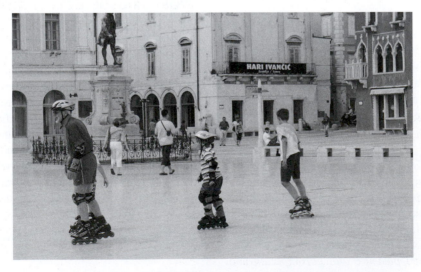

Concerns about health and fitness frequently lead people to engage in pleasure and participation sports such as in-line skating. In Piran, Slovenia, people young and old negotiate town streets and sidewalks on their skates. (*Source:* © Jay Coakley)

values and identities. Pleasure and participation sports today are popular to the extent that people define them as attractive alternatives to the more culturally dominant power and performance sports. Factors that motivate this search for alternatives today are (1) concerns about health and fitness; (2) participation preferences among the rapidly growing population of older people; (3) values and experiences brought to sports by women; and (4) groups seeking alternatives to highly structured, competitive sports that constrain their experiences.

Concerns About Health and Fitness   As health-care policies and programs emphasize prevention rather than expensive cures, people generally become more sensitive to health and fitness issues. In North America, health care and insurance companies now encourage strategies for staying well as they seek to cut costs and maximize profits. This encourages people to pursue activities with health benefits, and many pleasure and participation sports meet this need, whereas power and performance sports often undermine it with high injury rates.

When people realize that healthy exercise can be incorporated into challenging pleasure and participation sports that connect them with others and their environment and create enjoyment, they are likely to give higher priority to them—but this depends on how people choose to create the future for themselves and their families, and within their schools and communities.

Participation Preferences Among Older People   As the median age of the population increases in many societies and older people represent an increasingly larger proportion of the world's population, there will be more interest in sports that do not involve intimidation, physical force, the domination of opponents, and the risk of serious injuries.

As people age, they're less likely to risk physical well-being to establish a reputation in sports. Older people are more likely to see sports as social activities and make them inclusive rather than exclusive. They also realize that they have but one body, and it can be enjoyed only if they cultivate it

as though it were a garden rather than driving it as a performance machine.

People in the baby-boom generation in the United States are now in their fifties to late-sixties. They grew up playing and watching competitive sports and are not likely to abandon them as they age, but most of them will avoid participation in power and performance sports that have high injury rates. Instead, they'll redefine what it means to be an athlete and they will play modified versions of competitive activities in which rules emphasize the pleasure of movement, connections between people, and controlled challenges (Dionigi et al., 2013; Klostermann and Nagel, 2012; Tulle, 2007). Additionally, pleasure and participation sports will also be sites where older people challenge the notion that aging always involves increasing dependency and incapacity. "Seniors" and Masters sport programs will increase as people demand them. As a result, images of older people who are fit, healthy, and accomplished athletes will become more visible and serve as models for others seeking pleasure and participation.

Values and Experiences Brought to Sports by Women   As women gain more power and resources, many will revise or reject traditional power and performance sports. For instance, when women play sports such as rugby, soccer, and hockey, they often emphasize inclusiveness and support for teammates and opponents in explicit ways that are less common in men's versions of these sports. The "in-your-face" power and performance orientation exhibited by some men is replaced by a more cooperative orientation that highlights connections between participants.

Women often face difficulties when recruiting corporate sponsors for pleasure and participation sports, although this is beginning to change as people in corporations see that these sports can make employees healthier and create new realms of consumption for which products and services can be sold.

Groups Seeking Alternative Sports   People who reject certain aspects of power and performance sports have a history of creating alternative sports and unique sport cultures organized around them (Thorpe and Wheaton, 2013). Studies of skateboarders, snowboarders, surfers, BMX riders, in-line skaters, and others show that some people in these sports resist turning them into commercialized, competitive forms (Honea, 2004, 2007 Gilchrist and Wheaton, 2011; Storey, 2013; Thorpe and Wheaton, 2011a, 2011b; Wheaton, 2013). Even in official, formally sponsored contests, skaters have deliberately subverted the power and performance dimensions of events. Unregistered skaters have crashed the events. Registered skaters have pinned their competition numbers upside down on their shirts, boycotted award ceremonies, and focused on expressing themselves and supporting "opponents." Mass demonstrations have been staged at a few events where nonconforming athletes were disqualified for their actions. Of course, none of this is shown on television broadcasts that are edited to attract young viewers, but they are indicative of resistance to events organized around a power and performance model (Honea, 2014).

After skateboarding had been turned into a traditional competitive sport by the X Games, legendary skater Tony Hawk declared that "it's about time the riders took the competitions into their own hands" because others were destroying many of the expressive and pleasurable elements of boarding (in Higgins, 2005). Hawk organized his Boom Boom HuckJam tour in 2002 to preserve the spirit of action and lifestyle sports in a format that could generate revenues to support elite athletes as well as media coverage to grow the sports. Similarly, Terje Haakonsen and other snowboarders created "Ticket To Ride" (www.ttrworldtour.com/) in 2002—a series of rider-controlled events designed to preserve the ethos of their sports through "a movement connected to the core of snowboarding's identity [and an emphasis on a] sense of fun and friendship, the appreciation of nature, the travel and the unique experiences, the freedom and creativity. . . ." These alternative sport events have remained commercially successful. Although they now have sponsorship deals with corporations,

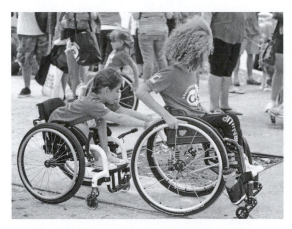

Athletes with a disability are participating in sports in greater numbers. Creatively designed equipment permits new forms of sports involvement for people of all ability levels, as shown by these young wheelchair racers. (*Source:* © Rich Cruse/Photo courtesy of the Challenged Athletes Foundation, http://www .challengedathletes.org)

they have not been reorganized around a power and performance model (Thorpe and Wheaton, 2011a).

People with physical or intellectual disabilities have also developed alternative sports or adapted dominant sports to fit their interests and needs. Although some of these sports emphasize elements of power and performance, most emphasize pleasure and participation. Concern and support for teammates and opponents, as well as inclusiveness related to physical abilities, characterize these sports.

The International Gay Games, the World Outgames, and the EuroGames provide examples of alternative sport forms emphasizing participation, support, inclusiveness, and the enjoyment of physical movement. The ninth quadrennial International Gay Games were hosted by Cleveland and Akron, Ohio, in 2014. More than 10,000 athletes participated—about the same number of athletes that participate in the Summer Olympic Games. The third World Outgames were hosted in 2013 by Antwerp, where over 12,000 athletes participated, and the 2017 games will be hosted by Miami, where record-breaking crowds

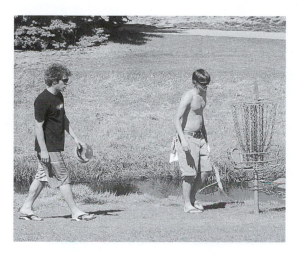

Disc golf, invented in the 1960s, initially used lampposts and fire hydrants as "holes." Since then it has become less "alternative," but it continues to attract people seeking a sport without coaches, schedules, referees, and other constraints that limit freedom and creativity. (*Source:* © Jay Coakley)

are expected. The EuroGames draw nearly 3000 athletes annually, similar to the number of athletes at other regional games that bring together gay men, lesbians, bisexuals, and transsexuals (GLBTs) in sports emphasizing inclusion and other aspects of the pleasure and participation model. GLBTs also organize sports at the community level to provide experiences free of the homophobia that can destroy enjoyment in other sports (Ravel and Rail, 2007; Travers and Deri, 2011).

The range of sports that incorporate elements of the pleasure and participation model grows as more people realize that sports are social constructions that can be created to fit even temporary interests and passing situations. This has been illustrated by people forming local adult kickball leagues and freerunning groups, and joining with others to surf on sand, play bike polo, go streetsurfing, and create uncounted other sports.

Although it often is a challenge to find corporate sponsors, various pleasure and participation sports usually survive because people are creative enough to find resources to maintain them. Furthermore,

corporate or media sponsors are needed only when a sport hires administrators, stages national and international tournaments, and involves expensive equipment and travel expenses. When a sport exists simply for pleasure and participation, the primary resources needed are people wishing to play it and spaces in which it can be played.

FACTORS INFLUENCING TRENDS TODAY

When we're creating futures it's useful to know about factors that influence current trends. This enables us to anticipate possibilities, prevent or overcome resistance, and make more informed decisions as we participate in social worlds.

Many factors influence trends in sports, but the discussion here is limited to five: (1) a widespread commitment to organization and rationalization; (2) a cultural emphasis on commercialism and consumption; (3) the widespread use of telecommunications and electronic media; (4) the growth of technology; and (5) the changing demographic composition of communities and societies.

Organization and Rationalization

Sports today focus on planning and productivity. "Fun" is associated with achieving goals rather than physical expression and joy. Process is now secondary to product, and the journey is secondary to the destination.

People in post-industrial societies live with the legacy of industrialization. They emphasize organization based on rational principles. Being organized and making plans to accomplish goals is so important that spontaneity, expression, creativity, and joy—the elements of play—are given low priority or may even be considered frivolous by event planners, coaches, and spectators. The implications of this emphasis on organization and rationalization were noted by legendary snowboarder Terje Haakonsen when he announced that he would not participate in the Olympics even though many people saw him as the best in the world. His explanation of the snowboarding experience provides interesting insights about sports:

> That was a fun time . . . I was always learning new tricks, figuring out ways to get better. When I'm having fun snowboarding, it's like meditation. I'm not thinking about anything but what I'm doing right now. No past, no future. . . . [But today, too many] people get stuck and all they do the whole year is pipe, and that's too bad for them. They do the same routine over and over, get the moves down. It becomes like this really precise, synchronized movement, like they're little ballerinas or something. It's no longer this spontaneous sport, like when you're a kid screwing around (Greenfeld, 1999).

Haakonsen felt that fun and effort merge together in sports when they are done on terms set by participants. This merger breaks down when sports are done for judges using criteria that ignore the subjective experience of participation.

These are important things to keep in mind when we think about what we'd like sports to be in the future. Many people today assume that sports should be organized primarily for the purpose of rationally assessing skills and performances. Haakonsen suggests that mastering a skill to expand possibilities for new experiences is one thing, but spending years perfecting a specialized skill to conform to single definition of technical perfection is another. Once this distinction becomes clear in our own sport participation, we become more creative when thinking about the future.

Commercialism and Consumption

Many people today are so deeply embedded in commercial culture that they think of themselves as customers rather than citizens. This changes the basis

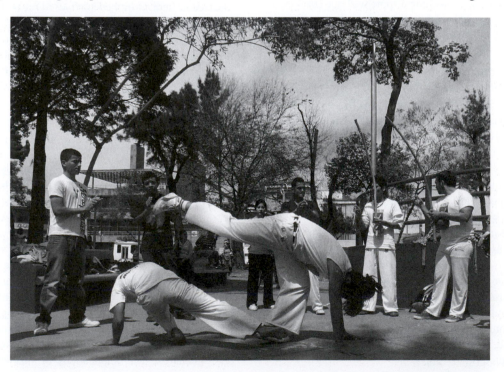

Trying to improve skills on your own terms is different from doing a routine over and over to meet someone else's idea of technical perfection. These practitioners of capoeira understand this distinction and use their sport to create new awareness and experiences. (*Source:* © Basia Borzecka)

for evaluating self, others, and experiences. When commercial ideology pervades sports, play becomes secondary to playoffs and payoffs; games, athletes, and sport participation become commodities—things bought and sold for bottom-line purposes. Participation then revolves around the consumption of equipment, lessons, clothing, nutritional supplements, gym and club memberships, and other material things. Identity is based on where you do sports, the equipment you use, and the clothing you wear—not the emotional joy and satisfaction gained through participation.

Many people are turned off by this approach, but unless they've experienced alternatives, it may be difficult to envision sports devoid of commercialism and consumption. This is why it's important to have public spaces where people can play sports that don't require fees, permits, or memberships. Creativity thrives in such spaces. In this sense, public policies at all levels of government can create or subvert possibilities for noncommercial sport futures.

Telecommunications and Electronic Media

Television, computers, the Internet, smart-phones and other handheld devices provide visual images and narratives that many people use to imagine future possibilities for sports; the same is true for video games. Some people even use electronic images to inform their choices about participation and formulate standards for assessing sport experiences. Therefore, media producers worldwide have considerable power to create the future. The events, athletes, and stories represented in the media influence popular discourse about sports, and it is out of that discourse that people form their ideas about what sports could and should be in the future.

To understand this process, imagine that football is the only sport you've ever seen on television. You would have a seriously limited sense of what sports are and what they could be. A version of this occurs as media companies select for coverage only those sports that generate profits. As a result, those are the sports that dominate popular discourse and

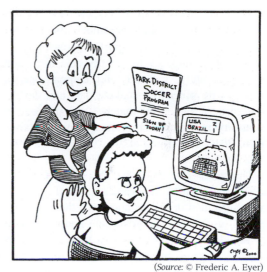

(*Source:* © Frederic A. Eyer)

"Oh, Mom! I'm not going outside to play when I can play on my virtual World Cup Team right here."

The future of sports is difficult to predict. Will children prefer video games and virtual sports over the dominant sport forms of today? Will playing virtual sports serve as a "gateway" into real-time sports by teaching children the rules and challenges that characterize real-time sports?

influence our visions for the future. If we realize this, we can seek images and narratives about sports that are not represented exclusively through commercial media. This expands our experience and enables us to think more creatively about the present and future. The more versions of sports we see and talk about, the more we can create futures to match our interests and circumstances.

Technology

Technology is the *application of scientific or other organized knowledge to solve problems, expand experiences, or alter the conditions of reality.* It is used to make sports safer, detect and treat injuries more effectively, assess physical limits and potential, expand the experiences available in sports. It is also used to train more efficiently, control athletes' bodies, increase the speeds at which bodies move, decrease the risks involved in sports, enhance the size and strength of bodies, and alter bodies to match the demands of particular sports. Increasingly, we depend on technology to identify rule infractions more accurately, measure and compare performances with precision, analyze data and develop strategies for games and matches, and improve the durability and functionality of equipment (Balmer et al., 2012; Futterman et al., 2012; Kwak, 2012; Wilson, 2012).

The major challenges we face with new technologies are how to assess and regulate them, and to make informed decisions about whether and when we will use them. The governing bodies of sports try to regulate the technologies used by coaches, officials, trainers, and athletes, but the rapid expansion of diverse, new technologies makes this difficult. Assessing the implications of particular technologies is not easy. Consistent and sensible decisions about them are made only when we know what we want sports to be in the future.

As a case in point, consider genetic-enhancement technologies. They can be used to improve human performance, heal injured bodies, and eliminate some physical impairments. If we want to create a future in which sports are organized around the power and performance model, we would assess, regulate, and make decisions about using a particular technology differently than we would if we want sports organized around a pleasure and participation model. This is why it is important to have a clear sense of what we want the meaning, purpose, and organization of sports to be in the future.

Changing Demographic Composition of Communities and Societies

Sports are social constructions, and some of the richest sport environments are those in which people have diverse cultural backgrounds and sport experiences. Even when people play the same sport, strategies and styles often vary with their cultural backgrounds. For example, Canadians created a secular and rationalized version of lacrosse that was different from the traditional, sacred game invented and played by Native Peoples in North America (King, 2007b). People in the United States took the sport of rugby as played in England and adapted it to fit their preferences; the result was American football, a game that is relatively unique in the world. In 2004 the New York Mets hired a Latino general manager, signed notable Latino players, and developed a style of play that was fast, assertive, and spirited. This style is now accepted in Major League Baseball and it influences everything from on-the-field strategy to marketing the game to Latinos in the United States and Latin America.

Although demographic diversity presents challenges, it also presents possibilities for creating new forms and versions of sports. As geographical mobility, labor migration, wars, and political turmoil push and pull people across national borders, there will be opportunities to borrow and blend different sports, styles of play, and game strategies. If people take advantage of those opportunities without systematically privileging games from one culture and marginalizing games from other cultures, it will be possible to envision and create sports that fit a wide range of interests and abilities.

BECOMING AGENTS OF CHANGE

Understanding connections between sports and social worlds is a prerequisite for becoming effective agents of change. This is because social change involves identifying goals, choosing a vantage point for making changes, and using social theories to create strategies for achieving goals.

Identifying Goals

Change means different things to different people because their goals for the future are different. For most people in sports, the primary goal is *growth*—strengthening and expanding what exists today. For others, the primary goal is *improvement*—eliminating problems and promoting justice and fairness in sports. And for a few people, the primary goal is *social transformation*—creating new sport forms that are healthy, inclusive, humane, and widely accessible.

Growth is a **conservative goal** based on the belief that sports are inherently positive activities that should be strengthened and expanded in their current forms. Accomplishing this goal requires using management and marketing techniques to expand and make sport organizations more efficient while maintaining the culture and structure of sports as they are. The belief is that increased efficiency will create resources that inevitably fuel growth. Most people in organized sports are dedicated to this goal for both ideological and personal reasons: they believe that the growth of sports as they now exist will improve society and increase opportunities to develop skills and achieve success.

Improvement is a **reformist goal** based on beliefs that sport participation produces positive consequences, that the ethical foundations of sports must be restored and maintained, and that participation

> **Exposing the gap between what is and what could be . . . remind[s] us that the world could be different.** —Michael Burawoy, president, International Sociological Association

opportunities must be increased. Accomplishing this goal requires changes that promote fair competition, responsible citizenship, and appropriate opportunities for everyone to participate. Cheating, deviance, and drug use must be controlled, discrimination must be eliminated from policies and programs, and participation must be made more accessible in schools and communities. Improvement is a widely accepted goal, although people may differ on the priorities for specific reforms. Reformist goals guided the people building "miracle fields," as described in Reflect on Sports, p. 524.

Transformation is a **radical goal** based on the belief that dominant forms of sports are systemically flawed and must be reorganized or replaced to create new meaning and purpose. Accomplishing this goal requires a critical assessment of dominant sports and the ability to create re-imagined or new sports in which previously disenfranchised people share power with others in determining policies, controlling sport resources and facilities, and developing opportunities that meet their needs and concerns. Few people associated with sports today are proponents of transformation, and those in positions of control usually are quick to use their resources to impede or undermine anyone who supports radical transformation.

My experience indicates that most people who read this book give priority to *growth,* with *reform* being an important but secondary goal. In the context of many sport organizations, reformists often are labeled as "anti-sport" and marginalized. Radicals seeking transformation of sports are especially unwelcome around sport organizations, although most radicals don't see this as a problem because their work focuses primarily on issues of poverty, homelessness, health care, education, accessible public transportation, full employment, and guaranteed minimum standards of living.

A few radicals have used sports as sites for challenging dominant definitions of masculinity and femininity, raising questions about the meaning of

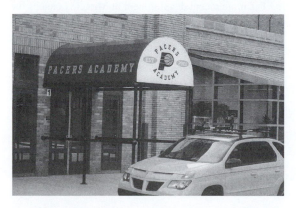

Professional sport teams sometimes fund community programs and services for children. The teams encourage players to be engaged in them. The NBA's Indiana Pacers help to sponsor the Pacers Academy Middle School and High School in central Indianapolis, where students receive focused attention in small classes. This is helpful, but it focuses on changing a few individuals rather than changing the social conditions that put thousands of children at risk. (*Source:* © Jay Coakley)

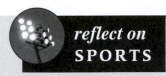

reflect on SPORTS

Miracle Field
Reforming Youth Sport Spaces

In 1997 a youth baseball coach in Conyers, Georgia, noticed that one of his five-year-old players came to every practice and game with his seven-year-old brother. The seven-year-old loved baseball, but there were no teams for children in wheelchairs. So the coach invited him to play.

This coach's action precipitated a series of events. The following season, local adults organized the Conyers "Miracle League" for children with disabilities. It was the first baseball league of its kind, and the rules were adapted to fit the players. For example, every player on a team would bat each inning, all base runners were safe, and every player scored a run. Able-bodied young people and volunteers served as buddies, assisting players when the need arose.

During the first year there were thirty-five players on four teams. Watching them play inspired Dean Alford, a former Georgia state representative and president of the local Rotary Club. He saw that a conventional ball field with grass, dirt, and elevated bases created barriers for players who were blind or using wheelchairs, walkers, and crutches. Alford worked with local Rotary Clubs to raise money to design and construct a rubberized turf playing field plus accessible restrooms, concession stand, and picnic area. Three other grass fields were designed so they could be converted to synthetic surfaces as the Miracle League grew.

The field, 25 miles east of Atlanta, opened in 2000. It attracted national media attention and interest among the families of more than 75,000 children with disabilities in the Atlanta area. In 2008 there were about 200 Miracle League organizations in the United States, Puerto Rico, and Canada.

When people hear of the Miracle League, visit websites, and watch games, their idealism often pushes them to think further outside the box of traditional parks and playing fields. Some communities have built universally accessible playgrounds adjacent to the smooth-surface baseball fields. Playground designers today are more likely to create environments that attract children with varying physical (dis)abilities. This type of design enables families and friends to play safely as they encounter physical challenges and have fun regardless of abilities.

When people see a Miracle League game played on a barrier-free field adjoining a barrier-free play area, they usually say: "This makes so much sense," and then they ask, "Why doesn't my community have one of these?" This response along with the development of more sport programs like the Miracle League is heartening for over 6 million U.S. children with physical impairments making it difficult or impossible to play sports in traditional programs that assume high ability among participants.

The more recent development of Miracle Leagues for adults is heartening to the thousands of veterans who returned from Iraq and Afghanistan with amputated limbs, sight and hearing impairments, and injuries that impede walking. Making sports accessible to them and others with a disability is both a political and a management challenge. It will require a revision of local priorities or the provision of incentives from state or federal government. *What do you think would be the most effective strategy for creating accessible facilities and leagues that meet the needs of people with a disability?*

race, exposing the poverty and inequalities that prevent meaningful participation in society, destroying stereotypes about (dis)abilities, and critiquing the antidemocratic, exclusive, and hierarchical structures that characterize most organized sports today. In the process, they inspire creative visions of what sports could be in the future and, in doing so, encourage others to critically assess sports and to become involved in progressive programs in which political

awareness and community activism are combined with playing sports (Zirin, 2005; 2008a).

Assessing Vantage Points

There are at least four vantage points or strategic positions for initiating changes in and through sports. We can work inside sport organizations, join opposition groups to resist or undermine certain sport forms, create new and alternative sports, or work outside of sports to create desired sport forms. Being aware of our personal vantage point is important because each comes with its own constraints and opportunities for making sports what we want them to be.

Working Inside Sport Organizations   An "insider" vantage point is constraining because promotions and job security generally depend on conforming to the values and culture of the organization where you work. This means that even though you may favor certain reforms or transformational goals, your commitment to change may decrease as you move up the organization into positions of power. Once people reach those positions, they tend to become more conservative and focus on growth and efficiency more than transforming a sport. This isn't inevitable, but it's customary.

On the other hand, an insider vantage point provides information about the structure and culture of sport organizations and enables a person to directly intervene in the processes that affect the meaning, purpose, and organization of sports. If a person reaches a position of power in a sport organization, the opportunities to make and influence changes increase.

Joining "Opposition" Groups   History shows that the future often is influenced by groups that oppose the status quo and promote policies and programs that alter the organization of social life. For example, opposition groups in recent years have effectively lobbied against using public funds to build costly stadiums that primarily serve the interests of privileged people (Boykoff, 2014b; Coakley and Souza, 2013; Delaney and Eckstein, 2003, 2007). Opposition groups have been less effective in opposing plans to host mega-events, such as the Olympics, but these groups will be more effective in the future as research continues to document the debts and other problems that come with hosting such events.

Local groups opposing specific policies and programs have often been effective, whether it be to promote gender equity, build a new skatepark or disc golf course, or reserve public spaces for pleasure and participation sports. As these groups alter the sport landscape they create more diverse sports that meet people's needs more effectively.

Creating New or Alternative Sports   Altering the future of sports also occurs when people reject dominant power and performance sports and develop new sports grounded in alternative ideas about what sports should be. This is not easy to do because resources are seldom available to entrepreneurs who are not in the mainstream of sports programs and organizations. However, working from this outsider vantage point can be effective when it influences others to consider and participate in alternatives to existing sport forms. Canadian Bruce Kidd, a former Olympian with a deep knowledge of sports history, says that creating "alternatives to the commercial sport culture [is] . . . an uphill fight," but he also notes that efforts to create these alternatives "have a long, rich, and proud history" (1997, p. 270).

When new or alternative sports are successfully created, commercial interests usually try to convert them into commodified forms of power and performance sports. Resisting this co-optation is difficult and not always successful, but the process of creating new and alternative sports is needed to inspire creative changes in the meaning, purpose, and organization of sports.

Working Outside Sports   Creating the future of sports from outside vantage points requires foresight and a good grasp of how social change occurs. For example, when feminists created the women's movement during the 1960s it provided an opportunity for activists, educators, and progressive politicians to draft Title IX as part of the Education Amendments to the Civil Rights Restoration Act. When this act became law in 1972 it changed the legal context in which sports were organized, sponsored, and played. In turn, this dramatically altered the future of sports.

Similarly, people working in military veterans' organizations today may effectively change how "disabilities" are defined in U.S. culture and, in the process, encourage others to draft laws and create programs that provide equal opportunities for people with a disability to play sports. In this sense, anyone who works to eliminate social injustice and create opportunities for new voices to be expressed and taken seriously in social worlds also lays the groundwork for creating more humane and accessible sports in the future.

Using Theories

Throughout this book it is noted that sociologists study and explain social worlds in terms of culture, interaction, and social structure. Theories related to each of these dimensions of social worlds are useful when thinking about the future and developing strategies to change or transform sports and achieve particular goals. Theories provide systematic interpretive frameworks that make it possible to improve the odds of accurately anticipating and even predicting the consequences of change-oriented strategies, regardless of the goals a person wants to achieve. In this sense, good theories are like road maps for navigating your way into desired futures.

Cultural Theories   People who wish to be agents of change can use cultural theories to understand the processes through which social worlds are produced, reproduced, and transformed. These theories indicate that to change sports, we must change the symbols, values, norms, vocabularies, beliefs, and ideologies that people use to make sense of and give meaning to sports and sport experiences. For example, the process of creating gender equity in sports has involved, among many things, changing the vocabulary used by media announcers covering women's sports. In the past, female athletes were identified by their first names, which gave the impression that their sports were not as serious as those played by men. As this habit was identified, often by researchers in the sociology of sport, announcers changed how they talked about women athletes. This was a relatively minor change, but it altered narratives so that women's sports were presented more seriously.

> The very passion we invest in sports can transform it from a kind of mindless escape into a site of resistance. It can become an arena where the ideas of our society are not only presented but also challenged. —Dave Zirin, sport journalist (2005)

Overall, cultural theories focus attention on issues of ideology, representation, and power dynamics in society. They explain how people use power to maintain cultural practices and social structures that represent their interests, and they identify how people resist or oppose those practices and structures. This is important to know when developing effective strategies for changing sports.

Research using cultural theories helps us envision sports that are inclusive and empowering. Goals based on cultural theories usually are reformist, seldom conservative, and occasionally radical. For this reason, cultural theories may be seen as threatening by many people who want only to expand sports as they are currently defined and organized.

Interactionist Theories   When people use interactionist theories, they focus on processes of social learning and development and the relationships through which people come to know and give meaning to the world. Interactionist theories explain that changing sports involves changing socialization processes, self-concepts and identities, and the priorities given to particular role models and significant others. For example, people often resist reformist and radical changes because their identities are grounded in and supported by the current culture and organization of sports. This is useful to know because it helps us anticipate that people will often be personally defensive in the face of efforts to change sports. Changes threaten their identities and provoke resistance. Therefore, strategies must be presented tactfully, based on clear research evidence, and implemented to include as allies those currently working in sports. Changing sports in this way requires patience, persistence, and a keen awareness of how others perceive and identify themselves with and through sports.

Interactionist theories can be used to support conservative, reformist, or radical goals, but they generally emphasize the need to include multiple voices and perspectives in the change process. The assumption underlying these theories is that when voices are effectively represented in social worlds, the organization of those worlds is more likely to support their interests and concerns. However, those using a critical approach usually combine interactionist theory with cultural theory and focus on power as well as representation. This often takes them in the direction of reform and transformation (Denzin, 2007).

Structural Theories   When people use structural theories, they focus on social organization and who has access to power, authority, material resources, and economic opportunities. Structural theories explain that changing sports involves changing the context in which social relationships exist. Functionalism is a form of structural theory based on the assumption that all social worlds are organized around shared values and ultimately become more efficient and socially integrated. This approach appeals to people with vested interests in the status quo because it supports an emphasis on growth and minor reforms. As a result it is consistent with conservative and only slightly reformist goals.

Conflict theory, grounded in the ideas of Karl Marx, is another form of structural theory. It identifies the economic factors that create social-class divisions in society and determine life chances and lifestyles among people in all social classes. Conflict theory is most consistent with reformist or radical goals such as redistributing power and economic resources so that relationships are more egalitarian and social policies are more responsive to people with the greatest needs in society. When strategies for changing sports are based on conflict theory, they identify the racism, sexism, nationalism, and militarism that distort the meaning, purpose, and organization of sports and they seek to eliminate the profit motive in sport organizations so that sports can be reorganized around the needs of those who play them rather than those who own them.

Social theories can be used to achieve conservative, reformist, or radical goals. But people interested in the sociology of sport are more likely than others, especially those working in sport organizations, to use a critical approach that focuses on reform and transformation (Donnelly et al, 2011, 2015). They focus on what can be done to make sports more democratic, accessible, and humane so that physical activities serve the needs of all people rather than simply expanding what already exists and more efficiently achieving the goals of those who currently control sports.

THE CHALLENGE OF TRANSFORMING SPORTS

Working to bring about changes that achieve conservative goals can be difficult, but people with power and resources often provide support for such goals, such as fostering growth and increasing efficiency. Creating changes to achieve reformist goals is more difficult and often contentious. Reform is often routinely resisted by people with a vested interest in the status quo or by those who fear the uncertainty involved when the status quo changes.

When existing forms of social organization or rules and traditions support a system of privilege for people involved in a sport, they see change as a threat to the benefits and privileges they define as normal (Travers, 2013a). We continue to see this in public schools, where achieving gender equity requires that people revise or abandon the ideological perspectives that they have used in the past to predict, interpret, and guide the feelings, thoughts, and actions of males and females. Similar resistance occurs when change requires revisions of racial ideology or ideas and beliefs about ethnicity, nationality, social class, age, and ability. Even reforms designed to *simply* "level the playing field" become complex and contentious when people privileged by the status quo see the playing field as already level.

Challenges become even greater when changes require transforming the structure of sport, changing rules, roles, relationships, and reward systems in the process. Even talk about transformation creates defensiveness and resistance that is grounded in identities and lifestyles. This is especially the case when people believe the great sport myth. They feel that sport is essentially pure and good and organized as it was meant to be organized. Even minor transformations are tenaciously resisted (Travers, 2013b).

This can be seen by going to a meeting of Little League coaches and telling them that research shows that, to protect the developing arms of ten- to twelve-year-olds who throw existing "official" balls thousands of times each year, the size of the ball must be reduced to better fit the youngsters' hand size. Or try telling hockey coaches that players under thirteen years old should no longer be allowed to body check and that children under ten should play on smaller cross-rink surfaces instead of the full-length surface. For the most definitive evidence of resistance to transforming sports, tell youth and high school football coaches that tackle football is being replaced by flag football for all children under fourteen years old until we know more about the consequences of repetitive head trauma and concussions on young, developing brains.

Changing sports is so difficult that people who want different sport experiences find it easier to create new sports. This was done in 2005 by students at Middlebury College in Vermont when they created Quidditch for Muggles, a Harry Potter–inspired game that now has annual international tournaments with teams from dozens of countries (Cohen and Peachey, 2015). It was also done by two students in a Harvard business class who created "Tough Mudder" obstacle course events—these mandated that all participants must pledge to, among other things, "put teamwork and camaraderie before my course time" and "help my fellow Mudders complete the course" (http://toughmudder.com/about/; Murphy, 2013; Weedon, 2015). Today there are hundreds of "Tough Mudder" events worldwide.

> Athletes who speak out on issues of social justice invariably pay a price. It's a problem that powerful commercial interests control the language of sports . . . because sports culture shapes other cultural attitudes, norms and power arrangements.
> —The Editors, *The Nation* (2011)

Athletes as Change Agents

Some people think that athletes should and could be effective agents of change because they are highly visible and popular in society. Athletes have a ready-made platform from which they can announce goals and promote strategies to achieve them. But things are not so simple.

The visibility and popularity of athletes depends heavily on media coverage and overall public image. Leagues, teams, and corporations use athletes' images to promote events and products, but this does not mean that athletes can readily convert their celebrity status into power related to serious social, political, or economic issues in sports or society.

The social context of sport celebrity limits the extent to which athletes can be effective agents of change. If the words and actions of athletes don't match the interests of those who control their images, they risk losing the coverage and support that sustains their celebrity. Team owners and corporate sponsors usually avoid relationships with athletes who speak out on social issues; neither owners nor corporations want to alienate fans and consumers.

Adonal Foyle, a social and political activist who played in the NBA from 1997 through 2009, notes that few athletes speak out, even though many have strong thoughts and feelings on certain issues. He says that they're "cautious because they don't want to stand out of the crowd and be controversial in that way" (in Zirin, 2004).

It's not surprising that socially concerned athletes select conservative strategies, often focusing on helping individual children. Building playgrounds, visiting children in hospitals, promoting literacy, and delivering anti-drug messages in high schools are also noncontroversial because they reaffirm dominant societal values and strengthen the status quo.

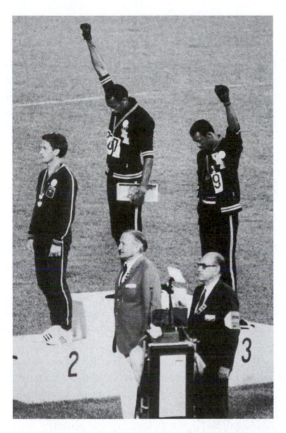 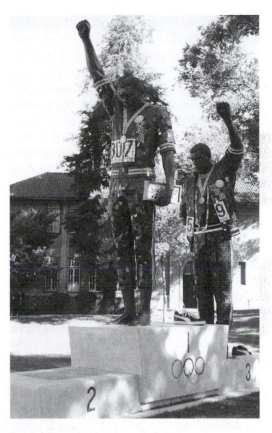

Tommy Smith and John Carlos took off their shoes and raised gloved fists to protest poverty and racism as they stood on the victory podium during the 1968 Olympic Games in Mexico City (*Source:* © Bettmann/Corbis). This action caused them to be expelled from the U.S. team and sent back to the United States, where they were widely criticized and demeaned for more than twenty years. Nearly four decades later–in 2005–they received honorary doctorates from San Jose State University, where a 23-foot-high statue (right) commemorates their commitment to the transformative goals of racial justice and the elimination of poverty. (*Source:* © Jay Johnson)

Individual athletes have occasionally resisted the sports establishment or advocated progressive changes, but they have usually endured negative consequences unless they have done it as part of a larger group of athletes that have relatively widespread public support. Evidence suggests that athletes can lessen the risks of promoting reformist and radical goals by working in or through established organizations that provide them with cover, support, and resources connecting them with larger efforts to promote change.

Former NBA player Adonal Foyle realized the importance of having this form of institutional legitimacy and support when he established his foundation, Democracy Matters (www.democracymatters.org) while playing for the Golden State Warriors. Through the foundation he speaks out on selected issues, but he also uses it to recruit college students to become involved in political efforts to reduce government corruption and increase democratic participation.

More recently, between 2009 and 2016 a few athletes have spoken out and taken stands in support of gay rights and gay marriage, Black Lives Matter, and protests against the racist treatment of students of color at the University of Missouri (Zirin, 2013h, 2013i, 2015a, 2015b, 2015c, 2015d). In some cases, these athletes were attacked by powerful people who wanted their teams and leagues to sanction them. But when people in the general public came to their defense, they escaped sanctions and even had an impact on the issues that they supported. This does not mean that players can now speak their minds freely on important issues and the need for social justice and progressive change but it does suggest that when players know that organizations and individuals will come to their defense, they may be able to advocate for significant changes without ending their careers (Lipsyte, 2011). However, their agents and lawyers will continue to encourage them to focus on conservative goals (Henderson, 2009; G. Smith, 2012).

College athletes, regardless of their media profiles, take a big risk if they speak out, because they have no players' association to protect them and they lack formal power in both the NCAA and the university. Scholarships and team membership are completely dependent on coaches, and future opportunities to play professionally or even to obtain jobs outside of sports could be jeopardized if they advocate an unpopular position. Despite recent cases in which groups of athletes have spoken out or taken a stand on a controversial issue, most college athletes, even in Division II and III sports, have little time to become involved in change-oriented efforts (Cunningham and Regan, 2011).

A Final Word About Change

Regardless of one's vantage point or theories used to develop strategies to change sports, being an effective agent of change always requires the following qualities:

1. Visions of what sports and social life *could* and *should* be like
2. Willingness to work hard on the strategies needed to turn visions into realities

3. Political abilities to rally the resources that make strategies effective in producing changes

Bringing these qualities together requires individual and collective efforts. If we don't make these efforts, the meaning, purpose, and organization of sports will be based on the interests of those who currently control and organize them.

summary

WHAT DO WE WANT SPORTS TO BE?

Sports are social constructions. This means that we play a role in making them what they are today and what they will be in the future. We can play this role actively by envisioning what we'd like sports to be and then working to make them so, or we can play it passively by doing nothing and allowing others to shape sports as they want them to be.

This chapter emphasized that the meaning, purpose, and organization of sports will become increasingly diverse in the future, and that power and performance sports will remain dominant because they continue to attract wealthy and powerful sponsors. Pleasure and participation sports will grow in connection with demographic trends and ideological changes, but they will not attract as much sponsorship as is enjoyed by power and performance sports.

Sports at all levels of participation are sites for struggles over who should play and how sports should be organized. Current trends suggest that pleasure and participation sports are supported by concerns about health and fitness, the participation preferences of older people whose influence will increase in the future, the values and experiences brought to sports by women, and groups seeking alternative sports.

Current trends are influenced by many factors, including values supportive of organization and rationalization, a cultural emphasis on commercialism and consumption, the media, new technologies, and the changing demographic composition of communities and societies.

Changing sports is a process that involves identifying goals, assessing what can be done from the vantage point that one occupies relative to sports in society, and using theories to plan effective strategies. Goals can be growth, reform, or transformation. Most people, especially those who are advantaged by the status quo, focus on the conservative goal of growth because they want to expand and strengthen sports as they are currently played and organized. Some people focus on the goal of reform because they want more people to enjoy the benefits that sports have to offer. And a few people focus on the radical goal of transformation because they want to remake sports with new meaning, purpose, and organization.

The effectiveness of people who want to be agents of change requires a clear understanding of the vantage point they occupy in the relationship between sports and society. The four major vantage points are in (a) sport organizations; (b) opposition groups; (c) groups that create new and alternative sport forms; and (d) groups working to transform the larger society in ways that will change sports.

Efforts to bring about change can utilize strategies based on cultural, interactionist, or structural theories, regardless of goals. Cultural theories emphasize that the future of sports is linked with the symbols, values, norms, and ideologies that people use as they organize and give meaning to sports and sport experiences. Interactionist theories emphasize that changes occur in connection with socialization processes, identities, and the influence of peers and significant others. Structural theories emphasize that changing sports requires changes in the larger context in which sports exist.

Social theories can support conservative, reformist, or radical goals. Scholars in the sociology of sport tend to be reformist and occasionally radical rather than conservative, and they often focus on making sports more democratic, accessible, inclusive, and humane.

Regardless of one's goals, vantage point, or theories used to develop strategies, being an effective agent of change requires a clear vision of what sports could and should be in the future, a willingness to work hard on turning visions into realities, and possessing the political abilities to initiate and maintain strategies that produce results. Unless we work to make sports into what we want them to be, they will reflect primarily the interests of those who want us to play on their terms and for their purposes.

This leaves us with an interesting choice: we can be consumers who accept sports as they are, or we can be citizens who actively work to make sports humane and sustainable. The goal of this book is to prepare people to be critically informed and active citizens.

SUPPLEMENTAL READINGS

Reading 1. Sport fans as agents of change
Reading 2. Technology and change in sports
Reading 3. Working for change: Charity versus social justice
Reading 4. Using sports to make change: Does it work?

SPORT MANAGEMENT ISSUES

- You are the new director of community sports and recreation in a city of 300,000 people. The motto of your department is *Sport for All—Play for Life.* The programs with the most participants are organized around a pleasure and participation model. In the face of budget cuts, you hope to convince a large company in the city to sponsor those programs. List and explain the main points you will make in your presentation to the company officials.
- Your sport management and development consulting firm has been hired by a major city to develop a proposal for building a Miracle Field and forming a Miracle League. The proposal will be used to convince voters that they should support a bond issue that will be the source of funding for these things. Outline and explain the points you will include in your proposal.
- You are an agent for five professional athletes—they all play different sports, but they

are all located in the same city. They come to you as a group and say that they want to be meaningfully involved in creating a culture of sport participation in their city. They look to you for guidance in setting goals, and for creating effective strategies to increase the

community's physical activity and sport participation. Using material from this chapter, identify the issues they should consider as they create specific goals and plan their strategies to achieve them. Additionally, what advice would you give them in their roles as change agents?

REFERENCES

AAA. 2006a. Science: 1680s–1800s: Early classification of nature. (http://www.understandingrace.org/history/science/early_class.html). In American Anthropological Association. *Race: Are we so different*. Online: http://www.understandingrace.org/about/index.html.

AAA. 2006b. 1770s–1850s: One race or several species. (http://www.understandingrace.org/history/science/one_race.html). In American Anthropological Association. *Race: Are we so different*. Online: http://www.understandingrace.org/about/index.html.

AAA. 2006c. 1830s–1890s: Race science exhibitions. (http://www.understandingrace.org/history/science/race_science_exhibit.html). In American Anthropological Association. *Race: Are we so different*. Online: http://www.understandingrace.org/about/index.html.

AAHPERD. 2013. Maximizing the benefits of youth sport. *Journal of Physical Education, Recreation and Dance* 84(7): 8–13.

Abad-Santos, Alexander. 2013. Everything you need to know about Steubenville High's football 'rape crew'. *The Atlantic Wire* (January 3): http://www.theatlanticwire.com/national/2013/01/steubenville-high-football-rape-crew/60554/ (retrieved 5-22-13).

Abdel-Shehid, Gamal, and Nathan Kalman-Lamb. 2011. *Out of left field: Social inequality and sport*. Black Point, Nova Scotia: Fernwood Publishing.

Abrams, Douglas E. 2013. Confronting the youth sports concussion crisis: A central role for responsible local enforcement of playing rules. *Mississippi Sports Law Review* 2(1): 75–114.

Abrams, Lindsey. 2012. Sex doesn't always sell: Why female Olympians fail in advertisements. *The Atlantic* (August 3): http://www.theatlantic.com/health/archive/2012/08/sex-doesnt-always-sell-why-female-olympians-fail-in-advertisements/260658/.

Ackerman, Kathryn E., and Madhusmita Misra. 2011. Bone health and the Female Athlete Triad in adolescent athletes. *The Physician and Sportsmedicine* 39: 131–141.

Acosta, R. Vivian. 1999. Hispanic women in sport. *Journal of Physical Education, Recreation and Dance* 70(4): 44–46.

Acosta, Vivien, and Linda Jean Carpenter. 2012. *Women in Intercollegiate Sport: A Longitudinal, National Study Thirty–Five Year Update*. See www.AcostaCarpenter.org.

Adair, Daryl, Tracy Taylor, and Simon Darcy. 2010. Managing ethnocultural and 'racial' diversity in sport: Obstacles and opportunities. *Sport Management Review* 13(2): 307–312.

Adams, Adi, and Eric Anderson. 2011. Exploring the relationship between homosexuality and sport among the teammates of a small, Midwestern Catholic college soccer team. *Sport, Education and Society* 17(3): 347–363.

Adams, Adi. 2011. "Josh wears pink cleats:" 'Doing gender' on a U.S. college men's soccer team. *Journal of Homosexuality* 58(5): 579–596.

Adams, Mary Louise. 2006. The game of whose lives? Gender, race and entitlement in Canada's 'national' game. In David Whitson and Richard Gruneau, eds., *Artificial ice: Hockey, culture, and commerce* (pp. 71–84). Peterborough, Ontario: Broadview Press.

Adams, Natalie, Auson Schmitke, and Amy Franklin. 2005. Tomboys, dykes, and girly girls: Interrogating the subjectivities of adolescent female athletes. *Women's Studies Quarterly* 33(1/2): 17–34.

Addams, Jane. 1909. *The spirit of youth and the city streets*. New York: Macmillan.

Adelman, Miriam & Lennita Ruggi. 2015. The sociology of the body. *Current Sociology* (Online first, September 7): DOI: 0011392115596561.

Adler, Patricia A., and Peter Adler. 1991. *Backboards and blackboards: College athletes and role engulfment*. New York: Columbia University Press.

Adler, Patricia A., and Peter Adler. 1999. College athletes in high-profile media sports: The consequences of glory. In Jay Coakley & Peter Donnelly, eds., *Inside sports* (pp. 162–170). London: Routledge.

Adler, Patricia A., and Peter Adler. 2003. The promise and pitfalls of going into the field. *Contexts* 2(2): 41–47.

Age Concern. 2006. *Ageism: A benchmark of public attitudes in Britain*. London: Age Concern.

Agyemang, Kwame JA. 2012. Black male athlete activism and the link to Michael Jordan: A transformational leadership and social cognitive theory analysis. *International Review for the Sociology of Sport* 47(4): 433–445.

Agyemang, Kwame, John N. Singer, and Joshua DeLorme. 2010. An exploratory study of black male college athletes' perceptions on race and athlete activism. *International Review for the Sociology of Sport* 45: 419–435.

Ahlberg, Matthew, Cliford J. Mallet, and Richard Tinning. 2008. Developing autonomy supportive coaching behaviors: An action research approach to coach development. *International Journal of Coaching Science* 2(2): 3–22.

Ahmad, Aisha. 2011. British football: Where are the Muslim female footballers? Exploring the connections between gender, ethnicity and Islam. *Soccer & Society* 12(3): 443–456.

Ahmed, Nadia. 2013. Paralympics 2012 legacy: Accessible housing and disability equality or inequality? *Disability & Society* 28(1): 129–133.

Albergotti, Reed. 2011. The footage the NFL won't show you. *Wall Street Journal* (November 4): http://online.wsj.com/article/SB10001424052970203716204577015903150731054.html.

Algazeera. 2006. Glory for Al Ghasara. *Algazeera.net* (December 11): http://english.aljazeera.net/NR /exeres/A3E2CB0F-A9CA-4327-A07B-4675C98E13C7.htm.

Allain, Kristi A. 2008. "Real fast and tough": The construction of Canadian hockey masculinity. *Sociology of Sport Journal* 25(4): 462–481.

Allan, Elizabeth J., and Mary Madden. 2008. Hazing in view: College students at risk. University of Maine, College of Education and Human Development.

Allen, James T., Dan D. Drane, Kevin K. Byon, and Richard S. Mohnb. 2010. Sport as a vehicle for socialization and maintenance of cultural identity: International students attending American universities. *Sport Management Review* 13(4): 421–434.

Alpert, Geoff, Jeff Rojek, Andy Hansen, Randy L. Shannon, and Scott H. Decker. 2011. *Examining the prevalence and impact of gangs in college athletic programs using multiple sources.* Bureau of Justice Assistance, the Office of Justice Programs, the U.S. Department of Justice (2008-F3611-SC-DD).

Alpert, Rebecca T. 2011. *Out of left field: Jews and black baseball.* Oxford, UK: Oxford University Press.

Altice, Chelsea. 2012. Lingerie football touches down in Abbotsford. *ctvbc.ca* (Feb. 9): http://www.ctvbc.ctv.ca/servlet/an/local/CTVNews/20120209/bc_lingerie_league_abbotsford_120209.

Amara, Mahfoud. 2007. An introduction to the study of sport in the Muslim world. In Barrie Houlihan, ed., *Sport and society: A student introduction* (2nd edition). London: Sage.

Amara, Mahfoud. 2008. The Muslim world in the global sporting arena. *The Brown Journal of World Affairs* 14(2): 67–76. Online: http://www.bjwa.org/article.php?id=lA4qNzhx371AQ441HNfY3nD8L4nal9j135l80fMc.

Amara, Mahfoud. 2010. Sport development in the Arab world: Between tradition and modernity. In Barrie Houlihan & Mick Green, eds., *A handbook of sport development* (pp. 114–126). New York/London: Routledge.

Amara, Mahfoud. 2013. Sport, Islam, and Muslims in Europe: In between or on the margin? *Religions* 4(4): 644–656.

Amick, Sam. 2014. For NBA teams, religion can be unifying or divisive. *USA Today* (May 4): http://www.usatoday.com/story/sports/nba/2014/05/03/nba-clippers-warriors-doc-rivers-mark-jackson-monty-williams-religion/8658755/.

Anderson, Eric. 2014. *21st Century jocks: Teamsport athletes and modern heterosexuality.*

Anderson, Eric, and Mark McCormack. 2015. Cuddling and spooning: Heteromasculinity and homosocial tactility among student-athletes. *Men and Masculinities* 18(2): 214–230.

Anderson, Eric, and Rachael Bullingham. 2015. Openly lesbian team sport athletes in an era of decreasing homohysteria. *International Review for the Sociology of Sport* 50(6): 647–660.

Anderson, Eric. 2015. *21st century jocks: Sporting men and contemporary heterosexuality.* Palgrave Macmillan.

Anderson, Eric. 2015. Assessing the sociology of sport: On changing masculinities and homophobia *International Review for the Sociology of Sport* 50(4–5): 363–367.

Anderson, Denise. 2009. Adolescent girls' involvement in disability sport: Implications for identity development. *Journal of Sport and Social Issues* 33(4): 427–449.

Anderson, Eric. 2005b. Orthodox, and inclusive masculinity: Competing masculinities among heterosexual men in a feminized terrain. *Sociological Perspectives* 48: 337–355.

Anderson, Eric. 2008a. "Being masculine is not about who you sleep with . . .": Heterosexual athletes contesting masculinity and the one-time rule of homosexuality. *Sex Roles* 58: 104–115.

Anderson, Eric. 2008b. "I used to think women were weak": Orthodox masculinity, gender segregation, and sport. *Sociological Forum* 23: 257–280.

Anderson, Eric. 2009a. The maintenance of masculinity among the stakeholders of sport. *Sport Management Review* 12(1): 3–14.

Anderson, Eric. 2009b. *Inclusive masculinity: The changing nature of masculinities.* New York: Routledge.

Anderson, Eric. 2011a. Inclusive masculinities of university soccer players in the American Midwest. *Gender and Education* 23(6): 729–744.

Anderson, Eric. 2011b. Masculinities and sexualities in sports and physical cultures: Three decades of evolving research. *Journal of Homosexuality* 58(5): 565–578.

Anderson, Eric. 2011c. The rise and fall of western homohysteria. *Journal of Feminist Scholarship* 1(1): 80–94.

Anderson, Eric. 2011d. Updating the outcome: Gay athletes, straight teams, and coming out at the end of the decade. *Gender & Society* 25(2): 250–268.

Anderson, Eric. 2013. i9 and the transformation of youth sports. *Journal of Sport and Social Issues* 37(1): 97–111.

Anderson, Eric, and Edward M. Kian. 2012. Examining media contestation of masculinity and head trauma in the National Football League. *Men and Masculinities* 15(2): 152–173.

Anderson, Eric, and Rhidian McGuire. 2010. Inclusive masculinity and the gendered politics of men's rugby. *Journal of Gender Studies* 19: 249–261.

Anderson, Eric, and Rachael Bullingham. 2013. Openly lesbian team sport athletes in an era of decreasing homohysteria. *International Review for the Sociology of Sport;* online, June 10, 2013 1012690213490520.

Andrews, David L., ed. 1996a. Deconstructing Michael Jordan: Reconstructing postindustrial America. *Sociology of Sport Journal* 13(4): special issue.

Andrews, David L. 1996b. The fact(s) of Michael Jordan's blackness: Excavating a floating racial signifier. *Sociology of Sport Journal* 13(2): 125–158.

Andrews, David L., ed. 2001. *Michael Jordan, Inc.: Corporate sport, media culture, and late modern America.* Albany, NY: State University of New York Press.

Andrews, David L. 2007. Sport as spectacle. In George Ritzer, ed., *Encyclopedia of sociology* (pp. 4702–4704). London/New York: Blackwell.

Andrews, David L., and Steven J. Jackson. 2001. *Sport stars: The cultural politics of sporting celebrity.* London/New York: Routledge.

Andrews, David L., and Michael L. Silk, eds. 2011. Physical cultural studies. *Sociology of Sport Journal* 28(1): special issue.

Anshel, Mark H., and Mitchell Smith. 2013. The role of religious leaders in promoting healthy habits in religious communities. *Journal of Religion and Health;* Online-First: doi: 10.1007/s10943-013-9702-5.

Antunovic, Dunja & Marie Hardin. 2012. Activism in women's sport blogs: Fandom and feminist potential. International Journal of Sport Communication 5(3): 305–322.

Antunovic, Dunja, and Marie Hardin. 2013. Women bloggers: Identity and the conceptualization of sports. *New Media & Society* 15(8): 1374–1392.

Antunovic, Dunja & Marie Hardin. 2015. Women and the blogosphere: Exploring feminist approaches to sport. *International Review for the Sociology of Sport* 50(6): 661–677.

AP. 2013. Facing class action threat, NCAA responds on concussions. *USA Today* (July 20): http://www.usatoday.com/story/sports/college/2013/07/20/ncaa-concussion-suit-and-response/2572071/.

Apelmo, Elisabet. 2012. Falling in love with a wheelchair: Enabling/disabling technologies. *Sport in Society* 15(3): 399–408.

Apostolis, Nicolas, and Audrey R. Giles. 2011. Portrayals of women golfers in the 2008 issues of *Golf Digest. Sociology of Sport Journal* 28(2): 226–238.

Appleby, Joyce. 2011. The wealth divide. *Los Angeles Times* (November 7): http://www.latimes.com/news/opinion/commentary/la-oe-appleby-wealth-versus-income-20111107%2C0%2C5865891.

Araki Kaori, Iky Kodani, Nidhi Gupta, and Diane L. Gill. 2013. Experiences in sport, physical activity, and physical education among Christian, Buddhist, and Hindu Asian adolescent girls. *Journal of Preventive Medicine and Public Health* 46(1): 43–49.

Archer, Louise, Sumi Hollingworth, and Anna Halsall. 2007. 'University's not for me—I'm a Nike person': Urban, working-class young people's negotiations of 'style,' identity and educational engagement. *Sociology* 41(2): 219–237.

Armstrong, Gary. 1998. *Football hooligans: Knowing the score.* Oxford: Berg.

Armstrong, Gary. 2007. Football hooliganism. In George Ritzer, ed., *Encyclopedia of sociology* (pp. 1767–1769). London/New York: Blackwell.

Armstrong, Gary, and Alberto Testa. 2010. *Football, fascism and fandom: The UltraS of Italian football.* A and C Black Publishers Ltd.

Aschwanden, Christie. 2012. The top athletes looking for an edge and the scientists trying to stop them. *Smithsonian* (July–August): http://www.smithsonianmag.com/science-nature/The-Top-Athletes-Looking-for-an-Edge-and-the-Scientists-Trying-to-Stop-Them-160284335.html.

Aspen Institute. 2015. *Project play report.* Washington, DC: Aspen Institute.

Assael, Shaun. 2008. Who is Martin Führer and why does he make the tennis world so nervous? *ESPN The Magazine* 11.04 (February 25): 82–88.

Associated Press. 2012. Sidebar quote. *Denver Post* (January 29): 2C.

Atencio, Matthew, and Becky Beal. 2011. Beautiful losers: The symbolic exhibition and legitimization of outsider masculinity. *Sport in Society* 14(1): 1–16.

Atencio, Matthew, and Jan Wright. 2008. "We be killin' them": Hierarchies of black masculinity in urban basketball spaces. *Sociology of Sport Journal* 25(2): 263–280.

Atencio, Matthew, Emily Chivers Yochim, and Becky Beal. 2013. "It ain't just black kids and white kids": The representation and reproduction of authentic "skurban" masculinities. *Sociology of Sport Journal* 30(2):153–172.

Atkinson, Michael. 2009. Parkour, anarcho-environmentalism, and poiesis. *Journal of Sport and Social Issues* 33(2): 169–194.

Atkinson, Michael, and Kevin Young. 2008. *Deviance and social control in sport.* Champaign, IL: Human Kinetics.

Atkinson, Michael, and Kevin Young. 2012. Shadowed by the corpse of war: Sport spectacles and the spirit of terrorism. *International Review for the Sociology of Sport* 47(3): 286–306.

Aubel, Olivier, and Brice Lefèvre. 2013. The comparability of quantitative surveys on sport participation in France (1967–2010). *International Review for the Sociology of Sport* 1012690213492964, first published on July 17, 2013 as doi: 10.1177/1012690213492964.

Axon, Rachel. 2013a. Does NCAA face more concussion liability than NFL? *USA Today* (July 25): http://www.usatoday.com/story/sports/ncaaf/2013/07/25/ncaa-concussion-lawsuit-adrian-arrington/2588189/.

Axon, Rachel. 2013b. Fifth concussion lawsuit filed against NCAA. *USA Today* (November 15): http://www.usatoday.com/story/sports/college/2013/11/15/ncaa-concussion-lawsuit-class-action-christopher-powell/3594003/.

Azimirad, Javad, and Mohammad Jalilvand. 2012. Relationship between spiritual transcendence and competitive anxiety in male athletes. *European Journal of Experimental Biology* 2(4): 1095–1097.

Baade, Robert A., Robert W. Baumann, and Victor A. Matheson. 2008. Assessing the economic impact of college football games on local economies. *Journal of Sports Economics* 9(6): 628–643.

Bachman, Rachel. 2012. Schools that train the enemy. *Wall Street Journal* (June 5): http://online.wsj.com/article/SB10001424052702303830204577448620436755502.html.

Bacon, Victoria L., and Pamela J. Russell. 2004. Addiction and the college athlete: The Multiple Addictive Behaviors Questionnaire (MABQ) with college athletes. *The Sport Journal* 7(2): unpaginated.

Badenhausen, Kurt. 2015. Michael Jordan Leads The Highest-Paid Retired Athletes 2015. *Forbes.com* (March 11): http://www.forbes.com/sites/kurtbadenhausen/2015/03/11/michael-jordan-leads-the-highest-paid-retired-athletes-2015/#21d7e538155e.

Bain-Selbo, Eric. 2008. Ecstasy, joy, and sorrow: The religious experience of southern college football.

Journal of Religion and Popular Culture 20 (Fall): http://www.usask.ca/relst/jrpc/articles20.html

Bain-Selbo, Eric. 2009. *Game day and God: Football, faith, and politics in the American South.* Macon, GA: Mercer University Press.

Baird, Julia. 2004. Privacy, a forgotten virtue. *Newsweek* (December 14): 29.

Bairner, Alan, and Dong-Jhy Hwang. 2011. Representing Taiwan: International sport, ethnicity and national identity in the Republic of China. *International Review for the Sociology of Sport* 46(3): 231–248.

Baker, Al. 2013. Culture warrior, gaining ground. *New York Times* (September 27): http://www.nytimes.com/2013/09/28/books/e-d-hirsch-sees-his-education-theories-taking-hold.html.

Baker, Phyllis L., and Douglas R. Hotek. 2011. Grappling with gender: Exploring masculinity and gender in the bodies, performances, and emotions of scholastic wrestlers. *Journal of Feminist Scholarship* 1 (Fall): 4–64. Online: http://www1.umassd.edu/jfs/issue1/pdfs/bakerhotek.pdf.

Baker, Stephanie Alice, and David Rowe. 2012. Mediating mega events and manufacturing multiculturalism: The cultural politics of the world game in Australia. *Journal of Sociology* published 25 July 2012.

Baker, William J. 2007. *Playing with God: Religion and modern sport.* Cambridge, MA: Harvard University Press.

Balmer, Nigel, Pascoe Pleasence, and Alan Nevill. 2012. Evolution and revolution: Gauging the impact of technological and technical innovation on Olympic performance. *Journal of Sports Sciences* 30(11): 1075–1083.

Balyi, Istvan, Richard Way, and Colin Higgs. 2013. *Long-term athlete development.* Champaign, IL USA: Human Kinetics.

Bandow, Doug. 2003. *Surprise: Stadiums don't pay after all!* Cato Institute Report (October 19). Washington, DC: Cato Institute.

Bank, Hannah. 2012. *Straight: The surprisingly short history of heterosexuality.* Beacon Press.

Banet-Weiser, Sarah. 1999. Hoop dreams: Professional basketball and the politics of race and gender. *Journal of Sport and Social Issues* 23(4): 403–420.

Banton, Michael. 2012. The colour line and the colour scale in the twentieth century. *Ethnic and Racial Studies* 35(7): 1109–1131.

Barnett, Lisa M., Eric Van Beurden, Philip J. Morgan, Lyndon O. Brooks, and John R. Beard. 2008. Does childhood motor skill proficiency predict adolescent fitness? *Medicine and Science in Sports and Exercise* 40(12): 2137–2144.

Barr, John. 2009. Athletes and evangelists cross paths. *ESPN Outside the Lines* (April 17): http://sports.espn.go.com/espn/otl/news/story?id=4076585.

Bartholomaeus, Clare. 2012. 'I'm not allowed wrestling stuff': Hegemonic masculinity and primary school boys. *Journal of Sociology* 48(3): 227–247.

Bartoluci, Sunčica, and Benjamin Perasović. 2009. National identity and sport: The case of Croatia. In Mojca Doupona Topič & Simon Ličen, eds., *Sport, culture & society: An account of views and perspectives on social issues in a continent (and beyond)* (pp. 187–191). Ljubljana, Slovenia: University of Ljubljana.

Baruth, Meghan, Sara Wilcox, Ruth P. Saunders, Steven P. Hooker, James R. Hussey, and Steven N. Blair. 2013. Perceived environmental church support and physical activity black church members. *Health Education and Behavior* 40(6): 712–720.

Bass, Amy 2002. *Not the triumph but the struggle: The 1968 Olympics and the making of the black athlete.* Minneapolis, MN: University of Minnesota Press.

Battista, Judy. 2012. N.F.L. Super Bowl ad will stress safety. *New York Times* (January 31): http://www.nytimes.com/2012/01/31/sports/football/nfl-to-address-head-injuries-in-commercial.html

Bauer, Olivier. 2011. *Hockey as a religion: The Montreal Canadiens.* Champaign, IL: Common Ground Publishing-Sport and Society.

Bauer, Thomas, and Tony Froissart. 2011. Jacques Morneve: Narrative glorification of Catholic sport. *The International Journal of the History of Sport* 28(14): 2047–2060.

BBC. 2012a. London 2012: Olympics women's boxing skirts issue to be decided. *BBC.co.uk* (January 24): http://news.bbc.co.uk/sport2/hi/boxing/16608826.stm.

BBC. 2012b. Olympics judo: Saudi Arabia judoka could pull out in hijab row. *BBC.co.uk* (July 30): http://www.bbc.co.uk/sport/0/olympics/19046923.

BBC. 2013. Nigeria 'lesbian football ban' reports examined by Fifa. *BBC.co.uk* (March7): http://www.bbc.co.uk/sport/0/football/21702308.

Beal, Becky. 1995. Disqualifying the official: An exploration of social resistance through the subculture of skateboarding. *Sociology of Sport Journal* 12(3): 252–267.

Beal, Becky. 1997. The Promise Keeper's use of sport in defining "Christ-like" masculinity. *Journal of Sport and Social Issues* 21(3): 274–284.

Beal, Becky, and Lisa Weidman. 2003. Authenticity in the skateboarding world. In Robert E. Rinehart & Synthia Sydnor, eds., *To the extreme: Alternative sports, inside and out* (pp. 337–352). Albany: State University of New York Press.

Beals, Katherine A., and Amanda K. Hill. 2006. The prevalence of disordered eating, menstrual dysfunction, and low bone mineral density among US collegiate athletes. *International Journal of Sport Nutrition and Exercise Metabolism* 16(1): 1–23.

Beamish, Rob, and Ian Ritchie. 2006. *Fastest, highest, strongest: A critique of high-performance sport.* New York and London: Routledge.

Beamish, Rob. 2011. *Steroids: A new look at performance-enhancing drugs.* Santa Barbara, CA: Praeger.

Beamon, Krystal, and Patricia A. Bell. 2006. Academics versus athletics: An examination of the effects on background and socialization on African American male student athletes. *The Social Science Journal* 43(3): 393–403.

Bearak, Barry. 2011. U.F.C. Dips a toe into the mainstream. *New York Times* (November 11): http://www.nytimes.com/imagepages/2011/11/12/sports/12ufc1.html.

Beaton, Anthony A., Daniel C. Funk, Lynn Ridinger, and Jeremy Jordan. 2011. Sport involvement: A conceptual and empirical analysis. *Sport Management Review* 14: 126–140.

Beauchamp-Pryor, Karen. 2011. Impairment, cure and identity: 'Where do I fit in?' *Disability & Society* 26(1): 5–17.

Beaver, Travis D. 2012. "By the skaters, for the skaters" The DIY ethos of the roller derby revival. *Journal of Sport and Social Issues* 36(1): 25–49.

Beck, Howard, and John Branch. 2013. With the words 'I'm gay,' an N.B.A. center breaks a barrier. *New York Times* (April 29): http://www.nytimes.com/2013/04/30/sports/basketball/nba-center-jason-collins-comes-out-as-gay.html.

Becker, Howard. 1998. *Tricks of the trade: How to think about your research while you're doing it.* Chicago: University of Chicago Press.

Beckman, E. et al. 2009. Towards evidence-based classification in Paralympic athletics: Evaluating the validity of activity limitation tests for use in classification of Paralympic running events. *British Journal of Sports Medicine* 43(13): 1067–1072.

Bell, Jarrett. 2013b. Diversity study: Black head coaches rarely get second chances. *USA Today* (May 1): http://www.usatoday.com/story/sports/nfl/2013/05/01/coaching-diversity-rooney-rule-central-florida-keith-harrison/2127051/.

Bell, Nathan T., Scott R. Johnson, and Jeffrey C. Petersen. 2011. Strength of religious faith of athletes and non-athletes at two NCAA Division III institutions. *The Sport Journal* 14: (January 7): http://thesportjournal.org/article/strength-of-religious-faith-of-athletes-and-nonathletes-at-two-ncaa-division-iii-institutions/.

Belson, Ken. 2014. Brain trauma to affect one in three players, N.F.L. agrees. *New York Times* (September 13): http://www.nytimes.com/2014/09/13/sports/football/actuarial-reports-in-nfl-concussion-deal-are-released.html.

Belson, Ken, and Joe Drape. 2015. N.F.L.'s forays to London muddle its stance on sports betting. *New York Times* (October 29): http://www.nytimes.com/2015/10/29/sports/football/nfls-forays-into-london-muddle-its-stance-on-sports-betting.html.

Belson, Ken, and Mary Pilon. 2012. Concern raised over painkiller's use in sports. *New York Times* (April 13): http://www.nytimes.com/2012/04/14/sports/wide-use-of-painkiller-toradol-before-games-raises-concerns.html?_r=0.

Belson, Matthew. 2002. Assistive technology and sports. In Artemis A.W. Joukowsky, III & Larry Rothstein, eds., *Raising the bar* (pp. 124–129). New York: Umbrage.

Benedict, Jeff, and Armen Keteyian. 2011. Straight outta Compton. *Sports Illustrated* 115(22, December 5): 88.

Benedict, Jeff, and Armen Keteyian. 2013. *The system: The glory and scandal of big-time college football.* New York: Doubleday.

Benn, Tansin, Gertrud Pfister, and Haifaa Jawad, eds. 2010. *Muslim women and sport.* Abingdon/NY: Routledge.

Benn, Tansin, Symeon Dagkas, and Haifaa Jawad. 2011. Embodied faith: Islam, religious freedom and educational practices in physical education, *Sport, Education and Society* 16(1): 17–34.

Bennett, Dylan. 2013. Harm reduction and NFL drug policy. *Journal of Sport and Social Issues* 37(2): 160–175.

Benton, Nigel 2010. Fair game? Is the grorevensky within online betting a threat to Australian sport? *Australasian Leisure Management* 78 Jan/Feb: 56, 58.

Berger, Ida E., Norman O'Reilly, Milena M. Parent, Benoit Séguin, and Tony Hernandez. 2008. Determinants of sport participation among Canadian adolescents. *Sport Management Review* 11(3): 277–307.

Berger, Jody. 2002. Pain game. *Rocky Mountain News* (February 23): 6S.

Berkowitz, Steve. 2013. NCAA had record $71 million surplus in fiscal 2012. *USA Today* (May 2): http://www.usatoday.com/story/sports/college/2013/05/02/ncaa-financial-statement-surplus/2128431/.

Berkowitz, Steve, and Jodi Upton. 2013. NCAA member revenue, spending increase. *USA Today* (July 1): http://www.usatoday.com/story/sports/college/2013/05/01/ncaa-spending-revenue-texas-ohio-state-athletic-departments/2128147/.

Berkowitz, Steve, Jodi Upton, and Erik Brady. 2013. Most NCAA Division I athletic departments take subsidies. *USA Today* (May 10): http://www.usatoday.com/story/sports/college/2013/05/07/ncaa-finances-subsidies/2142443/.

Bernache-Assollant, Iouri, Patrick Bouchet, Sarah Auvergne, and Marie-Françoise Lacassagne. 2011. Identity crossbreeding in soccer fan groups: A social approach. The case of Marseille (France). *Journal of Sport and Social Issues* 35(1): 72–100.

Bernhard, Laura M. 2014. "Nowhere for me to go:" Black Female Student-Athlete Experiences on a Predominantly White Campus. *Journal for the Study of Sports and Athletes in Education* 8(2): 67–76.

Bernstein, Samuel B., and Michael T. Friedman. 2013. Sticking out in the field: No, ma'am, I do not work for the governor. *Sociology of Sport Journal* 30(3): 274–295.

Berra, Lindsey. 2005. This is how they roll. *ESPN The Magazine* (December 5): 104–111.

Berri, David J., and Rob Simmons. 2009. Race and the evaluation of signal callers in the National Football League. *Journal of Sports Economics* 10(1): 23–43.

Bhanoo, Sindya N. 2012. For young athletes, good reasons to break the fast-food habit. *New York Times* (September 14): http://well.blogs.nytimes.com/2012/09/14/for-young-athletes-good-reasons-to-break-the-fast-food-habit/.

Bickenbach, Jerome. 2011. The world report on disability. *Disability & Society* 26(5): 655–658.

Biderman, David. 2010a. Announcers weren't always so chatty. *Wall Street Journal* (May 28): D4.

Biderman, David. 2010b. The anatomy of a baseball broadcast. *Wall Street Journal* (October 6): D8.

Bilger, Burkhard. 2004. The height gap. *New Yorker* (April 5): 38–45.

Billings, Andrew C., Natalie A. Brown, Kenon A. Brown, Guoqing, Mark A. Leeman, Simon Ličen, David R. Novak, and David Rowe. 2013. From pride to smugness and the nationalism between: Olympic media consumption effects on nationalism across the globe. *Mass Communication and Society* 16(6): 910–932.

Bimper, Albert Y., Jr., and Louis Harrison, Jr. 2011. Meet me at the crossroads: African American athletic and racial identity. *Quest* 63(3): 275–288.

Bimper, Albert Y. Jr. 2014. Lifting the veil: Exploring colorblind racism in black student athlete experiences. *Journal of Sport and Social Issues* 39(3): 225–243.

Bimper, Albert Y. Jr. 2015. Mentorship of Black student-athletes at a predominately White American university: critical race theory perspective on student-athlete development. *Sport, Education and Society,* DOI: 10.1080/13573322.2015.1022524.

Birchwood Diane, Ken Roberts, and Gary Pollock. 2008. Explaining differences in sport participation rates among young adults: Evidence from the South Caucasus. *European Physical Education Review* 14(3): 283–298.

Biscomb, Kay, and Gerald Griggs. 2012. 'A splendid effort!': Print media reporting of England's women's performance in the 2009 Cricket World Cup. *International Review for the Sociology of Sport* 47(1): 99–111.

Bissinger, H.G. 1990. *Friday night lights.* Reading, MA: Addison-Wesley.

Black, Mathew. 2012. Winner's curse? The economics of hosting the Olympic Games. *CBC News* (July 30): http://www.cbc.ca/news/canada/story/2012/07/18/f-olympic-host-city-economy.html.

Black, Victoria. 2012. The payoff from winning an Olympic medal. *BusinessWeek.com* (August 8): http://www.businessweek.com/articles/2012-08-08/the-payoff-from-winning-an-olympic-medal.

Blades, Nicole. 2005. Lucia Rijker. *ESPN The Magazine* (June 6): 96–97.

Blair, Roger D., and Jessica S. Haynes. 2009. Comment on "A stadium by any other name: The value of naming rights." *Journal of Sports Economics* 10(2): 204–206.

Blazer, Annie. 2015. *Playing for God: Evangelical women and the unintended consequences of sports ministry.* Albany NY: New York University Press.

Blitz, Roger. 2010. Sport organisers play high-stakes game. *Financial Times* (September 28): 7. Online: http://www.ft.com/cms/s/0/d8c14b38-cb26-11df-95c0-00144feab49a.html (see file and hard copy of article).

Blodgett, Amy T., Robert J. Schinke, Duke Peltier, Leslee A. Fisher, Jack W. Watson, and Mary Jo Wabano. 2011. May the circle be unbroken: The research recommendations of Aboriginal community members engaged in participatory action research with university academics. *Journal of Sport and Social Issues* 35(3): 264–283.

Bloodworth, Andrew, Mike McNamee, and Richard Bailey. 2012. Sport, physical activity and well-being: An objectivist account. *Sport, Education and Society* 17(4): 497–514.

Bloom, Benjamin S. 1985. *Developing talent in young people.* New York: Ballantine Books.

Bloom, John. 2000. *To show what an Indian can do: Sports at Native American boarding schools.* Minneapolis: University of Minnesota Press.

Blumenthal, Ralph. 2004. Texas tough, in lipstick, fishnet and skates. *New York Times,* section 1 (August 1): 14.

Blumstein, Alfred & Jeff Benedict. 1999. Criminal violence of NFL players compared to the general population. *Chance* 12(3): 12–15.

Bobswern. 2013. Saez & Piketty income inequality update: Top 1% have received 121% of income gains since 2009. *Dailly Kos* (February 13): http://www.dailykos.com/story/2013/02/13/1186890/-Saez-Piketty-Income-Inequality-Update-Top-1-Have-Received-121-of-Income-Gains-Since-2009.

Bogdanich, Walt, James Glanz, and Agustin Armendariz. 2015. Cash drops and keystrokes: The dark reality of sports betting and daily fantasy games. *New York Times* (October 15): http://www.nytimes.com/interactive/2015/10/15/us/sports-betting-daily-fantasy-games-fanduel-draftkings.html.

Bolaño, Tomás 2013, *Theology of Sport: Object, Sources and Method.* http://www.bubok.com/books/205597/Theology-of-sport-Object-Sources-and-Method.

Booth, Douglas. 2011. Olympic city bidding: An exegesis of power. *International Review for the Sociology of Sport* 46(4): 367–386.

Bopp, Melissa, and Elizabeth A. Fallon. 2011. Individual and institutional influences on faith-based health and wellness programming. *Health Education Research* 26(6): 1107–1119.

Bopp, Melissa, and Elizabeth A. Fallon. 2013. Health and wellness programming on faith-based organizations: A description of a nationwide sample. *Health Promotion Practice* 14(1): 122–131.

Bopp, Melissa, and Benjamin L. Webb. 2013. Factors associated with health promotion on megachurches: Implications for prevention. *Public Health Nursing;* Online-First: doi: 10.1111/phn.12045.

Bopp, Melissa, Diana Lattimore, Sara Wilcox, Marilyn Laken, Lottie McClorin, Rosetta Swinton, Octavia Gethers, and Deborah Bryant. 2007. Understanding physical activity participation in members of an African American church: A qualitative study. *Health Education Research* 22(6): 815–826.

Bopp, Melissa, Meghan Baruth, Jane A. Peterson, and Benjamin L. Webb. 2013. Leading their flocks to health? Clergy health and the role of clergy in faith-based health promotion interventions. *Family Community Health* 36(3): 182–192.

Bopp, Melissa, J.A. Peterson, and Benjamin L. Webb. 2013. A comprehensive review of faith-based physical activity interventions. *American Journal of Lifestyle Medicine* 6(6): 460–478.

Bopp, Melissa, Benjamin L. Webb, M. Baruth, and J.A. Peterson. 2013. The role of pastor support in a faith-based health promotion intervention. *Family Community Health* 36(3): 204–214.

Borden, Sam. 2012. For bettors, Masters is a major event, too. *New York Times* (April 4): http://www.nytimes.com/2012/04/05/sports/golf/masters-is-a-major-event-for-bettors-too.html.

Borden, Sam. 2013. A U.S. soccer star's declaration of independence. *New York Times* (April 10): http://www.nytimes.com/2013/04/11/sports/soccer/megan-rapinoe-does-it-her-way-in-us-and-in-france.html.

Borgers, Julie, Erik Thibaut, Hanne Vandermeerschen, Bart Vanreusel, Steven Vos, and Jeroen Scheerder. 2013. Sports participation styles revisited: A time-trend study in Belgium from the 1970s to the 2000s. *International Review for the Sociology of Sport* 1012690212470823, first published on January 29, 2013 as doi: 10.1177/1012690212470823.

Borland, John F., and Jennifer E. Bruening. 2010. Navigating barriers: A qualitative examination of the underrepresentation of Black females as head coaches in collegiate basketball. *Sport Management Review* 13: 407–420.

Bose, Christine E. 2012. Intersectionality and global gender inequality. *Gender & Society* 26(1): 67–72.

Bourdieu, Pierre. 1986a. *Distinction: A social critique of the judgment of taste*. London: Routledge.

Bourdieu, Pierre. 1986b. The forms of capital. In J. G. Richards, ed., *Handbook of theory and research for the sociology of education* (pp. 242–258). New York: Greenwood Press.

Bourdieu, Pierre. 1998. The essence of neoliberalism (trans. by Jeremy J. Shapiro). *Le Monde diplomatique* (December): http://mondediplo.com /1998/12/08bourdieu.

Bowen, William G., and Sarah Levine. 2003. *Reclaiming the game: College sports and educational values*. Princeton, NJ: Princeton University Press.

Bowen, William G., Martin A. Kurzweil, Eugene M. Tobin, and Suzanne C. Pichler. 2005. *Equity and excellence in American higher education*. Charlottesville, VA: University Press of Virginia.

Boykoff, Jules. 2014a. *Celebration capitalism and the Olympic Games*. London: Routledge.

Boykoff, Jules. 2014b. *Activism and the Olympics*. New Brunswick NJ: Rutgers University Press.

Boylan, Jennifer Finney. 2008. The XY games. *New York Times* (August 3): http://www.nytimes.com /2008/08/03/opinion/03boylan.html.

Boyle, Raymond, and Richard Haynes. 2009. *Power play: Sport, the media and popular culture*. Edinburgh, Scotland: Edinburgh University Press Ltd.

Boyle, Raymond. 2013. Reflections on communication and sport: On journalism and digital. *Communication & Sport* 1(1/2): 88–99.

Boyle, Raymond. 2014. Television sport in the age of screens and content. *Television & New Media* 15(8): 746–751.

Boyle, Robert H. 1970. Oral Roberts: Small but OH MY. *Sports Illustrated* (November 30): 64–66.

Brackenridge, Celia, and Kari Fasting. 2009. The grooming process in sport: Case studies of sexual harassment and abuse. In H. Humana, ed., *KINE 1000 socio-cultural perspectives in kinesiology*. Toronto: McGraw-Hill Ryerson Limited.

Brackenridge, Celia H., Daz Bishopp, and Sybille Moussalli. 2008. The characteristics of sexual abuse in sport: A multidimensional scaling analysis of events described in media reports. *International Journal of Sport and Exercise Psychology* 6(4): 385–406.

Brackenridge, Celia, Kari Fasting, S. Kirby, Trisha Leahy, Sylvie Parent, and Trond Svela Sand. 2010a. *The place of sport in the UN Study on Violence against Children*. Florence, Italy: UNICEF Innocenti Research Centre, IRC Stock No. 595U, Innocenti Discussion Papers, IDP 2010–01.

Brackenridge, Celia, Kari Fasting, S. Kirby, and Trisha Leahy. 2010b. *Protecting Children from Violence in Sport: A review with a focus on industrialized countries*. Florence: United Nations Innocenti Research Centre Review.

Brackenridge, Celia, and Daniel J. A. Rhind, eds. 2010. *Elite child athlete welfare: International perspectives*. London: Brunel University Press. ISBN: 978-1-902316-83-3 (open access, http://www .brunel.ac.uk/about/acad/sse/sseres/sseresearchcentres /youthsport/birnaw) (retrieved 6-26-13).

Bradbury, Steven. 2011. From racial exclusions to new inclusions: Black and minority ethnic participation in football clubs in the East Midlands of England. *International Review for the Sociology of Sport* 46(1): 23–44.

Bradley, Graham L. 2010. Skate parks as context for adolescent development. *Journal of Adolescent Research* 25(2): 288–323.

Bradley, Jeff. 2011. Force out. *ESPN The Magazine* (February 7): 98–103.

Brady, Erik, and Josh Barnett. 2015. Stretching the season: Up to 16-game seasons spark debate on player safety. *USA Today* (December 18): 1C.

Brake, Deborah L. 2010. *Getting in the game: Title IX and the women's sports revolution*. NY: New York University Press.

Branch, John. 2010. Playing with fire, barbed wire and beer. *New York Times* (April 28): http://www .nytimes.com/2010/04/29/sports/29mudder.html.

Branch, John. 2011. Site provides a rare forum for gay athletes. *New York Times* (April 7): http://www.nytimes.com/2011/04/08/sports/08outsports.html.

Branch, John. 2011b. Derek Boogaard: Blood on the ice. *New York Times* (December 4): http://www.nytimes.com/2011/12/05/sports/hockey/derek-boogaard-blood-on-the-ice.html.

Branch, John. 2014. *Boy on ice: The life and death of Derek Boogaard.* Norton.

Brand, Noah, and Ozy Frantz. 2012. What about the men? Why our gender system sucks for men, too. *AlterNet.org* (July 11): http://www.alternet.org/reproductivejustice/156194/What_About_the_Men%3F_Why_Our_Gender_System_Sucks_for_Men%2C_Too/.

Braun, Robert, and Rens Vliegenthart. 2008. The contentious fans: The impact of repression, media coverage, grievances and aggressive play on supporters violence. *International Sociology* 23(6): 796–818.

Braun, Robert, and Rens Vliegenthart. 2010. Two cheers for Spaaij and Anderson: A rejoinder. *International Sociology* 25(4): 581–588.

Braye, Stuart, Kevin Dixon, and Tom Gibbons. 2012. 'A mockery of equality': An exploratory investigation into disabled activists' views of the Paralympic Games. *Disability & Society.* Published online 12/21/2012.

Braye, Stuart, Kevin Dixon, and Tom Gibbons. 2013. 'A mockery of equality': An exploratory investigation into disabled activists' views of the Paralympic Games. *Disability & Society* 28(7): 984–996.

Breckinridge, R.Saylor, and Pat Rubio Goldsmith. 2009. Spectacle, distance, and threat: Attendance and integration of Major League Baseball, 1930–1961. *Sociology of Sport Journal* 26(2): 296–319.

Brennan, Christine. 2012. A healthy concern about some NFL players. *USA Today* (January 5): 3C. Online: http://usatoday30.usatoday.com/sports/columnist/brennan/story/2012-01-04/brennan/52380468/1.

Brenner, Michael & Gideon Reuveni, eds. 2006. *Emancipation through muscles: Jews and sports in Europe.* Lincoln: University of Nebraska Press.

Bretón, Marcos. 2000. Field of broken dreams: Latinos and baseball. *ColorLines* 3(1): 13–17.

Bretón, Marcos, and José Luis Villegas. 1999. *Away games: The life and times of a Latin baseball player.* Albuquerque: University of New Mexico Press.

Bridges, Tristan S. 2009. Gender capital and male bodybuilders. *Body and Society* 15(1): 83–107.

Briggs, Bill. 2002. A heavy burden: Way of life leads to early death for many NFL linemen. *Denver Post* (October 20): 1J, 8J.

Briggs, David. 2011. In God NFL players trust: Teams, pubic pave path to deviance. *TheArda.com*: http://blogs.thearda.com/trend/featured/in-god-nfl-players-can-trust-teams-public-pave-path-to-deviance/.

Briggs, David. 2013. The Final Four, Travel Teams and Empty Pews: Research on Sports and Religion. *Association of Religion Data Archives.* Available online: http://blogs.thearda.com/trend/featured/the-final-four-travel-teams-and-empty-pews-research-on-sports-and-religion/.

Brissonneau, Christophe. 2010. Doping in France (1960–2000): American and Eastern bloc influences. *Journal of Physical Education and Sport* 27(2): 33–38.

Brissonneau, Christophe. 2013. Was Lance Armstrong a cheater or an overconformist? Presentation at the University of Colorado, Colorado Springs (April 10).

Brissonneau, Christophe, and F. Depiesse. 2006. Doping and doping control in French sport. In Giselher Spitzer, ed., *Doping and doping control in Europe.* Aachen, Germany: Meyer and Meyer.

Brissonneau, Christophe, and Fabien Ohl. 2010. The genesis and effect of French anti-doping policies in cycling. *International Journal of Sport Policy* 2: 173–187.

Brittain, Ian. 2004a. The role of schools in constructing self-perceptions of sport and physical education in relation to people with disabilities. *Sport, Education and Society* 9(1): 75–94.

Brittain, Ian. 2004b. Perceptions of disability and their impact upon involvement in sport for people with disabilities at all levels. *Journal of Sport and Social Issues* 28(4): 429–452.

Brittain, Ian. 2012a. *From Stoke Mandeville to Stratford: A history of the Summer Paralympic Games.* Champaign, IL: Common Ground Publishing (Sport and Society).

Brittain, Ian. 2012b. The Paralympic Games as a force for peaceful coexistence. *Sport in Society* 15(6): 855–868.

Brooks, David. 2012. The Jeremy Lin problem. *New York Times* (February 16): http://www.nytimes.com/2012/02/17/opinion/brooks-the-jeremy-lin-problem.html.

Brooks, David. 2012. The opportunity gap. *New York Times* (July 9): A21. Online: http://www.nytimes.com/2012/07/10/opinion/brooks-the-opportunity-gap.html.

Brown, David Hugh Kendall. 2013. Seeking spirituality through physicality in schools: Learning from 'Eastern movement forms.' *International Journal of Children's Spirituality* 18(1): 30–45.

Brown, Gary. 2010. Hitting greens with regulation. *Champion* (Summer): 61–62.

Brown, Gary. 2013. An older league of their own. (NCAA) *Champion* 6(3): 65–66.

Brown, Katrina J., and Catherine Connolly. 2010. The role of law in promoting women in elite athletics: An examination of four nations. *International Review for the Sociology of Sport* 45(1): 3–21.

Brown, Kenneth H., and Lisa K. Jepsen. 2009. The impact of team revenues on MLB salaries. *Journal of Sports Economics* 10(2): 192–203.

Brown, Matthew, Mark Nagel, Chad McEvoy, and Daniel Rascher. 2004. Revenue and wealth maximization in the National Football League: The impact of stadia. *Sport Marketing Quarterly* 13(4): 227–236.

Brown, Seth. 2012. De Coubertin's Olympism and the laugh of Michel Foucault: Crisis discourse and the Olympic Games. *Quest* 64(3): 150–163.

Brown, Seth. 2015. Learning to be a 'goody-goody': Ethics and performativity in high school elite athlete programmes. *International Review for the Sociology of Sport* published 23 February 2015, 10.1177/1012690215571145.

Brownell, Susan. 2008. *Beijing's games: What the Olympics mean to China.* Lanham, MD: Rowman & Littlefield.

Browning, Blair, and Jimmy Sanderson. 2012. The positives and negatives of twitter: Exploring how student-athletes use Twitter and respond to critical tweets. *International Journal of Sport Communication* 5(4): 503–522.

Bruce, Steve. 2011. Defining religion: A practical response. *International Review of Sociology* 21(1): 107–120.

Bruce, Toni. 2013. Reflections on communication and sport: On women and femininities. *Communication & Sport* 1(1/2): 125–137.

Bruening, Jennifer E. 2004. Coaching difference: A case study of four African American female student-athletes. *Journal of Strength and Conditioning Research* 18(2): 242–251.

Bruening, Jennifer E. 2005. Gender and racial analysis in sport: Are all the women white and all the blacks men? *Quest* 57(3): 330–349.

Bruening, Jennifer E., and Marlene A. Dixon. 2007. Work-family conflict in coaching ll: Managing role conflict. *Journal of Sport Management* 21(4): 471–496.

Bruening, Jennifer E., and Marlene A. Dixon. 2008. Situating work-family negotiations within a life course perspective: Insights on the gendered experiences of NCAA Division I head coaching mothers. *Sex Roles: A Journal of Research* 58(1/2): 10–23.

Bruni, Frank. 2012. Pro football's violent toll. *New York Times* (December 3): http://www.nytimes.com/2012/12/04/opinion/bruni-pro-footballs-violent-toll.html (retrieved 5-25-13).

Bryant, Howard. 2013. More than words. *ESPN The Magazine* (June 24): 14.

Bryant, Howard. 2013. Smoke screen. *ESPN The Magazine* (December 23): 14.

Buffel, Tine, Chris Phillipson, and Thomas Scharf. 2012. Ageing in urban environments: Developing 'age-friendly' cities. *Critical Social Policy* 32(4): 597–617.

Buffett, Peter. 2013. The charitable-industrial complex. *New York Times* (July 26): http://www.nytimes.com/2013/07/27/opinion/the-charitable-industrial-complex.html.

Buffington, Daniel Taylor. 2012. Us and them: U.S. ambivalence toward the World Cup and American nationalism. *Journal of Sport and Social Issues* published 14 February 2012, 10.1177/0193723511433861.

Burawoy, Michael. 2004. Public sociologies: Contradictions, dilemmas and possibilities. *Social Forces* 82(4): 1603–1618.

Burawoy, Michael. 2005. For public sociology. *American Sociological Review* 70(1): 4–28.

Burkett, Brendan, Mike McNamee, and Wolfgang Potthast. 2011. Shifting boundaries in sports technology and disability: Equal rights or unfair advantage in the case of Oscar Pistorius? *Disability & Society* 26 (5—special issue: *Disability: Shifting frontiers and boundaries*): 643–654.

Burns, Elizabeth Booksh. 2013. When the Saints went marching in: Social identity in the world champion New Orleans Saints football team and its impact on their host city. *Journal of Sport and Social Issues* published 5 September 2013, 10.1177/0193723513499920.

Burnsed, Brian. 2014. Rates of excessive drinking among student-athletes falling. Champion 7(4): 21.

Burton, Laura J. 2015. Underrepresentation of women in sport leadership: A review of research. *Sport Management Review* 18(2): 155–165.

Burroughs, Benjamin, and W. Jeffrey Burroughs. 2012. The Masal Bugduv hoax: Football blogging and journalistic authority. *New Media and Society* 14(3): 476–491.

Busch, Angela. 2007. Cross country women keep running health risks. *Women's eNews* (January 25): http://www.womensenews.org/article.cfm/dyn/aid/3044/context/archive (retrieved 3-1-2008).

Burgos, Adrian. 2007. *Playing America's game: Baseball, Latinos, and the color line.* Berkeley: University of California Press.

Burstyn, Varda. 1999. *The rites of men: Manhood, politics, and the culture of sport.* Toronto, Ontario: University of Toronto Press.

Burton, Nsenga. 2012. "N—ger Cake" fl ap: Hottentot Venus 2.0. *The Root* (April 17): http://www.theroot.com/buzz/liljeroths-nger-cake-hottentot-venus-20.

Butler, Judith. 2004. *Undoing gender.* New York: Routledge.

Buts, Caroline, Cind Du Bois, Bruno Heyndels, and Marc Jegers. 2013. Socioeconomic determinants of success at the Summer Paralympics. *Journal of Sports Economics* 14(2): 133–147.

Butterworth, Michael L. 2011. Saved at home: Christian branding and faith nights in the 'church of baseball.' *Quarterly Journal of Speech* 97 (August): 309–333.

Butterworth, Michael L. 2013. The passion of the Tebow: Sports media and the heroic language in the tragic frame. *Critical Studies in Media and Communication* 30(1): 17–33.

Butterworth, Michael, and Karsten Senkbeil. 2015. Cross-cultural comparisons of religion as "character": Football and soccer in the United States and Germany. *International Review for the Sociology of Sport* published 28 May 2015, 10.1177/1012690215588214.

Buzinski, Jim. 2013. UFC's Rashad Evans comes out for gay marriage. *OutSports.com* (March 8): http://www.outsports.com/2013/3/8/4080284/rashad-evans-ufc-gay-marriage-supreme-court.

Cacciola, Scott. 2012. The long, arduous road to Indy. *Wall Street Journal* (May 25): D10.

Campaniello, Nadia. 2013. Mega events in sports and crime: Evidence from the 1990 football world cup. *Journal of Sports Economics* 14: 148-170.

Campbell, Bill, Colin Wilborn, Paul La Bounty. 2010. Supplements for strength-power athletes. *Strength and Conditioning Journal* 32(1): 93–100.

Campbell, Denis, and Daniel Boffey. 2012. Doctors turn on No. 10 over failure to curb obesity surge. *The Observer* (April 14): http://www.theguardian.com/society/2012/apr/14/obesity-crisis-doctors-fastfood-deals-ban.

Campbell, Paul, and John Williams. 2013. Can 'the ghetto' really take over the county? 'Race', generation & social change in local football in the UK. *International Review for the Sociology of Sport* published 4 December 2013, 10.1177/1012690213514740.

Capouya, John. 1986. Jerry Falwell's team. *Sport* 77(9): 72–81.

Card, David, and Gordon Dahl. 2009. *Family violence and football: The effect of unexpected emotional cues on violent behavior,* by National Bureau of Economic Research Working Papers, no. 15497. Online: http://www.nber.org/ (retrieved 5-27-13).

Carlson, C. 2013. The reality of fantasy sports: A metaphysical and ethical analysis. *Journal of the Philosophy of Sport,* published online first: doi: 10.1080/00948705.2013.785422.

Carlson, Deven, Leslie Scott, Michael Planty, and Jennifer Thompson. 2005. *Statistics in brief: What is the status of high school athletes 8 years after their senior year?* Washington, DC: U.S. Department of Education, Institute of Education Sciences, National Center for Educational Statistics (NCES 2005-303; http://nces.ed.gov/pubs2005/2005303.pdf).

Carpenter, Linda Jean, and R. Vivian Acosta. 2008. Women in intercollegiate sport, 1977–2008. Online: http://webpages.charter.net/womeninsport/.

Carrington, Ben. 2007. Sport and race. In George Ritzer, ed., *The Blackwell encyclopedia of sociology* (pp. 4686–4690). London: Blackwell Publishing.

Carrington, Ben. 2012. Introduction: Sport matters. *Ethnic and Racial Studies* 35(6): 961–970.

Carrington, Ben. 2013. The critical sociology of race and sport: The first fifty years. *Annual Review of Sociology* 39: 379–398.

Carrington, Ben, and Ian McDonald, eds. 2001. *"Race," sport, and British society.* New York/London: Routledge.

Carrington, Ben, and Ian McDonald, eds. 2008. *Marxism, cultural studies and sport.* Milton Park/NY: Routledge.

Carter, Akilah R., and Algerian Hart. 2010. Perspectives of mentoring: The Black female student-athlete. *Sport Management Review* 13: 382–394.

Carter, Akilah R., and Billy J. Hawkins. 2011. Coping strategies among African American female collegiate athletes' in the predominantly white institution. In K. Hylton, A. Pilkington, P. Warmington, and S. Housee, eds., *Atlantic Crossings: International Dialogues in Critical Race Theory* (pp. 61–92). Birmingham, United Kingdom: Sociology, Anthropology, Politics (C-SAP), The Higher Education Academy Network.

Carter, Eric. 2011. Religion and the NFL. *Research on Religion* (weekly podcast): http://www.researchonreligion.org/countries/united-states/eric-carter-on-religion-the-nfl.

Carter-Francique, Akilah R. 2014. The ethic of care: Black female college athlete development. In James L. Conyers, ed., *Race in American sports: Essays* (pp. 35–58). Jefferson, NC: McFarland and Company, Incorporated.

Carter-Francique, Akilah R., Malia Lawrence, and J. Eyanson. 2011. Racial episodes in sport: voices of African American female athletes. *Intellectbase International Consortium* 4(4): 1–18.

Carter, Neil, and John Williams. 2012. 'A genuinely emotional week': Learning disability, sport and television–notes on the Special Olympics GB National Summer Games 2009. *Media Culture & Society* 34(2): 211–227.

Carter, Thomas F. 2012. Re-placing sport migrants: Moving beyond the institutional structures informing international sport migration. *International Review for the Sociology of Sport* 47(1): 66–82.

Caruso-Cabrera, Michelle. 2012. US Olympic medal winners get bonuses and tax bill. *CNBC.com* (August 6): http://www.cnbc.com/id/48463442.

Cashmore, Ellis. 2008. Tiger Woods and the new racial order. *Current Sociology* 56(4): 621–634.

Cashmore, Ellis. 2012. *Beyond black: Celebrity and race in Obama's America.* Bloomsbury Books. Online: http://www.bloomsburyacademic.com/view/Beyond-Black/book-ba-9781780931500.xml.

Cassar, Robert. 2013. Gramsci and games. *Games and Culture* 8(5): 330–353.

Cavalier, Elizabeth S. 2011. Men at sport: Gay men's experiences in the sport workplace. *Journal of Homosexuality* 58(5): 626–646.

Cavallo, Dominick. 1981. *Muscles and morals: Organized playgrounds and urban reform, 1880–1920.* Philadelphia: University of Pennsylvania Press.

Cavanagh, Sheila, and Heather Sykes. 2006. Transsexual bodies at the Olympics: The International Olympic Committee's policy on transsexual athletes at the 2004 Summer Games. *Body and Society* 12(3): 75–102.

Cavar, Mile, Damir Sekulic, and Zoran Culjak. 2010. Complex interaction of religiousness with other factors in relation to substance use and misuse among female athletes. *Journal of Religion and Health,* published online first, May 6, doi: 10.1007/s10943-010-9360-9.

CDC. 2011. *The benefits of physical activity.* Atlanta, GA: Centers for Disease Control and Prevention. Online: http://www.cdc.gov/physicalactivity/everyone/health/index.html.

Cena, John. 2009. 7 things you should know about being a WWE superstar. *ESPN The Magazine* 12.08 (April 20): 26.

Chabin, Michelle. 2013. Maccabiah Games 2013: Athletes gather in Israel for 'Jewish Olympics'. *Huffington Post* (July 17): http://www.huffingtonpost.com/2013/07/17/maccabiah-games-2013_n_3606427.html.

Chafetz, Janet, and Joseph Kotarba. 1999. Little League mothers and the reproduction of gender. In Jay Coakley & Peter Donnelly, eds., *Inside sports* (pp. 46–54). London: Routledge.

Chappell, Robert. 2007. *Sport in developing countries.* Ewell, UK: International Sports Publications.

Chelladurai, Packianathan. 2008. Athletics IS education: A response to Kan, Leo, and Holleran's case study of University of Minnesota student-athletes. *Journal of Intercollegiate Sport* 1(1): 130–138.

Chen, Tzu-Hsuan. 2012. From the "Taiwan Yankees" to the New York Yankees: The glocal narratives of baseball. *Sociology of Sport Journal* 29(4): 546–558.

Cheng, Maria. 2012. UK doctors criticize McDonalds' Olympic sponsorship, say ads could worsen obesity epidemic. *Huffington Post* (May 1): http://www.huffingtonpost.ca/2012/05/01/uk-doctors-criticize-mcdo_n_1467323.html.

Cherrington, James. 2012. 'It's just superstition I suppose . . . I've always done something on game day': The construction of everyday life on a university basketball team. *International Review for the Sociology of Sport* published 16 October 2012, 10.1177/1012690212461632.

Cherrington, James. 2014 'It's just superstition I suppose . . . I've always done something on game day': The construction of everyday life on a university basketball team. *International Review for the Sociology of Sport* 49(5):509–525.

Cheslock, John. 2008. *Who's playing college sports? Money, race and gender.* Online: http://www .womenssportsfoundation.org/.

Chiang, Ying, and Tzu-hsuan Chen. 2013.Adopting the diasporic son: Jeremy Lin and Taiwan sport nationalism. *International Review for the Sociology of Sport* 1012690213491263, first published on June 18, 2013 as doi: 10.1177/1012690213491263.

Chiang, Ying, and Tzu-hsuan Chen. 2015. Adopting the diasporic son: Jeremy Lin and Taiwan sport nationalism. *International Review for the Sociology of Sport* 50(6): 705–721.

Child Trends. 2013. Participation in school athletics: Indicators on children and youth. *Child Trends Data Bank* (February): http://www.childtrendsdatabank.org.

Chimot, Caroline, and Catherine Louveau. 2010. Becoming a man while playing a female sport: The construction of masculine identity in boys doing rhythmic gymnastics. *International Review for the Sociology of Sport* 45(4): 436–456.

Chin, Christina. 2010. Gender dynamics within Japanese American youth basketball leagues. *CSW Update* (October): http://escholarship.org/uc/item/88h983x6.

Chin, Christina. 2012. *Hoops, history, and crossing over: Boundary making and community building in Japanese American youth basketball leagues.* A dissertation submitted in partial satisfaction of the requirements for the degree Doctor of Philosophy in Sociology, University of California, Los Angeles. Online: http://escholarship.org/uc /item/3g46x328#page-3.

Chin, Christina B. 2015. "Aren't you a little short to play ball?" Japanese American youth and racial microaggressions in basketball leagues. *Amerasian Journal* 41(2): 47–65.

Cho, Younghan. 2009. The glocalization of U.S. sports in South Korea. *Sociology of Sport Journal* 26(2): 320–334.

Cho, Younghan, Charles Leary, and Stephen J. Jackson. 2012. Glocalization and sports in Asia. *Sociology of Sport Journal* 29(4): 421–432.

Christakis, Erika, and Nicholas Christakis. 2010. Want to get your kids into college? Let them play. *CNN* (December 29): http://www.cnn.com/2010 /OPINION/12/29/christakis.play.children.learning /index.html (retrieved 6-20-13).

Christensen, Mette Krogh. 2009. "An eye for talent": Talent identification and the "practical sense" of top-level soccer coaches. *Sociology of Sport Journal* 26(3): 365–382.

Christianity Today. 2012. *Jeremy Linn, Tim Tebow, Josh Hamilton: Muscular Christianity's Newest Heroes: The New God Squad* (March 22): http:// www.christianitytoday.com/ct/2012/april/athletes-muscular-christianity.html.

Chudacoff, Howard. 2007. *Children at play: An American history.* New York: New York University Press.

Clammer, John. 2015. Performing ethnicity: Performance, gender, body and belief in the construction and signaling of identity. *Ethnic and Racial Studies* 38(13): 2159–2166.

Clarey, Christopher. 2012. For many athletes, one nation won't do. *New York Times* (July 31): http:// www.nytimes.com/2012/08/01/sports/olympics/for-many-athletes-one-nation-wont-do.html.

Clarey, Christopher. 2015. Every second counts in bid to keep sports fans. *New York Times* (February 28): http://www.nytimes.com/2015/03/01/sports/every-second-counts-in-bid-to-keep-sports-fans.html.

Clark, Kevin. 2013. How the Miami Dolphins fell apart. *Wall Street Journal* (November 14): D4.

Clarke, Kevin A., and David M. Primo. 2012. Overcoming 'physics envy.' *New York Times* (March 30): http://www.nytimes.com/2012/04/01 /opinion/sunday/the-social-sciences-physics-envy .html.

Clavio, Galen E. 2010. Introduction to this special issue of IJSC on New Media and Social Networking. *International Journal of Sport Communication* 3(4): 393–394.

Clayton, Ben. 2013. Initiate: Constructing the 'reality' of male team sport initiation rituals. *International Review for the Sociology of Sport* 48(2): 204–219.

Clayton, Ben, and Barbara Humberstone. 2006. Men's talk: A (pro)feminist analysis of male university football players' discourse. *International Review for the Sociology of Sport* 41(3–4): 295–316.

Cleland, Jamie. 2013. Discussing homosexuality on association football fan message boards: A changing cultural context. *International Review for the Sociology of Sport* published 18 February 2013, 10.1177/1012690213475437.

Cleland, Jamie. 2013. Racism, football fans, and online message boards: How social media has added a new dimension to racist discourse in English football. *Journal of Sport and Social Issues* 0193723513499922, first published on August 16, 2013 as doi: 10.1177/0193723513499922.

Cleland, Jamie, and Ellis Cashmore. 2013. Football fans' views of racism in British football. *International Review for the Sociology of Sport* published 22 October 2013, 10.1177/1012690213506585.

Clifford, Stephanie, and Matt Apuzzo. 2015. After indicting 14 soccer officials, U.S. vows to end graft in FIFA. *New York Times* (May 27): http://www.nytimes.com/2015/05/28/sports/soccer/fifa-officials-arrested-on-corruption-charges-blatter-isnt-among-them.html

Clopton, Aaron W. 2008. College sports on campus: Uncovering the link between team identification and sense of community. *International Journal of Sport Management* 9(4): 1–20.

Clopton, Aaron W. 2009. One for the team: The impact of community upon students as fans and academic and social integration. *Journal of Issues in Intercollegiate Athletics* (special issue): 24–61.

Clopton, Aaron. 2011. Social capital and college sport: In search of the bridging potential of intercollegiate athletics. *Journal of Intercollegiate Sport* 4(2): 174–189.

Clopton, Aaron W., and Bryan L. Finch. 2010. College sport and social capital: Are students 'bowling alone'? *Journal of Sport Behavior* 33(4): 333–366.

Clotfelder, Charles T. 2011. *Big-time sports in American universities.* New York: Cambridge University Press.

Cloud, John. 2010. Why genes aren't destiny. *Time* 175(2, January 18): 49–53. Online: http://www.time.com/time/health/article/0,8599,1951968,00.html.

Coakley, Jay. 1983a. Leaving competitive sport: Retirement or rebirth? *Quest* 35(1): 1–11.

Coakley, Jay. 1983b. Play, games and sports: Developmental implications for young people. In Janet C. Harris & Roberta J. Park, eds., *Play, games and sports in cultural contexts* (pp. 431–450). Champaign, IL: Human Kinetics.

Coakley, Jay. 1992. Burnout among adolescent athletes: A personal failure or social problem? *Sociology of Sport Journal* 9(3): 271–285.

Coakley, Jay. 2002. Using sports to control deviance and violence among youths: Let's be critical and cautious. In M. Gatz, M.A. Messner, & S.J. Ball-Rokeach, eds., *Paradoxes of youth and sport* (pp. 13–30). Albany: State University of New York Press.

Coakley, Jay. 2006. The good father: Parental expectations and youth sports. *Leisure Studies* 25(2): 153–163.

Coakley, Jay. 2008b. Studying intercollegiate sport: High stakes, low rewards. *Journal of Intercollegiate Sport* 1(1): 14–28.

Coakley, Jay. 2010. The "logic" of specialization: Using children for adult purposes. *Journal of Physical Education, Recreation and Dance* 81(8): 16–18, 25.

Coakley, Jay. 2011a. Sport specialization and its effects. In Sandra Spickard Prettyman & Brian Lampman, eds., *Learning culture through sports* (2nd edition, pp. 7–17). Lanham, MD: Rowman & Littlefield.

Coakley, Jay. 2011b. Youth sports: What counts as "positive development?" *Journal of Sport and Social Issues* 35(3): 306–324.

Coakley, Jay, and Doralice Lange Soouza. Sport mega-events: Can legacies and development be equitable and sustainable? *Motriz, Rio Claro* 19(3): 58–589. Online: http://www.pgedf.ufpr.br/downloads/Artigos%20PS%20Mest%202014/Doralice/COAKLEY;%20%20%20%20%20%20SOUZA.%20Sport%20Megaevents.pdf.

Coakley, Jay, and Anita White. 1999. Making decisions: How young people become involved and stay involved in sports. In Jay Coakley & Peter Donnelly, eds., *Inside sports* (pp. 77–85). London: Routledge.

Coalter, Fred. 2007. *A wider social role for sport: Who's keeping the score?* London, UK: Routledge.

Coalter, Fred. 2013. 'There is loads of relationships here': Developing a programme theory for sport-for-change programmes. *International Review for the Sociology of Sport* 48(5): 594–612.

Coalter, Fred (with John Taylor). 2010. *Sport-for-development impact study: A research initiative funded by Comic Relief and UK Sport and managed by International Development through Sport.* Stirling, UK: University of Stirling.

Coates, Corinne E., and David J. Berri. 2011. Skin tone and wages: Evidence from NBA free agents,

John Robst, Jennifer VanGilder. *Journal of Sports Economics* 12(2): 143–156.

Coelho, Morgado de Oliveira G., E. de Abreu Soares, and B.G. Ribeiro. 2010. Are female athletes at increased risk for disordered eating and its complications? *Appetite* 55: 379–387.

Coggon, Johm, Natasha Hammond, and Søren Holm. 2008. Transsexuals in sport: Fairness and freedom, regulation and law. *Sport, Ethics and Philosophy* 2(1): 4–17.

Cohen, Adam, and Jon Welty Peachey. 2015. Quidditch: Impacting and benefiting participants in a non-fictional manner. *Journal of Sport and Social Issues* 39(6): 521–544.

Cohen, Ben. 2013. A rich fantasy life: Sports fans dream of making a living off games. *Wall Street Journal* (June 28): A1, A7.

Cohen, Greta L. 1994. Media portrayal of the female athlete. In Greta L. Cohen, ed., *Women in sport: Issues and controversies* (pp. 171–184). Newbury Park, CA: Sage.

Cohen, Randy. 2015. Association of equipment worn and concussion injury rates in National Collegiate Athletic Association football practices: 2004-2005 to 2008-2009 Academic Years. *American Journal of Sport Medicine* 43(5): 1134–1141.

Cole, Cheryl L. 2000a. Body studies in the sociology of sport. In Jay Coakley & Eric Dunning, eds., *Handbook of sport studies* (pp. 439–460). London: Sage.

Cole, Cheryl. L. 2000b. The year that girls ruled. *Journal of Sport and Social Issues* 24(1): 3–7.

Cole, Cheryl. L. 2006. Nicole Franklin's double dutch. *Journal of Sport and Social Issues* 30(2): 119–121.

Cole, Teju. 2012. The white savior industrial complex. *The Atlantic* (March 21): http://www.theatlantic .com/international/archive/2012/03/the-white-savior -industrial-complex/254843/ (retrieved 9-15-13).

Coleman, B. Jay, J. Michael DuMond, and Allen K. Lynch. 2008. An examination of NBA MVP voting behavior: Does race matter? *Journal of Sports Economics* 9(6): 606–627.

Coles, Tony. 2009. Negotiating the field of masculinity: The production and reproduction of multiple dominant masculinities. *Men and Masculinities* 12(1): 30–44.

Collinet, Cécile, and Matthieu Delalandre. 2015. Physical and sports activities, and healthy and active ageing: Establishing a frame of reference for public action. *International Review for the Sociology of Sport* published 15 October 2015, 10.1177/1012690215609071.

Collins, Jason (with Franz Lidz). 2013. Why NBA center Jason Collins is coming out now. *Sports Illustrated* (May 6): http://sportsillustrated.cnn.com /magazine/news/20130429/jason-collins-gay-nba -player/ (retrieved 12-17-2013).

Collins, Malcolm. 2009. *Genetics and sports.* Basel, Switzerland: Karger Publishers (*Medicine and Sport Science* Vol. 54).

Collins, Patricia Hill. 2005. *Black sexual politics.* New York/London: Routledge.

Combeau-Mari, E. 2011. The Catholic mission, sport and renewal of elites: St Michel de Tananarive Jesuit College (1906–1975). *The International Journal of the History of Sport* 28(12): 1647–1672.

Comeaux, Eddie, and Marcia V. Fuentes. 2015. Cross-racial interaction of Division I athletes: The campus climate for diversity. In Eddie Comeaux, ed., *Introduction to intercollegiate athletics* (pp. 179–192). Baltimore MD: Johns Hopkins University Press.

Conatser, Phillip, Keith Naugle, Mark Tillman, and Christine Stopka. 2009. Athletic trainers' beliefs toward working with Special Olympic athletes. *Journal of Athletic Training* 44(3): 279–285.

Conn, David. 2012. London 2012 euphoria has died, but will the Olympic legacy live on? *The Guardian* (August 14): http://www.guardian.co.uk/uk/2012 /aug/14/london-2012-olympic-legacy.

Conn, Jordan Ritter. 2015. The lingerie football trap. *Grantland.com* (July 23): http://grantland.com /features/legends-football-league-womens-lingerie-football-league-mitchell-mortaza/

Conneeley, Rob, and Roscoe Kermode 1996. Tribal law surfriders code of ethics. Downloaded October 25, 2008 at www.surfrider.org.au/initiatives/education_ rb/06_01_surf_etiquette_2php.

Connell, Raewyn. 2008. Masculinity construction and sports in boys' education: A framework for thinking about the issue. *Sport, Education and Society* 13(2): 131–145.

Connell, Raewyn. 2011. Sociology for the whole world. *International Sociology* 26(3): 288–291.

Connolly, John. 2015. Civilising processes and doping in professional cycling. *Current Sociology* 63(7): 1037–1057.

Connolly, John, and Paddy Dolan. 2012. Sport, media and the Gaelic Athletic Association: The quest for the 'youth' of Ireland. *Media Culture Society* 34(4): 407–423.

Conway, Steven Craig. 2009. Starting at "Start": An exploration of the nondiegetic1 in soccer video games. *Sociology of Sport Journal* 26(1): 67–88.

Conroy, Pat. 1986. *The prince of tides*. Boston: Houghton Mifflin.

Coogan, Daniel. 2015. *Understanding racial portrayals in the sports media*. Champaign IL: Common Ground Publishing.

Cooke, Graham. 2008. Parent coaches: A tough balancing act. *Sports Coach* 30(2): 18–19.

Cooky, Cheryl. 2004. Raising the bar?: Urban girls' negotiations of structural barriers in recreational sports. Paper presented at the annual meeting of the American Sociological Association, San Francisco, CA, Aug. 14.

Cooky, Cheryl. 2006. Strong enough to be a man, but made a woman: Discourses on sport and femininity in *Sports Illustrated for Women*. In Linda K. Fuller, ed., *Sport, rhetoric, and gender* (pp. 97–106). New York: Palgrave Macmillan.

Cooky, Cheryl. 2009. "Girls just aren't interested": The social construction of interest in girls' sport. *Sociological Perspectives* 52(2): 259–284.

Cooky, Cheryl, and Mary G. McDonald. 2005. 'If you let me play': Young girls' inside-other narratives of sport. *Sociology of Sport Journal* 22(2): 158–177.

Cooky, Cheryl, Michael Messner, and Michela Musto 2015. "It's dude time!": A quarter century of excluding women's sports in televised news and highlight shows. *Communication and Sport* 3(3): 261–287.

Cooky, Cheryl, Michael A. Messner, and Robin H. Hextrum. 2013. Women play sport, but not on TV: A longitudinal study of televised news media. *Communication & Sport* 1(3): 203–230.

Cooky, Cheryl, Ranissa Dycus, and Shari L. Dworkin. 2013. "What makes a woman a woman?" Versus "Our first lady of sport": A comparative analysis of the United States and the South African media coverage of Caster Semenya. *Journal of Sport and Social Issues* 37(1): 31–56.

Cooley, Will. 2010. "Vanilla Thrillas": Modern boxing and white-ethnic masculinity. *Journal of Sport and Social Issues* 34(4): 418–437.

Coontz, Stephanie. 2012. The myth of male decline. *New York Times* (September 29): http://www

.nytimes.com/2012/09/30/opinion/sunday/the-myth-of-male-decline.html.

Coontz, Stephanie. 2013. Why gender equality stalled. *New York Times* (February 16): http://www.nytimes.com/2013/02/17/opinion/sunday/why-gender-equality-stalled.html.

Coop, Graham, Joseph K. Pickrell, John Novembre, Sridhar Kudaravalli, Jun Li, Devin Absher, Richard M. Myers, Luigi Luca Cavalli-Sforza, Marcus W. Feldman, and Jonathan K. Pritchard. 2009. The role of geography in human adaptation. *Plos Genetics*. Online: http://www.plosgenetics.org/article/info%3Adoi%2F10.1371%2Fjournal.pgen.1000500.

Corbett, Doris, and William Johnson. 2000. The African American female in collegiate sport: Sexism and racism. In D. Brooks & R. Althouse, eds., *Racism in college athletics: The African American athlete's experience* (pp. 199–226). Morgantown, WV: Fitness Information Technology.

Cornelissen, Scarlett. 2009. A delicate balance: Major sport events and development. In Roger Levermore & Aaron Beacom, eds., *Sport and international development* (pp. 76–97). New York: Palgrave MacMillan.

Cornelissen, Scarlett. 2010. Football's tsars: Proprietorship, corporatism and politics in the 2010 FIFA World Cup. *Soccer & Society* 11(1–2): 131–143.

Corsello, Andrew. 1999. Hallowed be thy game. *Gentlemen's Quarterly* (September): 432–440.

Costa, Brian. 2015. The CEO who gets to hand out World Series rings. *Wall Street Journal* (February 23): R4.

Cote, J. 2008. Coaching children: Five elements of expertise for coaches. *Coaching Edge* 14 (Winter): 32–33.

Côté, Jean. 2011. *More than a game: The power of soccer for youth development*. Montreal: BMO Financial Group and Queen's University, Kingston, Ontario.

Côté, Jean, and Jessica L. Fraser-Thomas. 2007. Youth involvement in sport. In P.R.E. Crocker, ed., *Introduction to sport psychology: A Canadian perspective* (pp. 266–294). Toronto: Pearson Prentice Hall.

Cotton, Anthony. 2013. Driving new revenue with athletics. *Denver Post* (July 28): 10B.

Couser, G. Thomas. 2000. The empire of the "normal": A forum on disability and self-representation—introduction. *American Quarterly* 52(2): 305–310.

Couser, G. Thomas. 2009. *Signifying bodies: Disability in contemporary life writing*. Ann Arbor: University of Michigan Press.

Cover, Rob. 2013. Suspended ethics and the team: Theorising team sportsplayers' group sexual assault in the context of identity. *Sexualities* 16: 300–318.

Cox, Barbara, and Richard Pringle. 2011. Gaining a foothold in football: A genealogical analysis of the emergence of the female footballer in New Zealand. *International Review for the Sociology of Sport* (11 April, 2011).

Coyne, Christopher J., Justin P. Isaacs, and Jeremy T. Schwartz. 2010. Comment on Hanssen and Meehan, "Who integrated major league baseball faster winning teams or losing teams?" *Journal of Sports Economics* 11: 227–231.

Coyte Cooper. 2013. Team segmentation at the Big Ten Wrestling Championships. *The impact of sports on Team Performance Management* 15(3/4): 117–127.

Cranley, Travis. 2009. Court sports: What exactly is the court of arbitration for sport and how much power does it really have? More than you might think. *Inside Sport* 208 (Apr): 38–42, 45.

Crawford, Garry. 2004. *Consuming sport: Fans, sport, and culture.* London/New York: Routledge.

Crawford, Garry. 2015. Is it in the game? Reconsidering play spaces, game definitions, theming, and sports video games. *Games and Culture* 10(6): 571–592.

Crawford, Garry, and Victoria K. Gosling. 2009. More than a game: Sports-themed video games and player narratives. *Sociology of Sport Journal* 26(1): 50–66.

Creaney, Leon. 2009. Growth factors, athletes and an anti-doping muddle. *Sports Injury Bulletin* 79: 1–3.

Crissey, Joy. 1999. *Corporate cooptation of sport: The case of snowboarding.* Master's thesis, Sociology Department, Colorado State University, Ft. Collins, CO.

Crissey, Sarah R., and Joy Crissey Honea. 2006. The relationship between athletic participation and perceptions of body size and weight control in adolescent girls: The role of sports. *Sociology of Sport Journal* 23(3): 248–272.

Critical Bogle. 2007. The social construction of disability: Struggles for definitions of the victims of language. In *Essays, Poems and Blogs of a Disabled Everyman* (September 11): http://criticalbogle .blogspot.com/2007/09/social-construction-of -disability.html.

Crocket, Hamish. 2012. 'This is men's ultimate': (Re) creating multiple masculinities in elite open Ultimate Frisbee. *International Review for the Sociology of Sport* 48(3): 318–333.

Crosset, Todd. 1999. Male athletes' violence against women: A critical assessment of the athletic affiliation, violence against women debate. *Quest* 52(3): 244–257.

Crouse, Karen. 2007. Torres is getting older, but swimming faster. *The New York Times* (November 18). Online: HYPERLINK "http://www.nytimes .com/2007/11/18/sports/othersports/18torres .html" www.nytimes.com/2007/11/18/sports /othersports/18torres.html .

Crow, Graham, and Catherine Pope. 2008. The importance of class. *Sociology* 42(6): 1045–1048.

CS4L 2013. Long-Term Athlete Development (LTAD) Stages. *Canadian Sport for Life* (CS4L): http:// canadiansportforlife.ca/learn-about-canadian-sport-life/ltad-stages.

Cullen, Fergus. 2013. Those "guest worker' of the NBA and NHL. *Wall Street Journal* (June 19): A13.

Cunningham, George B. 2007a. *Diversity in sport organizations.* Scottsdale, AZ: Holcomb Hathaway Publishers.

Cunningham, George B. 2007b. Opening the black box: The influence of perceived diversity and a common in-group identity in diverse groups. *Journal of Sport Management* 21: 58–78.

Cunningham, George B. 2009. Understanding the diversity-related change process: A field study. *Journal of Sport Management* 23(4): 407–428.

Cunningham, George B. 2012. Diversity issues in academic reform. *Journal of Intercollegiate Sport* 5(1): 54–59.

Cunningham, George B., and Janet S. Fink. 2006. Diversity issues in sport and leisure. *Journal of Sport Management* 20(4): 455–465.

Cunningham, George B., Kathi Miner, and Jennifer McDonald. 2013. Being different and suffering the consequences: The influence of head coach–player racial dissimilarity on experienced incivility. *International Review for the Sociology of Sport* 48(6): 689–705.

Cunningham, George B., and Michael R. Regan, Jr. 2011. Political activism, racial identity and the commercial endorsement of athletes: Athlete activism. *International Review for the Sociology of Sport* 47(6): 657–669.

Cunningham, George B., and Michael Sagas. 2005. Access discrimination in intercollegiate athletics.

Journal of Sport and Social Issues 29(2): 148–163.

Cunningham, George B., and Michael Sagas. 2008. Gender and sex diversity in sport organizations: Introduction to the special issue. *Sex Roles: A Journal of Research* 58(1–2): 3–9.

Cunningham, Phillip Lamarr. 2009. "Please don't fine me again!!!!!": Black athletic defiance in the NBA and NFL. *Journal of Sport and Social Issues* 33(1): 39–58.

Cuperman, Ronen, Rebecca L. Robinson, and William Ickes. 2014. On the malleability of self-image in individuals with a weak sense of self. *Self and Identity* 13(1): 1–23.

Curi, Martin, Jorge Knijnik, and Gilmar Mascarenhas. 2011. The Pan American Games in Rio de Janeiro 2007: Consequences of a sport mega-event on a BRIC country. *International Review for the Sociology of Sport* 46(2): 140–156.

Curry, christina, and Light, Richard. 2009. Children's reasons for joining sport clubs and staying in them: A case study of a Sydney soccer club. *ACHPER Healthy Lifestyles Journal* 56(1): 23–27.

Curry, Timothy J., Kent P. Schwirian, and Rachael Woldoff. 2004. *High stakes: Big time sports and downtown redevelopment.* Columbus: Ohio State University Press.

Curtis, Henry S. 1913. *The reorganized school playground.* Washington, DC: U.S. Bureau of Education, No. 40.

Curtis, Vanessa A., and David B. Allen. 2011. Boosting the late-blooming boy: Use of growth-promoting agents in the athlete with constitutional delay of growth and puberty. *Sports Health: A Multidisciplinary Approach* 3: 32–40.

Dagkasa, Symeon, Tansin Benn, and Haifaa Jawad. 2011. Multiple voices: Improving participation of Muslim girls in physical education and school sport. *Sport, Education and Society* 16(2): 223–239.

Dahmen, Nicole S., and Raluca Cozma, eds. 2009. *Media takes: On aging.* Sacramento, CA: International Longevity Center/Aging Services of California.

Dal Lago, Alessandro, and Rocco De Biasi. 1994. Italian football fans: Culture and organization. In Richard Giulianotti, Norman Bonney & Mike Hepworth, eds., *Football, violence and social identity* (pp. 21–86). London & New York: Routledge.

Damon, Arwa. 2009. Iraqi women wrestle with social barriers. *CNN.com:* http://ibnlive.in.com /videos/98766/iraqi-women-wrestle-with-social -barriers.html.

Daniels, Dayna B. 2009. *Polygendered and ponytailed: The dilemma of femininity and the female athlete.* Toronto, ON: Women's Press.

Daniels, Elizabeth A. 2009. Sex objects, athletes, and sexy athletes: How media representations of women athletes can impact adolescent girls and college women. *Journal of Adolescent Research* 24(4): 399–422.

Dannheisser, Ralph. 2008. Baseball, once just an American game, extends reach worldwide. Online: http://iipdigital.usembassy.gov/st/english /article/2008/03/20080331164120zjsredna0.6307947 .html#axzz48Mq14bVJ.

Darby, Paul. 2011. The Gaelic Athletic Association, transnational identities and Irish-America. *Sociology of Sport Journal* 27(4): 351–370.

Darcy, Simon, and Leanne Dowse. 2012. In search of a level playing field–the constraints and benefits of sport participation for people with intellectual disability. *Disability & Society* doi: 10.1080/0968759 9.2012.714258.

Darnell, Simon C. 2010a. Sport, race, and bio-politics: Encounters with difference in "Sport for Development and Peace" internships. *Journal of Sport and Social Issues* 34(4): 396–417.

Darnell, Simon C. 2010b. Power, politics and sport for development and peace: Investigating the utility of sport for international development. *Sociology of Sport Journal* 27(1): 54–75.

Darnell, Simon C. 2012. *Sport for development and peace: A critical sociology.* New York: Bloomsbury Academic.

Dart, Jon. 2014. New media, professional sport and political economy. *Journal of Sport and Social Issues* 38(6): 528–547.

Dart, Jon J. 2012. New media, professional sport and political economy. *Journal of Sport and Social Issues* published 6 December 2012, 10.1177/0193723512467356.

Dashper, Katherine. 2013. Getting better: An autoethnographic tale of recovery from sporting injury. *Sociology of Sport Journal* 30(3): 323–329.

Davenport, Elizabeth M., et al. 2014. Abnormal white matter integrity related to head impact exposure in a season of high school varsity football. *Journal of Neurotrauma* 31:327–338.

Davids, Keith, and Joseph Baker. 2007. Genes, environment and sport performance: Why the nature-nurture dualism is no longer relevant. *Sports Medicine* 37(11): 961–980.

Davidson, Patricia M., Michelle DeGiacomo, and Sarah J. McGrath. 2011. The feminization of aging: How will this impact on health outcomes and services? *Health Care for Women International* 32(12): 1031–1045.

Davies, Steven. 2011. Why I am coming out now. *UK Daily Telegraph* (28 February): http://www .telegraph.co.uk/news/newsvideo/8350711/Steven -Davies-why-I-am-coming-out-now.html.

Davis, F. James. 2001. *Who is black: One nation's definition.* University Park, PA: Penn State University Press.

Davis, Georgiann. 2011. DSD is a perfectly fine term: Reasserting medical authority through a shift in intersex terminology. In P.J. McGann & D.J. Hutson, eds., *Sociology of diagnosis* (pp. 155–182). Bingley, UK: Emerald.

Davis-Delano, Laurel R. 2007. Eliminating Native American mascots. *Journal of Sport and Social Issues* 31(4): 340–373.

Davis-Delano, Laurel R., and Todd Crosset. 2008. Using social movement theory to study outcomes in sport-related social movements. *International Review for the Sociology of Sport* 43(2): 115–134.

De Souza, Adriano, and Judy Oslin. 2008. A player-centered approach to coaching. *Journal of Physical Education, Recreation and Dance* 79(6): 24–30.

de Visser, Richard O. 2009. "I'm not a very manly man": Qualitative insights into young men's masculine subjectivity. *Men and Masculinities* 11(3): 367–371.

deMause, Neil. 2011. Why do mayors love sports stadiums? *The Nation* (August 15–22): http://www .thenation.com/article/why-do-mayors-love-sports-stadiums/?nc=1.

deMause, Neil, and Joanna Cagan. 2008. *Field of schemes: How the great stadium swindle turns public money into private profit* (revised/expanded edition). Lincoln: University of Nebraska Press.

Deardorff, Donald Lee, and John White, eds. 2008. *The image of God in the human body: Essays on Christianity and sports.* Lewiston, NY: Edwin Mellen Press.

Delaney, Kevin J., and Rick Eckstein. 2003. The devil is in the details: Neutralizing critical studies of publicly subsidized stadiums. *Critical Sociology* 29(2): 189–210.

Delaney, Kevin J., and Rick Eckstein. 2007. *Public dollars, private stadiums: The battle over building sports stadiums.* Piscataway, NJ: Rutgers University Press.

Delaney, Kevin, and Rick Eckstein. 2008. Local media coverage of sports stadium initiatives. *Journal of Sport and Social Issues* 32(1): 72–93.

Demerath, Nicholas J., and Philip Hammond. 1969. *Religion in social context: Tradition and transition.* New York: Random House.

Denham, Bryan. 2010. Correlates of pride in the performance success of United States athletes competing on an international stage. *International Review for the Sociology of Sport* 45(4): 457–473.

Denham, Bryan. 2011. Alcohol and marijuana use among American high school seniors: Empirical associations with competitive sports participation. *Sociology of Sport Journal* 28(3): 362–279.

Denzin, Norman K. 2007. *Symbolic interactionism and cultural studies: The politics of interpretation.* Oxford, UK: Wiley-Blackwell.

Department of Health. 2004. *At least five a week: Evidence on the impact of physical activity and its relationship to health.* A report from the Chief Medical Officer. Online: http://webarchive .nationalarchives.gov.uk/+/www.dh.gov .uk/en/publicationsandstatistics/publications /publicationspolicyandguidance/dh_4080994.

Desrochers. Donna M. 2013. *Academic spending versus athletic spending: Who wins?* Washington, DC: Delta Cost Project, American Institutes for Research.

Deutscher, Christian. 2010. The payoff to leadership in teams. *Journal of Sports Economics* 11(3): 358–360.

Dewan, Shaila. 2013. Has 'Caucasian' lost its meaning? *New York Times* (July 6): http://www.nytimes .com/2013/07/07/sunday-review/has-caucasian-lost-its-meaning.html

Dey, Ian. 1993. *Qualitative data analysis: A user-friendly guide for social scientists.* London: Routledge.

Diaz-Orueta, Unai, David Facal, Henk Herman Nap, and Myrto-Maria Ranga. 2012. What is the key for older people to show interest in playing digital learning games? Initial qualitative findings from the LEAGE Project on a multicultural European sample. *Games for Health Journal* 1(2): 124–128.

Digance, Justine and Kristine Toohey. 2011. Pilgrimage to Fallen Gods from Olympia: The cult of sporting celebrities. *Australian Religion Studies Review* 24(3): 374–375

Dionigi, Rylee. 2006. Competitive sport and aging: The need for qualitative sociological research. *Journal of Aging and Physical Activity* 14: 365–379.

Dionigi, Rylee. 2010. Masters sport as a strategy for managing the ageing process. In J. Baker, S. Horton, & P. Weir, eds., *The Masters athlete: Understanding the role of sport and exercise in optimizing aging* (pp. 137–156). London: Routledge.

Dionigi, Rylee. 2011. Older athletes: Resisting and reinforcing discourses of sport and aging. In Sandra Spikard Prettyman & Brian Lampman, eds., *Learning culture through sports* (2nd edition). Lanham, MD: Rowman & Littlefield Publishers, Inc.

Dionigi, Rylee, and Gabrielle O'Flynn. 2007. Performance discourses and old age: What does it mean to be an older athlete? *Sociology of Sport Journal* 24(4): 359–377.

Dionigi, Rylee A., Sean Horton, and Joseph Baker. 2011. Seniors in sport: The experiences and practices of older world masters games competitors. *The International Journal of Sport and Society* 1(1): 55–68.

Dionigi, Rylee A., Sean Horton, and Joseph Baker. 2013. Negotiations of the ageing process: Older adults' stories of sports participation. *Sport, Education and Society* 18(3): 370–387.

Dixon, Kevin. 2012. Learning the game: Football fandom culture and the origins of practice. *International Review for the Sociology of Sport* 48(3): 334–348.

Dixon, Kevin. 2013. The football fan and the pub: An enduring relationship. *International Review for the Sociology of Sport* published 18 November 2013, 10.1177/1012690213501500.

Dixon, Marlene A., and Jennifer E. Bruening. 2005. Perspectives on work–family conflict: A review and integrative approach. *Sport Management Review* 8: 227–254.

Dixon, Marlene A., and Jennifer E. Bruening. 2007. Work–family conflict in coaching I: A top-down perspective. *Journal of Sport Management* 21: 377–406.

Dixon, Marlene A., and Michael Sagas. 2007. The relationship between organizational support, work–family conflict, and the job-life satisfaction of university coaches. *Research Quarterly for Exercise and Sport* 78: 236–247.

Dixon, Marlene A., Stacy M. Warner, and Jennifer E. Bruening. 2008. More than just letting them

play: Parental influence on women's lifetime sport involvement. *Sociology of Sport Journal* 25(4): 538–559.

Dóczi, Tamás. 2012. Gold fever(?): Sport and national identity–The Hungarian case. *International Review for the Sociology of Sport* 47(2): 165–182.

Dohrmann, George, and Jeff Benedict. 2011. Rap sheets, recruits, and repercussions. *Sports Illustrated* 114(March 7): 32–39.

Dohrmann, George, and Thayer Evans. 2013a. How you go from very bad to very good very fast. *Sports Illustrated* 119(11, September 16): 30–41.

Dohrmann, George, and Thayer Evans. 2013c. Special report on Oklahoma State football: Part 2—The academics. *Sports Illustrated* (September 11): http://sportsillustrated.cnn.com/college-football /news/20130911/oklahoma-state-part-2-academics/.

Dohrmann, George, and Thayer Evans. 2013d. Special report on Oklahoma State football: Part 3—The drugs. *Sports Illustrated* (September 12): http://sportsillustrated.cnn.com/college-football /news/20130912/oklahoma-state-part-3-drugs/.

Dohrmann, George, and Thayer Evans. 2013e. Special report on Oklahoma State football: Part 4—The sex. *Sports Illustrated* (September 13): http://sportsillustrated.cnn.com/college-football /news/20130913/oklahoma-state-part-4-the-sex/.

Dohrmann, George, and Thayer Evans. 2013f. Special report on Oklahoma State football: Part 5–The fallout. *Sports Illustrated* 119(12, September 23): 60–71.

Doidge, Mark. 2013. 'If you jump up and down, Balotelli dies': Racism and player abuse in Italian football. *International Review for the Sociology of Sport* published 27 March 2013, 10.1177/1012690213480354.

Donnelly, Michele K. 2013. Drinking with the derby girls: Exploring the hidden ethnography in research of women's flat track roller derby. *International Review for the Sociology of Sport* published 16 December 2013, 10.1177/1012690213515664.

Donnelly, Michele K., Mark Norman, and Peter Donnelly. 2015. *The Sochi 2014 Olympics: A Gender Equality Audit.* Centre for Sport Policy Studies Research Report. Toronto: Centre for Sport Policy Studies, Faculty of Kinesiology and Physical Education, University of Toronto.

Donnelly, Peter (with Simon Darnell, Sandy Wells, and Jay Coakley). 2007. *The use of sport to foster child and youth development and education.* In Sport for Development and Peace, International Working Group (SDP/IWG): Literature reviews on sport for development and peace (pp. 7–47). Toronto, Ontario, Canada: University of Toronto, Faculty of Physical Education and Health.

Donnelly, Peter. 2008. *Opportunity knocks!: Increasing sport participation in Canada as a result of success at the Vancouver Olympics.* Toronto: Centre for Sport Policy Studies, University of Toronto.

Donnelly, Peter. 2015. Assessing the sociology of sport: On public sociology of sport and research that makes a difference. *International Review for the Sociology of Sport* 50(4/5): 419–423.

Donnelly, Peter, and Jay Coakley. 2003. *The role of recreation in promoting social inclusion.* Monograph in the Working Paper Series on Social Inclusion published by the Laidlaw Foundation, Toronto, Ontario.

Donnelly, Peter, and Kevin Young. 1999. Rock climbers and rugby players: Identity construction and confirmation. In Jay Coakley & Peter Donnelly, eds., *Inside sports* (pp. 67–76). London: Routledge.

Donnelly, Peter, and Leanne Petherick. 2004. Workers' playtime?: Child labour at the extremes of the sporting spectrum. *Sport in Society* 7(3): 301–321.

Donnelly, Peter, and Jean Harvey. 2007. Social class and gender: Intersections in sport and physical activity. In Kevin Young & Philip White, eds., *Sport and gender in Canada* (2nd edition, pp. 95–119). Don Mills, Ontario: Oxford University Press.

Donnelly, Peter, Michael Atkinson, Sarah Boyle, and Courtney Szto. 2011. Sport for development and peace: A public sociology perspective. *Third World Quarterly* 32(3): 589–601.

Donnelly, Peter, and Michele K. Donnelly. 2013a. *Sex testing, naked inspections and the Olympic Games: A correction to The London 2012 Olympics: A gender equality audit.* Centre for Sport Policy Studies Research Report. Toronto: Centre for Sport Policy Studies, Faculty of Kinesiology and Physical Education, University of Toronto.

Donnelly, Peter, and Michele K. Donnelly. 2013b. *The London 2012 Olympics: A gender equality audit.* Centre for Sport Policy Studies Research Report. Toronto: Centre for Sport Policy Studies, Faculty of Kinesiology and Physical Education, University of Toronto.

Dorgan, Byron. 2013. Broken promises. *New York Times* (July 10): http://www.nytimes.com /2013/07/11/opinion/broken-promises.html.

Dorsey, James M. 2012. Ultra violence: How Egypt's soccer mobs are threatening the revolution. *Foreign Policy* (February 2): http://www.foreignpolicy.com /articles/2012/02/01/ultra_violence (retrieved 5-29-13); http://mideastsoccer.blogspot.com/2013/06 /soccer-threaten-to-spark-protests-as.html.

Dorsey, James M. 2013a. Fan culture—a social and political indicator. *The Turbulent World of Middle East Soccer* (February 4): http://mideastsoccer .blogspot.com/2013/02/fan-culture-social-and-political.html (retrieved 5-30-13).

Dorsey, James M. 2013b. Football: A sporting barometer of European integration policies. *International Centre for Sport Security Journal* 1(2): http://icss-journal.newsdeskmedia.com /football-a-sporting-barometer-of-European -integration-policies.

Dorsey, James M. 2013b. Soccer fans defy emergency rule, force work stoppage in Port Said. *The Turbulent World of Middle East Soccer* (February 18): http://mideastsoccer.blogspot.com/2013/02/soccer-fans-defy-emergency-rule-force.html (retrieved 5-30-13).

Dorsey, James M. 2013c. Soccer emerges as focal point of dissent in Saudi Arabia. *The Turbulent World of Middle East Soccer* (May 12): http://mideastsoccer .blogspot.com/2013/05/soccer-emerges-as-focal -point-of.html (retrieved 5-30-13).

Dorsey, James M. 2013d. Algeria: Middle East's next revolt if soccer is a barometer. *The Turbulent World of Middle East Soccer* (May 19): http:// mideastsoccer.blogspot.com/2013/05/algeria-middle -easts-next-revolt-if.html (retrieved 5-30-13).

Dorsey, James M. 2013e. Soccer threatens to spark protests as Iran goes to the polls. *The Turbulent World of Middle East Soccer* (June 10): http:// mideastsoccer.blogspot.com/2013/06/soccer -threaten-to-spark-protests-as.html.

Dorsey, James M. 2013f. *Wahhabism vs. Wahhabism: Qatar Challenges Saudi Arabia.* The RSIS Working Paper series. No. 262. Singapore: S. Rajaratnam School of International Studies.

Dorsey, James M. 2013g. Qatar 2022–A mixed blessing. *The Turbulent World of Middle East Soccer* (August 30): http://mideastsoccer.blogspot .com/2013/08/qatar-2022-mixed-blessing.html.

Dorsey, James M. 2015. Women's sporting rights: The battle is in Philadelphia. . . and Riyadh. *The Turbulent World of Middle East Soccer* (February 7): http://mideastsoccer.blogspot .sg/2015/01/womens-sporting-rights-battle-is-in .html.

Dorsey, James M. 2016. Turkish stadiums: A contested political battleground. *The Turbulent World of Middle East Soccer* (May 3): http://mideastsoccer .blogspot.sg/2016/05/turkish-stadiums-contested-political.html

Dortants, Marianne, and Annelies Knoppers. 2013. Regulation of diversity through discipline: Practices of inclusion and exclusion in boxing. *International Review for the Sociology of Sport* 48(5): 535–549.

Dowling, Sandra, Roy McConkey, David Hassan, and Sabine Menke. 2010. *'Unified gives us a chance': An evaluation of Special Olympics Youth Unified Sports® Programme in Europe/Eurasia.* Washington, DC: Special Olympics International (and the University of Ulster in Northern Ireland).

Draper, Electa. 2011. For Ed McVaney, Valor Christian High School is labor of love. *Denver Post* (December 5): http://www.denverpost.com/preps /ci_19471245.

Dreger, Alice. 2009. Where's the rulebook for sex verification? *New York Times* (August 21): http:// www.nytimes.com/2009/08/22/sports/22runner.html.

Dreger, Alice. 2012. Media advisory on sex verification in sports. *alicedreger.com* http://www.alicedreger .com/media_advisory_01.html

Dretzin, Rachel. 2011. *Football high: Bigger and faster, but safer? Frontline* (PBS documentary). Online: http://www.pbs.org/wgbh/pages/frontline/football -high/.

Drew, Dr. 2012. Concussion hazards in youth football (video). *HLN* (January 17): http://www.youtube .com/watch?v=XnIRso_04Ks.

Drummond, Murray. 2010. The natural: An autoethnography of a masculinized body in sport. *Men and Masculinities* 12(3): 374–389.

DuBois, William Edward Burghardt. 1935. *Black reconstruction in America.* New York: Harcourt, Brace.

Dubrow, Joshua Kjerulf, and Jimi Adams. 2012. Hoop inequalities: Race, class and family structure background and the odds of playing in the National Basketball Association. *International Review for the Sociology of Sport* 47(1): 43–59.

Dumais, Susan A. 2008. Cohort and gender differences in extracurricular participation: The relationship between activities, math achievement, and college expectations. *Sociological Spectrum* 29(1): 72–100.

Duncan, Arne. 2013. We must provide equal opportunity in sports to students with disabilities. *U.S. Department of Education* (January 25): http:// www.ed.gov/blog/2013/01/we-must-provide-equal -opportunity-in-sports-to-students-with-disabilities/.

Duncan, Greg J., and Richard J. Murnane, eds. 2011. The American dream, then and now. In Greg J. Duncan & Richard J. Murnane, eds., *Whither opportunity? Rising inequality, schools, and children's life chances* (pp. 3–26). New York: The Rusell Sage Foundation.

Duncan, Margaret C., Michael A. Messner, and Nicole Willms. 2005. *Gender in televised sports: News and highlights shows, 1989–2004.* Los Angeles, CA: Amateur Athletic Foundation of Los Angeles. Online: http://www.aafla.org/11pub/over_frmst.htm.

Dunning, Eric. 1999. *Sport matters: Sociological studies of sport, violence and civilization.* London: Routledge.

Dunning, Eric, Patrick Murphy, Ivan Waddington, and Antonios E. Astrinakis, eds. 2002. *Fighting fans: Football hooliganism as a world phenomenon.* Dublin: University College Dublin Press.

Dunning, Eric, Patrick Murphy, and John Williams. 1988. *The foots of football hooliganism: An historical and sociological study.* London: Routledge and Kegan Paul.

Dworkin, Shari L., and Faye Linda Wachs. 2009. *Body panic: Gender, health, and the selling of fitness.* Albany: New York University Press.

Dyer, Bryce T.J., Siamak Noroozi, Sabi Redwood, and Philip Sewell. 2010. The design of lower-limb sports prostheses: Fair inclusion in disability sport. *Disability & Society* 25(5): 593–602.

Dyke, Noel. 2012. *Fields of play: An ethnography of children's sports.* North York, Ontario: University of Toronto Press.

Dzikus, Lars, S. Waller, and R. Hardin. 2010. Collegiate sport chaplaincy: Exploration of an emerging profession. *Journal of Contemporary Athletics* 5(1): 21–42.

Dziubiński, Zbigniew. 2011. Social aspects of physical education and sport in schools. *Physical Culture and Sport. Studies and Research* 52: 49–60.

Early, Gerald. 1998. Performance and reality: Race, sports and the modern world. *The Nation* 267(5): 11–20.

Eberle, Lucas. 2012. Interview with Orlando Cruz 'I couldn't accept being gay because I was too afraid.' *Spiegel.de* (November 9): http://www.spiegel.de /international/world/interview-with-first-openly-gay -boxer-orlando-cruz-a-866052.html.

Eder, Steve, Richard Sandomir, and James Andrew Miller. 2013. At Louisville, athletic boom is rooted in ESPN partnership. *New York Times* (August 25): http://www.nytimes.com/2013/08/26/sports/at-louisville-an-athletic-boom-made-for-and-by-tv.html.

Edwards, Harry. 2000. The decline of the black athlete (as interviewed by D. Leonard). *ColorLines* 3(1): 24–29.

Edwards, Harry. 2011. Transformational development at the interface of race, sport, and the collegiate arms race in the age of globalization. *Journal of Intercollegiate Sports* 4(1): 18–31.

Edwards, Michael B., Jason N. Bocarro, and Michael A. Kanters. 2013. Place disparities in supportive environments for extracurricular physical activity in North Carolina middle schools. *Youth and Society* 45(2): 265–285.

Edwards, Steven D. 2008. Should Oscar Pistorius be excluded from the 2008 Olympic Games? *Sport, Ethics and Philosophy* 2(2): 112–125.

EEOC. 2013. Nearly 100,000 job bias charges in fiscal year 2012. *Equal Employment Opportunity Commission* (January 28): http://www.eeoc.gov /eeoc/newsroom/release/1-28-13.cfm.

Eichberg, Henning. 2011. The normal body— anthropology of bodily otherness. *Physical Culture and Sport Studies and Research* 51: 5–14.

Eickelkamp, Ute. 2008. (Re)presenting experience: A comparison of Australian Aboriginal children's sand play in two settings. *International Journal of Applied Psychoanalytic Studies* 5(1): 23–50.

Elias, Norbert. 1986. An essay on sport and violence. In Nobert Elias & Eric Dunning, eds., *Quest for excitement* (pp. 150–174). Oxford, UK: Blackwell.

Elias, Norbert, and Eric Dunning. 1986. *Quest for excitement.* New York: Basil Blackwell.

Eliasoph, Nina. 1999. "Everyday racism" in a culture of political avoidance: Civil society, speech, and taboo. *Social Problems* 46(4): 479–502.

el-Khoury, Laura J. 2012. 'Being while black': Resistance and the management of the self. *Social Identities* 18(1): 85–100.

Elkind, David. 2007. *The hurried child.* Cambridge, MA: Da Capo Lifelong Books.

Elkind, David. 2008. *The power of play: Learning what comes naturally.* Cambridge, MA: Da Capo Lifelong Books.

Ellin, Abby. 2008. The high price of raising an Olympian. *MSN.com* (August 4): http://articles.moneycentral .msn.com/Investing/StockInvestingTrading /TheHighPriceOfRaisingAnOlympian.aspx (retrieved August 20, 2008).

Ellin, Abby. 2009. Exercise tailored to a hijab. *New York Times* (September 10): http://www.nytimes .com/2009/09/10/health/nutrition/10fitness.html.

Elling, Agnes, and Jacco van Sterkenburg. 2008. Respect: Ethnic bonding and distinction in team sports careers. *European Journal for Sport and Society* 5(2): 153–167.

Elling, Agnes, and Jan Janssens. 2009. Sexuality as a structural principle in sport participation negotiating sports spaces. *International Review for the Sociology of Sport* 44(1): 71–86.

Elling, Agnes, Ivo Van Hilvoorde, and Remko Van Den Dool. 2012. Creating or awakening national pride through sporting success: A longitudinal study on macro effects in the Netherlands. *International Review for the Sociology of Sport* August 22, 2012, doi: 10.1177/1012690212455961.

Elling, Agnes, Ivo Van Hilvoorde, and Remko Van Den Dool. 2014. Creating or awakening national pride through sporting success: A longitudinal study on macro effects in the Netherlands. *International Review for the Sociology of Sport* 49(2): 129–151.

Elliott, Richard. 2013. New Europe, new chances? The migration of professional footballers to Poland's Ekstraklasa. *International Review for the Sociology of Sport* 48(6): 736–750.

Elliott, Richard, and Gavin Weedon. 2011. Foreign players in the English Premier Academy League: 'Feet-drain' or 'feet-exchange'? *International Review for the Sociology of Sport* 46(1): 61–75.

Elliott, Richard, and Joseph A. Maguire. 2008. "Thinking outside of the box": Exploring a conceptual synthesis for research in the area of athletic labor migration. *Sociology of Sport Journal* 25(4): 482–497.

Empfield, Dan. 2007. Scott Tinley: His body sidelined, his brain in the game. *Slowtwitch.com* (December 28): http://www.slowtwitch.com/Interview/Scott_Tinley_

his_body_sidelined_his_brain_in_the_game_166
.html.

Engh, Mari Haugaa, and Sine Agergaard. 2013. Producing mobility through locality and visibility: Developing a transnational perspective on sports labour migration. *International Review for the Sociology of Sport* 1012690213509994, first published on November 18, 2013 as doi: 10.1177/101269021350999.

Engh, Mari Haugaa, and Sine Agergaard. 2015. Producing mobility through locality and visibility: Developing a transnational perspective on sports labour migration. *International Review for the Sociology of Sport* 50(8): 974–992.

Epstein, David. 2009. Well, is she or isn't she? *Sports Illustrated* 111(9, September 7): 24–25. Online: http://www.si.com/vault/2009/09/07/105854299/well-is-she-or-isnt-she.

Epstein, David. 2010. Sports genes. *Sports Illustrated* 112(21, May 17): 53–65.

Epstein, David. 2011. Sports medicine's new frontiers. *Sports Illustrated* 115(5, August 8): 47–66.

Epstein, David. 2013. *The sports gene: Inside the science of extraordinary athletic performance.* New York: Penguin Group.

Erčulj, Frane, and Mojca Doupona Topič. 2008. Media coverage of women's basketball in Slovenia. In Mojca Doupona Topič & Simon Ličen, eds., *Sport, culture & society: An account of views and perspectives on social issues in a continent (and beyond)* (pp. 104–108). Ljubljana, Slovenia: University of Ljubljana.

Erhart, Itir. 2011. Ladies of Besiktas: A dismantling of male hegemony at Inönü Stadium. *International Review for the Sociology of Sport* 47(1): 83–98.

Ericsson, K. Anders. 2012. Training history, deliberate practice and elite sports performance: An analysis in response to Tucker and Collins review—what makes champions? *British Journal of Sports Medicine* 47: 533–555.

Ericsson, K. Anders, Michael J. Prietula, and Edward T. Cokely. 2007. The making of an expert. *Harvard Business Review* (July-August): 1–7. Online: http://www.uvm.edu/~pdodds/files/papers/others/2007/ericsson2007a.pdf.

Erturan, E. Esra, Natasha Brison, and Tiffany Allen. 2012. Comparative analysis of university sports in the U.S. and Turkey. *Sport Management International Journal* 8(1): 5–24.

ESPN. 2011. Recruiting confidential. *ESPN The Magazine* (February 7): 64–83.

ESPN. 2012. NFL: Saints defense had 'bounty' fund. *ESPN.go.com* (March 4): http://espn.go.com/nfl/story/_/id/7638603/new-orleans-saints-defense-had-bounty-program-nfl-says (retrieved 5-25-13).

Estep, Tyler. 2015. Carroll schools investigating 'mass baptism' at football practice. *Atlanta Journal-Constitution* (September 2): http://www.ajc.com/news/news/local/carroll-schools-investigating-mass-baptism-at-foot/nnW2B/.

Etchison, William C., Elizabeth A. Bloodgood, Cholly P. Minton, Nancy J. Thompson, Mary Ann Collins, Stephen C. Hunter, and Hongying Dai. 2011. Body mass index and percentage of body fat as indicators for obesity in an adolescent athletic population. *Sports Health: A Multidisciplinary Approach* 3(3): 249–252.

Evans, Adam B., and David E. Stead. 2012. 'It's a long way to the Super League': The experiences of Australasian professional rugby league migrants in the United Kingdom. *International Review for the Sociology of Sport* published 4 December 2012, 10.1177/1012690212464700.

Evans, Ashley B., Kristine E. Copping, Stephanie J. Rowley, and Beth Kurtz-Costes. 2011. Academic self-concept in black adolescents: Do race and gender stereotypes matter? *Self and Identity* 10(2): 263–277.

Evans, Mark. 2011. A generation after Nike 'Let me play' ads, female athletes are totally cool. *Sequoyah County Times* (June 18): http://www.sequoyahcountytimes.com/view/full_story/14362433/article-A-generation-after-Nike-%E2%80%98Let-me-play%E2%80%99-ads—female-athletes-are-totally-cool.

Ewald, Keith, and Robert M. Jiobu. 1985. Explaining positive deviance: Becker's model and the case of runners and bodybuilders. *Sociology of Sport Journal* 2(2): 144–156.

Eyler, J. 2013. The athletes of Christ: Spiritual athleticism in early English Christian thought. *International Journal of Religion and Sport* 2: 21–32.

Fagan, Kate, and Luke Cyphers. 2012. Thanks but no thanks. *ESPN The Magazine* (June 11): 90–91.

Fainaru-Wada, Mark, and Steve Fainaru. 2013. *The NFL, concussions and the battle for truth.* New York: Crown Archetype.

Fair, Brian. 2011. Constructing masculinity through penetration discourse: The intersection of misogyny and homophobia in high school wrestling. *Men and Masculinities* 14(4): 491–504.

Falcous, Mark, and Christopher McLeod. 2012. Anyone for tennis? Sport, class and status in New Zealand. *New Zealand Sociology* 27(1): 13–30.

Falcous, Mark, and Joshua I. Newman. 2013. Sporting mythscapes, neoliberal histories, and post-colonial amnesia in Aotearoa/New Zealand. *International Review for the Sociology of Sport* published 18 November 2013, 10.1177/1012690213508942.

Falk, David. 2012. A Nobel sport: The racial football rhetoric of Mandela, Obama, and Martin Luther King Jr. *Journal of Sport and Social Issues* 36(4): 361–386.

Faris, Robert, and Diane Felmlee. 2011. The corner and the crew: The influence of geography and social networks on gang violence. *American Sociological Review* 76(1): 48–73.

Farooq, Sumaya, and Andrew Parker. 2009. Sport, physical education, and Islam: Muslim independent schooling and the social construction of masculinities. *Sociology of Sport Journal* 26(2): 277–295.

Farrey, Tom. 2005. Baby you're the greatest: Genetic testing for athletic traits. *ESPN The Magazine* 8.03 (February 14)**:** 80–87. Online: http://sports.espn .go.com/espn/news/story?id=2022781.

Farrey, Tom, 2008. *Game on: The All-American race to make champions of our children.* New York: ESPN Books.

Farrey, Tom. 2011. Men: AAU ex-CEO sexually abused them. *ESPN* (retrieved 12-9-2011): http://espn .go.com/espn/otl/story/_/id/7332846/ex-players-say -aau-bobby-dodd-sexually-abused-youths.

Farrey, Tom. 2012a. Outside the Lines: A fight for faith. *ESPN* (April 8): see video at espn.go.com/video/clip /clip?id=7784413.

Farrey, Tom. 2012b. Too high a price to play. *ESPN. go.com* (June 7): http://espn.go.com/espnw /title-ix/7986414/too-high-price-play.

Farrington, Neil, Daniel Kilvington, John Price, and Amir Saeed. 2012. *Race, Racism and Sports Journalism. Abingdon,* UK: Routledge, 2012.

Fasting, Kari, and Celia Brackenridge. 2009. Coaches, sexual harassment and education. *Sport, Education and Society* 14(1): 21–35. Online: http://bura.brunel .ac.uk/handle/2438/3207.

Fasting, Kari, Celia Brackenridge, and G. Kjølberg. 2011. Using court reports to enhance knowledge of sexual abuse in sport. *Brunel University Research Archive:* http://bura.brunel.ac.uk/handle /2438/5001.

Fasting, Kari, Celia Brackenridge, and Nada Knorre. 2010. Performance level and sexual harassment prevalence among female athletes in the Czech Republic. *Women in Sport and Physical Activity Journal* 19(1): 26–32. Online: http://bura.brunel .ac.uk/handle/2438/3248 (retrieved 6-26-13).

Fasting, Kari, Celia Brackenridge, Katherine Miller, and Don Sabo. 2008. Participation in college sports and protection from sexual victimization. *International Journal of Sport and Exercise Psychology* 16(4): 427–441.

Fasting, Kari, Celia Brackenridge, and Jorunn Sundgot-Borgen. 2004. Prevalence of sexual harassment among Norwegian female elite athletes in relation to sport type. *International Review for the Sociology of Sport* 39(4): 373–386.

Fausto-Sterling, Anne. 2000a. The five sexes, revisited. *Sciences* 40(4): 18–23.

Fausto-Sterling, Anne. 2000b. *Sexing the body: Gender politics and the construction of sexuality.* New York: Basic Books.

Fawcett, Joby. 2012. Injuries becoming biggest concern in football. *Scranton Times-Tribune* (August 26): http://thetimes-tribune.com/sports /football-2012-injuries-becoming-biggest-concern-in -football-1.1362411.

FCA. 2012. U.S. athletes in the 2012 London Olympics. *Fellowship of Christian Athletes.*

Feddersen, Arne, and Wolfgang Maennig. 2009. Arenas versus multifunctional stadiums: Which do spectators prefer? *Journal of Sports Economics* 10(2): 180–191.

Federico, Bruno, Lavinia Falese, Diego Marandola, and Giovanni Capelli. 2013. *Socioeconomic* 31(4): 451–458.

Feezell, R. 2013. Sport, religious belief, and religious diversity. *Journal of the Philosophy of Sport* 40(1): 135–162.

Feldman, Bruce. 2007. A recruiting pitch of another kind. *ESPN The Magazine* (May 28): http://espn .go.com/gen/s/2002/0527/1387550.html.

Fellowship of Christian Athletes. 2008. *Serving: True champions know that success takes surrender.* Ventura, CA, USA: Regal, From Gospel Light.

Fenstermaker, Sarah, and Candace West, eds. 2002. *Doing gender, doing difference: Inequality, power, and institutional change.* New York: Routledge.

Ferguson, Niall. 2013. The end of the American dream? *Newsweek* (June 26): http://www.newsweek.com/2013/06/26/niall-ferguson-end-american-dream-237614.html.

Ferkins, Lesley, David Shilbury, and Gael McDonald. 2009. Board involvement in strategy: Advancing the governance of sport organizations. *Journal of Sport Management* 23(3): 245–277.

Ferriter, Meghan M. 2009. "Arguably the greatest": Sport fans and communities at work on Wikipedia. *Sociology of Sport Journal* 26(1): 127–154.

Fertman, Carl I. 2008. *Student-athlete success: Meeting the challenges of college life.* Sudbury, MA: Jones and Bartlett Publishers.

Fields, Sara. K. 2012. Are we asking the right questions? A response to the academic reforms research by Todd Petr and Tom Paskus. *Journal of Intercollegiate Sport* 5(1): 60–64.

Findlay, Leanne C., Rochelle E. Garner, and Dafna E. Kohen. 2009. Children's organized physical activity patterns from childhood into adolescence. *Journal of Physical Activity & Health* 6(6): 708–715.

Finger, Dave. 2004. Before they were next. *ESPN The Magazine* 7.12 (June 7): 83–86.

Fink, Janet S., and George B. Cunningham. 2005. The effects of racial and gender dyad diversity on work experiences of university athletics personnel. *International Journal of Sport Management* 6: 199–213.

Fleming, David. 2007. Does God want John Kitna to win? *ESPN The Magazine* 10.20 (October 8): 48–54.

Fleming, David. 2013. No prayer. *ESPN The Magazine* (June 10): 70–75.

Fleming, Scott, and Alan Tomlinson. 2007. Racism and xenophobia in English football. In Alan Tomlinson, ed., *The sport studies reader* (pp. 304–315). London/New York: Routledge.

Fletcher, Thomas. 2011. 'Who do "they" cheer for?': Cricket, diaspora, hybridity and divided loyalties amongst British Asians. *International Review for the Sociology of Sport* published online before print July 29, 2011, doi: 10.1177/1012690211416556.

Fletcher, Thomas. 2012. 'Who do "they" cheer for?': Cricket, diaspora, hybridity and divided loyalties amongst British Asians. *International Review for the Sociology of Sport* 47(5): 612–631.

Flint, John, and John Kelly, eds. 2013. *Bigotry, football and Scotland.* Edinburgh, Scotland: Edinburgh University Press.

Flintoff, Anne. 2008. Targeting Mr. Average: Participation, gender equity and school sport partnerships. *Sport, Education and Society* 13(4): 393–411.

Florio, Mike. 2012. NFL's "magic potion" has risks, players like Urlacher don't care. *NBCSports.com* (January 24): http://profootballtalk.nbcsports.com/2012/01/24/nfls-magic-potion-has-risks-players-like-urlacher-dont-care/.

Foer, Franklin. 2004. *How soccer explains the world: An unlikely theory of globalization.* New York: HarperCollins.

Foer, Franklin, and Chris Hughes. 2013. Barack Obama is not pleased: The president on his enemies, the media, and the future of football. *New Republic* (January 27): http://www.newrepublic.com/article/112190/obama-interview-2013-sit-down-president# (retrieved 5-25-13).

Fogel, Curtis. 2011. Sporting masculinity on the gridiron: Construction, characteristics, and consequences. *Canadian Social Science* 7(2): 1–14.

Foley, Douglas E. 1990a. *Learning capitalist culture.* Philadelphia: University of Pennsylvania Press.

Foley, Douglas E. 1990b. The great American football ritual: Reproducing race, class, and gender inequality. *Sociology of Sport Journal* 7(2): 111–135.

Foley, Douglas E. 1999a. High school football: Deep in the heart of south Tejas. In Jay Coakley & Peter Donnelly, eds., *Inside sports* (pp. 133–138). London: Routledge.

Foley, Douglas E. 1999b. Jay White Hawk: Mesquaki athlete, AIM hellraiser, and anthropological informant. In Jay Coakley & Peter Donnelly, eds., *Inside sports* (pp. 156–161). London: Routledge.

Foote, Chandra J., and Bill Collins. 2011. You know, Eunice, the world will never be the same after this. *International Journal of Special Education* 26(3): 285–295.

Forde, Shawn D. 2013. Fear and loathing in Lesotho: An autoethnographic analysis of sport for development and peace. *International Review for the Sociology of Sport.* Published online before print September 10, 2013, doi: 10.1177/1012690213501916.

Forney, Craig A. 2007. *The holy trinity of American sports: Civil religion in football, baseball, and basketball.* Macon, GA: Mercer University Press.

Foster, William M., and Marvin Washington. 2013. Organizational structure and home team performance. *The impact of sports on Team Performance Management* 15(3/4): 158–171.

Foucault, Michel. 1961/1967. *Madness and civilization.* London: Travistock.

Fox Sports. 2011. FA report: Suarez kept using 'Negro'. *FoxSports.com* (December 31): http://www .foxsports.com/soccer/story/luis-suarez-patrice-evra-racism-incident-negro-seven-times-123111.

Fox, Claudia K., Daheia Barr-Anderson, Dianne Neumark-Sztainer, and Melanie Wall. 2010. Physical activity and sports team participation: Association with academic outcomes in middle school and high school students. *Journal of School Health* 80: 31–37.

Fox, Jon. 2012. Of colors and scales. *Ethnic and Racial Studies* 35(7): 1151–1156.

Foxworth, Domonique. 2005. Ties that bind team begin with prayer. *Denver Post* (October 19): 2D.

Francombe, Jessica Margaret. 2013. Methods that move: A physical performative pedagogy of subjectivity. *Sociology of Sport Journal* 30(3): 256–273.

Fraser-Thomas, Jessica, Jean Coté, and Janice Deakin. 2008. Examining adolescent sport dropout and prolonged engagement from a developmental perspective. *Journal of Applied Sport Psychology* 2(3): 318–333.

Frederick, Evan L., Choong Hoon Lim, Clavio, Galen, Walsh, Patrick. 2012. Why we follow: An examination of parasocial interaction and fan motivations for following athlete archetypes on Twitter. *International Journal of Sport Communication* 5(4): 481–503.

Fredrickson, Barbara L., and Kristen Harrison. 2005. Throwing like a girl: Self-objectification predicts adolescent girls' motor performance. *Journal of Sport and Social Issues* 29(1): 79–101.

Fredrickson, George M. 2003. *Racism: A short history.* Princeton, NJ: Princeton University Press.

Freeh Sporkin and Sullivan. 2012. *Report of the Special Investigative Counsel Regarding the Actions of the Pennsylvania State University Related to the Child Sexual Abuse Committed by Gerald A. Sandusky.* July 12.

Freeman, Mike. 1998. A cycle of violence, on the field and off. *New York Times,* section 8 (September 6): 1.

Friedman, Michael T., and David L. Andrews. 2011. The built sport spectacle and the opacity of democracy. *International Review for the Sociology of Sport* 46(2): 181–204.

Friedman, Michael T., David L. Andrews, and Michael L. Silk. 2004. Sport and the façade of redevelopment in the postindustrial city. *Sociology of Sport Journal* 21(2): 119–139.

Frontline. 2011. Football high (video). *PBS.org* (April 12): http://video.pbs.org/video/1880045332/.

Frontline. 2013. League of denial: The NFL's concussion crisis (video). *PBS.org* (October 8): http://video.pbs.org/video/2365093675/.

Frosch, Dan. 2012. Unified teams take Special Olympics approach to school sports. *New York Times* (February 12): http://www.nytimes .com/2012/02/13/sports/unified-sports-teams-open-doors-for-special-education-students.html.

Fry, Hap. 2006. Boosters take different roads to same goal. *The Coloradoan* (January 27): A1, A2.

FSTA. 2013. Industry demographics. Fantasy Sports Trade Association: http://fsta.org/research/industry -demographics/.

Fulks, Daniel L. 2012a. *NCAA revenues and expenses of division II intercollegiate athletics programs report fiscal years 2004 through 2011.* Indianapolis, IN: The National Collegiate Athletic Association.

Fulks, Daniel L. 2012b. *NCAA revenues and expenses of division III intercollegiate athletics programs report fiscal years 2004 through 2011.* Indianapolis, Indiana: The National Collegiate Athletic Association.

Fullinwider, Robert K. 2006. *Sports, youth and character: A critical survey.* Circle Working Paper 44, The Center for Information and Research on Civic Learning and Engagement. College Park, MD: University of Maryland.

Futterman, Matthew. 2013. NFL to charge New York prices. *Wall Street Journal* (September 17): http:// online.wsj.com/news/articles/SB1000142412788732 4665604579079424146436620.

Futterman, Matthew, Jonathan Clegg, and Geoffrey A. Fowler. 2012. An Olympics built for records. *Wall Street Journal* (August 10): D1-2.

Gabay, Danielle. 2013. Black female student-athletes in Canadian higher education. Ph.D. Dissertation, Department of Theory and Policy Studies in Education, Ontario Institute for Studies in Education of the University of Toronto, Toronto, Ontario, Canada.

Gabriel, Trip. 2010. To stop cheats, colleges learn their trickery. *New York Times* (July 5): http://www .nytimes.com/2010/07/06/education/06cheat.html (retrieved 6-26-13).

Gaffney, Gary R., and Robin Parisotto. 2007. Gene doping: A review of performance-enhancing genetics. *Pediatric Clinics of North America* 54(4): 807–822.

Gaither, Sarah E., and Samuel R. Sommers. 2012. Honk if you like minorities: Vuvuzela attitudes predict outgroup liking. *International Review for the Sociology of Sport* 48(1): 54–65.

Galanter, Seth M. 2013. "Dear Colleague" letter. Washington, DC: United States Department of Education, Office for Civil Rights.

Galily, Yair. 2014. When the medium becomes "well done": Sport, television, and technology in the twenty-first century. *Television & New Media* 15(8): 717–724.

Galily, Yair and Ilan Tamir. 2014. A match made in heaven?! Sport, television, and new media in the beginning of the third millennia. *Television & New Media* 15(8): 699–702.

Gantz, Walter. 2013. Reflections on communication and sport: On fanship and social relationships. *Communication & Sport* 1(1/2): 176–187.

Gantz, Walter, and Nicky Lewis. 2014. Sports on traditional and newer digital media: Is there really a fight for fans? *Television & New Media* 15(8): 760–768.

Garcia, Beatrice. 2012. *The Olympic Games and cultural policy.* London: Routledge.

Garber, Greg. 2007a. The Dominican Republic of the NFL. *ESPN The Magazine* (May 28): http://espn.go.com/gen/s/2002/0527/1387626.html.

Garber, Greg. 2007b. They might be giants. *ESPN The Magazine* (May 28): http://espn.go.com/gen/s/2002/0527/1387627.html.

Gates, Henry Louis, Jr. 2007. *Finding Oprah's roots: Finding your own.* New York: Crown.

Gates, Henry Louis, Jr. 2011. What it means to be 'Black in Latin America'. *NPR, Fresh Air from WHYY* (July 27): http://www.npr.org/2011/07/27/138601410/what-it-means-to-be-black-in-latin-americaandsc=nlandcc=es-20110731.

Gatti, Claudio. 2013. Looking upstream in doping cases. *New York Times* (January 15): http://www.nytimes.com/2013/01/16/sports/cycling/critics-take-a-look-upstream-in-doping-scandals.html?_r=0.

Gaunt, Kyra D. 2006. *The games black girls play.* New York: New York University Press.

Gavora, Jessica. 2002. *Tilting the playing field: Schools, sports, sex and Title IX.* San Francisco: Encounter Books.

Gay, Jason. 2011. Nobody suffers like Jens Voigt. *Wall Street Journal* (July 19): http://online.wsj.com/news/articles/SB10001424052702303661904576454451021920040.

Gay, Jason. 2013. The meaning of football tough. *Wall Street Journal* (November 11): B8.

Gee, Sarah, Steven J Jackson, and Mike Sam. 2014. Carnivalesque culture and alcohol promotion and consumption at an annual international sports event in New Zealand. *International Review for the Sociology of Sport* published 20 February 2014, 10.1177/1012690214522461.

Gelles, David, and Andrew Edgecliffe-Johnson. 2011. Television: Inflated assets. *Financial Times* (March 24): http://www.ft.com/cms/s/0/d2a693b2-5653-11e0-82aa-00144feab49a.html#axzz1HdO79lVX.

George, Christopher A., James P. Leonard, and Mark R. Hutchinson. 2011. The female athlete triad: A current concepts review. *South African Journal of Sports Medicine* 23: 50–56.

George, Rachel. 2013. Snowmobile athletes defined risks. *USA Today* (January 30): 8C. Online: http://www.usatoday.com/story/sports/olympics/2013/01/29/snowmobile-athletes-x-games-caleb-moore-levi-lavallee/1875447/ (retrieved 6-21-2013).

Gerber, Charlotte, 2015. Colleges that offer adaptive sports programs for their students. *About Health* (December 11): http://disability.about.com/od/CareerDecisionsAndCollege/tp/College-Adaptive-Sports-Programs.htm.

Ghanem, Sharifa. 2012. Iran says no to women watching Euro 2012. *Bikyamasr.com* (June 12): http://bikyamasr.com/69684/iran-says-no-to-women-watching-euro-2012/.

Gianfreda, Anna. 2011. Religious offences in Italy: Recent laws concerning blasphemy and sport. *Ecclesiastical Law Journal* 13(2): 182–197.

Giardina, Michael D., and Norman K. Denzin. 2013. Confronting neoliberalism: Toward a militant pedagogy of empowered citizenship. *Cultural Studies <=> Critical Methodologies* published 17 September 2013, 10.1177/1532708613503767.

Giardina, Michael D., and Jason Laurendeau. 2013. Truth untold? Evidence, knowledge, and research practice(s). *Sociology of Sport Journal* 30(3): 237–255.

Gibbons, Tom. 2014. *English national identity and football fan culture: Who are ya?* Surrey, Ashgate.

Gibbs, Chad. 2012. *Love thy rival: What sports' greatest rivalries teach us about loving our enemies.* Clearwater, FL, USA: Blue Moon Books.

Gieseler, Carly. 2014. Derby drag: Parodying sexualities in the sport of roller derby. *Sexualities* 17(5–6): 758–776.

Gilchrist, Paul, and Belinda Wheaton. 2011. Lifestyle sport, public policy and youth engagement: Examining the emergence of parkour. *International Journal of Sport Policy and Politics* 3(1): 109–131.

Giles, Audrey. 2004. Kevlar®, Crisco®, and menstruation: "Tradition" and Dene games. *Sociology of Sport Journal* 21(1): 18–35.

Gilldenpsenning, Sven. 2001. *Sport: Kritik und eigensinn: Der sport der gesellescahft.* Sankt Augustin: Academia.

Gilmour, Callum, and David Rowe. 2012. Sport in Malaysia: National imperatives and Western seductions. *Sociology of Sport Journal* 29(4): 485–505.

Ginsburg, Kenneth R. 2007. The importance of play in promoting healthy child development and maintaining strong parent-child bonds. *Pediatrics* 119(1): http://www.aap.org/pressroom/playFINAL.pdf.

Giulianotti, Richard. 2009. Risk and sport: An analysis of sociological theories and research agendas. *Sociology of Sport Journal* 26(4): 540–556.

Giulianotti, Richard, and Francisco Klauser. 2010. Security governance and sport mega-events: Toward an interdisciplinary research agenda. *Journal of Sport and Social Issues* 34(1): 49–61.

Giulianotti, Richard, and Francisco Klauser. 2012. Sport mega-events and 'terrorism': A critical analysis. *International Review for the Sociology of Sport* 47(3): 307–323.

Glanville, Doug. 2008. In baseball, fear bats at the top of the order. *The New York Times* (January 16): www.nytimes.com/2008/01/16/opinion/16glanville.html.

Glanz, James, Agustin Armendariz, and Walt Bogdanich. 2015a. Finding 'who' and 'where' within the sports cyber-betting universe. *New York Times* (October 15): http://www.nytimes.com/2015/10/16/us/finding-who-and-where-within-the-sports-cyber-betting-universe.html.

Glanz, James, Agustin Armendariz, and Walt Bogdanich.2015b. The offshore game of online sports betting. *New York Times* (October 25): http://www.nytimes.com/2015/10/26/us/pinnacle-sports-online-sports-betting.html.

Glenn, Evelyn Nakano, ed. 2009. *Shades of difference: Why skin color matters.* Stanford, CA: Stanford University Press.

Glenn, Nicole M., Camilla J. Knight, Nicholas L. Holt, and John C. Spence. 2013. Meanings of play among children. *Childhood* 20(2): 185–199.

Glennie, Elizabeth J., and Elizabeth Stearns. 2012. Opportunities to play the game: The effect of individual and school attributes on participation in sports. *Sociological Spectrum: Mid-South Sociological Association* 32(6): 532–557.

Glickman, Charlie. 2011. A perfect illustration of the act like a man box. *Adult Sexuality Education* (November 17): http://www.charlieglickman.com/2011/11/a-perfect-illustration-of-the-act-like-a-man-box/.

Gluck, Jeff. 2015. Real sport or circus sideshow? *USA Today* (November 2): 7C.

Godoy-Pressland, Amy. 2014. 'Nothing to report': S semi-longitudinal investigation of the print media coverage of sportswomen in British Sunday newspapers. *Media Culture & Society* 36(5): 595–609.

Goff, Brian L., and Robert D. Tollison. 2009. Racial integration of coaching: Evidence from the NFL. *Journal of Sports Economics* 10(2): 127–140.

Goff, Brian L., and Robert D. Tollison. 2010. Who integrated major league baseball faster: Winning teams or losing teams? A comment. *Journal of Sports Economics* 11(3): 236–238.

Goffman, Erving. 1961. *Asylums: Essays on the social situation of mental patients and other inmates.* New York: Anchor Books.

Goldsmith, Belinda. 2012. Battle of the sexes swings from ring to pool. *Reuters.com* (July 5): http://www.reuters.com/article/oly-sports-equality-idUSL6E8HSIQH20120705.

Goodley, Dan, and Katherine Runswick-Cole. 2010. Emancipating play: dis/abled children, development and deconstruction. *Disability & Society* 25(4): 499–512.

Goodman, Cary. 1979. *Choosing sides: Playground and street life on the lower east side.* New York: Schocken Books.

Gordon, Ian. 2007. Caught looking. *ESPN The Magazine* 10.11 (June 4): 100–104.

Gore, Will. 2011. "I pray for my opponents before fights." *The Catholic Herald* (September 16): 7.

Graham, Stephen. 2012. Olympics 2012 security. *City: Analysis of Urban Trends, Culture, Theory, Policy, Action* 16(4): 446–451.

Grainey, Timothy F., and Brittany Timko. 2012. *Beyond bend it like Beckham: The global phenomenon of women's soccer.* University of Nebraska Press.

Gramsci, Antonio. 1971. *Selections from the prison notebook* (Q. Hoare & G.N. Smith, trans). New York: International Publishers (original work published in 1947).

Gramsci, Antonio. 1988. D. Forgacs, ed. *Selected writings: 1918–1935.* New York: Shocken.

Graves, Joseph L., Jr. 2002. *The emperor's new clothes: Biological theories of race at the millennium.* New Brunswick, NJ: Rutgers University Press.

Graves, Joseph L., Jr. 2004. *The race myth: Why we pretend race exists in America.* New York: Penguin Books.

Gray, Caroline. 2009. Narratives of disability and the movement from deficiency to difference. *Cultural Sociology* 3(2): 317–332.

Green, Ken. 2012. London 2012 and sports participation: The myths of legacy. *Significance* 9(3): 2–48.

Green, Kyle, and Doug Hartmann. 2012. Politics and sports: Strange, secret bedfellows. *The Society Pages* (February 3): http://thesocietypages.org/papers/politics-and-sport/.

Green, Mick. 2006. From "sport for all" to not about "sport" at all?: Interrogating sport policy interventions in the United Kingdom. *European Sport Management Quarterly* 6(3): 217–238.

Green, Mick, and Barrie Houlihan. 2004. Advocacy coalitions and elite sport policy change in Canada and the United Kingdom. *International Review for the Sociology of Sport* 39(4): 387–403.

Greenfeld, Karl Taro. 1999. Adjustment in mid-flight. *Outside* (February): http://outside.away.com/magazine/0299/9902terje_2.html.

Greenfield, Karl Taro. 2012. ESPN: Everywhere sports profit network. *BusinessWeek.com* (August 30): http://www.businessweek.com/articles/2012-08-30/espn-everywhere-sports-profit-network.

Greenlees, Ian, Alex Leyland, Richard Thelwell, and William Filby. 2008. Soccer penalty takers' uniform colour and pre-penalty kick gaze affect the impressions formed of them by opposing goalkeepers. *Journal of Sports Sciences* 26(6): 569–576.

Gregory, Michele Rene. 2009. Inside the locker room: Homosociability in the advertising industry. *Gender, Work and Organization* 16(3): 323–347.

Gregory, Michele Rene. 2010. Slam dunk: Strategic sport metaphors and the construction of masculine embodiment at work. In Marcia Texler Segal, ed., *Advances in gender research,* Vol. 14, *Interactions and intersections of gendered bodies at work, at home, and at play* (pp. 297–318). Emerald Group Publishing Ltd.

Gregory, Sean. 2012. No more tears. *Time* 179(6): 61. Online: http://www.time.com/time/magazine/article/0,9171,2105962,00.html#ixzz1llGgknq1.

Gregory, Sean. 2013a. Final four for the 4-foot set. *Time* 182(4 July 22): 44–48.

Gregory, Sean. 2013b. Should this kid be making $225,047 a year for playing college football? *Time* 182(12, September 16): 36–42.

Gregory, Sean. 2015. U.S. ranks worst in sports homophobia study. *Time* (May 9): http://time.com/3852611/sports-homophobia-study/.

Greider, William. 2006. Olympic swagger. *The Nation* (February 28): http://www.thenation.com/doc/20060313/greider2.

Griffin, Pat. 1998. *Strong women, deep closets: Lesbians and homophobia in sport.* Champaign, IL: Human Kinetics.

Griffin, Pat, and Helen J. Carroll. 2012. *On the team: Equal opportunity for transgender student athletes.* National Center for Lesbian Rights and the Women's Sports Foundation. Online: http://www.transyouthequality.org/documents/TransgenderStudentAthleteReport.pdf.

Griffin, Pat, and Hudson Taylor. 2012. *Champions of respect: Inclusion of LGBTQ student-athletes and staff in NCAA programs.* Indianapolis, IN: National Collegiate Athletic Association. Online: http://www.ncaapublications.com/p-4305-champions-of-respect-inclusion-of-lgbtq-student-athletes-and-staff-in-ncaa-programs.aspx.

Griggs, Gerald, and Tom Gibbons. 2014. 'Harry walks, Fabio runs': A case study on the current relationship between English national identity, soccer and the English press. *International Review for the Sociology of Sport* 49(5): 536–549.

Groothuis, Peter A., and James Richard Hill. 2013. Pay discrimination, exit discrimination or both? Another look at an old issue using NBA data. *Journal of Sports Economics* 14: 171–185.

Group of Experts. 2014. *Gender equality in sport: Proposal for strategic actions 2014–2020.* Brussels: Education and Culture of the European Commission.

Grow, Helene Mollie, Brian E. Saelens, Jacqueline Kerr, Nefertiti H. Durant, Gregory J. Norman, and James F. Sallis. 2008. Where are youth active? Roles of proximity, active transport, and built environment. *Medicine and Science in Sports and Exercise* 40(12): 2071–2079.

Grundy, Pamela, and Susan Shackelford. 2005. *Shattering the glass: The remarkable history of women's basketball.* New York: The New Press.

Grünenberg, Kristina, Line Hillersdal, Hanne Kjærgaard Walker, and Hanne Bess Boelsbjerg. 2013. Doing wholeness, producing subjects: Kinesiological sensemaking and energetic kinship. *Body and Society* 19(4): 92–119.

Guest, Andrew, and Barbara Schneider. 2003. Adolescents' extracurricular participation in context: The mediating effects of schools, communities, and identity. *Sociology of Education* 76(2): 89–109.

Guiliano, Jennifer. 2011. Chasing objectivity? Critical reflections on history, identity, and the public performance of Indian mascots. *Cultural Studies < = > Critical Methodologies* 11: 535–543.

Guimarães, Antonio Sérgio Alfredo. 2012. The Brazilian system of racial classification. *Ethnic and Racial Studies* 35(7): 1157–1162.

Güldenpfenning, Sven. 2001. *Sport: Kritik und eigensinn: Der sport der gesellescahft.* Sankt Augustin: Academia.

Gulick, Luther Halsey. 1906. Athletics do not test womanliness. *American Physical Education Review* 11(3): 158–159.

Gulick, Luther Halsey. 1920. *A philosophy of play.* Washington, DC: McGrath.

Gustafsson, Henrik, Peter Hassmén, and Leslie Podlog. 2010. Exploring the relationship between hope and burnout in competitive sport. *Journal of Sports Sciences* 28(14): 1495–1504.

Guttmann, Allen. 1978. *From ritual to record: The nature of modern sports.* New York: Columbia University Press.

Guttmann, Allen. 1986. *Sport spectators.* New York: Columbia University Press.

Guttmann, Allen. 1988. *A whole new ball game: An interpretation of American sports.* Chapel Hill: University of North Carolina Press.

Guttmann, Allen. 1998. The appeal of violent sports. In J. Goldstein, ed., *Why we watch: The attractions of violent entertainment* (pp. 7–26). New York: Oxford University Press.

Guttmann, Allen. 2004. *Sports: The first five millennia.* Amherst: University of Massachusetts Press.

Hadden, Jeffrey. K. 2000. Religious movements. In E.F. Borgotta & R.J.V. Montgomery, eds., *Encyclopedia of sociology* (pp. 2364–2376). New York: Macmillan Reference.

Hall, C. Michael. 2006. Urban entrepreneurship, corporate interests and sports mega-events: The thin policies of competitiveness within the hard outcomes of neoliberalism. *The Sociological Review* 54 (Supplement 2): 59–70.

Hall, C. Michael. 2012. Sustainable mega-events: Beyond the myth of balanced approaches to mega-event sustainability. Revision of a paper presented at the Global Events Congress IV, Leeds, July 14, 2010; accessed at http://canterbury-nz.academia.edu /CMichaelHall/Papers (retrieved 9-13-2012).

Halldorsson, Vidar, Thorolfur Thorlindsson, and Inga Dora Sigfusdottir. 2013. Adolescent sport participation and alcohol use: The importance of sport organization and the wider social context. *International Review for the Sociology of Sport* published 30 October 2013, 10.1177/1012690213507718.

Hallinan, Chris, and Steven J. Jackson, eds. 2008. *Social and cultural diversity in a sporting world.* Bingley, UK: Emerald.

Hamish, Crocket. 2013. 'This is men's ultimate': (Re) creating multiple masculinities in elite open Ultimate Frisbee. *International Review for the Sociology of Sport* 48(3): 318–333.

Hammersley, Martyn. 2007. Ethnography. In George Ritzer, ed., *Encyclopedia of sociology* (pp. 1479–1483). London/New York: Blackwell.

Hamrick, Jeff, and John Rasp. 2013. The connection between race and called strikes and balls. *Journal of Sports Economics* published 28 October 2013, 10.1177/1527002513509817.

Hannah, Katharine. 2011. Reconstructing fame: Sport, race, and evolving reputations. *Sociology of Sport Journal* 28(2): 254–256.

Hanssen, F. Andrew, and James W. Meehan, Jr. 2009. Who integrated Major League Baseball faster: Winning teams or losing teams? *Journal of Sports Economics* 10(2): 141–154.

Haraway, Donna. 1991. A cyborg manifesto: Science, technology, and socialist-feminism in the late twentieth century. Online: faculty.georgetown.edu /irvinem/theory/Haraway-CyborgManifesto-1.pdf articles/donna-haraway-a-cyborg-manifesto/.

Hardin, Marie, and Erin Elizabeth Whiteside. 2009. The power of "small stories:" Narratives and notions of gender equality in conversations about sport. *Sociology of Sport Journal* 26(2): 255–276.

Hardin, Marie, Erin Whiteside, and Erin Ash. 2012. Ambivalence on the front lines? Attitudes toward Title IX and women's sports among Division I sports information directors. *International Review for the Sociology of Sport* published 13 July 2012.

Hardy, Louise L., Michael Booth, Timothy Dobbins, and Anthony D. Okely. 2008. Physical activity among adolescents in New South Wales (Australia): 1997 and 2004. *Medicine & Science in Sports & Exercise* 40(5): 835–841.

Hardy, Stephen, John Loy, and Douglas Booth. 2009. The material culture sport: Toward a typology. *Journal of Sport History* 36(1): 129–152.

Hargreaves, Jennifer. 2000. *Heroines of sport: The politics of difference and identity.* London: Routledge.

Hargreaves, Jennifer, and Patricia Anne Vertinsky, eds. 2006. *Physical culture, power and the body.* Abingdon/New York: Routledge.

Harper, Catherine. 2007. *Intersex.* New York: Berg.

Harper, Shaun. 2013. Black male student-athletes and the 2014 Bowl Championship Series. University of Pennsylvania, Graduate school of Education, Center for the Study of Race and Equity in Education (December 9): http://www.gse.upenn.edu/news /black-male-student-athletes-and-2014-bowl -championship-series.

Harper, Shaun. R. Collin D. Williams, Jr. and Horatio W. Blackman. 2013. *Black male student-athletes and racial inequities in NCAA Division I college sports.* Philadelphia: University of Pennsylvania, Center for the Study of Race and Equity in Education.

Harpur, Paul. 2009. Sexism and racism, why not ableism? Calling for a cultural shift in the approach to disability discrimination. *Alternative Law Journal* (Melbourne: Legal Service Bulletin Co-operative Ltd) 34(3): 163–167.

Harpur, Paul. 2012. From disability to ability: Changing the phrasing of the debate. *Disability and Society* 27(3): 325–337.

Harris, Andrew. 2013. Students' concussion suits against NCAA, unlike NFL suits, defy grouping. *Insurance Journal* (December 6): http://www .insurancejournal.com/news/national/2013/12/06 /313236.htm.

Harris, Harry. 2011. PFA chief wants Rooney Rule (September 6): http://soccernet.espn.go.com/news /story/_/id/953246/pfa-chief-executive-gordon-taylor -wants-rooney-rule.

Harrison, Anthony Kwame. 2013. Black skiing, everyday racism, and the racial spatiality of whiteness. *Journal of Sport and Social Issues* 37(4) 315–339.

Harrison, C. Keith. 1998. Themes that thread through society: Racism and athletic manifestation in the African-American community. *Race, Ethnicity and Education* 1(1): 63–74.

Harrison, C. Keith, and Associates. 2013. *Coaching mobility* (Volume I in the Good Business Series). A Report for the NFL Diversity and Inclusion Series. Online: http://www.nfl.com/DrHarrison /goodbusinessvolume1/diversityinclusionbestpractices.

Harrison, C. Keith (with Sharon Yee). 2007. *The big game in sport management and higher education: The hiring practices of Division IA and IAA head football coaches.* Indianapolis: Black Coaches and Administrators.

Harrison, C. Keith, and Suzanne Malia Lawrence. 2004. College students' perceptions, myths, and stereotypes about African American athletes: A qualitative investigation. *Sport, Education and Society* 9(1): 33–52.

Harrison, C. Keith, Suzanne Malia Lawrence, and Scott J. Bukstein. 2011. White college students' explanations of white (and black) athletic performance: A qualitative investigation of white college students. *Sociology of Sport Journal* 28(3): 347–361.

Harrison, C. Keith, Jeff Stone, Jenessa Shapiro, Sharon Yee, Jean A. Boyd, and Vashti Rullan. 2009. The role of gender identities and stereotype salience with the academic performance of male and female college athletes. *Journal of Sport and Social Issues* 33(1): 78–96.

Harrison, Louis, Jr., and Leonard Moore. 2007. Who am I? Racial identity, athletic identity, and the African American athlete. In D. Brooks & R. Althouse, eds., *Diversity and social justice in college sports: Sport management and the student athlete* (pp. 243–260). Morgantown, WV: Fitness Information Technology.

Harrison, Louis, Gary Sailes, Willy K. Rotich, and Albert Y. Bimper. 2011. Living the dream or awakening from the nightmare: Race and athletic identity. *Race, Ethnicity and Education* 14(1): 91–103.

Hart, M. Marie. 1981. On being female in sport. In M.M. Hart & S. Birrell, eds., *Sport in the socio-cultural process* (pp. 291–301). Dubuque, IA: Brown.

Hartill, Mike. 2009. The sexual abuse of boys in organized male sports. *Men and Masculinities* 12(2): 225–249.

Hartmann, Douglas. 2003. The sanctity of Sunday afternoon football: Why men love sports. *Contexts* 2(4): 13–21.

Hartmann, Douglas. 2008. *High school sports participation and educational attainment: Recognizing, assessing, and utilizing the relationship.* Report to the LA84 Foundation. Los Angeles: Amateur Athletic Foundation. Online: http://www.la84foundation.org/3ce /HighSchoolSportsParticipation.pdf .

Hartmann, Douglas. 2012. Beyond the sporting boundary: The racial significance of sport through midnight basketball. *Ethnic and Racial Studies* 35(6): 1007–1022.

Hartmann, Douglas, Joseph N. Cooper, Joey Gawrysiak, and Billy Hawkins. 2013. Racial perceptions of baseball at historically black colleges and universities. *Journal of Sport and Social Issues* 37(2): 196–221.

Hartmann, Douglas, and Brooks Depro. 2006. Rethinking sports-based community crime prevention: A preliminary analysis of the relationship between midnight basketball and urban crime rates. *Journal of Sport and Social Issues* 30(2): 180–196.

Hartmann, Douglas, and Michael Massoglia. 2007. Re-assessing high school sports participation and deviance in early adulthood: Evidence of enduring, bifurcated effects. *The Sociological Quarterly* 48(3): 485–505.

Hartmann, Douglas, John Sullivan, and Toben Nelson. 2012. The attitudes and opinions of high school sports participants: An exploratory empirical examination. *Sport, Education and Society* 17(1): 113–132.

Harvey, Jean, John Horne, and Parissa Safai. 2009. Alterglobalization, global social movements, and the possibility of political transformation through sport. *Sociology of Sport Journal* 26(3): 383–403.

Harvey, Jean, Maurice Levesque, and Peter Donnelly. 2007. Sport volunteerism and social capital. *Sociology of Sport Journal* 24(2): 206–223.

Harwood, Chris, and Camilla Knight. 2009. Understanding parental stressors: An investigation of British tennis-parents. *Journal of Sports Sciences* 27(4): 339–351.

Hassan, David. 2012. Sport and terrorism: Two of modern life's most prevalent themes. *International Review for the Sociology of Sport* 47(3): 263–267.

Hattery, Anglea. 2012. Title IX at 40: More work needs to be done. *USA Today* (June 21): 7A.

Haudenhuyse, Reinhard Paul, Marc Theeboom, and Fred Coalter. 2012. The potential of sports-based social interventions for vulnerable youth: Implications for sport coaches and youth workers. *Journal of Youth Studies* 15(4): 437–454.

Hawkins, Billy. 2010. *The new plantation: Black athletes, college sports and predominately white NCAA institutions.* Palgrave Macmillan.

Hayes, Chris. 2012. Wall Street, Penn State and institutional corruption. *MSNBC.com* (June 16): http://www.msnbc.com/up-with-chris-hayes /watch/wall-street-penn-state-and-institutional -corruption-44107331875.

Hayhurst, Dirk. 2014. An inside look into the harsh conditions of minor league baseball. (May 14): http:// bleacherreport.com/articles/2062307-an-inside-look- into-the-harsh-conditions-of-minor-league-baseball

Healy, Michelle. 2013. Young athletes sidelined in ER. *USA Today* (August 6): 3A.

Hearn, Jeff, Marie Nordberg, Kjerstin Andersson, Dag Balkmar, Lucas Gottzén, Roger Klinth, Keith Pringle, and Linn Sandberg. 2012. Hegemonic masculinity and beyond: 40 years of research in Sweden. *Men and Masculinities* 15(1): 31–55.

Heckert, Alex, and Druann Heckert. 2002. A new typology of deviance: Integrating normative and reactivist definitions of deviance. *Deviant Behavior* 23: 449–479.

Heckert, Druann Maria, and Daniel Alex Heckert. 2007. Positive deviance. In George Ritzer, ed., *Encyclopedia of sociology* (pp. 3542–3544). London/ New York: Blackwell.

Hédi, Csaba. 2011. Global, national, and local factors in the management of university sport: The Hungarian case. *Physical Culture and Sport. Studies and Research* 53: 39–47.

Hehir, Thomas. 2002. Eliminating ableism in education. *The Harvard Educational Review* 72(1): 1–32.

Helmrich, Barbara H. 2010. Window of opportunity? Adolescence, music, and algebra. *Journal of Adolescent Research* 25(4) 557–577.

Henderson, Simon. 2009. Crossing the line: Sport and the limits of civil rights protests. *The International Journal of the History of Sport* 26(1): 101–121.

Hendley, Alexandra, and Denise D. Bielby. 2012. Freedom between the lines: Clothing behavior and identity work among young female soccer players. *Sport, Education and Society* 17(4): 515–533.

Henricks, Thomas S. 2006. *Play reconsidered: Sociological perspectives on human expression.* Urbana: University of Illinois Press.

Hennessy E., S. Hughes, J. Goldberg, R. Hyatt, and C. Economos. 2010. Parent–child interactions and objectively measured child physical activity: A cross sectional study. *International Journal of Behavioural Nutrition and Physical Activity* 7(1): 71–85.

Henning, April Dawn. 2009. Book Review: *Equal Play: Title IX and Social Change* edited by Nancy Hogshead-Makar & Andrew Zimbalist. Philadelphia: Temple University Press, 2007. *Gender & Society* 23(3): 422–424.

Henry, Ian, and Leigh Robinson. 2010. *Gender equality and leadership in Olympic bodies.* Lausanne, Switzerland: International Olympic Committee.

Hepler, Teri, and Deborah Feltz. 2008. Coaching efficacy: A review examining implications for women in sport. *International Journal of Coaching Science* 2(1): 25–41.

Hershow, Rebecca Beth, Katherine Gannett, Jamison Merrill, Elise Braunschweig Kaufman, Chris Barkley, Jeff DeCelles, and Abigail Harrison. 2015. Using soccer to build confidence and increase HCT uptake among adolescent girls: A mixed-methods study of an HIV prevention programme in South Africa. *Sport in Society: Cultures, Commerce, Media, Politics* DOI: 10.1080/17430437.2014.997586.

Hesse, David, and David Lavallee. 2010. Career transitions in professional football coaches. *Insight* 12(2): 41–43.

Hickey, Christoper. 2008. Physical education, sport and hyper-masculinity in schools. *Sport, Education and Society* 13(2): 147–161.

Hickey, Christopher, and Peter Kelly. 2008. Preparing to not be a footballer: Higher education and professional sport. *Sport, Education and Society* 13(4): 477–494.

Hickey, Christopher, Sue Cormack, Peter Kelly, Jo Lindsey, and Lyn Harrison. 2009. Sporting clubs, alcohol and young people: Enduring tensions and emerging possibilities. *ACHPER Healthy Lifestyles Journal* 56(1): 17–21.

Higgins, Eleanor L, Marshall H. Rashkind, Roberta J. Goldberg, and Kenneth L. Herman. 2002. Stages of acceptance of a learning disability: The impact of labeling. *Learning Disabilities Quarterly* 25(1): 3–18.

Higgins, George E., Richard Tewksbury, and Elizabeth Ehrhardt Mustaine. 2007. Sports fan binge drinking: An examination using low self-control and peer association. *Sociological Spectrum* 27(4): 389–404.

Higgins, Matt. 2005. A sport so popular, they added a second boom. *New York Times* (July 25): http://www.nytimes.com/2005/07/25/sports/othersports/a-sport-so-popular-they-added-a-second-boom.html?_r=0.

Higgins, Matt. 2007. It's a kids' world on the halfpipe. *New York Times* (July 15): http://www.nytimes.com/2007/07/15/sports/othersports/15skate.html.

Higgs, Robert J. 1995. *God in the stadium: Sports and religion in America.* Lexington: University of Kentucky Press.

Hill, Andrew P., and Paul R. Appleton. 2011. The predictive ability of the frequency of perfectionistic cognitions, self-oriented perfectionism, and socially prescribed perfectionism in relation to symptoms of burnout in youth rugby players. *Journal of Sports Sciences* 29(7): 695–703.

Hill, Andrew P., Paul R. Appleton, and Howard K. Hall. 2009. Relations between multidimensional perfectionism and burnout in junior-elite male athletes. *Psychology of Sport and Exercise* 10(4): 457–465.

Hill, Michael. 2007. Achievement and athletics: Issues and concerns for state boards of education. *State Education Standard* 8(1): 22–31.

Hirose, Akihiko, and Kay Kei-ho Pih. 2010. Men who strike and men who submit: Hegemonic and marginalized masculinities in mixed martial arts. *Men and Masculinities* 13(2): 190–209.

Hite, Carolyn Elizabeth. 2012. *Superheldchen: The creation, perfection and exportation of the GDR model of elite youth sport development.* Senior Thesis Submitted in Partial Fulfillment of the German Major, Pomona College; April 12th, 2012.

Hoberman, John M. 1992. *Mortal engines: The science of performance and the dehumanization of sport.* New York: Free Press.

Hoberman, John M. 1994. The sportive-dynamic body as a symbol of productivity. In T. Siebers, ed., *Heterotopia: Postmodern utopia and the body politic* (pp. 199–228). Ann Arbor: University of Michigan Press.

Hoberman, John M. 2005. *Testosterone dreams: Rejuvenation, aphrodisia, doping.* Berkeley: University of California Press.

Hobson, Janell. 2005. The "batty" politic: Toward an aesthetic of the black female body. *AfricanAmerica.org* (March 15): http://www.africanamerica.org/topic/serena-and-hottentot-venus.

Hobson, Will, and Steven Rich. 2015. Playing in the red. *Washington Post* (November 23): http://www.washingtonpost.com/sf/sports/wp/2015/11/23/running-up-the-bills/.

Hochman, Benjamin, and Ryan Casey. 2011a. Private schools defining Colorado prep sports' shift in power. *Denver Post* (December 4): 1A, 22–23A. Online: http://www.denverpost.com/preps/ci_19465830.

Hochman, Benjamin, and Ryan Casey. 2011b. Youth leagues the new target of high school football programs. *Denver Post* (December 4): http://www.denverpost.com/preps/ci_19465159.

Hochman, Benjamin, and Ryan Casey. 2011c. Valor Christian rockets to success and gains its share of detractors. *Denver Post* (December 5): http://www.denverpost.com/preps/ci_19471426.

Hochman, Benjamin, and Ryan Casey. 2011d. High school powers that offer solutions to public, private problem. *Denver Post* (December 6): http://www.denverpost.com/preps/ci_19478018.

Hochman, Benjamin. 2013. Inside the locker room. *Denver Post* (November 27): 1A, 17A.

Hochschild, Thomas R., Jr. 2013. Cul-de-sac kids. *Childhood* 20(2): 229–243.

Hodge, S.R., F.M. Kozub, A.D. Dixson, J.L. Moore, III., and K. Kambon. 2008. A comparison of high school students' stereotypic beliefs about intelligence and athleticism. *Educational Foundations* 22(1/2): 99–119.

Hoffer, Richard. 2013. Book it, dude. *Sports Illustrated* 118(14, April 1): 39–42.

Hoffman, Jay R, William Kraemer, Shalender Bhasin, Thomas Storer, Nicholas A. Ratamess, G. Gregory Haff, Darryn Willoughby, and alan Rogol. 2009. Position stand on androgen and human growth hormone use. *Journal of Strength and Conditioning Research* 23(Suppl 5): S1–S59.

Hoffman, John P. 2006. Extracurricular activities, athletic participation, and adolescent alcohol use: Gender-differentiated and school-contextual effects. *Journal of Health and Social Behavior* 47(3): 275–290.

Hoffman, Shirl James. 2010. *Good game: Christianity and the culture of sports.* Waco, TX: Baylor University Press.

Holden, Will C. 2013. NFL brass want women; NFL players want them to 'shut up' and 'clean toilets.' KDVR.com (November 21): http://kdvr.com/2013/11/21/holden-nfl-brass-wants-women-nfl-players-want-them-to-shut-up-clean-toilets/

Holmes, Rachel. 2007. *African queen: The real life of the Hottentot Venus.* New York: Random House.

Holt, Nicholas L., ed. 2008. *Positive youth development through sport.* New York, NY: Routledge.

Holt, Nickolas L., ed. 2016. *Positive youth development through sport* (2nd edition). New York: Routledge.

Holt, Nicholas L., Bethan C. Kingsley, Lisa N. Tink, and Jay Scherer. 2011. Benefits and challenges associated with sport participation by children and parents from low-income families. *Psychology of Sport and Exercise* 12: 490–499.

Honea, Joy. 2004. *Youth cultures and consumerism: Sport subcultures and possibilities for resistance.* Ph.D. dissertation, Sociology Department, Colorado State University; Fort Collins, CO.

Honea, Joy Crissey. 2007. Sport, alternative. In George Ritzer ed., *The Blackwell encyclopedia of sociology* (pp. 4653–4656). Malden, MA: Blackwell Publishing.

Honea, Joy. 2014. Beyond the alternative vs. mainstream dichotomy: Olympic BMX and the future of action sports. *Journal of Popular Culture* 46(6): 1253–1275.

Hong, Fan, Duncan Mackay, and Karen Christensen, eds. 2008. *China gold: China's quest for global power and Olympic glory.* Great Barrington, MA: Berkshire Pub Group.

Hoogenboom, B.J., J. Morris, C. Morris, and K. Schaefer. 2009. Nutritional knowledge and eating behaviours of female, collegiate swimmers. *North American Sports Physical Therapy* 4: 139–148.

Hopsicker, Peter M. 2009. Miracles in sport: Finding the 'ears to hear' and the 'eyes to see'. *Sport, Ethics and Philosophy* 3(1): 75–93.

Horky, Thomas, and Jörg-Uwe Nieland. 2011. *International sports press survey.* Cologne: German Sport University.

Horne, John D. 2007. The four 'knowns' of sports mega-events. *Leisure Studies* 26(1): 81–96.

HoSang, Daniel Martinez, Oneka LaBennett, and Laura Pulido, eds. 2012. *Racial formation in the twenty-first century.* Berkeley, CA: University of California Press.

Houlihan, Barrie. 2000. Politics and sport. In Jay Coakley and Eric Dunning, eds., *Handbook of sport studies* (pp. 213–227). London: Sage.

Houlihan, Barrie, and Mick Green, eds. 2007. *Comparative elite sport development: Systems, structures and public policy.* Amsterdam/Boston: Elsevier/Butterworth-Heinemann.

Hourcade, Jack J. 1989. Special Olympics: A review and critical analysis. *Therapeutic Recreation Journal* 23: 58–65.

Howard, Johnette. 2013. What to make of recent women's sports milestones. *ESPN.go.com* (February 27): http://espn.go.com/espnw/news-commentary/article/8994771/espnw-make-recent-milestones-women-sports.

Howe, P. David. 2004. *Sport, professionalism and pain: Ethnographies of injury and risk.* London/New York: Routledge.

Hoye, Russell, Matthew Nicholson, and Kevin Brown. 2012. Involvement in sport and social connectedness. *International Review for the Sociology of Sport* first published on November 27, 2012 as doi: 10.1177/1012690212466076.

Hruby, Patrick. 2012a. We should have known better. *Sports on Earth* (October 12): http://www.sportsonearth.com/article/39977734/.

Hruby, Patrick. 2012b. Looking for an edge. *Sports on Earth* (December 3): http://www.patrickhruby.net/2012/12/looking-for-edge.html.

Hruby, Patrick. 2012c. Maintaining appearances. *Sports on Earth* (December 13): http://www.sportsonearth.com/article/40628020/ (retrieved 5-29-13).

Hruby, Patrick. 2012d. Game over. *Sports on Earth* (August 29): http://www.sportsonearth.com/article/37580666/ (retrieved 5-29-13).

Hruby, Patrick. 2013a. Why wouldn't NBA players use PEDs? *Sports on Earth* (February 15): http://www.sportsonearth.com/article/41666640.

Hruby, Patrick. 2013b. Head games. *Sports on Earth* (January 16): http://www.sportsonearth.com/article/40980196/ (retrieved 5-29-13).

Hruby, Patrick. 2013c. The NFL: Forever backward. *Sports on Earth* (February 8): http://www.patrickhruby.net/2013/02/subhead-here-drop-cap-here-suppose-you.html.

Hruby, Patrick. 2013d. The myth of safe football. *Sports on Earth* (March 28): http://www.patrickhruby.net/2013/04/the-myth-of-safe-football.html.

Hruby, Patrick. 2013e. Heads Up: What Roger Goodell's youth football safety letter leaves out. Online: http://www.patrickhruby.net/2013/04/heads-up-their.html.

Hruby, Patrick. 2013g. Sports and terror: Q & A with Bill Braniff. Online: http://www.start.umd.edu/news/start-in-the-news/rotation-sports-and-terror-q-bill-braniff.

Hruby, Patrick. 2013h. Haven't got a clue. Online: http://www.patrickhruby.net/2013/07/havent-got-clue.html.

Hruby, Patrick. 2013i. Herbal remedy. Online: http://www.patrickhruby.net/2013/04/herbal-remedy.html.

Hu, Elise. 2013. Digital seen surpassing TV in capturing our time. *National Public Radio* (August 4): http://www.npr.org/blogs/alltechconsidered/2013/08/04/208353200/digital-seen-surpassing-tv-in-capturing-our-time.

Huang, Chin-Ju, and Ian Brittain. 2006. Negotiating identities through disability sport. *Sociology of Sport Journal* 23(4): 352–375.

Hubbert, Jennifer. 2013. Of menace and mimicry: The 2008 Beijing Olympics. *Modern China* 39: 408–437.

Huening, Drew. 2009. Olympic gender testing: A historic review of gender testing and its influence on current IOC policy. *drewhuening.com*: http://drewhuening.com/PDFs/drew_huening_olympic.pdf.

Hughes, Bill, and Kevin Paterson. 1997. The social model of disability and the disappearing body: Towards a sociology of impairment. *Disability & Society* 12(3): 325–340.

Hughes, David. 2013. 'Organised crime and drugs in sport': Did they teach us about that in medical school? *British Journal of Sport Medicine* 47(11): 661–662.

Hughes, Robin L. 2015. For colored girls who have considered Black feminist thought when feminist discourse and Title IX weren't enough. In Eddie Comeaux, ed., *Introduction to intercollegiate athletics* (pp. 2017–218). Baltimore MD: Johns Hopkins University Press.

Hughes, Robin, and James Satterfield, Jr., eds. 2012. Understanding the experiences of LGBT sport participants. *Journal for the Study of Sports and Athletes in Education* 6(1): special issue.

Hughey, Matthew W. 2012. Black guys and white guise: The discursive construction of white masculinity. *Journal of Contemporary Ethnography* 41(1): 95–124.

Hulley, Agela, Alan Currie, Frank Njenga, and Andrew Hill. 2007. Eating disorders in female distance runners: Effects of nationality and running environment. *Psychology of Sport and Exercise* 8(4): 521–533.

Huma, Ramogi, and Ellen J. Staurowsky. 2011. *The price of poverty in big-time college sports.* National College Players Association and Drexel University. Online: http://assets.usw.org/ncpa/The-Price-of-Poverty-in-Big-Time-College-Sport.pdf.

Huma, Ramogi, and Ellen J. Staurowsky. 2012. *The $6 billion heist: Robbing college athletes under the guise of amateurism.* A report collaboratively produced by the National College Players Association and Drexel University Sport Management. Online: http://www.ncpanow.org.

Hunt, H. David. 2005. The effect of extracurricular activities in the educational process: Influence on academic outcomes? *Sociological Spectrum* 25(4): 417–445.

Hunt, Thomas M. 2011. *Drug games: The International Olympic Committee and the politics of doping, 1960–2008.* Austin: University of Texas Press.

Hunter, Margaret L. 2005. *Race, gender, and the politics of skin tone.* London/New York: Routldge.

Huntington, Samuel P. 1997. *The clash of civilizations and the remaking of world order.* New York: Touchstone.

Hutchins, Brett. 2013. Sport on the move: The unfolding impact of mobile communications on the media sport content economy. *Journal of Sport and Social Issues* published 13 September 2012, 10.1177/0193723512458933.

Hutchins, Brett, and David Rowe. 2009. From broadcast scarcity to digital plenitude: The changing dynamics of the media sport content economy. *Television and New Media* 10(4): 354–370.

Hutchins, Brett, David Rowe, and Andy Ruddock. 2009. "It's fantasy football made real": Networked media sport, the internet, and the hybrid reality of MyFootballClub. *Sociology of Sport Journal* 26(1): 89–106.

Hutchinson, Nichola. 2008. Disabling beliefs? Impaired embodiment in the religious tradition of the West. *Body and Society* 12(4): 1–23.

Hwang, Junwook, Minki Hong, Seung-Yeol Yee, and Sang-Min Lee. 2012. Impact of sports' characteristics on the labor market. *International Review for the Sociology of Sport* 47(1): 60–76.

Hwang, Seunghyun, Deborah L. Feltz, Laura A. Kietzmann, and Matthew A. Diemer. 2013. Sport involvement and educational outcomes of high school students: A longitudinal study. *Youth and Society* published 6 December 2013, 10.1177/0044118X13513479.

Hyland, Drew A. 2008. Paidia and paideia: The educational power of athletics. *Journal of Intercollegiate Sport* 1(1): 66–71.

Hylton, Kevin. 2008. *Race and sport: Critical race theory.* London/NY: Routledge.

Hyman, Mark. 2009. *Until it hurts: America's obsession with youth sports and how it harms our kids.* Boston: Beacon Press.

Hyman, Mark. 2012. Why kids under 14 should not play tackle football. *Time* (November 6): http://ideas.time.com/2012/11/06/why-kids-under-14-should-not-play-tackle-football/.

IAAF. 2007. A first for Bahrain. *IAAF Magazine* (Issue 1, June 1): http://www.iaaf.org/news/news/a-first-for-bahrain.

IAAF. 2011. IAAF regulations governing eligibility of females with hyperandrogenism to compete in women's competitions (In force as from 1st May 2011). Online: http://www.iaaf.org/about-iaaf/documents/medical

Ingham, Alan, and Alison Dewar. 1999. Through the eyes of youth: "Deep play" in peewee ice hockey. In Jay Coakley & Peter Donnelly, eds., *Inside Sports* (pp. 7–16).

Intrator, Sam M., and Donald Siegel. 2008. Project coach: Youth development and academic achievement through sport. *Journal of Physical Education, Recreation and Dance* 79(7): 17–23.

IOC. 2012. *IOC Regulations on female hyperandrogenism: Games of the XXX Olympiad in London, 2012.* IOC Medical and Scientific Department, Lausanne, Switzerland.

IPC. 2007a. *Layman's guide to Paralympic classification.* Bonn, Germany: International Paralympic Committee. Online: http://www.paralympic.org/sites/default/files/document/120716152047682_ClassificationGuide_2.pdf.

IPC. 2007b. *IPC classification code and international standards.* Bonn, Germany: International Paralympic Committee. Online: http://www.paralympic.org/sites

/default/files/document/120201084329386_2008_2_ Classification_Code6.pdf.

IPC. 2008. *IPC position statement on IAAF's commissioned research on Oscar Pistorius.* International Paralympic Committee. Online: http://www.paralympic.org/release/Main_Sections_Menu /News/Press_Releases/2008_01_14_a.html.

Jack, Andrew. 2012. Lifestyle conditions increase the pains for medical systems. *The Financial Times* (August 1): 4.

Jackson, Nate. 2011. No pain, no gain? Not so fast. *New York Times* (December 13): http://www.nytimes .com/2011/12/14/opinion/painkillers-for-nfl-players- not-so-fast.html.

Jackson, Steven J., and David L. Andrews, eds. 2004. *Sport, culture and advertising: Identities, commodities and the politics of representation.* London/New York: Routledge.

Jackson, Susan A., and Mihaly Csikszentmihalyi. 1999. *Flow in sports.* Champaign, IL: Human Kinetics.

Jacobson, David. 2010. Insights from softball star Jennie Finch on playing multiple sports. *Positive Coaching Alliance Connector* (August 17): 1.

Jamieson, Katherine. 1998. Navigating the system: The case of Latina student-athletes in women's collegiate sports. Paper presented at the annual conference of the American Alliance for Health, Physical Education, Recreation and Dance, Reno, NV (April).

Jamieson, Katherine. 2003. Occupying a middle space: Toward a Mestiza sport studies. *Sociology of Sport Journal* 1(1): 1–16.

Jamieson, Katherine. 2005. "All my hopes and dreams": Families, schools, and subjectivities in collegiate softball. *Journal of Sport and Social Issues* 29(2): 133–147.

Jamieson, Katherine M. 2007. Advance at your own risk: Latinas, families, and collegiate softball. In Jorge Iber & Samuel O. Regalado, eds., *Mexican Americans and sports: A reader on athletics and barrio life* (pp. 213–232). College Station: Texas A&M University Press.

Jarvie, Grant, Dong-Jhy Hwang, and Mel Brennan, eds. 2008. *Sport, revolution and the Beijing Olympics.* Oxford/NY: Berg.

Jarvis, Nigel. 2013. The inclusive masculinities of heterosexual men within UK gay sport clubs. *International Review for the Sociology of Sport* published 11 April 2013, 10.1177/1012690213482481.

Jarvis, Nigel. 2015. The inclusive masculinities of heterosexual men within UK gay sport clubs.

International Review for the Sociology of Sport 50(3): 283–300.

Jenkins, Chris. 2005. Steroid policy hits Latin Americans. *USA Today* (May 6): 7C.

Jenkins, Sally. 2013. Women's basketball needs to work to earn an audience. *Washington Post* (May 31): http://www.washingtonpost.com/sports/othersports /womens-basketball-needs-to-work-to-earn-an -audience/2013/05/31/b4bc8f46-ca0f-11e2-8da7 -d274bc611a47_story.html.

Jenkins, Tricia. 2013. The militarization of American professional sports: How the sports–war intertext influences athletic ritual and sports media. *Journal of Sport and Social Issues* 37(3): 245–260.

Jennings, Andrew. 1996a. *The new lords of the rings.* London: Pocket Books.

Jennings, Andrew. 1996b. Power, corruption, and lies. *Esquire* (May): 99–104.

Jennings, Andrew. 2006. *Foul! The secret world of FIFA—bribes, vote rigging, and ticket scandals.* New York, NY: HarperSport.

Jennings, Andrew. 2011. Investigating corruption in corporate sport: The IOC and FIFA. *International Review for the Sociology of Sport* 46: 387–398.

Jennings, Andrew. 2012. Blatter bribes Warner with TV bonanza. *Transparency in Sport News* (January 29): http://www.transparencyinsport.org /When_Blatter_gave_Warner_secret_TV_rights /when_blatter_gave_warner_secret_tv_rights.html.

Jennings, Andrew. 2013a. DavosMan takes control at FIFA. *Transparency in Sport News* (April 8): http://transparencyinsportblog.wordpress.com /2013/04/08/davosman-takes-control-at-fifa/.

Jennings, Andrew. 2013b. Have the FBI got FIFA's bribe emails and offshore bank accounts? *Transparency in Sport News* (July 25): http:// transparencyinsportblog.wordpress.com/page/2/.

Jennings, Andrew, and Clare Sambrook. 2000. *The great Olympic swindle: When the world wanted its games back.* New York: Simon and Schuster.

Jijon, Isabel. 2013. The glocalization of time and space: Soccer and meaning in Chota Valley, Ecuador. *International Sociology* 28(4): 373–390.

Jiwani, Nisara, and Geneviève Rail. 2010. Islam, hijab and young Shia Muslim Canadian women's discursive constructions of physical activity. *Sociology of Sport Journal* 7(3): 251–267.

Jobey, Liz. 2012. Everything to play for. *Financial Times* (July 13): Life and Arts, 1–2. Online: http://

www.ft.com/cms/s/2/2cf282dc-cbb4-11e1-911e
-00144feabdc0.html#axzz215J4cFTL.

John, Alastair, and Steve Jackson. 2011. Call me
loyal: Globalization, corporate nationalism and
the America's Cup. *International Review for the
Sociology of Sport* 46(4): 399–417.

Johns, David. 2004. Weight management as sport
injury: Deconstructing disciplinary power in the
sport ethic. In Kevin Young, ed., *Sporting bodies,
damaged selves: Sociological studies of sports-
related injury* (pp. 117–133). Amsterdam: Elsevier.

Johns, David P., and Jennifer S. Johns. 2000.
Surveillance, subjectivism and technologies of
power. *International Review for the Sociology of
Sport* 35(2): 219–234.

Johnson, Allan G. 2006. *Privilege, power, and
difference* (2nd edition). New York: McGraw-Hill.

Johnson, Allan. 2013. Fatal distraction: Manhood,
guns, and violence. *Male Voice* (January 13): http://
voicemalemagazine.org/fatal-distraction-manhood
-guns-and-violence/#more-1143%27.

Johnson, Mark. 2012. University of Texas professor
explores cultural phenomenon of doping. *VeloNews.
competitor.com* (November 16): http://velonews
.competitor.com/2012/11/analysis/university-of
-texas-professor-explores-cultural-phenomenon-of
-doping_265230.

Jona, N., and F.T. Okou. 2012. Sports and religion.
*Asian Journal of Management Science and
Education* 2(1): 46–54.

Jonas, Scott. 2005. Should women play sports? Online:
http://www.jesus-is-savior.com/Womens%20Page
/christian_women_and_sports.htm (retrieved
7-8-2005).

Jones, Clive Martin, and Gershon Tenenbaum. 2009.
Adjustment disorder: A new way of conceptualizing
the overtraining syndrome. *International Review of
Sport and Exercise Psychology* 2(2): 181–197.

Jordan, Bryant. 2013. NFL research yields possible
TBI breakthrough. *Military.com* (February 27):
http://www.military.com/daily-news/2013/02/27
/nfl-research-yields-possible-tbi-breakthrough.html
(retrieved 5-25-13).

Jordan-Young, Rebecca, and Katrina Karkazis. 2012.
You say you're a woman? That should be enough.
New York Times (June 17): http://www.nytimes
.com/2012/06/18/sports/olympics/olympic-sex-
verification-you-say-youre-a-woman-that-should-be-
enough.html.

Joseph, Drew. 2012. Stanford analyzes athletes'
concussions. *Sfgate.com* (November 20): http://
www.sfgate.com/collegesports/article/Stanford
-analyzes-athletes-concussions-4055088.php
(retrieved 5-25-13).

Joseph, Janelle. 2012a. The practice of capoeira:
Diasporic black culture in Canada. *Ethnic and Racial
Studies* 35(6): 1078–1095.

Joseph, Janelle. 2012b. Culture, community,
consciousness: The Caribbean sporting
diaspora. *International Review for the Sociology
of Sport* published 12 December 2012,
0.1177/1012690212465735.

Joseph, Janelle. 2014. Culture, community,
consciousness: The Caribbean sporting diaspora.
International Review for the Sociology of Sport
49(6): 660–687.

Joukowsky, Artemis A.W., III, and Larry Rothstein.
2002. *Raising the bar.* New York: Umbrage
Editions.

Jowett, Sophia, Melina Timson-Katchis, and Rachel
Adams. 2008. Too close for comfort? Dependence in
the dual role parent/coach-child/athlete relationship.
International Journal of Coaching Science 1(1):
59–78.

Juncà, Alberto. 2008. Sport and national identity
discourses in the Catalan/Spanish press. In Mojca
Doupona Topič & Simon Ličen, eds., *Sport, culture
& society: An account of views and perspectives on
social issues in a continent (and beyond)* (pp. 99–
103). Ljubljana, Slovenia: University of Ljubljana.

Kahma, Nina. 2012. Sport and social class: The case of
Finland. *International Review for the Sociology of
Sport* 47(1): 113–130.

Kane, Emily W. 2000. Racial and ethnic variations in
gender-related attitudes. *Annual Review of Sociology*
26: 419–439.

Kane, Emily W. 2006. "No way my boys are going to be
like that!": Parents' responses to children's gender
nonconformity. *Gender & Society* 20(2): 149–176.

Kane, Mary Jo. 2011. Sex sells sex, not women's sports.
The Nation (August 15–22; Special issue, *Sports:
Views from left field*): http://www.thenation.com
/article/sex-sells-sex-not-womens-sports/.

Kane, Mary Jo, and Nicole M. LaVoi. 2007. *The
2007 Tucker Center Research Report, Developing
physically active girls: An evidence-based
multidisciplinary approach.* University of
Minnesota, Minneapolis, MN.

Kane, Mary Jo, Perry Leo, and Lynn K. Holleran. 2008. Issues related to academic support and performance of Division I student-athlete: A case study at the University of Minnesota. *Journal of Intercollegiate Sport 1*(1): 98–129.

Kanemasu, Yoko, and Gyozo Molnar. 2013. Pride of the people: Fijian rugby labour migration and collective identity. *International Review for the Sociology of Sport* 48(6): 720–735.

Kang, Jiyeon, Jae-On Kim, and Yan Wang. 2013. Salvaging national pride: The 2010 taekwondo controversy and Taiwan's quest for global recognition. *International Review for the Sociology of Sport* published 7 February 2013.

Kang, Jiyeon, Jae-On Kim, and Yan Wang. 2015. Salvaging national pride: The 2010 taekwondo controversy and Taiwan's quest for global recognition. *International Review for the Sociology of Sport* 50(1): 98–114.

Karkazis, Katrina. 2008. *Fixing sex: Intersex, medical authority, and lived experience.* Duke University Press.

Karkazis, Katrina, Rebecca Jordan-Young, Georgiann Davis, and Silvia Camporesi. 2012. Out of bounds? A critique of the new policies on hyperandrogenism in elite female athletes. *The American Journal of Bioethics* 12(7): 3–16.

Karp, Hannah. 2009. The NFL doesn't want your bets. *Wall Street Journal* (June 16): D16.

Karp, Hannah. 2011. In English soccer, the bettors rule. *Wall Street Journal* (March 8): D6.

Kassimeris, Christos. 2008. *European football in black and white: Tackling racism in football.* Lanham, MD: Lexington Books.

Kassimeris, Christos. 2009. *Anti-racism in European football: Fair play for all.* Lanham, MD: Lexington Books.

Kassing, Jeffrey W., and Jimmy Sanderson. 2013. Playing in the new media game or riding the virtual bench: Confirming and disconfirming membership in the community of sport. *Journal of Sport and Social Issues* published 13 September 2012, 10.1177/0193723512458931.

Kassouf, Jeff. 2013. A quick look at NWSL salaries. *The Equalizer* (April 11): http://equalizersoccer.com/2013/04/11/nwsl-salaries-national-womens-soccer-league/.

Kaufman, Peter, and Eli A. Wolff. 2010. Playing and protesting: Sport as a vehicle for social change. *Journal of Sport and Social Issues* 34(2): 154–175.

Kay, Tess. 2006. Daughters of Islam: Family influences on Muslim young women's participation in sport. *International Review for the Sociology of Sport* 41(3/4): 357–374.

Kaye, Andrew H., and Paul McCrory. 2012. Does football cause brain damage? *Medical Journal of Australia* 196(9): 547–549. Online: https://www.mja.com.au/journal/2012/196/9/does-football-cause-brain-damage (retrieved 5-25-13).

Kearney, Mary Celeste. 2011. Tough girls in a rough game. *Feminist Media Studies* 11(3): 283–301.

Keating, Peter. 2011. Next level. *ESPN The Magazine* (July 25): 20; http://espn.go.com/espn/story/_/id/6777581/importance-athlete-background-making-nba.

Keats, Patrice A., and William R. Keats-Osborn. Overexposed: Capturing a secret side of sports photography. *International Review for the Sociology of Sport* 48: 643–657.

Kechiche, Abdellatif. 2005. *Back Venus (Vénus noire).* Paris: MK2 Productions (film released, 2010). Online: http://www.youtube.com/watch?feature=player_embedded&v=_PD5aAd7HPc#at=33.

Keller, Josh. 2007. As football players get bigger, more of them risk a dangerous sleep disorder. *Chronicle of Higher Education* 53(27, March 9): 43.

Kelley, Bruce, and Carl Carchia. 2013. "Hey, data data—swing!" The hidden demographics of youth sports. *ESPN The Magazine* (July 11): http://espn.go.com/espn/story/_/id/9469252/hidden-demographics-youth-sports-espn-magazine.

Kelly, Jason. 2014. The money games. *Notre Dame Magazine* 43(2): 25–29.20.

Kelly, John. 2011. 'Sectarianism' and Scottish football: Critical reflections on dominant discourse and press commentary. *International Review for the Sociology of Sport* 46: 418–435.

Kelly, Laura. 2011. 'Social inclusion' through sports-based interventions? *Critical Social Policy* 31(1): 126–150.

Kennedy, Eileen, and Pirkko Markula, eds. 2010. *Women and exercise: The body, health and consumerism.* London: Routledge.

Kenny, Jeannine. 2012. *Plaintiffs' Master Administrative Long-Form Complaint* In Re:

National Football Players' Concussion Injury Litigation (United States District Court, No. 2:12-md-02323-AB MDL No. 2323, June 7): http://www.washingtonpost.com/wp-srv/sports/NFL-master-complaint.html (retrieved 5-25-13).

Keown, Tim. 2004. World of hurt. *ESPN The Magazine* (August 2): 57–77.

Kerr, Gretchen A., and Ashley Stirling. 2008. Child protection in sport: Implications of an athlete-centered philosophy. *Quest* 60(2): 307–323.

Kerr, Zachary Y.; Johna K. Register-Mihalik, Emily Kroshus, Christine M. Baugh & Stephen W. Marshall. 2016. Motivations associated with nondisclosure of self-reported concussions in former collegiate athletes. *American Journal of Sport Medicine* 44(1): 220–225.

Kerr, Zachary Y. Ross Hayden, Thomas P. Dompier, and Randy Cohen. 2015. Association of equipment worn and concussion injury rates in National Collegiate Athletic Association football practices: 2004-2005 to 2008-2009 Academic Years. *American Journal of Sport Medicine* 43(5): 1134–1141.

Kian, Edward M., Eric Anderson, John Vincent, and Ray Murray. 2013. Sport journalists' views on gay men in sport, society and within sport media. *International Review for the Sociology of Sport* published 2 October 2013, 10.1177/1012690213504101.

Kian, Edward M., John Vincent, and Michael Mondello. 2008. Masculine hegemonic hoops: An analysis of media coverage of March madness. *Sociology of Sport Journal* 25(2): 223–242.

Kidd, Bruce. 1996. Taking the rhetoric seriously: Proposals for Olympic education. *Quest* 48(1): 82–92.

Kidd, Bruce. 1997. *The struggle for Canadian sport.* Toronto: University of Toronto Press.

Kidder, Jeffrey L. 2013. Parkour, masculinity, and the city. *Sociology of Sport Journal* 30(1): 1–23.

Kids Sports. 2008. Canadian Social Trends, No. 85 (Summer): 54–61.

Kilgannon, Corey. 2011. Rugby it's not, but watch the teeth. *New York Times* (April 22): http://www.nytimes.com/2011/04/24/nyregion/mens-field-hockey-isnt-rugby-but-watch-the-teeth.html.

Kim, Kyoung-yim. 2013. Translation with abusive fidelity: Methodological issues in translating media texts about Korean LPGA players. *Sociology of Sport Journal* 30(3): 340–358.

King, Anthony. 2013. The naked female athlete: The case of Rebecca Romero. *International Review for the Sociology of Sport* 48(5): 515–534.

King, C. Richard, ed. 2004a. *Native Americans in sports.* Armonk, NY: Sharpe Reference.

King, C. Richard. 2004b. Reclaiming Indianness: Critical perspectives on Native American mascots. *Journal of Sport and Social Issues* 28(1): special issue.

King, C. Richard. 2007a. Postcolonialism and sports. In George Ritzer, ed., *Encyclopedia of sociology* (pp. 3547–3548). London/New York: Blackwell.

King, C. Richard. 2007b. Sport and ethnicity. In George Ritzer, ed., *Encyclopedia of sociology* (pp. 4681–4684). London/New York: Blackwell.

King, C. Richard. 2007c. Staging the White Olympics. *Journal of Sport and Social Issues* 31(1): 89–94.

King, C. Richard. 2016. *Redskins: Insult and brand.* Lincoln NE: University of Nebraska Press.

King, Peter. 2004. Painful reality. *Sports Illustrated* (October 11): 6063.

King, Peter. 2012. Way out of bounds. *Sports Illustrated* 116(11, March 12): 34–39.

King, Samantha. 2014. Beyond the war on drugs? Notes on prescription opioids and the NFL. *Journal of Sport and Social Issues* 38(2): 184–193.

King, Samantha, R. Scott Carey, Naila Jinnah, Rob Millington, Andrea Phillipson, Carolyn Prouse, and Matt Ventresca. 2014. When is a drug not a drug? Troubling silences and unsettling painkillers in the National Football League. *Sociology of Sport Journal* 31(3): 249–266.

King-White, Ryan. 2013. I am not a scientist: Being honest with oneself and the researched in critical interventionist ethnography. *Sociology of Sport Journal* 30(3): 296–322.

Klarevas, Louis. 2011. Do the wrong thing: Why Penn State failed as an institution. *Huffington Post* (November 14): http://www.huffingtonpost.com/louis-klarevas/penn-state-scandal_b_1087603.html (retrieved 6-26-13).

Klein, Alan. 1991. *Sugarball: The American game, the Dominican dream.* New Haven, CT: Yale University Press.

Klein, Alan. 2006. *Growing the game: The globalization of major league baseball.* New Haven, CT: Yale University Press.

Klein, Alan. 2008a. Anti-semitism and anti-somatism: Seeking the elusive sporting Jew. In Alan Klein, ed.,

American sports: An anthropological approach (pp. 1120–1137). New York/London: Routledge (also published in *Sociology of Sport Journal* 17(3): 213–228).

Klein, Alan. 2008b. Progressive ethnocentrism: Ideology and understanding in Dominican baseball. *Journal of Sport and Social Issues* 32(2): 121–138.

Klein, Alan. 2012. Chain reaction: Neoliberal exceptions to global commodity chains in Dominican baseball. *International Review for the Sociology of Sport* 47(1): 27–42.

Klemko, Robert. 2011. Elway able to spiral things his way on Twitter. *Denver Post* (January 20): 3C.

Klostermann, Claudia, and Siegfried Nagel. 2012. Changes in German sport participation: Historical trends in individual sports. *International Review for the Sociology of Sport* 1012690212464699, first published on November 19, 2012 as doi: 10.1177/1012690212464699.

Knapp, Bobbi A. 2013. Garters on the gridiron: A critical reading of the lingerie football league. *International Review for the Sociology of Sport* published 18 February 2013, 10.1177/1012690212475244.

Knapp, Bobbi A. 2014. Smash mouth football: Identity development and maintenance on a women's tackle football team. *Journal of Sport and Social Issues* 38(1): 51–74. Published 26 December 2012, 10.1177/0193723512468759.

Kniffin, Kevin M., Brian Wansink, and Mitsuru Shimizu. 2015. Sports at work: Anticipated and persistent correlates of participation in high school athletics. *Journal of Leadership & Organizational Studies* 22(2): 217–230.

Knijnik, Jorge. 2013. Visions of gender justice: Untested feasibility on the football fields of Brazil. *Journal of Sport and Social Issues* 37(1): 8–30.

Knudson, Mark. 2005. The Mark: The whole IX yards. *Mile High Sports Magazine* (May): 21–23.

Kobayashi, Koji. 2012. Globalization, corporate nationalism and Japanese cultural intermediaries: Representation of bukatsu through Nike advertising at the global–local nexus. *International Review for the Sociology of Sport* 47(6): 724–742.

Kochhar, Rakesh, Richard Fry, and Paul Taylor. 2011. *Wealth gaps rise to record highs between Whites, Blacks, Hispanics.* Washington, DC: Pew Research Center.

Koehlinger, A. 2012. *Rosaries and rope burns: Boxing and manhood in American Catholicism, 1890–1970.* Princeton, NJ, USA: Princeton University Press.

Komlos, John, and Benjamin E. Lauderdale. 2007. Underperformance in affluence: The remarkable relative decline in U.S. heights in the second half of the 20th century. *Social Science Quarterly* 88(2): 283–305.

Kortekaas, Vanessa. 2012. Sports participation: Uphill task turning inspiration into perspiration. *The Financial Times* (August 19): http://www.ft.com/intl/cms/s/0/5486b32c-d7df-11e1-9980-00144feabdc0.html.

Kosiewicz, Jerzy. 2008. Sociology of sport in Europe: Historical and research perspective—a report with a focus on the Polish contribution. In Mojca Doupona Topič and Simon Ličen, eds., *Sport, culture & society: An account of views and perspectives on social issues in a continent (and beyond)* (pp. 39–43). Ljubljana, Slovenia: University of Ljubljana.

Kossakowski, Radosław. 2015. Where are the hooligans? Dimensions of football fandom in Poland. *International Review for the Sociology of Sport* published 27 October 2015, 10.1177/1012690215612458.

Koukouris, Konstantinos. 1994. Constructed case studies: Athletes' perspectives of disengaging from organized competitive sport. *Sociology of Sport Journal* 11(2): 114–139.

Koukouris, Konstantinos. 2005. Premature athletic disengagement of elite Greek gymnasts. *European Journal for Sport and Society* 2(1): 35–56.

Kraaykamp, Gerbert, Marloes Oldenkamp, and Koen Breedveld. 2012. Starting a sport in the Netherlands: A life-course analysis of the effects of individual, parental and partner characteristics. *International Review for the Sociology of Sport* 489(2): 153–170.

Krane, Vicki., Pricilla Y.L. Choi, Shannon M. Baird, Christine M. Aimar, and Kerrie J. Kauer. 2004. Living the paradox: Female athletes negotiate femininity and muscularity. *Sex Roles* 50(5/6): 315–329.

Krattenmaker, Tom. 2010. *Onward Christian athletes: Turning ballparks into pulpits and players into preachers.* Rowman and Littlefield.

Krattenmaker, Tom. 2012. Can faith help an Olympian? *USA Today* (August 6): 7A.

Krattenmaker, Tom. 2013. NFL violence a moral thorn for Christians. *USA Today* (October): http://

www.usatoday.com/story/opinion/2013/10/09/nfl
-concussions-football-christians-column/2955997/.

Krautmann, Anthony C., and James Ciecka. 2009.
The postseason value of an elite player to a
contending team. *Journal of Sports Economics*
10(2): 168–179.

Kreager, Derek A. 2007. Unnecessary roughness?
School sports, peer networks, and male adolescent
violence. *American Sociological Review* 72(5):
705–724.

Kreager, Derek A., and Jeremy Staff. 2009. The sexual
double standard and adolescent peer acceptance.
Social Psychology Quarterly 72(2): 143–164.

Kretsedemas, Philip. 2008. Redefining 'race' in North
America. *Current Sociology* 56(6): 826–844.

Krieger, Jörg. 2013. Fastest, highest, youngest?
Analysing the athlete's experience of the Singapore
Youth Olympic Games. *International Review for the
Sociology of Sport* 48(6): 706–719.

Kristal, Nicole. 2005. "Tutoring" rich kids cost me my
dreams. *Newsweek* (April 11): 19.

Kristiansen, Elsa, and Glyn C. Roberts. 2007. Religion
as a coping strategy for stress among elite wrestlers.
In Hannu ltkonen, Anna-Katriina Salmikangas &
Eileen McEvoy, eds., *The changing role of public,
civic and private sectors in sport culture*
(pp. 224–227). Proceedings of the 3rd Conference
of the European Association for Sociology of Sport,
Jyvaskyla, Finland.

Kristiansen, Elsa, Dag Vidar Hanstad, and Glyn
Roberts. 2011. Coping with the media at the
Vancouver Winter Olympics: "We all make a living
out of this." *Journal of Applied Sport Psychology*
23(4): 443–458.

Kruschwitz, Robert B. 2008. *Sports.* Baylor University,
TX, USA: The Centre for Christian Ethics. Available
online: http://www.baylor.edu/content/services
/document.php/75224.pdf.

Kruse, David, and Brooke Lemmen. 2009. Spine
injuries in the sport of gymnastics. *Current Sports
Medicine Reports* 8(1): 20–28.

Kruse, Holly. 2011. Multimedia use in a sport setting:
Communication technologies at off-track betting
facilities. *Sociology of Sport Journal* 27(4):
413–427.

Kuchler, Hannah. 2013. Sports groups lack women
in boardrooms. *Financial Times* (March 4): http://
www.ft.com/cms/s/2/2cea863e-8290-11e2-8404
-00144feabdc0.html#axzz2MfymjOsS.

Kuper, Simon. 2010. South Africa's football lesson.
Financial Times (October 30): http://www.ft.com
/cms/s/2/64d78af2-e16f-11df-90b7-00144feabdc0
.html.

Kuper, Simon. 2012. Gold rush. *The Financial Times*
(July 7): Life & Arts, p. 14.

Kurková, Petra, Hana Válková, and Nanci Scheetz.
2011. Factors impacting participation of European
elite deaf athletes in sport. *Journal of Sports
Sciences* 29(6): 607–618.

Kusz, Kyle. 2007a. *Revolt of the white athlete: Race,
media and the emergence of extreme athletes in
America.* New York: Peter Lang Publishing.

Kusz, Kyle W. 2007b. From NASCAR nation to Pat
Tillman: Notes on sport and the politics of white
cultural nationalism in post-9/11 America. *Journal
of Sport and Social Issues* 30(1): 77–88.

Kwak, Sarah. 2012. Innovation games. *Sports
Illustrated* (July 30): http://www.si.com/vault
/2012/07/30/106216162/innovation-games.

Laberge, Suzanne, and Mathieu Albert. 1999.
Conceptions of masculinity and of gender
transgressions in sport among adolescent boys:
Hegemony, contestation, and social class dynamic.
Men and Masculinities 1(3): 243–267.

Ladd, Tony, and James A. Mathisen. 1999. *Muscular
Christianity: Evangelical Protestants and the
development of American sport.* Grand Rapids, MI:
Baker Books.

Lagaert, Susan & Henk Roose. 2014. Exploring the
adequacy and validity of 'sport': Reflections on a
contested and open concept. *International Review
for the Sociology of Sport* published 8 April 2014,
10.1177/1012690214529295.

Laine, Kate. 2012. Gender equality and the 2012
Olympic Games. International Working Group on
Women and Sport (IWG). Online: http://www.iwg
-gti.org/catalyst/july-2012/gender-equality-and-the
-2012-oly/.

Lake, Robert J. 2012. 'They treat me like I'm scum':
Social exclusion and established-outsider relations
in a British tennis club. *International Review for the
Sociology of Sport* 47(1): 112–128.

Lamb, Penny & Esther Priyadharshini. 2015. The
conundrum of C/cheerleading. *Sport, Education and
Society* 20(7): 889–907.

Lämmer, Manfred, Maureen Smith, and Thierry Terret.
2009. Sport and religion. *Stadion: International
Journal of the History of Sport* 35: 1–39.

Landale, Sarah, and Martin Roderick. 2013. Recovery from addiction and the potential role of sport: Using a life-course theory to study change. *International Review for the Sociology of Sport* published 22 October 2013, 10.1177/1012690213507273.

Lang, Melanie. 2010. Surveillance and conformity in competitive youth swimming. *Sport, Education and Society* 15(1): 19–37.

Langton, Chris. 2015. Top 15 deadliest sports riots of all time. *TheSportster.com* (June 2): http://www.thesportster.com/entertainment/top-15-deadliest-sports-riots-of-all-time/

Lantz, Lawrence 2008. Reasons the Kenyans dominate long distance running. *Track Coach* 185 (Fall): 5897–5899.

Lapchick, Richard. 2005. *2004 racial and gender report card.* Orlando, FL: The Institute for Diversity and Ethics in Sports, University of Central Florida.

Lapchick, Richard E. 2007. Asian American athletes: Past, present and future. *ESPN The Magazine* (May 1): http://espn.go.com/gen/s/2002/0430/1376346.html.

Lapchick, Richard. 2008a. Games could have lasting impact for Asian-Americans. *Sports Business Journal* 11(17, August 25–31): 29.

Lapchick, Richard. 2008b. *NCAA graduation rates* (21 online reports, 2003–2008). Orlando, FL: The Institute for Diversity and Ethics in Sports (University of Central Florida).

Lapchick, Richard. 2008c. *"Scoring the hire": A hiring report for NCAA Division I women's basketball head coaching positions.* Indianapolis, IN: Black Coaches and Administrators. Online: http://bcasports.cstv.com/auto_pdf/p_hotos/s_chools/bca/genrel/auto_pdf/0406-report-card.

Lapchick, Richard E. 2010. *100 campeones: Latino groundbreakers who paved the way in sport.* Morgantown: Fitness Information Technology.

Lapchick, Richard. 2010. The effect of economic downturn on college athletics and athletic departments on issues of diversity and inclusion. *Journal of Intercollegiate Sport* 3(1): 81–95.

Lapchick, Richard. 2012a. *The 2012 Associated Press sports editors racial and gender report card.* The Institute for Diversity and Ethics in Sport, University of Central Florida, Orlando, FL. Online: http://www.tidesport.org/apse-rgrc.html.

Lapchick, Richard E. 2013. Despite progress, diversity hiring in sports media still poor. *Sports Business Daily* (February 25): http://www.sportsbusinessdaily.com/Journal/Issues/2013/02/25/Opinion/Richard-Lapchick.aspx

Lapchick, Richard. 2015. *Regression throughout collegiate athletic leadership: Assessing diversity among campus and conference leaders for Football Bowl Subdivision (FBS) schools in the 2015–16 academic year.* The Institute for Diversity and Ethics in Sport, University of Central Florida.

Lapointe, Joe. 2008. Michigan stadium will expand seating for disabled fans. *New York Times* (March 11): http://www.nytimes.com/2008/03/11/sports/ncaafootball/11michigan.html.

Laqueur, Thomas. 1990. *Making sex.* Cambridge, MA: Harvard University Press.

Lardner, James, and David A. Smith, eds. 2005. *Inequality matters: The growing economic divide in America and its poisonous consequences.* New York: The New Press.

Laskas, Jeanne Marie. 2015. *Concussion.* New York: Random House.

Laslett, Peter. 1987. The emergence of the Third Age. *Ageing and Society* 7(2): 133–160.

Laslett, Peter. 1996. *A fresh map of life: The emergence of the Third Age* (2nd edition). New York: Palgrave Macmillan.

Latimer, Joanna. 2013. Rewriting bodies, portraiting persons? The new genetics, the clinic and the figure of the human. *Body and Society* 19(1): 3–31.

Laurendeau, Jason. 2008. "Gendered risk regimes": A theoretical consideration of edgework and gender. *Sociology of Sport Journal* 25(3): 293–309.

Laurendeau, Jason, and Nancy Sharara. 2008. "Women could be every bit as good as guys." Reproductive and resistant agency in two "action" sports. *Journal of Sport and Social Issues* 32(1): 24–47.

Laurson, Kelly R., and Joey C. Eisenmann. 2007. Prevalence of overweight among high school football linemen. *Journal of the American Medical Association* 297(4, January 24/31): http://jama.ama-assn.org/cgi/content/full/297/4/363.

Lavign, Paula. 2012. Concussion news worries parents. *ESPN.com* (August 26): http://espn.go.com/espn/otl/story/_/id/8297366/espn-survey-finds-news-coverage-concussions-leads-majority-parents-less-likely-allow-sons-play-youth-football-leagues (retrieved 5-25-13).

Lavoie, Marc. 2000. Economics and sport. In J. Coakley and E. Dunning, eds., *Handbook of sports studies* (pp. 157–170). London: Sage.

Lawrence, Heather J., and Christopher R. Moberg. Luxury suites and team selling in professional sport. *Team Performance Management* 15(3/4): 185–201.

Lawrence, Marta. 2011. Transgender policy approved. *NCAA.org* (September): http://fs.ncaa.org/Docs /NCAANewsArchive/2011/september /transgender+policy+approveddf30.html.

Layden. Tim. 2010a. American flyers. *Sports Illustrated* 112(9, March 1): 30–35.

Layden, Tim. 2010b. Crash course. *Sports Illustrated* 113(6, August 23): 42–46.

Le Batard, Dan. 2005. Open look: Is it cheating if you don't understand the rules? *Es posible. ESPN The Magazine* 8.10 (May 23): 14.

Le Batard, Dan. 2013. Jason Taylor's pain shows NFL's world of hurt. *Miami Herald* (January 13): http:// www.miamiherald.com/sports/article1946293.html.

Le Clair, Jill M., ed. 2012. *Disability in the global sport arena: A sporting chance.* London: Routledge.

Leahy, Michael. 2008. The pain game. *Washington Post* (February 3): W08. Online: http://www .washingtonpost.com/wp-dyn/content/article /2008/01/29/AR2008012904015.html.

Leahy, Trisha. 2011. Safeguarding child athletes from abuse in elite sport systems: The role of the sport psychologist. In David Gilbourne & Mark Andersen, eds., *Critical essays in applied sport psychology* (Essay 15). Champaign, IL: Human Kinetics.

Leal, Wanda, Marc Gertz, Alex R. Piquero. 2015. The National Felon League?: A comparison of NFL arrests to general population arrests. *Journal of Criminal Justice* 43(5): 397–403.

Leavy, Jane. 2012. The woman who would save football. *Grantland.com* (August 17): http:// grantland.com/features/neuropathologist-dr-ann-mckee-accused-killing-football-be-sport-only-hope/.

Lebel, Katie, and Karen Danylchuk. 2012. How tweet it is: A gendered analysis of professional tennis players' self-presentation on twitter. *International Journal of Sport Communication* 5(4): 461–481.

Lederman, Doug. 2010. Reversing Bush on Title IX (Update). *InsideHigherEd.com* (April 20): http:// www.insidehighered.com/news/2010/04/20/titleix.

Lee, C. 1915. A brief history of the playground movement in America. *The Playground* 9(1): 2–11, 39–45.

Lee, Hedwig. 2013. The role of parenting in linking family socioeconomic disadvantage to physical activity in adolescence and young adulthood. *Youth & Society* published 1 January 2013, 10.1177/0044118X12470431.

Lee, Jessica, Doune Macdonald, and Jan Wright. 2009. Young men's physical activity choices: The impact of capital, masculinities, and location. *Journal of Sport and Social Issues* 33(1): 59–77.

Lee, Jung Woo, and Joseph Maguire. 2009. Global festivals through a national prism: The global— national nexus in South Korean media coverage of the 2004 Athens Olympic Games. *International Review for the Sociology of Sport* 44(1): 5–24.

Lee-St. John, Jenine. 2006. The meaning of white. *Time* 168(11, September): 21. Online: http://content.time.com/time/magazine/article /0,9171,1531296,00.html.

Leeds, Eva Marikova, Michael A. Leeds, and Irina Pistolet. 2009. Response to Blair and Haynes. *Journal of Sports Economics* 10(2): 207–208.

Leeds, Michael A., Cristen Miller, and Judith Stull. 2007. Interscholastic athletics and investment in human capital. *Social Science Quarterly* 88(3): 729–744.

Leek, Leek, Desiree; Jordan A. Carlson, Kelli L. Cain, Sara Henrichon, Dori Rosenberg, Kevin Patrick, and James F. Sallis. 2011. Physical activity during youth sports practices. *Archives of Pediatric and Adolescent Medicine* 165(4): 294–299.

Legg, David, Claudia Ernes, David Stewart, and Robert Steadway. 2004. Historical overview of the Paralympics, Special Olympics and Deaflympics. Online: http://www.thefreelibrary.com /Historical+overview+of+the+Paralympics,+ Special+Olympics,+and...-a0114366604.

Legg, David, and Keith Gilbert. 2011. *Paralympic legacies.* Champaign, IL: Common Ground Publishing (Sport and Society).

Leng, Ho Keat, Tzu-Yin Kuo, Grain Baysa-Pee, and Josephine Tay. 2014. Make me proud! Singapore 2010 Youth Olympic Games and its effect on national pride of young Singaporeans. *International Review for the Sociology of Sport* 49(6): 745–760.

Lenskyj, Helen Jefferson. 2008. *Olympic industry resistance: Challenging Olympic power and propaganda.* Albany, NY: State University of New York Press.

Leonard, David J. 2010. Jumping the gun: Sporting cultures and the criminalization of Black masculinity. *Journal of Sport and Social Issues* 34(2): 252–262.

Leonard, David J. 2013. A super failure: Domestic violence and football's big game. *TheFeministWire.com* (February 3): http://thefeministwire.com /2012/02/3460/.

Leonard, David J., and C. Richard King. 2010. *Commodified and criminalized: New racism and African Americans in contemporary sports.* Lanham, MD: Rowman and Littlefield.

Leonard, David J., and C. Richard King. 2011. Lack of black opps: Kobe Bryant and the difficult path of redemption. *Journal of Sport and Social Issues* 35(2): 209–223.

Levy, Ariel. 2009. Either/Or: Sports, sex, and the case of Caster Semenya. *The New Yorker* (November 30): http://www.newyorker.com/reporting /2009/11/30/091130fa_fact_levy.

Lewandowski, Joseph. 2007. Boxing: The sweet science of constraints. *Journal of the Philosophy of Sport* 34(1): 26–38.

Lewandowski, Joseph. 2008. On social poverty: Human development and the distribution of social capital. *Journal of Poverty* 12(1): 27–48.

Lewis, Frank W. 2010. In Cleveland, sports fans cheer until it hurts. *New York Times* (May 14): http://www.nytimes.com/2010/05/15/sports /basketball/15cleveland.html.

Lewis, Jerry. 2007. *Sports fan violence in North America.* New York: Rowman & Littlefield.

Li, Jun. 2009. Forging the future between two different worlds: Recent Chinese immigrant adolescents tell their cross-cultural experiences. *Journal of Adolescent Research* 24(4): 477–504.

Liang, Limin. 2013. Television, technology and creativity in the production of a sports mega event. *Media, Culture & Society* 35(4): 472–488.

Liang, Ursula. 2007. The emphasis is not on 'Asian' but 'American.' *ESPN The Magazine* (May 1): http:// espn.go.com/gen/s/2002/0429/1375733.html.

Ličen, Simon, and Andrew C. Billings. 2013. Affirming nationality in transnational circumstances: Slovenian coverage of continental franchise sports competitions. *International Review for the Sociology of Sport* 48(6): 751–767.

Liechty, Toni, Careen Yarnal, and Deborah Kerstetter. 2012. 'I want to do everything!': Leisure innovation among retirement-age women. *Leisure Studies* 31(4): 389–408.

Lifschitz, Arik, Michael Sauder, and Mitchell L. Stevens. 2014. Football as a status system in U.S. higher education. *Sociology of Education* 87(3) 204–219.

Light, Richard. 2008a. Learning masculinities in a Japanese high school rugby club. *Sport, Education and Society* 13(2): 163–179.

Light, Richard. 2008b. *Sport in the lives of young Australians.* Sydney: University of Sydney Press.

Light, Richard L. 2010. Children's social and personal development through sport: A case study of an Australian swimming club. *Journal of Sport and Social Issues* 34(4): 379–395.

Light, Richard, Stephen Harvey, and Daniel Memmert. 2013. Why children join and stay in sports clubs: Case studies in Australian, French and German swimming clubs. *Sport, Education and Society* 18(4): 550–566.

Light, Richard, and Louise Kinnaird. 2002. Appeasing the Gods: Shinto, sumo and "true" Japanese spirit. In T. Magdalinski & T.J.L. Chandler, eds., *With God on their side: Sport in the service of religion* (pp. 139–159). London/New York: Routledge.

Lindo, Jason M., Isaac D. Swensen, and Glen R. Waddell. 2012. Are big-time sports a threat to student achievement? *American Economic Journal: Applied Economics, American Economic Association* 4(4): 254–274.

Lipscomb, Stephen. 2006. Secondary school extracurricular involvement and academic achievement: A fixed effects approach. *Economics of Education Review* 26(4): 463–472.

Lipsyte, Robert. 1996. One fell swoosh: Can a logo conquer all? *New York Times,* section B (February 7): 9.

Lipsyte, Robert. 2011. Why can't athletes have opinions? *USA Today* (May 17): 9A.

Lipsyte, Robert. 2015. Goodbye to Grantland, ESPN's home for actual sports journalism. *The Nation* (November 2): http://www.thenation.com/article /goodbye-grantland-espns-home-for-actual-sports-journalism/.

Liston, Katie, Dean Reacher, Andy Smith, and Ivan Waddington. 2006. Managing pain and injury in non-elite rugby union and rugby league: A case study of players at a British university. *Sport in Society* 9(3): 388–402.

Little, Anita. 2012. Serena Williams, the Hottentot Venus and accidental racism. *Ms Magazine* (December 15): http://msmagazine.com/blog

/2012/12/15/serena-williams-the-hottentot-venus-and-accidental-racism/.

Little, Daniel. 2012. Why a sociology major? *Huffington Post* (July 3): http://www.huffingtonpost.com/daniel-little/college-sociology-major_b_1641546.html.

Liu, Zhengjia, and Dan Berkowitz. 2013. "Love sport, even when it breaks your heart again": Ritualizing consumerism in sports on Weibo. *International Journal of Sport Communication* 6(3): 258–273.

Ljungqvist Arne, and Joe Leigh Simpson. 1992. Medical examination for health of all athletes replacing the need for gender verification in international sports. *JAMA* 267(6): 850–852.

Llopis-Goig, Ramon. 2013. Racism, xenophobia and intolerance in Spanish football: Evolution and responses from the government and the civil society. *Soccer & Society* 14(2): 262–276.

Lomax, Michael E., ed. 2008. *Sports and the racial divide: African American and Latino experience in an era of change.* Jackson: University Press of Mississippi.

Long, Breanne, and Marni Goldenberg. 2010. A means-end analysis of Special Olympics volunteers. *Leisure/ Loisir* 34(2): 145–167; postprint copy at http://digitalcommons.calpoly.edu/rpta_fac/9/.

Long, Jonathan, Ben Carrington, and Karl Spracklin. 2007. 'Asians cannot wear turbans in the scrum': Explorations of racist discourse within professional rugby league. In Alan Tomlinson, ed., *The sport studies reader* (pp. 283–288). London/New York: Routledge.

Longman, Jeré. 1996. Slow down, speed up. *New York Times* (May 1): B11.

Longman, Jeré. 2007a. An amputee sprinter: Is he disabled or too-abled? *New York Times* (May 15): http://www.nytimes.com/2007/05/15/sports/othersports/15runner.html.

Longman, Jeré. 2007b. Putting on weight for football glory. *New York Times* (November 30): http://www.nytimes.com/2007/11/30/sports/30obesity.html.

Longman, Jeré. 2011a. N.F.L. linemen tip the scales. *New York Times* (January 28): http://www.nytimes.com/2011/01/29/sports/football/29weight.html.

Longman, Jeré. 2011c. Lionel Messi: Boy genius. *New York Times* (May 21): http://www.nytimes.com/2011/05/22/sports/soccer/lionel-messi-boy-genius.html.

Longman, Jeré. 2012a. Football team keeps mill town's heart beating. *New York Times* (November 21): http://www.nytimes.com/2012/11/22/sports/in-clairton-pa-a-high-school-football-team-keeps-a-towns-heart-beating.html.

Longman, Jeré. 2012b. For Lolo Jones, everything is image. *New York Times* (August 4): http://www.nytimes.com/2012/08/05/sports/olympics/olympian-lolo-jones-draws-attention-to-beauty-not-achievement.html.

Longman, Jeré. 2013a. A push to invigorate women's basketball. *New York Times* (June 17): http://www.nytimes.com/2013/06/18/sports/ncaabasketball/official-offers-ways-to-invigorate-womens-basketball.html.

Longman, Jeré. 2013b. Far from reservation, sisters lead Louisville. *New York Times* (April 6): http://www.nytimes.com/2013/04/07/sports/ncaabasketball/final-four-for-louisville-american-indian-sisters-inspire.html.

López, Bernat. 2011. Creating fear: The social construction of human growth hormone as a dangerous doping drug. *International Review for the Sociology of Sport* 48(2): 220–237.

Lorber, Judith. 2007. Sports: The playing grounds of gender. Keynote address, Annual Conference of the International Sociology of Sport Association, Copenhagen, Denmark (August 4).

Los Angeles Municipal Code. 2013a. Chapter IV, General welfare; Article 6, Public hazards; SEC. 56.15. Bicycle riding-sidewalks. Online: http://www.amlegal.com/nxt/gateway.dll/California/lamc/municipalcode?f=templates$fn=default.htm$3.0$vid=amlegal:losangeles_ca_mc.

Los Angeles Municipal Code. 2013b. Chapter IV, General welfare; Article 6, Public hazards; SEC. 56.16. Streets—Sidewalks—Playing ball or games of sport. Online: http://www.amlegal.com/nxt/gateway.dll/California/lamc/municipalcode?f=templates$fn=default.htm$3.0$vid=amlegal:losangeles_ca_mc.

Loucks, A.B. 2007. Refutation of the myth of the female athlete triad. *British Journal Sports Medicine* 41: 55–57.

Love, Adam, and Kimberly Kelly. 2011. Equity or essentialism? U.S. courts and the legitimation of girls' teams in high school sport. *Gender & Society* 25(2): 227–249.

Love, Adam, and Matthew W. Hughey. 2015. Out of bounds? Racial discourse on college basketball message boards. *Ethnic and Racial Studies* 38(6): 877-893.

Lowe, Bob. 2013. Prosthetic arm is no obstacle for Berry athlete. *NCAA Champion* 6(3): 28.

Lowrey, Annie. 2013. Wealth gap among races widened since recession. *New York Times* (April 28): http://www.nytimes.com/2013/04/29/business/racial-wealth-gap-widened-during-recession.html.

Loy, John W., Fiona McLachlan, and Douglas Booth. 2009. Connotations of female movement and meaning: The development of women's participation in the Olympic Games. *Olympika* 18: 1–24.

Løyland, Knut, and Vidar Ringstad. 2009. On the price and income sensitivity of the demand for sports: Has Linder's disease become more serious? *Journal of Sports Economics* 10(6): 601–618.

Lund, Anker Brink. 2007. The political economy of mass mediated sports. Keynote address at the ISHPES and ISSA Joint World Congress, Copenhagen (August 3).

Lüschen, Günther. 1967. The interdependence of sport and culture. *International Review of Sport Sociology* 2: 127–141.

MacKay, Steph, and Christine Dallaire. 2009. Campus newspaper coverage of varsity sports: Getting closer to equitable and sports-related representations of female athletes? *International Review for the Sociology of Sport* 44(1): 25–40.

MacKay, Steph, and Christine Dallaire. 2012. Skirtboarder net-a-narratives: Young women creating their own skateboarding (re)presentations. *International Review for the Sociology of Sport* 48(2): 171–195.

Mackin, Robert Sean, and Carol S. Walther. 2011. Race, sport and social mobility: Horatio Alger in short pants? *International Review for the Sociology of Sport* 47(6): 670–689.

MacLeod, Calum. 2007. Stars keep medals but not all the gold. *USA Today* (June 14): 6A.

Macur, Juliet. 2013. In Florida state case, a tangle of questions. *New York Times* (December 13): http://www.nytimes.com/2013/12/14/sports/ncaafootball/no-one-wins-in-florida-state-case.html.

Macur, Juliet, and Nate Schweber. 2012. Rape case unfolds on web and splits city. *New York Times* (December 16): http://www.nytimes.com/2012/12/17/sports/high-school-football-rape-case-unfolds-online-and-divides-steubenville-ohio.html (retrieved 5-25-13).

Macy, Sue. 2011. *Wheels of change: How women rode the bicycle to freedom.* Washington, DC: National Geographic Society.

Madalozzo, Regina, and Rodrigo Berber Villar. 2009. Brazilian football: What brings fans to the game? *Journal of Sports Economics* 10(6): 639–650.

Madden, Janice Fanning, and Matthew Ruther. 2011. Has the NFL's Rooney rule efforts "leveled the field" for African American head coach candidates? *Journal of Sports Economics* 12(2): 127–142.

Madianou, Mirca, and Daniel Miller. 2013. Polymedia: Towards a new theory of digital media in interpersonal communication. *International Journal of Cultural Studies* 16(2): 169–187.

Magee, Jonathan, ed. 2007. *Women, football and Europe: Histories, equity and experiences.* Oxford/NY: Meyer & Meyer Sport.

Magrath, Rory, Eric Anderson, and Steven Roberts. 2013. On the door-step of equality: Attitudes toward gay athletes among academy-level footballers. *International Review for the Sociology of Sport.*

Maguire, Brendan. 2005. American professional wrestling: Evolution, content, and popular appeal. *Sociological Spectrum* 25(2): 155–176.

Maguire, Jennifer Smith. 2006. Exercising control: Empowerment and the fitness discourse. In Linda K. Fuller, ed., *Sport, rhetoric, and gender* (pp. 119–130). New York: Palgrave Macmillan.

Maguire, Jennifer Smith. 2008. *Fit for consumption: Sociology and the business of fitness.* London/New York: Routledge.

Maguire, Joseph. 1999. *Global sport: Identities, societies, civilizations.* Cambridge, England: Polity Press.

Maguire, Joseph, ed. 2005. *Power and global sport: Zones of prestige, emulation and resistance.* London/New York: Routledge.

Maguire, Joseph A., Katie Butler, Sarah Barnard, and Peter Golding. 2008. Olympism and consumption: An analysis of advertising in the British media coverage of the 2004 Athens Olympic Games. *Sociology of Sport Journal* 25(2): 167–186.

Maguire, Joseph A., and Mark Falcous, eds. 2010. *Sport and migration.* London/NY: Routledge.

Mahiri, Jabari, and Derek Van Rheenen. 2010. *Out of bounds: When scholarship athletes become academic scholars.* New York: Peter Lang.

Majumdar, Boria, and Nalin Mehta. 2010. *Sellotape legacy: Delhi & the Commonwealth Games.* New Delhi: Harper Collins.

Makdissi, Michael, Paul McCrory, Antony Ugoni, David Darby, and Peter Brukner. 2009. A prospective study of postconcussive outcomes after return to play in Australian football. *The American Journal of Sports Medicine* 37(5): 877–883.

Malcolm, Dominic. 2009. Medical uncertainty and clinician–athlete relations: The management of concussion injuries in Rugby Union. *Sociology of Sport Journal* 26(2): 191–210.

Malcolm, Dominic, Alan Bairner, and Graham Curry. 2010. "Woolmergate": Cricket and the representation of Islam and Muslims in the British press. *Journal of Sport and Social Issues* 34(2): 215–235.

Malone, Keith D., Jim F. Couch, and J. Douglas Barrett. 2008. Differences in the success of NFL coaches by race: A different perspective. *Journal of Sports Economics* 9(6): 663–670.

Mandela, Nelson. 2000. Speech by Nelson Mandela at the Inaugural Laureus Lifetime Achievement Award, Monaco 2000. *Nelson Mandela Centre of Memory*: http://www.sweetspeeches.com/s/2474-nelson-mandela-speech-by-nelson-mandela-at-the-inaugural-laureus-lifetime-achievement-award-monaco-2000.

Mansfield, Louise. 2009. Fitness cultures and environmental (in)justice? *International Review for the Sociology of Sport* 44(4): 345–362.

Maraniss, David. 2008. *Rome 1960: The Olympics that changed the world.* NY: Simon & Schuster.

Marcellinia, Anne, Sylvain Fereza, Damien Issanchoua, Eric De Léséleuca, and Mike McNameeb. 2012. Challenging human and sporting boundaries: The case of Oscar Pistorius. *Performance Enhancement & Health* 1(1): 3–9.

Marchi, Nicola, Jeffrey J. Bazarian, Vikram Puvenna, Mattia Janigro, Chaitali Ghosh, Jianhui Zhong, Tong Zhu, Eric Blackman, Desiree Stewart, Jasmina Ellis, Robert Butler, and Damir Janigro. 2013. Consequences of repeated blood-brain barrier disruption in football players. *PLOS One.* Online: http://journals.plos.org/plosone/article?id=10.1371/journal.pone.0056805#abstract0.

Marklein, Mary Beth. 2013. Division I schools spend more on athletes than education. *USA Today* (January 16): 3A. Online: http://www.usatoday.com/story/sports/ncaaf/2013/01/15/division-i-colleges-spend-more-on-athletes-than-education/1837721/.

Markula, Pirkko, ed. 2009. *Olympic women and the media: International perspectives.* NY: Palgrave Macmillan.

Marlett, Jeffrey. 2012. Don't give me no lip: The cultural and religious roots of Leo Durocher's competitiveness. *A Journal of Baseball History and Culture* 20(2): 43–54.

Marriott, Michel. 2005. Cyberbodies: Robo-legs. *New York Times* (June 20): F1.

Marsh, Herbert W., and Sabina Kleitman. 2002. Extracurricular school activities: The good, the bad, and the nonlinear. *Harvard Educational Review* 72(4): 464–511.

Marsh, Herbert W., and Sabina Kleitman. 2003. School athletic participation: Mostly gain with little pain. *Journal of Sport and Exercise Psychology* 25(2): 205–228.

Marshall, Barbara L., and Momin Rahman. 2015. Celebrity, ageing and the construction of 'third age' identities. *International Journal of Cultural Studies* 18(6): 577–593.

Martin, Brandon E., C. Keith Harrison, Jeffrey Stone, and S. Malia Lawrence. 2010. Athletic voices and academic victories: African American male student–athlete experiences in the Pac-Ten. *Journal of Sport and Social Issues* 34(2): 131–153.

Martin, Michel. 2013. Should parents nix after-school sports? *National Public Radio, Tell Me More* (September 24): http://www.npr.org/2013/09/24/225747074/should-parents-nix-after-school-sports.

Martín, Montserrat. 2012. The (im)possible sexual difference: Representations from a rugby union setting. *International Review for the Sociology of Sport* 47(2): 183–199.

Martin, Renee. 2009. Is Serena Williams the new Sarah Baartman? *Global Comment* (July 8): http://globalcomment.com/is-serena-williams-the-new-sarah-baartman/.

Marty, Martin E., and R. Scott Appleby, eds. 1995. *Fundamentalisms comprehended* (vol. 5 of *The fundamentalism project*). Chicago: University of Chicago Press.

Maseko, Zola. 1998. *The life and times of Sarah Baartman: "The Hottentot Venus."* Brooklyn, NY: Icarus Films.

Mason, Bryan C., and Mark Lavallee. 2012. Emerging supplements in sports. *Sports Health: A Multidisciplinary Approach* 4(2): 142–146.

Mason, Garu. 2011. The sad, painful truth about the Vancouver rioters' true identities. *Globe and Mail* (June 18): http://www.theglobeandmail.com/news

/british-columbia/the-sad-painful-truth-about-the-vancouver-rioters-true-identities/article625374/.

Massao, Prisca Bruno, and Kari Fasting. 2010. Race and racism: Experiences of black Norwegian athletes. *International Review for the Sociology of Sport* 45(2): 147–162.

Matz, Eddie. 2011. Stick route. *ESPN The Magazine* (November 17): http://espn.go.com/nfl/story/_/id/7243606/nfl-players-tony-romo-ronde-barber-rely-new-painkiller-toradol.

Maxwell, Hazel, and Tracy Taylor. 2010. A culture of trust: Engaging Muslim women in community sport organizations. *European Sport Management Quarterly* 10(4): 465–483.

May, Caroline. 2012. Saudi sports commentator: 'Allah slaughter me' before Saudi women enter Olympics. *The Daily Caller* (April 23): http://dailycaller.com/2012/04/23/saudi-sports-commentator-allah-slaughter-me-before-saudi-women-enter-olympics/.

May, Reuben A. Buford. 2008. *Living through the hoop: High school basketball, race, and the American dream.* New York: New York University Press.

May, Reuben A. Buford. 2009. The good and bad of it all: Professional black male basketball players as role models for young black male basketball players. *Sociology of Sport Journal* 26(3): 443–461.

McCallum, Jack. 2003. Thank God it's Friday. *Sports Illustrated* (September 29): 40–42.

McCann, Sean. 2008. At the Olympics, everything is a performance issue. *International Journal of Sport and Exercise Psychology* 6(3): 267–276.

McCarthy, Brigid. 2013. Consuming sports media, producing sports media: An analysis of two fan sports blogospheres. *International Review for the Sociology of Sport* 48(4): 421–434.

McCarthy, Cameron, Michael Giardina, Susan Harewood, and Jin-Kyung Park. 2005. Contesting culture. In Cameron McCarthy, Warren Crichlow, Greg Dimitriadis & Nadine Dolby, eds., *Race, identity and representation in education* (pp. 153–178). New York: Routledge.

McCarthy, Claudine. 2012. Law firm report finds institutional failures that led to Penn State scandal. *College Athletics and the Law* (September 14): http://www.collegeathleticslaw.com/article-detail-print/law-firm-report-finds-institutional-failures-that-led-to-penn-state-scandal.aspx.

McClusky, Mark. 2012. One one-hundredth of a second faster: Building better Olympic athletes. *Wired.com* (July 25): http://www.wired.com/playbook/2012/06/ff_superhumans/all/.

McCormack, Jane B., and Laurence Chalip. 1988. Sport as socialization: A critique of methodological premises. *Social Science Journal* 25(1): 83–92.

McCormack, Mark. 2012. *The declining significance of homophobia: How teenage boys are redefining masculinity and heterosexuality.* New York: Oxford University Press.

McCree, Roy Dereck. 2011. The death of a female boxer: Media, sport, nationalism, and gender. *Journal of Sport and Social Issues* 35(4): 327–249.

McCurry, Justin. 2011. Sumo wrestling hit by match-fixing scandal. *The Guardian* (February 2): http://www.theguardian.com/world/2011/feb/02/japan-sumo-wrestling-match-fixing.

McDonald, Brent Douglas. 2009. Learning masculinity through Japanese university rowing. *Sociology of Sport Journal* 26(3): 425–442.

McDonald, Brent, and Kate Sylvester. 2013. Learning to get drunk: The importance of drinking in Japanese university sports clubs. *International Review for the Sociology of Sport* published 22 October 2013, 10.1177/1012690213506584.

McDonald, Ian. 1999. "Physiological patriots"?: The politics of physical culture and Hindu nationalism in India. *International Review for the Sociology of Sport* 34(4): 343–358.

McDonald, Mary. 2015. Imagining neoliberal feminisms? Thinking critically about the U.S. diplomacy campaign, 'Empowering women and girls through sports.' *Sport in Society: Cultures, Commerce, Media, Politics* 18(8): 909–922.

McDonald, Mary G., and David L. Andrews. 2001. Michael Jordan: Corporate sport and postmodern celebrityhood. In David L. Andrews & Steven J. Jackson, eds., *Sport stars: The cultural politics of sporting celebrity* (pp. 20–35). London/New York: Routledge.

McGrath, Shelly, and Ruth Chananie-Hill. 2009. "Big freaky-looking women": Normalizing gender transgression through bodybuilding. *Sociology of Sport Journal* 26(2): 235–254.

McHale, James P., Penelope G. Vindon, Loren Bush, Derek Richer, David Shaw, and Brienne Smith. 2005. Patterns of personal and social adjustment among sport-involved and noninvolved urban middle-school children. *Sociology of Sport Journal* 22(2): 119–136.

McHugh, Josh; Po Bronson and Ethan Watters, eds. *The Future of Sports*. Delaware North. Online, http://futureof.org/sports/

McIntyre, Doug. 2012. Foreign exchange. *ESPN The Magazine* (May 28): 90–91.

McKay, Jim, and Martin Roderick. 2010. 'Lay down Sally': Media narratives of failure in Australian sport. *Journal of Australian Studies* 34(3): 295–315.

McKnight, Kerbi, Kerry Bernes, Thelma Gunn, David Chorney, David Orr, and Angela Bardick. 2009. Life after sport: Athletic career transition and transferable skills. *Journal of Excellence* 13: 63–77.

McMichael, Christopher. 2012. Hosting the world. *City: Analysis of Urban Trends, Culture, Theory, Policy, Action* 16(5): 519–534.

McMullin, S. 2012. The secularization of Sunday: real or perceived competition for churches. *Review of Religious Research* 55: 43–49.

McNeil, Daniel. 2009. Lennox Lewis and Black Atlantic politics: The hard sell. *Journal of Sport and Social Issues* 33(1): 25–38. Online: http://jss.sagepub.com/cgi/content/abstract/33/1/25.

Mead, Chris. 1985. *Champion Joe Louis: Black hero in white America*. New York: Scribner.

Meadows, James A. 2006. 'X' marks the spot to party. *Rocky Mountain News* (January 27): 6A.

Mehus, Ingar. 2005. Distinction through sport consumption: Spectators of soccer, basketball and ski-jumping. *International Review for the Sociology of Sport* 40(3): 321–333.

Mehus, Ingar, and Arnulf Kolstad. 2011. Football team identification in Norway: Spectators of local and national football matches. *Social Identities* 17(6): 833–845.

Melendez, Mickey C. 2008. Black football players on a predominantly white college campus: Psychosocial and emotional realities of the Black college athlete experience. *The Journal of Black Psychology* 34(4): 423–451.

Melnick, Merrill, Kathleen E. Miller, Donald F. Sabo, Grace M. Barnes, and Michael P. Farrell. 2010. Athletic participation and seatbelt omission among U.S. high school students: A national study. *Health Education & Behavior* 37(1): 23–36.

Mendoza, Alexander. 2007. Beating the odds: Mexican American distance runners in Texas, 1950–1995. In Jorge Iber & Samuel O. Regalado, eds., *Mexican Americans and sports: A reader on athletics and barrio life* (pp. 188–191). College Station: Texas A&M University Press.

Mennesson, Christine. 2012. Gender regimes and habitus: An avenue for analyzing gender building in sports contexts. *Sociology of Sport Journal* 29(1): 4–21.

Merkel, Udo. 2012. Sport and physical culture in North Korea: Resisting, recognizing and relishing globalization. *Sociology of Sport Journal* 29(4): 506–525.

Merrill, Kenneth, Aidan Bryant, Emily Dolan, and Siying Chang. 2012. The male gaze and online sports punditry: Reactions to the Ines Sainz controversy on the sports blogosphere. *Journal of Sport and Social Issues* published 10 September 2012, 10.1177/0193723512455920.

Messner, Michael A. 1992. *Power at play*. Boston: Beacon Press.

Messner, Michael A. 1996. Studying up on sex. *Sociology of Sport Journal* 13(3): 221–237.

Messner, Michael A. 2000. Barbie girls versus sea monsters: Children constructing gender. *Gender & Society* 14(6): 765–784.

Messner, Michael A. 2002. *Taking the field: Women, men, and sports*. Minneapolis: University of Minnesota Press.

Messner, Michael A. 2007. *Out of play: Critical essays on gender and sport*. Albany, NY: State University of New York Press.

Messner, Michael A. 2009. *It's all for the kids: Gender, families, and youth sports*. Berkeley, CA: University of California Press.

Messner, Michael A. 2011. Gender ideologies, youth sports, and the production of soft essentialism. *Sociology of Sport Journal* 28(2): 151–170.

Messner, Michael A., Michele Dunbar, and Darnell Hunt. 2000. The televised sports manhood formula. *Journal of Sport and Social Issues* 24(4): 380–394.

Messner, Michael A., Margaret Carlisle Duncan, and Cheryl Cooky. 2003. Silence, sports bras, and wrestling porn: Women in televised sports news and highlights shows. *Journal of Sport and Social Issues* 27(1): 38–51.

Messner, Michael A., Darnell Hunt, and Michele Dunbar. 1999. *Boys to men: Sports media messages about masculinity*. Oakland, CA: Children Now.

Messner, Michael A., and Mark A. Stevens. 2002. Scoring without consent: Confronting male athletes' violence against women. In M. Gatz, M.A. Messner & S.J. Ball-Rokeach, eds., *Paradoxes of youth and sport* (pp. 225–240). Albany: State University of New York Press.

Meyer, Caroline, Lorin Taranis, Huw Goodwin, and Emma Haycraft. (2011). Compulsive exercise and eating disorders. *European Eating Disorder Review* 19: 174–189.

Michaelis, Vicki. 2011. Cougars come uncaged. *USA Today* (August 17): 1–2C.

Middleton, Richard T. 2008. Institutions, inculcation, and black racial identity: Pigmentocracy vs. the rule of hypodescent. *Social Identities* 14(5): 567–585.

Miguel, Edward, Sebastian Saiegh, and Shanker Satyanath. 2008. *National cultures and soccer violence.* Cambridge, MA: National Bureau of Economic Research.

Milcinski, Maja. 2008. Self-cultivation and the art of positive alienation. In Mojca Doupona Topič & Simon Ličen, eds., *Sport, culture & society: An account of views and perspectives on social issues in a continent (and beyond)* (pp. 167–172). Ljubljana, Slovenia: University of Ljubljana.

Miller, James Andrew, and Tom Shales. 2011. *Those guys have all the fun.* New York: Little, Brown & Company.

Miller, James Andrew, Steve Eder, and Richard Sandomir. 2013. College football's most dominant player? It's ESPN. *New York Times* (August 24): http://www.nytimes.com/2013/08/25/sports /ncaafootball/college-footballs-most-dominant-player-its-espn.html.

Miller, Kathleen E., Donald F. Sabo, Michael P. Farrell, Grace M. Barnes, and Merrill J. Melnick. 1998. Athletic participation and sexual behavior in adolescents: The different world of boys and girls. *Journal of Health and Social Behavior* 39: 108–123.

Miller, Kathleen E., Don Sabo, Michael Farrell, Grace Barnes, and Merrill Melnick. 1999. Sports, sexual behavior, contraceptive use, and pregnancy among female and male high school students: Testing cultural resource theory. *Sociology of Sport Journal* 16(4): 366–387.

Miller, Kathleen E., Merrill Melnick, Grace Barnes, Michael Farrell, Don Sabo. 2005. Untangling the links among athletic involvement, gender, race, and adolescent academic outcomes. *Sociology of Sport Journal* 22(2): 178–193.

Miller, Kathleen, and Joseph H. Hoffman. 2009. Mental well-being and sport-related identities in college students. *Sociology of Sport Journal* 26(2): 335–356.

Miller, Patrick B., and David K. Wiggins, eds. 2003. *Sport and the color line: Black athletes and race relations in twentieth-century America.* London/New York: Routledge.

Miller, Stephen A. 2012. The NCAA needs to let someone else enforce its rules. *The Atlantic* (October 23): http://www.theatlantic.com /entertainment/archive/2012/10/the-ncaa-needs-to-let-someone-else-enforce-its-rules/264012/ (retrieved 6-26-13).

Miller, Ted. 2007. American football, Samoan style. *ESPN The Magazine* (May 28): http://espn.go.com /gen/s/2002/0527/1387562.html.

Millington, Brad, and Brian Wilson. 2010. Media consumption and the contexts of physical culture: Methodological reflections on third generation study of media audiences. *Sociology of Sport Journal* 27(1): 30–53.

Millington, Brad. 2012. Use it or lose it: Ageing and the politics of brain training. *Leisure Studies* 31(4): 429–446.

Millington, Rob, and Simon C. Darnell. 2012. Constructing and contesting the Olympics online: The Internet, Rio 2016 and the politics of Brazilian development. *International Review for the Sociology of Sport* published 9 September 2012, 10.1177/1012690212455374.

Millington, Rob, and Simon C Darnell. 2014. Constructing and contesting the Olympics online: The internet, Rio 2016 and the politics of Brazilian development. *International Review for the Sociology of Sport* 49(2): 190–210.

Millman, Chad. 2010a. The insider. *ESPN The Magazine* 12.19 (September 21): 13–14.

Millman, Chad. 2010b. The insider. *ESPN The Magazine* 13.09 (May 3): 13–14.

Mills, C. Wright. 1951. *White collar: The American middle classes.* New York: Oxford University Press.

Mincyte, Diana, Monica J. Casper, and C.L. Cole. 2009. Sports, environmentalism, land use, and urban development. *Journal of Sport and Social Issues* 33(2): 103–110.

Mincyte, Diana, Monica J. Casper, and C.L. Cole, eds. 2009. Bodies of nature: Politics of wilderness, recreation, and technology. *Journal of Sport and Social Issues* 33(3): special issue.

Mirsafian, Hamidreza, and Azadeh Mohamadinejad. 2011. Overview of university sport in Iran.

Physical Culture and Sport. Studies and Research 52: 61–68.

Mishel, Lawrence, and Natalie Sabadish. 2013. *CEO pay in 2012 was extraordinarily high relative to typical workers and other high earners.* Washington, DC: Economic Policy Institute, Issue Brief #367 (June 26). Online: http://www.epi.org/files/2013 /ceo-pay-2012-extraordinarily-high.pdf.

Mitchell, Heather, Constantino Stavros, and Mark F. Stewart. 2011. Does the Australian Football League draft undervalue indigenous Australian footballers? *Journal of Sports Economics* 12(1): 36–54.

Mitchell, Nicole, and Lisa A. Ennis. 2007. *Encyclopedia of Title IX and sports.* Westport, CT: Greenwood Press.

Moehringer, J.R. 2012. Football is dead. Long live football. *ESPN The Magazine* (September 3): 46–60.

Moltz, David. 2010. Key Title IX ruling. *Inside Higher Ed* (July 22): http://www.insidehighered.com /news/2010/07/22/quinnipiac.

Mooney, Chris. 2003. Teen herbicide. *Mother Jones* (May–June): 18–22.

Moore, David Leon. 2012. Head games. *USA Today* (October 12): 1–2C.

Morgan, Robert. 1993. The 'Great Emancipator' and the issue of race. *The Journal for Historical Review* 13(5): 4. Online: http://www.ihr.org/jhr/v13 /v13n5p-4_Morgan.html.

Morgan, William J. 2012. The academic reform of intercollegiate athletics: The good, the problematic, and the truly worrisome. *Journal of Intercollegiate Sports* 5(1): 90–97.

Morris, David S. 2013. Actively closing the gap? Social class, organized activities, and academic achievement in high school. *Youth & Society* published 17 September 2012, 10.1177/0044118X12461159.

Moss, Frank. 2011. *The Sorcerers and their apprentices: How the digital magicians of the MIT Media Lab are creating the innovative technologies that will change our lives.* New York: Crown Business.

Moyo, Phatisani. 2009. She's a lady, man. *Mail and Guardian* (August 21): http://mg.co.za/article/2009 -08-21-shes-a-lady-man.

Mrozek, Donald J. 1983. *Sport and American mentality, 1880–1920.* Knoxville: University of Tennessee Press.

Muller, Frederick O., and Robert C. Cantu. 2010. *Football fatalities and catastrophic injuries: 1931–2008.* Carolina Academic Press.

Murnen, Sarah K., and Marla H. Kohlman. 2007. Athletic participation, fraternity membership, and sexual aggression among college men: A meta-analytic review. *Sex Roles* 57(1/2): 145–157.

Murphy, Jean. 2012. Getting 'whipped' into shape. *Wall Street Journal* (January 3): D2. Online: http://online .wsj.com/article/SB1000142405297020347910457 7124573567538192.html.

Murphy, Wendy. 2013. CNN Steubenville coverage did more good than harm. *WeNews* (March 22): http://womensenews.org/story/rape/130321/cnn -steubenville-coverage-did-more-good-harm#. UUzznzfuwek (retrieved 5-25-13).

Muscat, Anne C., and Bonita C. Long. 2008. Critical comments about body shape and weight: Disordered eating of female athletes and sport participants. *Journal of Applied Sport Psychology* 20(1): 1–24.

Musto, Michela. 2013. Athletes in the pool, girls and boys on deck: The contextual construction of gender in coed youth swimming. *Gender & Society* published 13 December 2013, 10.1177/0891243213515945.

Mwaniki, Munene F. 2012. Reading the career of a Kenyan runner: The case of Tegla Loroupe. *International Review for the Sociology of Sport* 47(4): 446–460.

Myers, J. 2000. *Afraid of the dark: What whites and blacks need to know about each other.* Chicago: Lawrence Hill Books.

Nabokov, Peter. 1981. *Indian running: Native American history and tradition.* Santa Fe, NM: Ancient City Press.

Nadolny, Tricia L. 2010. CPS challenged on scarcity of girls sports teams. *Chicago Tribune* (November 10): http://articles.chicagotribune.com/2010-11-10/news /ct-met-girls-sports-lawsuit-20101110_1_female-athletes-cps-neena-chaudhry.

Narcotta, Eileen M., Jeffrey C. Petersen, and Scott R. Johnson. 2013. Mentor functions in NCAA women's soccer coaching dyads. *The impact of sports on Team Performance Management* 15(3/4): 100–116.

Narimani, M., A.Z. Babolan, and S. Ariapooran. 2011. The role of spiritual transcendence on predictive of competitive anxiety and self-confidence in athletes. *World Applied Sciences Journal* 15(1): 136–141.

Nario-Redmond, Michelle R., Jeffrey G. Noel, and Emily Fern. 2013. Redefining disability, re-imagining the self: Disability identification predicts self-esteem and strategic responses to stigma. *Self and Identity* 12(5): 468–488.

Nash, Bruce, and Allan Zullo. 1989. *The baseball hall of shame(2)*. New York: Pocket Books.

NASPE. 2009. Choosing the right sport and physical activity program for your child. (Position Statement). Reston, VA: National Association for Sport and Physical Education.

NASPE. 2010. *Guidelines for participation in youth sport programs: Specialization versus multiple-sport participation* (Position Statement). Reston, VA: National Association for Sport and Physical Education.

NASPE. 2013. *Maximizing the benefits of youth sport* (Position Statement). Reston, VA: National Association for Sport and Physical Education.

Nattiv, A., A.B. Loucks, M.M. Manore, C.F. Sanborn, J. Sundgot-Borgen, and M.P. Warren. 2007. American College of Sports Medicine Position Stand: The female athlete triad. *Medical Science Sport Exercise* 39: 1867–1882.

NCAA. 2015. *2.3 or take a knee: 2016 NCAA Division I initial eligibility academic requirements*. NCAA Eligibility Center. http://www.ncaa.org /static/2point3/.

NCAA Research. 2012b. Estimated probability of competing in athletics beyond the high school interscholastic level. *NCAA.org* (September 17).

Neighmond, Patti. 2015. Playing youth sports takes a lot more green than it used to. *National Public Radio* (September 07): http://www.npr.org/sections/health -shots/2015/09/07/437000903/playing-youth-sports -takes-a-lot-more-green-than-it-used-to.

Nesbit, Todd M., and Kerry A. King-Adzima. 2011. Major league baseball attendance and the role of fantasy baseball. *Journal of Sports Economics* 13(5): 494–514.

Newcomb, Tim. 2012a. The hustle meter. *Sports Illustrated* 117(5, August 6): 23.

Newcomb, Tim. 2012b. Fast-tracking. *Sports Illustrated* (November 4): 20.

Newman, Joshua I. 2007b. Old times there are not forgotten: Sport, identity, and the Confederate flag in the Dixie South. *Sociology of Sport Journal* 24(3): 261–282.

Newman, Joshua. 2010. *Embodying Dixie: Studies of body pedagogics of Southern whites*. Champaign, IL: Common Ground Publishing.

Newman, Joshua. 2013. Arousing a [post] Enlightenment active body praxis. *Sociology of Sport Journal* 30(3): 380–407.

Newman, Joshua, and Adam S. Beissel. 2009. The limits to "NASCAR Nation": Sport and the "Recovery Movement" in disjunctural times. *Sociology of Sport Journal* 26(4): 517–539.

Newsday. 2013. Joe Paterno, Jerry Sandusky and the Penn State sex abuse scandal. *Newsday.com* (90-articles): (retrieved 6-26-13).

Newsweek. 1971. Are sports good for the soul? *Newsweek* (January 11): 51–52.

NFHS. 2013. *2012–13 High school athletics participation survey*. Indianapolis, IN: The National Federation of State High School Associations. Online: http://www.nfhs.org/content.aspx.

NFL Brief. 2012. Urlacher admits use of painkillers. *Denver Post* (January 24): 6C.

Ng, Shu Wen, and Barry M. Popkin. 2012. Time use and physical activity: A shift away from movement across the globe. *Obesity Reviews* 13(8): 659–680.

Nicholson, Matthew, and Russell Hoye, eds. 2008. *Sport and social capital*. Oxford: Butterworth-Heinemann.

Nicholson, Matthew, Russell Hoye, and David Gallant. 2011. The provision of social support for elite indigenous athletes in Australian football. *Journal of Sport Management* 25(2): 131–142.

Nielsen, A.C. 2012. *State of the media: The social media report*. New York: The Nielsen Company.

Nightengale, Bob. 2006. Team's rebuilding effort focuses on Christianity, character. *USA Today* (May 31): 1A–2A.

Niiya, Brian, ed. 2000. *More than a game: Sport in the Japanese American community*. Los Angeles: Japanese American National Museum.

Nike, Inc. 2012. *Designed to move: Framework for action*. Nike, Inc., Responsibility. Online: http:// www.designedtomove.org/en_US/?locale=en_US.

Niman, Neil B. 2013. The allure of games: Toward an updated theory of the leisure class. *Games and Culture* 8(1): 26–42.

Nixon, Howard. 2014. *The athletic trap: How college sports corrupted the academy*. Johns Hopkins University Press.

Nobles, Melissa. 2000. *Shades of citizenship: Race and the census in modern politics.* Stanford, CA: Stanford University Press.

Norman, Leanne. 2012. Gendered homophobia in sport and coaching: Understanding the everyday experiences of lesbian coaches. *International Review for the Sociology of Sport* 47: 705–723.

Norman, Leanne. 2013. Gendered homophobia in sport and coaching: Understanding the everyday experiences of lesbian coaches. *International Review for the Sociology of Sport* 16(1): 1326–1345.

Norman, Mark. 2012a. Saturday night's alright for tweeting: Cultural citizenship, collective discussion, and the new media consumption/production of Hockey Day in Canada. *Sociology of Sport Journal* 29(3): 306–324.

Norman, Mark. 2012b. Online community or electronic tribe? Exploring the social characteristics and spatial production of an internet hockey fan culture. *Journal of Sport and Social Issues* December 4, 2012, 0193723512467191.

Normana, Moss E., and Fiona Moolab. 2011. 'Bladerunner or boundary runner'?: Oscar Pistorius, cyborg transgressions and strategies of containment. *Sport in Society: Cultures, Commerce, Media, Politics* 14(9): 1265–1279.

NPR et al. 2015. *Sports and health in America.* A national poll sponsored by NPR, Robert Wood Johnson Foundation, and Harvard T.H. Chan School of Public Health. Online, http://www.rwjf.org/en/library/research/2015/06/sports-and-health-in-america.html

O'Brien, Anne. 2015. Producing television and reproducing gender. *Television New Media March* 16(3): 259-274.

O'Brien, Barbara. 2014. 34 other states view cheerleading as a sport. The Buffalo News (April 30): B,B 10.

O'Bryant, Camile. 2012. Academic performance programs: New directions and (dis)connections in academic reform. *Journal of Intercollegiate Sport* 5(1): 83–89.

Obama, Barack. 2012. Entitled to a fair shot: The president reflects on the impact of Title IX. *Newsweek* 160(1 & 2, July 2 & 9): 10–11.

Ogden, David C., and Joel Nathan Rosen, eds. 2008. *Reconstructing fame: Sport, race, and evolving reputations.* Jackson: University Press of Mississippi.

Ohl, Fabien, Bertrand Fincoeur, Vanessa Lentillon-Kaestner, Jacques Defrance, and Christophe Brissonneau. 2015. The socialization of young cyclists and the culture of doping. *International Review for the Sociology of Sport* 50(7): 865–882.

Okada, Chiaki, and Kevin Young. 2012. Sport and social development: Promise and caution from an incipient Cambodian football league. *International Review for the Sociology of Sport* 47(1): 5–26.

Olds, Tim, Jim Dollman, and Carol Maher. 2009.Adolescent sport in Australia: Who, when, where and what? *ACHPER Healthy Lifestyles Journal* 56(1): 11–15.

Oliver, Mike. 1983. *Social work with disabled people.* Basingstoke: Macmillan.

Oliver, Mike. 1990. The *politics of disablement.* Basingstoke: Macmillan.

Oliver, Mike. 2013. The social model of disability: Thirty years on. *Disability & Society* 28(7): 1024–1026.

Oliver, Mike, and Colin Barnes. 2012. The *new politics of disablement.* Basingstoke: Palgrave.

Olmsted, Larry, 2012. Olympic swag bags & freebies: Why every U.S. athlete came home a winner. *Forbes.com* (August 13): http://www.forbes.com/sites/larryolmsted/2012/08/13/olympic-swag-bags-freebies-why-every-u-s-athlete-came-home-a-winner/#1386dc34299c.

Omalu, Bennet. 2008. *Play hard die young: Football dementia, depression and death.* Lodi, CA: Neo Forenxis Books.

Omi, Michael, and Howard Winant. 1994. *Racial formation in the United States.* New York/London: Routledge.

Oppenheimer, Mark. 2013. In the fields of the lord. *Sports Illustrated* 118(4, February 4): 38–43.

O'Reilly, Heather. 2012. The soccer chronicles: Better training through technology. *New York Times* (July 9): http://london2012.blogs.nytimes.com/2012/07/09/heather-oreilly-post/.

O'Reilly, Lara. 2012. McDonald's, Coke defend Olympic choice. *Marketing Week* (July 10): http://www.marketingweek.com/2012/07/10/mcdonalds-coke-defend-olympic-choice/.

Orenstein, Peggy. 2008. The way we live now: Girls will be girls. *New York Times Magazine* (February 10): http://www.nytimes.com/2008/02/10/magazine/10wwln-lede-t.html.

Oriard, Michael. 2007. *Brand NFL: Making and selling America's favorite sport.* Chapel Hill, NC: University of North Carolina Press.

Oriard, Michael. 2012. NCAA academic reform: History, context and challenges. *Journal of Intercollegiate Sport* 5(1): 4–18.

Orwell, George. 1945. The sporting spirit. In *The complete works of George Orwell*. Online: http://www.george-orwell.org/The_Sporting_Spirit/0.html (retrieved 6-4-10).

Ostrander, Elaine A., Heather J. Huson, and Gary K. Ostrander. 2009. Genetics of athletic performance. *Annual Review* of *Genomics and Human Genetics* 10: 407–429.

Otto, Allison Ann. 2003. Scoring with Latinos. *Denver Post* (May 13): 1A.

Overman, Steven J. 2011. *The Protestant work ethic and the spirit of sport: How Calvinism and capitalism shaped American games.* Macon, GA: Mercer University Press.

Oxendine, Joseph B. 1988. *American Indian sports heritage.* Champaign, IL: Human Kinetics.

Pace, Enzo. 2007. Fundamentalism. In George Ritzer, ed., *Encyclopedia of sociology* (pp. 1813–1816). London/New York: Blackwell.

Packard, Josh. 2009. Running off-tackle through the last bastion: Women, resistance, and professional football. *Sociological Spectrum* 29(3): 321–345.

Page, Holly. 2009. *God's girls in sports: Guiding young girls through the benefits and pitfalls.* Milton Keynes, UK: Authentic.

Palmer, Catherine. 2014. Introduction to special issue on sport and alcohol: On the contemporary agenda of research on alcohol within the sociology of sport. *International Review for the Sociology of Sport* 49(3–4): 259–262.

Pappa, Evdokia, and Eileen Kennedy. 2013. 'It was my thought . . . he made it a reality': Normalization and responsibility in athletes' accounts of performance-enhancing drug use. *International Review for the Sociology of Sport* 48(3): 277–294.

Pappano, Laura. 2012. How big-time sports ate college life. *New York Times* (January 20): http://www.nytimes.com/2012/01/22/education/edlife/how-big-time-sports-ate-college-life.html.

Pappano, Laura, and Eileen McDonagh. 2008a. *Playing with the boys: Why separate is not equal in sports.* New York: Oxford University Press.

Pappas, Nick, Patrick McKenry, and Beth Catlett. 2004. "Athlete aggression on the rink and off the ice." *Men and Masculinities* 6: 291–312.

Paradis, Elise. 2012. Boxers, briefs or bras? Bodies, gender and change in the boxing gym. *Body and Society* 18(2): 82–109.

Paradiso, Eugenio. 2009. The social, political, and economic causes of violence in Argentine soccer. *The Canadian Student Journal of Anthropology* 21(July): 65–79.

Park, Jae-Woo, Seung-Yup Lim, and Paul Bretherton. 2012. Exploring the truth: A critical approach to the success of Korean elite sport. *Journal of Sport and Social Issues* 36(3): 245–267.

Parker, Andrew, and Stuart Weir. 2012. Sport, spirituality and religion: Muscular Christianity in the modern age. *Transmission* (Spring): 17–19. Online: http://www.veritesport.org/downloads/BiT_Spring_2012_Park_and_Weir.pdf.

Parker, Mitchum B., and Mathew D. Curtner-Smith. 2012. Sport education: A panacea for hegemonic masculinity in physical education or more of the same? *Sport, Education and Society* 17(4): 479–496.

Parry, Jim, N.J. Watson, and M.N. Nesti, eds. 2011. *Theology, ethics and transcendence in sports* (Foreword by Robert Higgs). New York: Routledge.

Paskus, Tom. 2010. NCAA takes a new look at gambling trends. *Champion* (Summer): 23.

Paskus, Thomas, and Jeffrey Derevensky. 2013. NCAA Student-Athlete Gambling Behaviors and Attitudes (2004–2012). Indianapolis, IN: National Collegiate Athletic Association. Online: http://fs.ncaa.org/Docs/public/pdf/ncaa_wagering_prelim_may2013.pdf (retrieved 6-26-13).

Pate, Russell. 2014. An inside view of the U.S. National Physical Activity Plan. *Journal of Physical Activity and Health* 11: 461–462.

Pate, Russell, and J.R. O'Neill. 2009. After-school interventions to increase physical activity among youth. *British Journal of Sports Medicine* 43(1): 14–18.

Patiño, Jorge Humberto Ruiz. 2011. Female football: A view from the public and private. *Revista da ALESDE* 1(1): http://ojs.c3sl.ufpr.br/ojs2/index.php/alesde/issue/view/1133/showToc.

Patrick, Dick. 2009. Naama Shafir, Toledo share a religious experience. *USA Today* (February 18): http://usatoday30.usatoday.com/sports/college/womensbasketball/2009-02-18-womens-ncaa-notes_N.htm.

Paule, Amanda. 2012. Recruiting high caliber athletes during difficult financial times: Coaches' perceptions of the recruitment process and the role of socioeconomic status. Unpublished paper, Bowling Green State University, School of Human Movement, Sport and Leisure Studies.

Pauline, Gina and Jeffrey S. Pauline. Volunteer motivation and demographic influences at a professional tennis event. *Team Performance Management* 15(3/4): 172–184.

Pavlidis, Adele, and Simone Fullagar. 2013. Becoming roller derby grrrls: Exploring the gendered play of affect in mediated sport cultures. *International Review for the Sociology of Sport* 48(6): 673–688.

Pavlidis, Adele, and Simone Fullagar. 2015. The pain and pleasure of roller derby: Thinking through affect and subjectification. *International Journal of Cultural Studies* September 18(5): 483–499.

PBS. 2006. *Race—The power of an illusion* (transcripts of Episodes I, II, III). Online: http://www.newsreel .org/nav/title.asp?tc=CN0149.

Pear, Robert. 2008. Plan seeks more access for disabled. *New York Times* (June 16): http://www.nytimes .com/2008/06/16/washington/16disabled.html.

Pearlman, Jeff. 2011. Talking sports beats watching it. *Wall Street Journal* (February 15): D8.

Pearson, Catherine. 2012. Brain injury study: A single season of hits may harm college athletes' ability to learn. *Huffington Post* (May 16): http://www .huffingtonpost.com/2012/05/16/brain-injury -concussion-college-athletes_n_1522145.html (retrieved 5-25-13).

Pearson, Eric. 2010. Benching the Title IX changes. *National Public Radio* (June 1): http://www.npr.org /templates/story/story.php?storyId=127306783.

Pearson, Jennifer, Sarah R. Crissey, and Catherine Riegle-Crumb. 2009. Gendered fields: Sports and advanced course taking in high school. *Sex Roles* 61(7–8): 519–535.

Pelissero, Tom. 2013. Stakes are high in bullying case. *USA Today* (November 15): 1C, 11C.

Pennington, Bill. 2004. Reading, writing and corporate sponsorships. *New York Times* (October 18): A1.

Pennington, Bill. 2012a. Cheating scandal dulls pride in athletics at Harvard. *New York Times* (September 18): http://www.nytimes.com/2012/09/19 /sports/ncaabasketball/harvard-cheating-scandal- revives-debate-over-athletics.html (retrieved 6-26-13).

Pennington, Bill. 2012b. In Virginia's hills, a football crusade. *New York Times* (November 10): http:// www.nytimes.com/2012/11/11/sports/ncaafootball /in-virginias-hills-a-football-crusade.html.

Pennington, Bill. 2013. Hidden threats to young athletes. *New York Times* (May 11): http://www .nytimes.com/2013/05/12/sports/safety-advocates- focus-on-hidden-threats-to-young-athletes.html.

Pennington, Bill. 2013. Treating concussions in young athletes. *New York Times* (May 5): http://www .nytimes.com/2013/05/06/sports/concussion-fears- lead-to-growth-in-specialized-clinics-for-young- athletes.html (retrieved 5-25-13).

Peretti-Watel, Patrick, Valérie Guagliardo, Pierre Verger, Patrick Mignon, Jacques Pruvost, and Yolande Obadia. 2004a. Attitudes toward doping and recreational drug use among French elite student-athletes. *Sociology of Sport Journal* 21(1): 1–17.

Peretti-Watel, Patrick, Valérie Guagliardo, Pierre Verger, Jacques Pruvost, Patrick Mignon, and Yolande Obadia. 2004b. Risky behaviours among young elite-student-athletes: Results from a pilot survey in South-Eastern France. *International Review for the Sociology of Sport* 39(2): 233–244.

Perks, Thomas. 2007. Does sport foster social capital? The contribution of sport to lifestyle of community participation. *Sociology of Sport Journal* 24(4): 378–401.

Pessi, Sonia, and Anna Paula Trussardi Fayh. 2011. Evaluation of the nutritional knowledge of professional track and field and triathlon athletes. *Revista Brasileira de Medicina do Esporte* 17: 242–245.

Peterson, Tomas, 2008. The professionalization of sport in the Scandinavian countries. *Nordic Sport Science Forum* (February 20): http://idrottsforum .org/articles/peterson/peterson080220.html (retrieved 7-20-2008).

Petr, Todd, Tom Paskus, and Michael Miranda. 2011. Examining the student-athletes experience through the NCAA GOALS and SCORE studies. Presentation to the NCAA Convention, San Antonio, January 13 (pdf available online).

Pew Global Attitudes Project. 2013. *The global divide on homosexuality.* Pew Research Center (June 4): http://www.pewglobal.org/2013/06/04/the-global- divide-on-homosexuality/.

Pfanner, Eric. 2012. BBC uses Olympics to give glimpse of TV's future. *New York Times* (August 5):

http://www.nytimes.com/2012/08/06/sports/olympics/bbc-uses-olympics-to-give-glimpse-of-tvs-future.html.

Pfister, Gertrud. 2012. It is never too late to win–sporting activities and performances of ageing women. *Sport in Society* 15(3): 369–384.

Pieper, Lindsay Parks. 2012. Gender regulation: Renée Richards revisited. *The International Journal of the History of Sport* 29(5): 675–690.

Piggin, Joe. 2009. Telling the truth in public policy: An analysis of New Zealand sport policy discourse. *Sociology of Sport Journal* 26(3): 462–482.

Piggin, Joe, Steven J. Jackson, and Malcolm Lewis. 2009. Knowledge, power and politics: Contesting 'evidence-based' national sport policy. *International Review for the Sociology of Sport* 44(1): 87–101.

Pike, Elizabeth C.J. 2004. Risk, pain, and injury: "A natural thing in rowing"? In Kevin Young, ed., *Sporting bodies, damaged selves: Sociological studies of sports-related injury* (pp. 151–162). Amsterdam: Elsevier.

Pike, Elizabeth C.J. 2005. "Doctors just say 'Rest and take ibuprofen,'": A critical examination of the role of "non-orthodox" health care in women's sport. *International Review for the Sociology of Sport* 40(2): 201–220.

Pike, Elizabeth C.J. 2010. Growing old (dis)gracefully? The gender/ageing/exercise nexus. In E. Kennedy & P. Markula, eds., *Women and exercise: The body, health and consumerism* (pp. 180–196). London: Routledge.

Pike, Elizabeth C.J. 2011. The active ageing agenda, old folk devils and a new moral panic. *Sociology of Sport Journal* 28(2): 209–225.

Pike, Elizabeth C.J. 2012. Aquatic antiques: Swimming off this mortal coil? *International Review for the Sociology of Sport* 47(4): 492–510.

Pike, Elizabeth C.J. 2013. The role of fiction in (mis)representing later life leisure activities. *Leisure Studies* 32(1): 69–87.

Pike, Elizabeth C.J., and Johnny Weinstock. 2014. Identity politics in the outdoor adventure environment. Unpublished paper, Department of Sports Studies and Management, University of Chichester.

Pitsch, Werner, and Eike Emrich. 2012. The frequency of doping in elite sport: Results of a replication study. *International Review for the Sociology of Sport* 47(5): 559–580.

Player X (Anonymous). 2009a. Will a player die on the field one day? It's certainly possible. *ESPN The Magazine* 12.21 (October 19): 21.

Player X (Anonymous). 2009b. The NFL can be like high school, but hazing has a real purpose. *ESPN The Magazine* 12.20 (October 5): 15.

Plotz, David. 2000. Does God care who wins the Super Bowl? *Denver Post* (February 13): 6G.

Plymire, Darcy Cree. 2009. Remediating football for the posthuman future: Embodiment and subjectivity in sport video games. *Sociology of Sport Journal* 26(1): 17–30.

Poli, Raffaele. 2010. Understanding globalization through football: The new international division of labour, migratory channels and transnational trade circuits. *International Review for the Sociology of Sport* 45(4): 491–506.

Polychroniou, D.J. 2013. Violence is deeply rooted in American culture: An interview with Henry A. Giroux. *Truth-Out* (January 17): http://truth-out.org/news/item/13982-violence-is-deeply-rooted-in-american-culture-interview-with-henry-a-giroux (retrieved 5-25-13).

Pomerantz, Shauna, Rebecca Rab, and Andrea Stefanik. 2013. Girls run the world? Caught between sexism and postfeminism in the school. *Gender & Society* 27(2): 185–207.

Poniatowska, Elena. 1975. *Massacre in Mexico* (original title *La noche de Tlatelolco;* translated by Helen R. Lane). New York: Viking Books.

Pontifical Council for the Laity. 2006. *The world of sport today: A field of Christian mission.* Proceedings, November 2005 Vatican Seminar. Vaticam: Libreria Editrice Vaticana.

Pontifical Council for the Laity. 2008. *Sport: An educational and pastoral challenge.* Proceedings, November 2007 Vatican Seminar. Vaticam: Libreria Editrice Vaticana.

Pontifical Council for the Laity. 2011. *Sport, education, faith: Towards a new season for Catholic sports associations.* Proceedings, November 2009 Vatican Seminar. Vaticam: Libreria Editrice Vaticana.

Pope Francis. 2013. *Address of Pope Francis to members of the European Olympic Committee.* Vatican City: Pontifical Council for Culture. Online: http://www.cultura.va/content/cultura/en/dipartimenti/sport/risorse/messaggiodelpapa/europeanolimpiccommittee.html.

Porat, Amir Ben. 2012. Who are we? My club? My people? My state? The dilemma of the Arab soccer fan in Israel. *International Review for the Sociology of Sport* published 27 November 2012, 10.1177/1012690212458506.

Pot, Niek, Neils Schenk, and Ivo van Hilvoore. 2014. School sports and identity formation: Socialisation or selection? *European Journal of Sport Science* 14(5): 484–491.

Potrac, Paul, and Robyn L. Jones. 2009. Micropolitical workings in semi-professional football. *Sociology of Sport Journal* 26(4): 557–577.

Powell-Wiley, Tiffany M., Kamakki Banks-Richard, Elicia Williams-King, Liyue Tong, Colby R. Ayers, James A. de Lemos, Nora Gimpel, Jenny J. Lee, and Mark J. DeHaven. 2013. Churches as targets for cardiovascular disease prevention: Comparison of genes, nutrition, exercise, wellness and spiritual growth (GoodNEWS) and Dallas county populations. *Journal of Public Health* 35(1): 99.

Powers-Beck, Jeffrey P. 2004. *The American Indian integration of baseball.* Lincoln: University of Nebraska Press.

Price, John, Neil Farrington, Daniel Kilvington, and Amir Saeed. 2012. Black, white and read all over: Institutional racism and the sports media. *The International Journal of Sport and Society* 3(2): 81–90.

Price, John, Neil Farrington, Daniel Kilvington, and Amir Saeed. 2013. Black, white and read all over: Institutional racism and the sports media. *The International Journal of Sport and Society* 3(2): 81–90.

Price, Monroe Edwin, and Daniel Dayan, eds. 2008. *Owning the Olympics: Narratives of the new China.* Ann Arbor: University of Michigan Press.

Pringle, Richard. 2009. Defamiliarizing heavy-contact sports: A critical examination of rugby, discipline, and pleasure. *Sociology of Sport Journal* 26(2): 211–234.

Project Play, 2015. *Sport for all, play for life.* Washington, D.C.: The Aspen Institute.

Pruscino, Cathryn, John R. Gregory, Bernard savage, and Troy R. Flanagan. 2008. Effects of sodium bicarbonate, caffeine, and their combination on repeated 200m freestyle performance. *International Journal of Sport Nutrition and Exercise Metabolism* 18(2): 116–130.

Purcell, L. 2009. What are the most appropriate return-to-play guidelines for concussed child athletes? *British Journal of Sports Medicine* 43(S1): i51–i55.

Purdue, David E.J. 2013. An (in)convenient truce? Paralympic stakeholders' reflections on the Olympic–Paralympic relationship. *Journal of Sport and Social Issues* 37(4): 384–402.

Purdue, David E.J., and P. David Howe. 2012. Empower, inspire, achieve: (Dis)empowerment and the Paralympic Games. *Disability & Society* 27(7): 903–916.

Putney, Clifford. 2003. *Muscular Christianity: Manhood and sports in Protestant America: 1880–1920.* Cambridge, MA: Harvard University Press.

Puzo, Mario. 1969. *The godfather.* New York: G.P. Putnam's Sons.

Quarmby, Thomas, and Symeon Dagkas. 2010. Children's engagement in leisure time physical activity: Exploring family structure as a determinant. *Leisure Studies* 29(1): 53–66.

Quart, Alissa. 2008. When girls will be boys. *New York Times* (March 16): http://www.nytimes .com/2008/03/16/magazine/16students-t.html.

Quenqua, Douglas. 2012. The fight club generation. *New York Times* (March 14): http://www.nytimes .com/2012/03/15/fashion/mixed-martial-arts-catches-on-with-the-internet-generation.html (retrieved 5-23-13).

Rago, Joseph. 2013. The liberating age of bionics. *Wall Street Journal* (July 17): A11.

Rand, Erica. 2012. *Red nails, black skates: Gender, cash, and pleasure on and off the ice.* Duke University Press.

Randall, Joseph. 2012. A changing game: The inclusion of transsexual athletes in the sports industry. *Pace. I.P. Sports & Entertainment Law Forum* 2(1): 198–209. Online: http://digitalcommons.pace.edu /pipself/vol2/iss1/9.

Randels, George D., and Becky Beal. 2002. What makes a man? Religion, sport and negotiating masculine identity in the Promise Keepers. In Tara Magdalinski & Timothy J.L. Chandler, eds., *With God on their side: Sport in the service of religion* (pp. 160–176). London: Routledge.

Rascher, Daniel A., Matthew T. Brown, Mark S. Nagel, and Chad D. McEvoy. 2012. Financial risk management: The role of a new stadium in minimizing the variation in franchise revenues. *Journal of Sports Economics* 13(4): 431–450.

Ratten, Vanessa. 2013. The impact of sports on team performance management. *Team Performance Management* 15(3/4): 97–99.

Rauscher, Lauren, Kerrie Kauer, and Bianca D.M. Wilson. 2013. The healthy body paradox: Organizational and interactional influences on preadolescent girls' body image in Los Angeles. *Gender & Society* 27(2): 208–230.

Ravel, Barbara, and Geneviève Rail. 2006. The lightness of being 'gaie': Discursive constructions of gender and sexuality in Quebec women's sport. *International Review for the Sociology of Sport* 41(3/4): 395–412.

Ravel, Barbara, and Geneviève Rail. 2007. On the limits of "gaie" spaces: Discursive constructions of women's sport in Quebec. *Sociology of Sport Journal* 24(4): 402–420.

Rawls, Anne W., Adam Jeffery, and David Mann. 2013. Locating the modern sacred: Moral/ social facts and constitutive practices. *Journal of Classical Sociology* published 18 November 2013, 10.1177/1468795X13497137.

Real, Michael. R. 1996. The postmodern Olympics: Technology and the commodification of the Olympic movement. *Quest* 48(1): 9–24.

Real, Michael. R. 1998. MediaSport: Technology and the commodification of postmodern sport. In L. A. Wenner, ed., *MediaSport* (pp. 14–26). London/New York: Routledge.

Reardon, Sean F., and Kendra Bischoff. 2011. *Growth in the residential segregation of families by income: 1970–2009.* New York: Russell Sage Foundation.

Reddy, Sumathi. 2014. Guidelines for young athletes to reduce injuries. *WSJ Wall Street Journal* (November 24): http://www.wsj.com/articles /guidelines-for-young-athletes-to-reduce-injuries-1416869652.

Reed, Ken. 2012. Youth football participation dropping. *League of Fans* (December 12): http://leagueoffans .org/2012/12/12/youth-football-participation-dropping/ (retrieved 5-25-13).

Regalado, Samuel O. 2008. *Viva Baseball! Latin major leaguers and their special hunger.* Urbana: University of Illinois Press.

Reid, S.M. 1996. The selling of the Games. *Denver Post* (July 21): 4BB.

Reilly, Rick. 2009. Life of Reilly. *ESPN The Magazine* 12(25, December 14): 68.

Resmovits, Joy. 2013. Students with disabilities have right to play school sports, Obama administration tells schools. *Huffington Post* (January 24): http:// www.huffingtonpost.com/2013/01/24/students -disabilities-school-sports-obama_n_2546057.html.

Rhoden, William C. 2012a. Head injuries pose a serious problem for the N.F.L. *New York Times* (September 5): http://fifthdown.blogs.nytimes .com/2012/09/05/head-injuries-pose-a-serious-problem-for-the-n-f-l/ (retrieved 5-25-13).

Rhoden, William C. 2012b. Football's future rests on parents as much as players. *New York Times* (September 2): http://www.nytimes.com/2012/09/03 /sports/football/footballs-future-rests-on-parents-as-much-as-players.html (retrieved 5-25-13).

Rhoden, William C. 2012c. Black and white women far from equal under Title IX. *New York Times* (June 10): http://www.nytimes.com/2012/06/11/sports /title-ix-has-not-given-black-female-athletes-equal-opportunity.html.

Rhodes, James. 2011. Fighting for "respectability": Media representations of the white, "working-class" male boxing "hero." *Journal of Sport and Social Issues* 35(4): 350–376.

Rial, Carmen. 2012. Banal religiosity: Brazilian athletes as new missionaries of the neo-pentecostal diaspora. *Vibrant: Virtual Brazilian Anthropology* 9(2): 130–158. Online: http://www.vibrant.org.br /downloads/v9n2_rial.pdf.

Rice, Ron (with David Fleming). 2005. Moment of impact. *ESPN The Magazine* (June 6): 82–83.

Richard, Joanne. 2010. How parents are destroying love of the game in their kids by being over-competitive. *lfpress.com* (January 25): http://www.lfpress.com /life/2010/01/25/12600666.html.

Ridgeway, Cecelia L. 2011. *Framed by gender: How gender inequality persists in the modern world.* New York: Oxford University Press.

Ridpath, David. 2012. *Tainted glory: Marshall University, the NCAA and one man's fight for justice.* Bloomington, IN: iUniverse Inc.

Riede, Paul. 2006. Athletic eligibility: Struggling to raise the bar. *The School Administrator* (June): http://www.aasa.org/SchoolAdministratorArticle .aspx?id=8084.

Riis, Jacob. (1902, later ed. 1913). *The battle with the slum.* New York: Macmillan.

Rinaldi, Ray Mark. 2015. At Aspen Ideas Festival 2015: Dwelling on the decline of America. *Denver Post*

(July 3): http://www.denverpost.com/news /ci_28429223/at-aspen-ideas-festival-2015-dwelling-decline-america

Rinehart, Robert E. 2000. Emerging arriving sport: Alternatives to formal sports. In Jay Coakley & Eric Dunning, eds., *Handbook of sports studies* (pp. 504–519). London: Sage.

Rinehart, Robert E., and Synthia Syndor, eds. 2003. *To the extreme: Alternative sports inside and out.* Albany, NY: State University of New York Press.

Ripley, Amanda. 2013a. *The smartest kids in the world, and how they got that way.* New York: Simon & Schuster. Online: http://www.amandaripley.com /books/the-smartest-kids-in-the-world.

Ripley, Amanda. 2013b. The case against high-school sports. *The Atlantic* (September 18): http://www .theatlantic.com/magazine/print/2013/10/the-case -against-high-school-sports/309447/.

Risman, Barbara J. 2004. Gender as a social structure: Theory wrestling with activism. *Gender & Society* 18(4): 429–451.

Risman, Barbara J., and Georgiann Davis. 2013. From sex roles to gender structure. *Current Sociology* 61(5/6): 733–755.

Risman, Barbara, and Pepper Schwartz. 2002. After the sexual revolution: Gender politics in teen dating. *Contexts* 1(1): 16–24.

Ritzer, George. 2005. *Enchanting a disenchanted world: Revolutionizing the means of consumption.* Thousand Oaks, CA: Pine Forge Press.

Rival, Deborah L. 2015. Athletes with disabilities: Where does empowerment end and disempowerment begin? *The International Journal of Sport and Society: Annual Review* 5:1–10.

Rivara, Frederick P., and Robert Graham. 2013. Sports-related concussion in youth: Report from the Institute of Medicine and National Research Council. JAMA. Published online November 01, 2013. doi: 10.1001/jama.2013.282985.

Robbins, Blaine G. 2012. Playing with fire, competing with spirit: Cooperation in the sport of Ultimate. *Sociological Spectrum* 32(3): 270–290.

Roberts, Daniel. 2013a. The fortunate 50. *Sports Illustrated* (*SI.com*): http://www.si.com/vault /2013/05/20/106324251/fortunate-50.

Roberts, Daniel. 2013b. The international 20. Fortune: http://fortune.com/international-20/.

Roberts, Selena. 2007a. College booster bias is delaying minority hiring. *New York Times* (January 28): http://select.nytimes.com/2007/01/28/sports /ncaafootball/28roberts.html.

Robinson, Joshua. 2013. Soccer match-fixing probe goes global. *Wall Street Journal* (February 5): A8.

Robinson, Patrick. 2009. *Jamaican athletics: A model for 2012 and the world.* London: BlackAmber.

Robson, Douglas. 2010. Gender issues in sport, court. *USA Today* (November 30): 1–2C.

Roderick, Martin J. 2012. An unpaid labor of love: Professional footballers, family life, and the problem of job relocation. *Journal of Sport and Social Issues* 36(3): 317–338.

Roderick, Martin. 2013. Domestic moves: An exploration of intra-national labour mobility in the working lives of professional footballers. *International Review for the Sociology of Sport* 48(4): 387–404.

Roenigk, Alyssa. 2006. Action sports insider. *ESPN The Magazine* 9.10 (May 22): 104.

Rollock, Nicola, David Gillborn, Carol Vincent, and Stephen Ball. 2011. The public identities of the black middle classes: Managing race in public spaces. *Sociology* 45(6): 1078–1093.

Rookwood, Joel, and Geoff Pearson. 2012. The hoolifan: Positive fan attitudes to football 'hooliganism.' *International Review for the Sociology of Sport* 47(2): 149–164.

Rose, Damon. 2004. Don't call me handicapped. *BBC News* (October 4): http://news.bbc.co.uk/2/hi /uk_news/magazine/3708576.stm.

Rosen, Daniel M. 2008. *Dope: A history of performance enhancement in sports from the nineteenth century to today.* Westport, CT: Praeger.

Ross, Philippe. 2011. Is there an expertise of production? The case of new media producers. *New Media Society* 13(6): 912–928.

Ross, Sally R., and Kimberly J. Shinew. 2008. Perspectives of women college athletes on sport and gender. *Sex Roles: A Journal of Research* 58(1/2): 40–57.

Rovell, Darren. 2012. Teams face workers' comp threat. *ESPN.com* (August 30): http://espn.go.com/espn /otl/story/_/id/8316657/nfl-teams-facing-large-bills -related-workers-compensation-claims-head-injuries (retrieved 5-25-13).

Rowe, David. 2009. Media and sport: The cultural dynamics of global games. *Sociology Compass* 3/4: 543–558.

Rowe, David. 2010. Stages of the global: Media, sport, racialization and the last temptation of Zinedine

Zidane. *International Review for the Sociology of Sport* 45(3): 355–371.

Rowe, David. 2013. Reflections on communication and sport: On nation and globalization. *Communication & Sport* 1(1/2): 18–29.

Ruck, Rob. 1987. *Sandlot seasons: Sport in black Pittsburgh.* Urbana: University of Illinois Press.

Ruihley, Brody J., and Andrew C. Billings. 2012. Infiltrating the boys' club: Motivations for women's fantasy sport participation. *International Review for the Sociology of Sport* 48(4): 435–452.

Ruihley, Brody J., and Andrew C. Billings. 2013. Infiltrating the boys' club: Motivations for women's fantasy sport participation. *International Review for the Sociology of Sport* 48(4): 435–452.

Rushin, Steve. 2013. SI's Power 50 list: Who sits atop our throne of games? *Sports Illustrated* (March 11): http://www.si.com/more-sports/2013/03/06/sis-50-most-powerful-people-sports.

Russell, Gordon W. 2008. *Aggression in the sports world: A social psychological perspective.* Oxford/NY: Oxford University Press.

Rynne, Steven. 2008. Coaching females: Is it different? *Sports Coach* 30(2): 38–39.

Sabo, Don, Kathleen E. Miller, Merrill J. Melnick, Michael P. Farrell, and Grace M. Barnes. 2005. High school athletic participation and adolescent suicide: A nationwide study. *International Review for the Sociology of Sport* 40(1): 5–23.

Sabo, Don, and Marj Snyder. 2013. *Progress and promise: Title IX at 40 white paper.* Ann Arbor, MI: SHARP Center for Women and Girls.

Sabo, Don, and Phil Veliz. 2008. *Go out and play: Youth sports in America.* East Meadow, NY: Women's Sports Foundation. Online: http://www.womenssportsfoundation.org/.

Sabo, Don, Phil Veliz, and Lisa Rafalson. 2013. *More than a sport: Tennis, education and health.* White Plains, NY: USTA Serves. Online: http://assets.usta.com/assets/822/15/More_than_a_Sport_Full_Report_2.27.13.pdf (retrieved 6-10-2013).

Sachs, Carolyn J., and Lawrence D. Chu. 2000. The association between professional football games and domestic violence in Los Angeles County. *Journal of Interpersonal Violence* 15: 1192–1201.

Sack, Allen, ed. 2008. *Counterfeit amateurs: An athlete's journey through the sixties to the age of academic capitalism.* University Park, PA: The Pennsylvania State University Press.

Saez, Emmanuel, and Thomas Piketty. 2006. The evolution of top incomes: A historical and international perspective. American Economic Association Papers and Proceedings. *Measuring and Interpreting Trends in Economic Inequality* 96(2): 200–205.

Safai, Parissa. 2003. Healing the body in the "culture of risk": Examining the negotiation of treatment between sport medicine clinicians and injured athletes in Canadian intercollegiate sport. *Sociology of Sport Journal* 20(2): 127–146.

Sailes, Gary, ed. 2010. *Modern sport and the African American experience.* San Diego: Cognella Academic Publishing.

Sailors, Pam R., Sarah Teetzel, and Charlene Weaving. 2012. The complexities of sport, gender, and drug testing. *The American Journal of Bioethics* 12(7): 23–25.

Sakamoto, Arthur, Isao Takei, and Hyeyoung Woo. 2012. The myth of the model minority myth. *Sociological Spectrum* 32(4): 309–321.

Samie, Samaya Farooq. 2013. Hetero-sexy self/body work and basketball: The invisible sporting women of British Pakistani Muslim heritage. *South Asian Popular Culture* 11(3): 257–270.

Samie, Sumaya Farooq & Sertaç Sehlikoglu. 2015. Strange, incompetent and out-of-place: Media, Muslim sportswomen and London 2012. *Feminist Media Studies* 15(3): 363–381.

Sammond, Nicholas, ed. 2005. *Steel chair to the head: The pleasure and pain of professional wrestling.* Durham, NC: Duke University Press.

Sanchanta, Mariko. 2011. Match-fixing claims hit sumo wrestlers. *Wall Street Journal* (February 3): http://online.wsj.com/news/articles/SB10001424052748703960804576119481319525882#printMode.

Sander, Libby. 2010. Is cheerleading a sport? *The Chronicle of Higher Education* (July 21): http://chronicle.com/blogPost/Is-Cheerleading-a-Sport-/25707/.

Sanderson, Jimmy. 2011. *It's a whole new ball-game: How social media is changing sports.* New York: Hampton Press.

Sanderson, Jimmy, and Jeffrey W. Kassing. 2011. Tweets and blogs: Transformative, adversarial, and integrative developments in sports media. In Andrew Billings, ed., *Sports media: Transformation, integration, consumption.* New York: Routledge.

Sandomir, Richard. 2013a. Time Warner faces suit after taking over Los Angeles sports market. *New York Times* (June 19): http://www.nytimes.com/2013/06/20/business/time-warner-faces-suit-after-taking-over-los-angeles-sports-market.html.

Sandomir, Richard. 2013b. ESPN quits film project on concussions in N.F.L. *New York Times* (August 22): http://www.nytimes.com/2013/08/23/sports/football/espn-exits-film-project-on-concussions.html.

Sandomir, Richard, James Andrew Miller, and Steve Eder. 2013. To protect its empire, ESPN stays on offense. *New York Times* (August 26): A1. Online: http://www.nytimes.com/2013/08/27/sports/ncaafootball/to-defend-its-empire-espn-stays-on-offensive.html.

SAPA (South African Press Association). 2009. SA lashes out at 'racist' world athletics body. *Mail and Guardian* (August 20): http://mg.co.za/article/2009-08-20-sa-lashes-out-at-racist-world-athletics-body.

Sapolsky, Robert M. 2000. Genetic hyping. *The Sciences* 40(2): http://www.panix.com/userdirs/jwinters/thesciences/Sapolsky_MA00/SapolskyFrame.html.

Saraceno, Jon. 2005. Native Americans aren't fair game for nicknames. *USA Today* (June 1): 10C.

Sartore, Melanie, and George Cunningham. 2010. The lesbian label as a component of women's stigmatization in sport organizations: An exploration of two health and kinesiology departments. *Journal of Sport Management* 24(5): 481–501.

Scalia, Vincenzo, and Anglia Ruskin. 2009. Just a few rogues? Football ultras, clubs and politics in contemporary Italy. *International Review for the Sociology of Sport* 44(1): 41–53.

Schantz, Otto J., and Keith Gilbert. 2012. *Heroes or zeros?—The media's perceptions of Paralympic sport.* Champaign, IL: Common Ground Publishing (Sport and Society).

Schausteck de Almeida, Barbara, Jay Coakley, Wanderley Marchi Júnior, and Fernando Augusto Starepravo. 2012. Federal government funding and sport: The case of Brazil, 2004–2009. *International Journal of Sport Policy and Politics* 4(3): 411–426.

Schausteck de Almeida, Barbara, Chris Bolsmann, Wanderley Marchi Júnior, and Juliano de Souza. 2013. Rationales, rhetoric and realities: FIFA's World Cup in South Africa 2010 and Brazil 2014.

International Review for the Sociology of Sport April 26, 2013, 1012690213481970.

Scheinin, Richard. 1994. *Field of screams: The dark underside of America's national pastime.* New York: Norton.

Scherer, Jay. 2007. Globalization, promotional culture and the production/consumption of online games: Engaging Adidas's 'Beat Rugby' Campaign. *New Media & Society* 9(3): 475–496.

Scherer, Jay, and Steven Jackson. 2008. Producing Allblacks.com: Cultural intermediaries and the policing of electronic spaces of sporting consumption. *Sociology of Sport Journal* 25(2): 187–205.

Scherer, Jay, and Judy Davidson. 2010. Promoting the 'arriviste' city: Producing neoliberal urban identity and communities of consumption during the Edmonton Oilers' 2006 playoff campaign. *International Review for the Sociology of Sport* 46(2): 157–180.

Scherer, Jay, and Steve Jackson. 2010. *Globalization, sport and corporate nationalism.* Pieterlen, Switzerland: Peter Lang AG.

Schiesel, Seth. 2007a. Flashy wrestling shows grab the world by the neck and flex. *New York Times* (April 4): http://www.nytimes.com/2007/04/04/arts/television/04mania.html.

Schiesel, Seth. 2007b. With famed players, game takes on Madden's turf. *New York Times* (September 17): http://www.nytimes.com/2007/09/17/technology/17game.html.

Schimmel, Kimberly S. 2012. Protecting the NFL/militarizing the homeland: Citizen soldiers and urban resilience in post-9/11 America. *International Review for the Sociology of Sport* 47(3): 338–357.

Schimmel, Kimberly. 2013. *Major sport events: Challenges and outlook.* Belo Horizonte, Brazil: UNICAMP- Advanced Studies Center, Collection CEAv Sport.

Schinke, Robert J., Amy T. Blodgett, Hope E. Yungblut, Mark A. Eys, Randy C. Battochio, Mary Jo Wabano, Duke Peltier, Stephen Ritchie, Patricia Pickard, and Danielle Recollet-Saikonnen. 2010. The adaptation challenges and strategies of adolescent Aboriginal athletes competing off reserve. *Journal of Sport and Social Issues* 34(4): 438–456.

Schirato, Tony. 2012. Fantasy sport and media interactivity. *Sport in Society* 15(1): 78–87.

Schneider, Robert C. 2011. Major college basketball in the United States: Morality, amateurism, and hypocrisies. *Physical Culture and Sport. Studies and Research* 52: 22–32.

Schrock, Douglas P., and Michael Schwalbe. 2009. Men, masculinity, and manhood acts. *Annual Review of Sociology* 35: 277–295.

Schroffel, Jesse L., and Christopher S.P. Magee. 2011. Own-race bias among NBA coaches. *Journal of Sports Economics* 13(2): 130–151.

Schrotenboer, Brent. 2013. Arrests of black NFL players point to profiling. *USA Today* (November 29): 1–2A.

Schull, Vicki, Sally Shaw, and Lisa A. Kihl. 2013. "If a woman came in . . . she would have been eaten up alive": Analyzing gendered political processes in the search for an athletic director. *Gender & Society* 27(1): 56–81.

Schultz, Brad, and Mary Lou Sheffer. 2010. An exploratory study of how Twitter is affecting sports journalism. *International Journal of Sport Communication* 3(2): 226–239.

Schultz, Katie. 2015. Do high school athletes get better grades during the off-season? *Journal of Sports Economics* published 14 January 2015, 10.1177/1527002514566279.

Schwartz, Daniel. 2011. Vancouver not typical sports riot, sociologist says. *CBC.ca* (June 16): http://www.cbc.ca/news/canada/british-columbia/story/2011/06/16/f-vancouver-riot-effect.html (retrieved 5-30-13).

Schwarz, Alan. 2007a. Concussions put college players in murky world. *New York Times* (November 29): http://www.nytimes.com/2007/11/29/sports/ncaafootball/29concussions.html.

Schwarz, Alan. 2007c. Girls are often neglected victims of concussions. *New York Times* (October 2): http://www.nytimes.com/2007/10/02/sports/othersports/02concussions.html.

Schwarz, Alan. 2007d. In high school football, an injury no one sees. *New York Times* (September 15): http://www.nytimes.com/2007/09/15/sports/football/15concussions.html.

Schyfter, Pablo. 2008. Tackling the 'body inescapable' in sport: Body—artifact kinesthetics, embodied skill and the community of practice in lacrosse masculinity. *Body and Society* 14(3): 81–103.

Scott, Robert A., Rachael Irving, Laura Irwin, Errol Morrison, Vilma Charlton, Krista Austin, Dawn Tladi, Michael Deason, Samuel A. Headley, Fred W. Kolkhorst, Nan Yang, Kathryn North, and Yannis P. Pitsiladis. 2010. ACTN3 and ACE genotypes in elite Jamaican and U.S. sprinters. *Medicine and Science in Sports and Exercise* 42(1): 107–112.

Scott, Sabrina. 2012. Wrong regulations: Shorter hems for women's hoopsters? *Slamonline.com* (April 5): http://sabrinascrossing.blogspot.com/2012/04/shorter-hems-for-womens-hoopsters.html.

Sean Dunne. 2013. The Irish bifocal and American sport: Exploring racial formation in the Irish diaspora. *International Review for the Sociology of Sport* 48(4): 405–420.

Seichepine, Daniel R., Julie M. Stamm, Daniel H. Daneshvar, David O. Riley, Christine M. Baugh, Brandon E. Gavett, Yorghos Tripodis, Brett Martin, Christine Chaisson, Ann C. McKee, Robert C. Cantu, Christopher J. Nowinski, and Robert A. Stern. 2013. Profile of self-reported problems with executive functioning in college and professional football players. *Journal of Neurotrauma* 30(July):1299–1304.

Sefiha, Ophir. 2010. Now's when we throw him under the bus: Institutional and occupational identities and the coverage of doping in sport. *Sociology of Sport Journal* 27(2): 200–218.

Sefiha, Ophir. 2012. Bike racing, neutralization, and the social construction of performance-enhancing drug use. *Contemporary Drug Problems* 39(Summer): 213–245.

Sehlikoglu-Karakas, Sertaç. 2012. Boundaries of a veiled female body. *Anthropology News* (August 17): http://www.anthropology-news.org/index.php/toc/an-table-of-contents-summer-2012-volume-536/.

Seifert, T., and C. Henderson. 2010. Intrinsic motivation and flow in skateboarding: An ethnographic study. *Journal of Happiness Studies* 11(3): 277–292.

Seifried, Chad. 2008. Examining punishment and discipline: Defending the use of punishment by coaches. *Quest* 60(3): 370–386.

Sekulic, Damir, Marko Ostojic, Miryana Vasilj, Slavica Coric, and Natasa Zenic. 2014. Gender-specific predictors of cigarette smoking in adolescents: An analysis of sport participation, parental factors and religiosity as protective/risk factors. *Journal of Substance Abuse* 19(1/2): 89–94.

Sellers, Robert, and S. Keiper. 1998. Opportunity given or lost? Academic support services for NCAA Division I student-athletes. Paper presented at the annual conference of the North American Society for the Sociology of Sport, Las Vegas (November).

Serazio, Michael. 2013. Just how much is sports fandom like religion? *The Atlantic* (January 29): http://www .theatlantic.com/entertainment/archive/2013/01/just -how-much-is-sports-fandom-like-religion/272631/.

Serrao, Holly F., Matthew P. Martens, Jessica L. Martin, and Tracey L. Rocha 2008. Competitiveness and alcohol use among recreational and elite collegiate athletes. *Journal of Clinical Sport Psychology* 2(3): 205–215.

Seung-Yup, Lim. 2012. *Racial and sexual discrimination occurring to Korean players on the LPGA Tour.* Ph.D. Dissertation, University of Tennessee–Knoxville.

Shachar, Ayelet. 2012. Serious moral quandaries. *New York Times* (July 27): http://www.nytimes.com /roomfordebate/2012/07/26/which-country-did-you- say-you-were-playing-for-in-the-olympics/serious- moral-quandries-in-the-olympic-passport-swap.

Shafer, Michael R. 2012. *A Christian theology of sport and the ethics of doping.* Ph.D. Thesis, University of Durham, UK. Full text available online: http:// etheses.dur.ac.uk/6398/1/A_Christian_Theology_ of_Sport_and_the_Ethics_of_Doping1.pdf.

Shakespeare, Tom, and Nicholas Watson. 2002. The social model of disability: An outdated ideology? *Research in Social Science and Disability* 2(1): 9–28.

Shakib, Sohaila, and Philip Veliz. 2013. Race, sport and social support: A comparison between African American and White youths' perceptions of social support for sport participation. *International Review for the Sociology of Sport* 48(3): 295–317.

Shakib, Sohaila, Philip Veliz, Michele D. Dunbar, and Donald Sabo. 2011. Athletics as a source for social status among youth: Examining variation by gender, race/ethnicity, and socioeconomic status. *Sociology of Sport Journal* 28(3): 303–328.

Shani, Roi, and Yechiel Michael Barilan. 2012. Excellence, deviance, and gender: Lessons from the XYY Episode. *The American Journal of Bioethics* 12(7): 27–30.

Shaw, Mark. 2002. Board with sports. Paper written in Introductory Sociology, University of Colorado, Colorado Springs, spring semester.

Sheffer, Mary Lou, and Brad Schultz. 2010. Paradigm shift or passing fad? Twitter and sports journalism. *International Journal of Sport Communication* 3(4): 472–484.

Sheil, Pat. 2000. Shed a tear or two . . . or else! Online: http://www.abc.net.au/paralympics/features /s201108.htm.

Sheinin, Dave. 2009. Set for life (a 5-part series on the retirement of professional athletes). *Washington Post* (May–September): http://www.washingtonpost.com /wp-srv/special/sports/setforlife/index.html.

Shields, David L.L., and Brenda J.L. Bredemeier. 1995. *Character development and physical activity.* Champaign, IL: Human Kinetics.

Shifrer, Dara, Jennifer Pearson, Chandra Muller, and Lindsey Wilkinson. 2013. College-going benefits of high school sports participation: Race and gender differences over three decades. *Youth & Society* published 7 October 2012, 10.1177/0044118X12461656.

Shifrer, Dara, Jennifer Pearson, Chandra Muller, and Lindsey Wilkinson. 2015. College-going benefits of high school sports participation: Race and gender differences over three decades. *Youth & Society* 47(3): 295–318.

Shipway, Richard, Immy Holloway, and Ian Jones. 2013. Organisations, practices, actors, and events: Exploring inside the distance running social world. *International Review for the Sociology of Sport* 48(3): 259–276.

Shor, Eran, and Yair Galily. 2012. Between adoption and resistance: Grobalization and glocalization in the development of Israeli basketball. *Sociology of Sport Journal* 29(4): 526–545.

Shor, Eran, and Yuval Yonay. 2011. 'Play and shut up': The silencing of Palestinian athletes in Israeli media. *Ethnic and Racial Studies* 34(2): 229–247.

Shostak, Sara, Jeremy Freese, Bruce G. Link, and Jo C. Phelan. 2009. The politics of the gene: Social status and beliefs about genetics for individual outcomes. *Social Psychology Quarterly* 72(1): 77–93.

Shurley, Jason P., and Janice S. Todd. 2012. Boxing lessons: An historical review of chronic head trauma in boxing and football. *Kinesiology Review* 1(1): 170–184.

Siemaszko, Corky. 2011. Iranian women's soccer team disqualified by FIFA from match for wearing hijab scarves, track suits. *New York Daily News* (June 7): http://www.nydailynews.com/news /world/2011/06/07/2011-06-07_iranian_womens_ soccer_team_disqualified_by_fifa_from_match_for_ wearing_hijab_sca.html.

Sifferlin, Alexandra. 2013a. Even football players without concussions show signs of brain injury. *Healthland.Time.com* (March 7): http://healthland.time.com/2013/03/07/even-football-players-without-concussions-show-signs-of-brain-injury/.

Sifferlin, Alexandra. 2013b. High school athletes continue to play despite concussion symptoms. *Healthland.Time.com* (May 7): http://healthland.time.com/2013/05/07/high-school-athletes-dont-report-concussion-symptoms/.

Silk, Michael L. 2004. A tale of two cities: The social production of sterile sporting space. *Journal of Sport and Social Issues* 28(4): 349–378.

Silk, Michael L. 2011. *The cultural politics of post-9/11 American sport: Power, pedagogy and the popular.* London: Routledge.

Silk, Michael L., and David L. Andrews. 2008. Managing Memphis: Governance and regulation in sterile spaces of play. *Social Identities: Journal for the Study of Race, Nation and Culture* 14(3): 395–414.

Silk, Michael L., and David L. Andrews. 2010. Managing Memphis: Governance and regulation in sterile spaces of play. *Social Identities: Journal for the Study of Race, Nation and Culture* 14(3): 395–414.

Silk, Michael L., and Andrew Manley. 2012. Globalization, urbanization & sporting spectacle in Pacific Asia: Places, peoples & pastness. *Sociology of Sport Journal* 29(4): 455–484.

Silva, Carla Filomena, and P. David Howe. 2012. The (in)validity of supercrip representation of Paralympian athletes. *Journal of Sport and Social Issues* 36(2): 174–194.

Simpson, Ian. 2013. U.S. launches study into youth sports concussions. *NBC News* (January 7): http://vitals.nbcnews.com/_news/2013/01/07/16399636-us-launches-study-into-youth-sports-concussions (retrieved 5-25-13).

Simpson, Joe Leigh, and Arne Ljungqvist. 1992. Medical examination for health of all athletes replacing the need for gender verification in international sports. *JAMA* 267: 850–852.

Simpson, Joe Leigh, Arne Ljungqvist, Malcolm A. Ferguson-Smith, Albert de la Chapelle, Louis J. Elsas II, A. A. Ehrhardt, Myron Genel, Elizabeth A. Ferris, and Alison Carlson. 2000. Gender verification in the Olympics. *JAMA* 284(12): 1568–1569. Online: http://jama.jamanetwork.com/article.aspx?articleid=193101.

Sinden, Jane Lee. 2013. The elite sport and Christianity debate: Shifting focus from normative values to the conscious disregard for health. *Journal of Religion and Health* 52(1): 335–349.

Sinden, Jane Lee. 2013. The sociology of emotion in elite sport: Examining the role of normalization and technologies. *International Review for the Sociology of Sport* 48(5): 613–628.

Sing, Susan Saint. 2013. *Play matters, so play as if it matters.* Phoenix, AZ: Tau Publishing.

Singer, John N. 2008. Benefits and detriments of African American male athletes' participation in a big time college football program. *International Review for the Sociology of Sport* 43(4): 399–408.

Singer, John N., and Akilah R. Carter-Francique. 2013. Representation, participation, and the experiences of racial minorities in college sport. In Gary Sailes, ed., *Sports in higher education: Issues and controversies in college athletics* (pp. 113–138). San Diego, CA: Cognella

Singer, John N., and George B. Cunningham. 2012. A case study of the diversity culture of an American university athletic department: Perceptions of senior level administrators. *Sport, Education and Society* 17(5): 647–669.

Singer, John N., and Reuben A. Buford May. 2011. The career trajectory of a Black male high school basketball player: A social reproduction perspective. *International Review for the Sociology of Sport* 46(3): 299–314.

Singh, Asha, and Deepa Gupta. 2012. Contexts of childhood and play: Exploring parental perceptions. *Childhood* 19: 235–250.

Singh, Vanessa, and Anita Ghai. 2009. Notions of self: Lived realities of children with disabilities. *Disability & Society* 24(2): 129–145.

Sirard, John R., Martha Y. Kubik, Jayne A. Fulkerson, and Chrisa Arcan. 2008. Objectively measured physical activity in urban alternative high school students. *Medicine and Science in Sports and Exercise* 40(12): 2088–2095.

Sisjord, Mari Kristi, and Elsa Kristiansen. 2009. Elite women wrestlers' muscles: Physical strength and a social burden. *International Review for the Sociology of Sport* 44(2/3): 231–246.

Skille, Eivind Å. 2010. Competitiveness and health: The work of sport clubs as seen by sport clubs representatives—a Norwegian case study. *International Review for the Sociology of Sport* 45(1): 73–85.

Smale, Will. 2011. Brazil confident World Cup will leave a lasting legacy. *BBC News* (December 1): http://www.bbc.co.uk/news/business-15981073.

Smedley, Audrey. 1997. Origin of the idea of race. *PBS. org:* http://www.pbs.org/race/000_About/002_04-background-02-09.htm.

Smedley, Audrey. 1999. Review of Theodore Allen. *The Invention of the White Race, vol. 2. Journal of World History* 10(1): 234–237.

Smedley, Audrey. 2003. PBS interview for the series, *Race—the power of an illusion.* Online: http://www.pbs.org/race/000_About/002_04-background-02-06.htm (retrieved June 2005).

Smith, Aaron, and Joanna Brenner. 2012. *Twitter use 2012. Pew Internet and American Life Project.* Online: http://www.pewinternet.org/2012/05/31/twitter-use-2012/.

Smith, Andrew, and Nigel Thomas. 2005. The inclusion of elite athletes with disabilities in the 2002 Manchester Commonwealth Games: An exploratory analysis of British newspaper coverage. *Sports, Education and Society* 10(1): 49–67.

Smith, Andy, and Nigel Thomas. 2012. The politics and policy of inclusion and technology in Paralympic sport: Beyond Pistorius. *International Journal of Sport Policy and Politics* 4(3): 397–410.

Smith, Brett. 2013. Sporting spinal cord injuries, social relations, and rehabilitation narratives: An ethnographic creative non-fiction of becoming disabled through sport. *Sociology of Sport Journal* 30(2): 132–152.

Smith, Brett, and Andrew Sparkes. 2002. Men, sport spinal cord injury and the construction of coherence: Narrative practice in action. *Qualitative Research* 2(2): 143–171.

Smith, Charlotte. 2015. 'Tour du Dopage: Confessions of doping professional cyclists in a modern work environment.' *International Review for the Sociology of Sport,* doi: 10.1177/1012690215572855.

Smith, Chris. 2012. United States tops Olympic medal list, but is third to China and Russia in bonus payouts. *Forbes.com* (August 13): http://www.forbes.com/sites/chrissmith/2012/08/13/united-states-olympic-committee-to-pay-5-million-in-medal-bonuses/#5e0c8c6156a5.

Smith, David. 2009. Semenya sex row causes outrage in SA. *Mail and Guardian* (August 23): http://allofusornone.org/pipermail/members_allofusornone.org/2009-September/000355.html.

Smith, Dennis. 2008. Editorial: Beyond greed, fear and anger. *Current Sociology* 56(3): 347–350. Online: http://csi.sagepub.com/cgi/reprint/56/3/347.

Smith, Dorothy E. 2009. Categories are not enough. *Gender & Society* 23(1): 76–80.

Smith, Earl. 2007. *Race, sport and the American dream.* Durham, NC: Carolina Academic Press.

Smith, Earl. 2009. *Race, sport and the American Dream.* 2nd ed. Durham, NC: Carolina Academic Press.

Smith, Gary. 2012. Why don't more athletes take a stand? *Sports Illustrated* 117(2, July 9): 50–65.

Smith, Hillary. 2010. Study: Women's sports aren't equal. *Nwi.com* (June 7): http://www.nwitimes.com/sports/columnists/hillary-smith/article_1353cfa2-8dca-5815-9e62-f636896caa9d.html.

Smith, J. Goosby. 2013. NFL head coaches as sensegiving change agents. *Team Performance Management* 15(3/4): 202–214.

Smith, Jason M., and Alan G. Ingham. 2003. On the waterfront: Retrospectives on the relationship between sport and communities. *Sociology of Sport Journal* 20(3): 252–274.

Smith, Jay M., and Mary Willingham. 2015. *Cheated: The UNC Scandal, the Education of Athletes, and the Future of Big-Time College Sports.* Lincoln NE: Potomac Books.

Smith, Justin E.H. 2013. The enlightenment's 'race' problem, and ours. *New York Times* (February 10): http://opinionator.blogs.nytimes.com/2013/02/10/why-has-race-survived/.

Smith, Lauren. 2007. NCAA proposal would let colleges cash in on player images. *The Chronicle of Higher Education* 54(6, October 5): A1. Online: http://chronicle.com/weekly/v54/i06/06a00102.htm.

Smith, Maureen, and Alison M. Wrynn. 2010. *Women in the 2010 Olympic and Paralympic Games: An analysis of participation, leadership and media opportunities.* East Meadow, NY: Women's Sports Foundation.

Smith, Michael. 1983. *Violence and sport.* Toronto: Butterworths.

Smith, R. Tyson. 2008. Passion work: The joint production of emotional labor in professional wrestling. *Social Psychology Quarterly* 71(2): 157–176.

Smith, Stephanie. 2011. Ex-Falcons lineman had brain disease linked to concussions. *CNN.com* (April 1): http://www.cnn.com/2011/HEALTH/04/01/brain.concussion.dronett/index.html.

Soebbing, Brian P., and Daniel S. Mason. Managing legitimacy and uncertainty in professional team sport: The NBA's draft lottery. *The impact of sports on Team Performance Management* 15(3/4): 141–157.

Soffian, Seth. 2012. Sports exclusive: Undercurrent of homophobia still shapes women's sports. *News-Press.com* (July 10): http://www.marcoislandflorida.com/article/20120710/SPORTS/307100002/Sports-exclusive-Undercurrent-homophobia-still-shapes-women-s-sports.

Solomon, Alisa. 2000. Our bodies, ourselves: The mainstream embraces the athlete Amazon. *The Village Voice* (April 19–25): http://www.villagevoice.com/news/our-bodies-ourselves-6395048.

Sorek, Tamir. 2007. *Arab soccer in a Jewish state: The integrative enclave.* Cambridge: Cambridge University Press.

Sorek, Tamir. 2011. The quest for victory: Collective memory and national identification among the Arab-Palestinian citizens of Israel. *Sociology* 45(3): 464–479.

Spaaij, Ramón. 2006. *Understanding football hooliganism: A comparison of six Western European football clubs.* Amsterdam: Amsterdam University Press.

Spaaij, Ramón. 2007. Football hooliganism as a transnational phenomenon: Past and present analysis: A critique–more specificity and less generality. *International Journal of the History of Sport* 24(4): 411–431.

Spaaij, Ramón, and Alastair Anderson. 2010. Soccer fan violence: A holistic approach. A Reply to Braun & Vliegenthart. *International Sociology* 25(4): 561–579.

SPARC. 2013. What does the science say about athletic development in children? A research brief prepared by the University of Florida Sport Policy & Research Collaborative for the Aspen Institute Sports & Society. Online: http://sparc.hhp.ufl.edu/.

Sparkes, Andrew, and Brett Smith. 2002. Sport, spinal cord injury, embodied masculinities, and the dilemmas of narrative identity. *Men and Masculinities* 4(3): 258–285.

Spencer-Cavaliere, Nancy, and Danielle Peers. 2011. "What's the difference?" Women's wheelchair basketball, reverse integration, and the question(ing) of disability. *Adapted Physical Activity Quarterly* 28(4): 291–309.

Spiegel, Alix. 2008. Old-fashioned play builds serious skills. *PBS, Morning Edition* (February 21): http://www.npr.org/templates/story/story.php?storyId=19212514 .

Spirou, Costas, and Larry Bennett. 2003. *It's hardly sporting: Stadiums, neighborhoods, and the new Chicago.* DeKalb: Northern Illinois University Press.

Sport England. 2013. *Active people survey.* London, Sport England.

St. Louis, Brett. 2010. Sport, genetics and the 'natural athlete': The resurgence of racial science. *Body and Society* 9(2): 75–95.

Starr, Mark. 1999. Voices of the century: Blood, sweat, and cheers. *Newsweek* (October 25): 44–73.

START. 2013. *Background report: Bombings at the Boston Marathon.* National Consortium for the Study of Terrorism and Responses to Terrorism. College Park, MD: University of Maryland.

Staurowsky, Ellen J. 2007. "You know, we are all Indian": Exploring white power and privilege in reactions to the NCAA Native American Mascot Policy. *Journal of Sport and Social Issues* 31(1): 61–76.

Staurowsky, Ellen J. 2014. College athletes' rights in the age of the super conference: The case of the All Players United campaign. *Journal of Intercollegiate Sport* 7(1): 11–34.

Staurowsky, Ellen J., and Erianne A. Weight. 2011. Title IX literacy: What coaches don't know and need to find out. *Journal of Intercollegiate Sport* 4(2): 190–209.

Steele, Claude. 2010. *Whistling Vivaldi and other clues to how stereotypes affect us.* New York: W.W. Norton & Company.

Stelter, Brian. 2013. Rising TV fees mean all viewers pay to keep sports fans happy. *New York Times* (January 25): http://www.nytimes.com/2013/01/26/business/media/all-viewers-pay-to-keep-tv-sports-fans-happy.html.

Stempel, Carl. 2005. Adult participation sports as cultural capital: A test of Bourdieu's theory on the field of sports. *International Review for the Sociology of Sport* 40(4): 411–432.

Stempel, Carl. 2006. Gender, social class and the sporting capital-economic capital nexus. *Sociology of Sport Journal* 23(3): 273–292.

Stephenson, Ben, and Sophia Jowett. 2009. Factors that influence the development of English youth soccer coaches. *International Journal of Coaching Science* 3(1): 3–16.

Stevens, Julie, and Carly Adams. 2013. "Together we can make it better": Collective action and governance in a girls' ice hockey association. *International Review for the Sociology of Sport* 48(6): 658–672.

Stevenson, Betsey. 2010. Beyond the classroom: Using Title IX to measure the return to high school sports. *The Review of Economics and Statistics* 92(2): 284–301.

Stiglitz, Joseph. 2012. *The price of inequality.* New York: W. W. Norton & Company.

Stockdale, Liam. 2012. More than just games: The global politics of the Olympic Movement. *Sport in Society: Cultures, Commerce, Media, Politics* 15(6): 839–854.

Stoddart, Brian. 2008. *Sport in Australian culture revisited.* London/NY: Routledge.

Stokvis, Ruud. 2012. Social stratification and sports in Amsterdam in the 20th century. *International Review for the Sociology of Sport* 47(4): 511–525.

Stone, Christian, and L. Jon Wertheim. 2013. Special investigation, Part 5: What it all means. *Sports Illustrated* 119(12, September 23): 70–71.

Storey, Keith. 2004. The case against Special Olympics. *Journal of Disability Policy Studies* 15: 35–42.

Storey, Keith. 2008. The more things change, the more they are the same: Continuing concerns with the Special Olympics. *Research and Practice for Persons with Severe Disabilities* 33(3): 134–142.

Storey, Samantha. 2013. Parkour, a pastime born on the streets, moves indoors and uptown. *New York Times* (August 8): http://www.nytimes.com/2013/08/09 /sports/parkour-a-pastime-born-on-the-streets- moves-indoors-and-uptown.html.

St-Pierre, Renée, Caroline E. Temcheff, Rina Gupta, Jeffrey Derevensky, and Thoma Paskus. 2013. Predicting gambling problems from gambling outcome expectancies in college student-athletes. *Journal of Gambling Studies.* Online first: http:// link.springer.com/journal/10899/onlineFirst/page/2 (retrieved 6-26-13).

Strachan, Maxwell. 2015. Historic transgender athlete opens up about what he hopes his story teaches others. *Huffington Post* (June 19): http://www .huffingtonpost.com/2015/06/19/chris-mosier- transgender_n_7622178.html.

Straume, Solveig, and Kari Steen-Johnsen. 2012. On the terms of the recipient? Norwegian sports development aid to Tanzania in the 1980s. *International Review for the Sociology of Sport* 47(1): 95–112.

Stuart, Hunter. 2014. School football coach ordered to stop praying with students. *Huffington Post* (February 5): http://www.huffingtonpost .com/2014/02/05/school-football-coach-baptism -prayer-ordered-to-stop-students_n_4725890.html.

Sugden, John. 2007. Inside the grafters' game: An ethnographic examination of football's underground economy. *Journal of Sport and Social Issues* 31(3): 242–258.

Sugden, John. 2012. Watched by the Games: Surveillance and security at the Olympics. *International Review for the Sociology of Sport* 47(3): 414–429.

Sugden, John, and Alan Tomlinson. 1998. *FIFA and the contest for world football: Who rules the peoples' game?* Cambridge, UK: Polity Press.

Suggs, Welch. 2001. Left behind. *Chronicle of Higher Education* 48(14): A35–A37.

Suggs, Welch. 2005. *A place on the team: The triumph and tragedy of Title IX.* Princeton, NJ: Princeton University Press.

Sullivan, Charley. 2012. "Why women can't coach football": Title IX turns 40. *GayGamesBlog* (July 6): http://gaygamesblog.blogspot.fi/2012/07/why -women-cant-coach-football-title-ix.html.

Sullivan, Claire F. 2011. Gender verification and gender policies in elite sport: Eligibility and "fair play." *Journal of Sport and Social Issues* 35(4): 400–419.

Summers, Amber, Amy R. Confair, Laura Flamm, Attia Goheer, Karlene Graham, Mwende Muindi, Joel Gittelsohn. 2013. Designing the healthy bodies, healthy souls church-based diabetes prevention program through a participatory process. *American Journal of Health Education* 44(2): 53–66.

Sundgot-Borgen, J., and M.K. Torsveit. 2010. Aspects of disordered eating continuum in elite high-intensity sports. *Scandinavian Journal of Medicine and Science in Sports* 20(Suppl 2): 112–121.

Surowiecki, James 2013. A call to action. *The New Yorker* (February 11): 36.

Sutherland, Allan. 1981. *Disabled we stand.* Bloomington, IN: Indiana University Press.

Swain, Derek. 1999. Moving on: Leaving pro sports. In Jay Coakley & Peter Donnelly, eds., *Inside sports* (pp. 223–231). London: Routledge.

Swanson, Jennifer, Amelie Ramirez, and Kipling J. Gallion. 2013. Salud America! Active spaces for Latino Kids. Princeton, NJ: The Robert Woods Johnson Foundation.

Swanson, Lisa. 2009. Soccer fields of cultural [re] production: Creating good boys in suburban America. *Sociology of Sport Journal* 26(3): 404–424.

Swartz, Leslie, and Brian Watermeyer. 2008. Cyborg anxiety: Oscar Pistorius and the boundaries of what it means to be human. *Disability & Society* 23(2): 187–190.

Sylwester, MaryJo. 2005a. Girls following in Ochoa's, Fernandez's sports cleats. *USA Today* (March 29): 4C.

Sylwester, MaryJo. 2005b. Hispanic girls in sports held back by tradition. *USA Today* (March 29): 1A–2A.

Sylwester, MaryJo. 2005c. Sky's the limit for Hispanic teen. *USA Today* (March 29): 4C.

Sze, Julie. 2009. Sports and environmental justice: "Games" of race, place, nostalgia, and power in neoliberal New York City. *Journal of Sport and Social Issues* 33(2): 111–129.

Tagg, Brendon. 2012. Transgender netballers: Ethical issues and lived realities. *Sociology of Sport Journal* 29(2): 151–167.

Taheri, Amir. 2004. Muslim women play only an incidental part in the Olympics. Online: http://www .benadorassociates.com/article/6651.

Tamir, Ilan. 2014. The decline of nationalism among football fans. *Television & New Media* 15(8): 741–745.

Tan, Tien-Chin, and Barrie Houlihan. 2012. Chinese Olympic sport policy: Managing the impact of globalization. *International Review for the Sociology of Sport* 48(2): 131–152.

Tanier, Mike. 2012. Big price tags attached to even the littlest leagues. *New York Times* (April 23): http:// www.nytimes.com/2012/04/24/sports/big-price-tags-attached-to-even-the-littlest-leagues.html.

Taniguchi, Hiromi, and Frances L. Shupe. 2014. Gender and family status differences in leisure-time sports/ fitness participation. *International Review for the Sociology of Sport* 49(1): 65–84.

Taub, Diane E., and Kimberly R. Greer. 2000. Physical activity as a normalizing experience for school-age children with physical disabilities: Implications for legitimating of social identity and enhancement of social ties. *Journal of Sport and Social Issues* 24(4): 395–414.

Tavernise, Sabrina. 2012. Survey finds rising perception of class tension. *New York Times* (January 11): http:// www.nytimes.com/2012/01/12/us/more-conflict-seen-between-rich-and-poor-survey-finds.html.

Taylor, Matthew J., and G.M. Turek. 2010. If only she would play? The impact of sports participation on self-esteem, school adjustment, and substance use among rural and urban African American girls. *Journal of Sport Behavior* 33(3): 315–336.

Taylor, Matthew J., Rachel A. Wamser, and Michelle E. Sanchez. 2010. The impact of sports participation on violence and victimization among rural minority adolescent girls. *Women in Sport and Physical Activity Journal* 19(1): 3–13.

Taylor, Matthew J., Tara L. Shoemaker, Desiree Z. Welch, and Maurice Endsley, Jr. 2010. Sports participation and delinquent peer associations: Implications for individual behavior of minority girls. *International Journal of Sport and Society* 1(3): 146–160.

Taylor, Nate. 2013. For Spurs, every game is a global summit. *New York Times* (June 9): http://www .nytimes.com/2013/06/10/sports/basketball/for-spurs-every-game-is-a-global-summit.html.

Temple, Kerry. 1992. Brought to you by . . . *Notre Dame Magazine* 21(2): 29.

Thamel, Pete, and Alexander Wolff. 2013. The institution has lost control. *Sports Illustrated* (June 17): 60–69.

Thangaraj, Stanley. 2012. Playing through differences: Black–white racial logic and interrogating South Asian American identity. *Ethnic and Racial Studies* 35(6): 988–1006.

Theberge, Nancy. 1999. Being physical: Sources of pleasure and satisfaction in women's ice hockey. In J. Coakley & P. Donnelly, eds., *Inside Sports* (pp. 146–155). London: Routledge.

Theberge, Nancy. 2000a. Gender and sport. In J. Coakley & E. Dunning, eds., *Handbook of sport studies* (pp. 322–333). London: Sage.

Theberge, Nancy. 2000b. *Higher goals: Women's ice hockey and the politics of gender.* Albany: State University of New York Press.

Theberge, Nancy. 2008. "Just a normal bad part of what I do": Elite athletes' accounts of the relationship between health and sport. *Sociology of Sport Journal* 25(2): 206–222.

The Daily Caller. 2013. 'A racial, derogatory slur': Congressmen call for Redskins to lose the 'R word.' *dailycaller.com* (May 29): http://dailycaller .com/2013/05/29/a-racial-derogatory-slur-congressmen-call-for-redskins-to-lose-the-r-word/.

The Editors. 2011. The sports issue: Views from left field. *The Nation* (August 15–22): http://www.thenation.com/article/sports-issue-views-left-field/.

Thelin, John R. 2008. Academics and athletics: A part and apart in the American campus. *Journal of Intercollegiate Sport* 1, 1: 72–81.

Thoennes, K. Erik. 2008. Created to play: Thoughts on play, sport, and the Christian life. In Donald Lee Deardorff & John White, eds., *The image of god in the human body: Essays on God Christianity and sports.* Lewiston, NY: Edwin Mellen Press.

Thomas, Katie. 2008a. Big game is no place for the average fan. *New York Times* (February 3): http://select.nytimes.com/mem/tnt.html?emc_tnt&tntget_2008/02/03/sports/football/03corporate.html.

Thomas, Katie. 2008b. A lab is set to test the gender of some female athletes. *New York Times* (July 30): http://www.nytimes.com/2008/07/30/sports/olympics/30gender.html.

Thomas, Katie. 2010a. Women's group cites 12 districts in Title IX complaint. *New York Times* (November 10): http://www.nytimes.com/2010/11/11/sports/11titleIX.html.

Thomas, Katie. 2010b. No tackling, but a girls' sport takes some hits. *New York Times* (May 15): http://www.nytimes.com/2010/05/16/sports/16flag.html.

Thomas, Katie. 2011. College teams, relying on deception, undermine gender equity. *New York Times* (April 25): http://www.nytimes.com/2011/04/26/sports/26titleix.html.

Thomas, Ryan J., and Mary Grace Antony. 2015. Competing constructions of British national identity: British newspaper comment on the 2012 Olympics opening ceremony. *Media, Culture & Society* 37(3): 493–503.

Thompson, Kirrilly, and Chanel Nesci. 2013. Over-riding concerns: Developing safe relations in the high-risk interspecies sport of eventing. *International Review for the Sociology of Sport* published 4 December 2013, 10.1177/1012690213513266.

Thompson, Wright. 2013. Generation June: Fury, anarchy, martyrdom—Why the youth of Brazil are (forever) protesting, and how their anger may consume the World Cup. *ESPN The Magazine* (December 23): 42–55.

Thomson, Rosemarie Garland. 2000. Staring back: Self-representations of disabled performance artists. *American Quarterly* 52(2): 334–338.

Thomson, Rosemarie Garland. 2002. Integrating disability, transforming feminist theory. *National Women's Studies Association Journal* 14(3): 1–32.

Thomson, Rosemarie Garland. 2009. *Staring: How we look.* New York: Oxford University Press.

Thornton, Grant. 2013. *Meta-evaluation of the impacts and legacy of the London 2012 Olympic Games and Paralympic Games* (July; Report 5: Post-Games Evaluation). London: Department for Culture, Media and Sport.

Thorpe, Holly. 2009a. Bourdieu, gender reflexivity and physical culture: A case of masculinities in the snowboarding field. *Journal of Sport and Social Issues* 34(2): 176–214.

Thorpe, Holly, and Belinda Wheaton. 2011a. 'Generation X Games,' action sports and the Olympic movement: Understanding the cultural politics of incorporation. *Sociology* 45(5): 830–847.

Thorpe, Holly, and Belinda Wheaton. 2011b. The Olympic movement, action sports and the search for Generation Y. In John Sugden & Alan Tomlinson, eds., *Watching the Olympics: Politics, power and representation* (pp. 182–200). London: Routledge.

Thorpe, Holly, and Belinda Wheaton. 2013. Dissecting action sport studies: Past, present and beyond. In David Andrews & Ben Carrington, eds., *Blackwell companion to sport* (pp. 341–358). Chichester, UK: Wiley-Blackwell.

Thualagant, Nicole. 2012. The conceptualization of fitness doping and its limitations. *Sport in Society* 15(3): 409–419.

Tigay, Chanan. 2011. Women and sports. *CQ Researcher* 21(March 25): 265–288. Online: http://library.cqpress.com/cqresearcher/ (retrieved 12-17-2013).

Timothy, David Ryan, and Michael Sagas. 2013. Relationships between pay satisfaction, work-family conflict, and coaching turnover intentions. *Team Performance Management* 15(3/4): 128–140.

Tinley, Scott P. 2012. *Seeing stars: Emotional trauma in athlete retirement: Contexts, intersections, and explorations.* Ph.D. dissertation, Claremont Graduate University, Claremont, CA.

Tinley, Scott. 2015a. *Racing the sunset How athletes survive, thrive, or fail in life after sport.* New York: Skyhorse Publishing.

Tinley, Scott. 2015b. *Finding triathlon.* New York: Hatherleigh Press.

Toffoletti, Kim. 2012. Iranian women's sports fandom: Gender, resistance, and identity in the football movie *Offside. Journal of Sport and Social Issues* published 26 December 2012, 10.1177/0193723512468758.

Toft, Ditte. 2011. New sports press survey: Newspapers focus narrowly on sports results. *Playthegame.org* (October 3): http://www.playthegame.org/news /detailed/new-sports-press-survey-newspapers-focus -narrowly-on-sports-results-5248.html.

Toma, J. Douglas. 2010. Intercollegiate athletics, institutional aspirations, and why legitimacy is more compelling than sustainability. *Journal of Intercollegiate Sport* 3(1): 51–68.

Tomc, Gregor. 2008. The nature of sport. In Mojca Doupona Topič & Simon Ličen, eds., *Sport, culture & society: An account of views and perspectives on social issues in a continent (and beyond)* (pp. 9–12). Ljubljana, Slovenia: University of Ljubljana.

Tomlinson, Alan. 2007. Sport and social class. In George Ritzer, ed., *Encyclopedia of sociology* (pp. 4695–4699). London/New York: Blackwell.

Tomlinson, Alan. 2008. *Gender, sport and leisure* (2nd edition). Aachen/Oxford: Meyer and Meyer Sport.

Toohey, Kristine, and Tracy Taylor. 2012. Surveillance and securitization: A forgotten Sydney Olympic legacy. *International Review for the Sociology of Sport* 47(3): 324–337.

Topič, Mojca Doupona, and Jay Coakley. 2010. Complicating the relationship between sport and national identity: The case of post-socialist Slovenia. *Sociology of Sport Journal* 27(4): 371–389.

Topič, Mojca Doupona, Otmar Weiss, Michael Methagl, and Simon Ličen. 2008. The role of sport in society. In Mojca Doupona Topič & Simon Ličen, eds., *Sport, culture & society: An account of views and perspectives on social issues in a continent (and beyond)* (pp. 60–64). Ljubljana, Slovenia: University of Ljubljana.

Torre, Pablo S., and David Epstein. 2012. The transgender athlete. *Sports Illustrated* 118(22, May 28): 66–73. Online: http://www.si.com/ vault/2012/05/28/106195901/the-transgender-athlete.

Torres, Kimberly. 2009. 'Culture shock': Black students account for their distinctiveness at an elite college. *Ethnic and Racial Studies* 32(5): 883–905.

Tozer, Malcolm. 2013. 'One of the worst statistics in British sport, and wholly unacceptable': The contribution of privately educated members of Team GB to the Summer Olympic Games, 2000–2012. *The International Journal of the History of Sport* 30(12): 1436–1454.

Tranter, Paul J., and Mark Lowes. 2009. Life in the fast lane: Environmental, economic, and public health outcomes of motorsport spectacles in Australia. *Journal of Sport and Social Issues* 33(2): 150–168.

Traub, Amy, and Catherine Ruetschlin. 2015. The racial wealth gap: Why policy matters. Demos.org (March 10): http://www.demos.org/publication /racial-wealth-gap-why-policy-matters.

Travers, Ann. 2006. Queering sport: Lesbian softball leagues and the transgender challenge. *International Review for the Sociology of Sport* 41(3/4): 431–446.

Travers, Ann. 2008. The sport nexus and gender injustice. *Studies in Social Justice* 2(1): 79–101.

Travers, Ann. 2011. Women's ski jumping, the 2010 Olympic Games, and the deafening silence of sex segregation, whiteness, and wealth. *Journal of Sport and Social Issues* 35(2): 126–145.

Travers, Ann. 2013. Thinking the unthinkable: Imagining an "Un-American," girl-friendly, women- and trans-inclusive alternative for baseball. *Journal of Sport and Social Issues* 37: 78–96.

Travers, Ann. 2013a. Transformative sporting visions. *Journal of Sport and Social Issues* 37(1): 3–7.

Travers, Ann. 2013b. Thinking the unthinkable: Imagining an "un-American," girl-friendly, women and trans-inclusive alternative for baseball. *Journal of Sport and Social Issues* 37(1): 78–96.

Travers, Ann, and Jillian Deri. 2011. Transgender inclusion and the changing face of lesbian softball leagues. *International Review for the Sociology of Sport* 46(4): 488–507.

Treviño, José Luis Pérez. 2013. Cyborgpersons: Between disability and enhancement. *Physical Culture and Sport. Studies and Research* 57: 12–21.

Troutman, Kelly, P., and Mikaela J. Dufur. 2007. From high school jocks to college grads assessing the long-term effects of high school sport participation on females' educational attainment. *Youth & Society* 38(4): 443–462.

Troutman, Parke. 2004. A growth machine's plan B: Legitimating development when the value-free growth ideology is under fire. *Journal of Urban Affairs* 26(5): 611–622.

Trulson, Michael E. 1986. Martial arts training: A novel "cure" for juvenile delinquency. *Human Relations* 39(12): 1131–1140.

Tucker, Ross, 2009. Truth about players playing injured. *SI.com* (December 2): http://www.si.com /more-sports/2009/12/02/concussions.

Tulle, Emmanuelle. 2007. Running to run: Embodiment, structure and agency amongst veteran elite runners. *Sociology* 41(2): 329–346.

Tulle, Emmanuelle. 2008a. Acting your age? Sports science and the ageing body. *Journal of Aging Studies* 22(4): 340–347.

Tulle, Emmanuelle. 2008b. The ageing body and the ontology of ageing: Athletic competence in later life. *Body and Society* 14(3): 1–19.

Tulle, Emmanuelle. 2008c. *Ageing, The body and social change.* Basingstoke: Palgrave MacMillan.

Tulle, Emmanuelle. 2014. Living by numbers: Media representations of sports stars' careers. *International Review for the Sociology of Sport* published 10 March 2014, 10.1177/1012690214525157.

Turk, Austin T. 2004. Sociology of terrorism. *Annual Review of Sociology* 30: 271–286.

Tynedal, Jeremy, and Gregor Wolbring. 2013. Paralympics and its athletes through the lens of the *New York Times*. *Sports* 1(1): 13–36.

U.S. Department of Labor. 2011. Disability employment statistics. Washington, DC: Office of Disability Employment Policy. Online: http://www.dol.gov /odep/topics/DisabilityEmploymentStatistics.htm.

U.S. News & World Report. 1983. A sport fan's guide to the 1984 Olympics. *U.S. News & World Report* (May 9): 124.

U.S. Department of Health and Human Services. 2008. Physical Activity Guidelines Advisory Committee Report Washington, DC. Online: health.gov/ paguidelines/report/pdf/committeereport.pdf.

UK Sport. 2013. Transsexual people and sport. London: Department for Culture, Media and Sport, Sport Division.

Unruh, David R. 1980. The nature of social worlds. *Pacific Sociological Review* 23(3): 271–296.

Vaczi, Mariann. 2013. "The Spanish Fury": A political geography of soccer in Spain. *International Review for the Sociology of Sport* published 25 February 2013, 10.1177/1012690213478940.

Vaczi, Mariann. 2015. "The Spanish Fury": A political geography of soccer in Spain. *International Review for the Sociology of Sport* 50(2):196–210.

Valenti, Jessica. 2013. Feminism, sexuality & social justice—With a sense of humor. *The Nation* (June 3): http://www.thenation.com/blog/174624/fuck-high-road-upside-sinking-their-level.

Vallerand, Robert J., Nikos Ntoumanis, Frederick Philippe, Genevieve Lavigne, Noemie Carbonneau, Arielle Bonneville, Camille Lagace-Labonte, and

Gabrielle Maliha. 2008. On passion and sports fans: A look at football. *Journal of Sport Sciences* 26(12): 1279–1293.

Van Amsterdam, Noortje, Annelies Knoppers, Inge Claringbould, and Marian Jongmans. 2012. A picture is worth a thousand words: Constructing (non-) athletic bodies. *Journal of Youth Studies* 15(3): 293–309.

Van de Walle, Guy. 2011. 'Becoming familiar with a world': A relational view of socialization. *International Review of Sociology* 21(2): 315–333.

Van Hilvoorde, Ivo, and Laurens Landeweerd, 2008. Disability or extraordinary talent—Francesco Lentini (Three Legs) versus Oscar Pistorius (No Legs). *Ethics, Dis/ability and Sport* 2(2): 97–111.

Van Hilvoorde, Ivo, Agnes Elling, and Ruud Stokvis. 2010. How to influence national pride? The Olympic medal index as a unifying narrative. *International Review for the Sociology of Sport* 45(1): 87–102.

van Houten, Jasper M.A., Gerbert Kraaykamp, and Koen Breedveld. 2015. When do young adults stop practising a sport? An event history analysis on the impact of four major life events. *International Review for the Sociology of Sport.* Published before print, December; DOI: 10.1177/1012690215619204.

Van Ingen, Kathy. 2011. Spatialities of anger: Emotional geographies in a boxing program for survivors of violence. *Sociology of Sport Journal* 28(2): 171–188.

Van Sterkenburg, Jacco, Annelies Knoppers, and Sonja De Leeuw. 2010. Race, ethnicity, and content analysis of the sports media: A critical reflection. *Media, Culture & Society* 32(5): 819–839.

van Sterkenburg, Jacco, Annelies Knoppers, and Sonja de Leeuw. 2012. Constructing racial/ethnic difference in and through Dutch televised soccer commentary. *Journal of Sport and Social Issues* 36(4): 422–442.

Van Tuyckom, Charlotte, Jeroen Scheerder, and Piet Bracke. 2010. Gender and age inequalities in regular sports participation: A cross-national study of 25 European countries. *Journal of Sports Sciences* 28(10): 1077–1084.

Van Valkenburg, Kevin. 2012a. Games of chance. *ESPN. com* (August 30): http://espn.go.com/espn/otl/story/_ /id/8307997/why-men-dave-coleman-jr-willing-risk -much-play-semi-pro-football (retrieved 2-20-13).

Vannini, April, and Barbara Fornssler. 2011. Girl, Interrupted: Interpreting Semenya's body, gender verification testing, and public discourse. *Cultural Studies—Critical Methodologies* 11(3): 243–257.

Vasquez, Jessica M., and Christopher Wetzel. 2009. Tradition and the invention of racial selves: Symbolic boundaries, collective authenticity, and contemporary struggles for racial equality. *Ethnic and Racial Studies* 32(9): 1557–1575.

Vecsey, George. 2012. Soccer is welcome at home of Sox. *New York Times* (July 25): http://www .nytimes.com/2012/07/26/sports/soccer/at-fenway-a-night-of-soccer-not-sox-totti-not-papi.html.

Veliz, Phil. 2012. *The role of interscholastic sport in public high schools: A zero-sum game or a bridge to success?* A dissertation, Faculty of the Graduate School of the University at Buffalo, State University of New York.

Veliz, Philip, John Schulenberg, Megan Patrick, Deborah Kloska, Sean Esteban McCabe, and Nicole Zarrett. 2015. Competitive sports participation in high school and subsequent substance use in young adulthood: Assessing differences based on level of contact. *International Review for the Sociology of Sport* published 17 May 2015, 10.1177/1012690215586998.

Veliz, Philip, and Sohaila Shakib. 2012. Interscholastic sports participation and school based delinquency: Does participation in sport foster a positive high school environment? *Sociological Spectrum: Mid-South Sociological Association* 32(6): 558–580.

Veri, Maria J., and Rita Liberti. 2013. Tailgate warriors: Exploring constructions of masculinity, food, and football. *Journal of Sport and Social Issues* published 25 January 2013, 10.1177/0193723512472897.

Vermillion, Mark. 2007. Sport participation and adolescent deviance: A logistic analysis. *Social Thought and Research* 28: 227–258.

Viloria, Hida Patricia, and Maria Jose Martinez-Patino. 2012. Reexamining rationales of "fairness": An athlete and insider's perspective on the new policies on hyperandrogenism in elite female athletes. *The American Journal of Bioethics* 12(7): 17–19.

Vivoni, Francisco. 2009. Spots of spatial desire: Skateparks, skateplazas, and urban politics. *Journal of Sport and Social Issues* 33(2): 130–149.

Volpi, Frederic. 2006. Politics. In Bryan S. Turner, ed., *The Cambridge dictionary of sociology* (pp. 445–447). Cambridge, UK: Cambridge University Press.

Volz, Brian. 2009. Minority status and managerial survival in Major League Baseball. *Journal of Sports Economics* 10(5): 522–542.

von Scheve, Christian, Manuela Beyer, Sven Ismer, Marta Kozlowska, and Carmen Morawetz. 2014. Emotional entrainment, national symbols, and identification: A naturalistic study around the men's football World Cup. *Current Sociology* 62(1): 3–23.

Vygotsky, L. 1978. *Thought and language.* London: MIT Press.

Vygotsky, Lev S. 1980. *Mind in society: The development of higher psychological processes.* (Original translation and editing supervised by Michael Cole.) Cambridge, MA: Harvard University Press.

Wacquant, Loïc J.D. 1992. The social logic of boxing in black Chicago: Toward a sociology of pugilism. *Sociology of Sport Journal* 9(3): 221–254.

Wacquant, Loïc J.D. 1995a. The pugilistic point of view: How boxers think and feel about their trade. *Theory and Society* 24: 489–535.

Wacquant, Loïc J.D. 1995b. Why men desire muscles. *Body and Society* 1(1): 163–179.

Wacquant, Loïc J.D. 2004. *Body and soul: Notebooks of an apprentice boxer.* Oxford, UK/New York: Oxford University Press.

WADA. 2009. *World Anti-Doping Code.* Montreal, Quebec, Canada: World Anti-Doping Agency. Online: http://www.wada-ama.org/en/World -Anti-Doping-Program/Sports-and-Anti-Doping -Organizations/The-Code/ (retrieved 6-26-13).

WADA. 2009. The guide (Edition 5). World Anti-Doping Agency. Online: http://www.wada-ama.org /en/Anti-Doping-Community/Athletes-/.

Waddington, Ivan. 2000a. Sport and health: A sociological perspective. In Jay Coakley & Eric Dunning, eds., *Handbook of sports studies* (pp. 408–421). London: Sage.

Waddington, Ivan. 2000b. *Sport, health and drugs: A critical sociological perspective.* London: Routledge.

Waddington, Ivan. 2007. Health and sport. In George Ritzer, ed., *Encyclopedia of sociology* (pp. 2091–2095). London: Blackwell.

Waddington, Ivan, and Andy Smith. 2009. *An introduction to drugs in sport: Addicted to winning?* London and New York: Routledge.

Wahlert, Lance, and Autumn Fiester. 2012. Gender transports: Privileging the "natural" in gender testing debates for intersex and transgender athletes. *The American Journal of Bioethics* 12(7): 19–21.

Walby, Sylvia. 2011. *The future of feminism.* Cambridge, UK: Polity Press.

Waldron, Jennifer J., and Christopher L. Kowalski. 2009. Crossing the line: Rites of passage, team aspects, and ambiguity of hazing. *Research Quarterly for Exercise and Sport* 80(2): 291–302.

Waldron, Jennifer J., Quinten Lynn, and Vikki Krane. 2011. Duct tape, icy hot & paddles: Narratives of initiation onto U.S. male sport teams. *Sport, Education and Society* 16(1): 111–125.

Walker, Marlon A. 2013. Leaders urge colleges to expand sports programs for students with disabilities. *Diverse Issues in Higher Education* (April 16): http://diverseeducation.com/article/52686/.

Walseth, Kristin. 2006. Sport and belonging. *International Review for the Sociology of Sport* 41(3/4): 447–464.

Warde, Alan. 2006. Cultural capital and the place of sport. *Cultural Trends* 15(2/3): 107–122.

Watermeyer, Brian. 2012. Is it possible to create a politically engaged, contextual psychology of disability? *Disability & Society* 27(2): 161–174.

Watson, Nick J., and Andrew Parker. 2013 A Christian theological analysis of the institutions and governance of sport: A case study of the modern Olympic Games. *Journal of Religion and Society* 15(1): 1–21. Online: http://moses.creighton.edu/JRS/2013/2013-22.pdf.

Watson, Nick J., and Brian Brock. 2014. Religion in the ring: Death, concussion and brain bleeds. *Theos, Public Theology Think-Tank.* London. http://www.theosthinktank.co.uk/comment/2014/12/15/religion-in-the-ring-death-concussion-and-brain-bleeds.

Weaver, Paul. 2005. Alma mater of Coe and Radcliffe brings sport to Muslim women. Online: https://www.theguardian.com/sport/2005/feb/22/highereducation.education.

Weber, Jonetta D., and Robert M. Carini. 2013. Where are the female athletes in *Sports Illustrated?* A content analysis of covers (2000–2011). *International Review for the Sociology of Sport* 48(2): 196–203.

Weber, Julia, and Natalie Barker-Ruchti. 2012. Bending, flirting, floating, flying: A critical analysis of female figures in 1970s gymnastics photographs. *Sociology of Sport Journal* 29(1): 22–41.

Weber, Max. 1922a/1968. *Economy and society: An outline of interpretive sociology* (trans. G. Roth and G. Wittich). New York: Bedminster Press.

Weber, Max. 1922b/1993. *The sociology of religion.* Boston, MA: Beacon Press.

Weber, Romana. 2009. Protection of children in competitive sport: Some critical questions for London 2012. *International Review for the Sociology of Sport* 44(1): 55–69.

Webster, Paul. 2000. France keeps a hold on Black Venus. *The Observer* (April 2): http://www.guardian.co.uk/world/2000/apr/02/paulwebster.theobserver1.

Wedgwood, Nikki. 2004. Kicking like a boy: Schoolgirl Australian rules football and bi-gendered female embodiment. *Sociology of Sport Journal* 21(2): 140–162.

Wedgwood, Nikki. 2013. Hahn versus Guttmann: Revisiting 'Sports and the Political Movement of Disabled Persons.' *Disability & Society* 29(1): 129–142.

Weedon, Gavin. 2012. 'Glocal boys': Exploring experiences of acculturation amongst migrant youth footballers in Premier League academies. *International Review for the Sociology of Sport* 47(2): 200–216.

Weedon, Gavin. 2013. The writing's on the firewall: Assessing the promise of open access journal publishing for a public sociology of sport. *Sociology of Sport Journal* 30(3): 359–379.

Weedon, Gavin. 2015. Camaraderie reincorporated: Tough Mudder and the extended distribution of the social. *Journal of Sport and Social Issues* 39(6): 431–454.

Weir, Patricia, Joe Baker, and Sean Horton. 2010. The emergence of Masters sport: Participatory trends and historical developments. In Joe Baker, Sean Horton & Patricia Weir, eds., *The Masters athlete: Understanding the role of sport and exercise in optimizing aging.* New York/London: Routledge.

Weir, Tom. 2006. Rookie always in a hurry. *USA Today* (June 30): C1–2.

Weisman, Larry. 2004. Propelled to think past NFL. *USA Today* (June 16): 1C.

Weiss, Maureen R., and Diane M. Wiese-Bjornstal. 2009. Promoting positive youth development through physical activity. *Research Digest of the President's Council on Physical Fitness and Sports* 10 (3, September).

Weiss, Windee M. 2008. Coaching your parents: Support vs. pressure. *Technique* 28(10): 18, 20–22.

Wellard, Ian. 2012. *Sport, masculinities and the body.* London: Routledge.

Wells, Steven. 2008. Bend it like Janiah. *Philadelphia Weekly* (January 23–29): http://philadelphiaweekly

.com/2007/jul/4/bend_it_like_janiah-38428359/#
.VzJYl75dvEY.

Wenner, Lawrence A. 2012. On roads traveled and journeys ahead for IRSS. *International Review for the Sociology of Sport* 47(1): 3–4.

Wenner, Lawrence A. 2013. Reflections on communication and sport: On reading sport and narrative ethics. *Communication & Sport* 1(1/2): 188–199.

Wenner, Lawrence A. 2014. On the limits of the new and the lasting power of the mediasport interpellation. *Television & New Media* 15(8): 732–740.

West, Brad. 2003. Synergies in deviance: Revisiting the positive deviance debate. *Electronic Journal of Sociology* (November): http://www.sociology.org/content/vol7.4/west.html.

Whannel, Garry. 2014. The paradoxical character of live television sport in the twenty-first century. *Television & New Media* 15(8): 769–776.

Wheatley, Sean, Saira Khana, Andrea D. Szekelyb, Declan P. Naughtona, and Andrea Petroczia. 2012. Expanding the Female Athlete Triad concept to address a public health issue. *Performance Enhancement & Health* 1(1): 10–27.

Wheaton, Belinda. 2004. Selling out? The commercialization and globalization of lifestyle sport. In Lincoln Allison, ed., *The global politics of sport: The role of global institutions in sport* (pp. 140–185). London: Routledge.

Wheaton, Belinda. 2004. *Understanding lifestyle sports: Consumption, identity and difference.* London/New York: Routledge.

Wheaton, Belinda. 2013. *The cultural politics of lifestyle sports.* London: Routledge.

Wheeler, Garry David, Robert D. Steadward, David Legg, Yesahayu Hutzler, Elizabeth Campbell, and Anne Johnson. 1999. Personal investment in disability sport careers: An international study. *Adapted Physical Activity Quarterly* 16(3): 219–237.

Wheeler, Sharon. 2012. The significance of family culture for sports participation. *International Review for the Sociology of Sport* 47(2): 235–252.

Wheeler, Sharon, and Ken Green. 2014. Parenting in relation to children's sports participation: Generational changes and potential implications. *Leisure Studies* 33(3): 267–284.

Wheelock, Darren, and Douglas Hartmann. 2007. Midnight basketball and the 1994 crime bill debates: The operation of a racial code. *The Sociological Quarterly* 48(2): 315–342.

White, Amanda M., and Constance T. Gager. 2007. Idle hands and empty pockets? Youth involvement in extracurricular activities, social capital, and economic status. *Youth and Society* 39(1): 75–111.

White, John. 2008. Idols in the stadium: Sport as an 'idol factory.' In Donald Lee Deardorff & John White, eds., *The image of God in the human body: Essays on Christianity and sports.* Lewiston, NY: Edwin Mellen Press.

White. Kerry. 2005. Breaking news, breaking boundaries. Online: http://www.womenssportsfoundation.org/http://www.womenssportsfoundation.org/Content/Articles/Careers/B/Breaking%20News%20Breaking%20Boundaries.aspx.

White, Paul. 2012. Cortisone: Is it worth the shot? *USA Today* (October 9): 1–2C. Online: http://www.usatoday.com/story/sports/mlb/2012/10/08/mlb-cortisone-shots/1621781/.

White, Philip, and William McTeer. 2012. Socioeconomic status and sport participation at different developmental stages during childhood and youth: Multivariate analyses using Canadian national survey data. *Sociology of Sport Journal* 29(2): 186–209.

White, Philip, and Kevin Young. 1997. Masculinity, sport, and the injury process: A review of Canadian and international evidence. *Avante* 3(2): 1–30.

Whiteside, Erin, and Marie Hardin. 2011. Women (not) watching women: Leisure time, television, and implications for televised coverage of women's sports. *Communication, Culture and Critique* 4(2): 122–143.

Wolverton, Brad. 2014. At meeting of Knight Commission, old ideas are new again. The Chronicle of Higher Education (September 9): http://chronicle.com/article/At-Meeting-of-Knight/148709/

World Health Organization. 2007. *Women and physical activity.* Geneva, Switzerland. Online: http://www.who.int/moveforhealth/advocacy/information_sheets/woman/en/index.html.

WHO. 2011. *World report on disability.* Geneva, Switzerland: World Health Organization.

WHO. 2013. *World health statistics, 2013.* Geneva, Switzerland: World Health Organization.

Wickersham, Seth, 2011. Is Gordon Gee serious? *ESPN* (August 8): http://espn.go.com/college-football/story/_/id/6843627/college-football-ohio-state-president-gordon-gee-recent-football-scandal-espn-magazine.

Wieberg, Steve. 2010. NCAA study: Athletes continue to disregard rules, gamble on sports. *USA Today* (November 13): http://www.usatoday.com/sports /college/2009-11-13-ncaa-gambling-study_N.htm (retrieved 6-26-13).

Wiedeman, Reeves. 2013. Football's hidden pains. *The New Yorker* (January 13): http://www.newyorker .com/online/blogs/sportingscene/2013/01/ footballs-hidden-pains.html (retrieved 5-25-13).

Wiederer, Dan. 2012. NFL and pain: League zeros in on one pain medication. *Minneapolis Star Tribune* (August 22): http://www.startribune.com/sports /vikings/166712256.html.

Wilcke, Christoph, ed. 2012. *"Steps of the devil:" Denial of women's and girls' rights to sport in Saudi Arabia.* Washington, DC: Human Right Watch.

Wilińska, Monika. 2010. Because women will always be women and men are just getting older: Intersecting discourses of ageing and gender. *Current Sociology* 58(6): 879–896.

Wilkins, Amy. 2012. Stigma and status: Interracial intimacy and intersectional identities among Black college men. *Gender & Society* 26(2): 165–189.

Wilkinson, Richard, and Kate Pickett. 2010. *The spirit level: Why greater equality makes societies stronger.* New York: Bloomsbury Press.

Will, George. 2011a. The NBA standoff pits the elite vs. the elite. *Washington Post* (October 14): http://www.washingtonpost.com/opinions/the -nba-standoff-pits-the-elite-vs-the-elite/2011/10/13 /gIQA2LkykL_story.html.

Willard, Frances. 1895. *Wheel within a wheel: A woman's quest for freedom.* Bedford, MA: Applewood Books.

Willett, Jennifer Beck, Bernie Goldfine, Todd Seidler, Andy Gillentine, and Scott Marley. 2014. Prayer 101: Deciphering the law. *Journal of Physical Education, Recreation & Dance* 85(9): 15–19.

Williams, Dana. 2007. Where's the honor? Attitudes toward the "Fighting Sioux" nickname and logo. *Sociology of Sport Journal* 24(4): 437–456.

Williams, Lovoria B., Richard W. Sattin, James Dias, Jane T. Garvin, Lucy Marion, Thomas Joshua, Andrea Kriska, M. Kaye Kramer, Justin B. Echouffo-Tcheugui, Arin Freeman, and K. M. Venkat Narayan. 2013. Design of a cluster-randomized controlled trail of diabetes prevention program within African-American churches: The fit body and soul study. *Contemporary Clinical Trials* 34(2): 336–347.

Williams, Patricia J. 2005. Genetically speaking. *The Nation* 280(24): 10.

Willmsen, Christine, and Maureen O'Hagan. 2003. Coaches continue working for schools and private teams after being caught for sexual misconduct. *Seattle Times* (December 14): http://old.seattletimes .com/news/local/coaches/news/dayone.html.

Wilson, Daniel H. 2012. Bionic brains and beyond. *Wall Street Journal* (June 2): C1–2.

Wilson, Noela C., and Selina Khoob. 2013. Benefits and barriers to sports participation for athletes with disabilities: The case of Malaysia. *Disability & Society* 28(8): 1132–1145.

Winant, Howard. 2001. *The world is a ghetto: Race and democracy since World War II.* New York: Basic Books.

Winant, Howard. 2004. *The new politics of race: Globalism, difference, justice.* Minneapolis: University of Minnesota Press.

Winant, Howard. 2006. Race and racism: Towards a global future. *Ethnic and Racial Studies* 29(5): 986–1003.

Winant, Howard. 2015. Race, ethnicity and social science. *Ethnic and Racial Studies* 38(13): 2176–2185.

Wise, Nicholas. 2015. Maintaining Dominican identity in the Dominican Republic: Forging a baseball landscape in Villa Ascensión. *International Review for the Sociology of Sport* 50(2):161–178.

Withycombe, Jenny Lind. 2011. Intersecting selves: African American female athletes' experiences of sport. *Sociology of Sport Journal* 28(4): 478–493.

Witkowski, Emma. 2012. On the digital playing field: How we "do sport" with networked computer games. *Games and Culture* 7(5): 349–374.

Wittebols, James H. 2004. *The soap opera paradigm: Television programming and corporate priorities.* Lanham, MD: Rowman & Littlefield.

Witz, Billy. 2013. Rogers says he's ready for a role as a pioneer. *New York Times* (May 25): http://www .nytimes.com/2013/05/26/sports/soccer/robbie-rogers-signs-with-galaxy-welcoming-pioneers-role.html.

Wolbring, Gregor. 2008a. The politics of ableism. *Development* 51(2): 252–258.

Wolbring, Gregor. 2008b. Oscar Pistorius and the future nature of Olympic, Paralympic and other sports. *SCRIPT-ed* 5(1): http://ucalgary.academia.edu

/GregorWolbring/Papers/80894/Oscar_Pistorius_
and_the_Future_Nature_of_Olympic_Paralympic_
and_Other_Sports.

Wolbring, Gregor. 2009. Innovation for whom?
Innovation for what? The impact of ableism.
2020science.org (December 14): http://2020science
.org/2009/12/14/wolbring/#ixzz1VTq8dZI7.

Wolbring, Gregor. 2012a. Paralympians outperforming
Olympians: An increasing challenge for Olympism and
the Paralympic and Olympic Movement. *Sport, Ethics
and Philosophy* 6(2): 251–266.

Wolbring, Gregor. 2012b. Leg-ism leaves some
Paralympic stars out on a limb. *TheConversation.com*
(August 29): https://theconversation.com/leg-ism
-leaves-some-paralympic-stars-out-on-a-limb-9008.

Wolbring, Gregor. 2012c. Superhip to supercrip:
the 'trickle-down' effect of the Paralympics.
TheConversation.com (August 31): https://
theconversation.com/superhip-to-supercrip-the
-trickle-down-effect-of-the-paralympics-9009.

Wolbring, Gregor. 2012d. To define oneself as less able:
A prerequisite for a Paralympian? *TheConversation.
com* (September 1): https://theconversation.com
/to-define-oneself-as-less-able-a-prerequisite-for-a
-paralympian-9241.

Wolbring, Gregor. 2012e. Where will it end:
Enhancement-lympics? *TheConversation.com*
(September 8): https://theconversation.com/where
-will-it-end-enhancement-lympics-9426.

Wolbring, Gregor, David Legg, and Frank W.
Stahnisch. 2010. Meaning of inclusion throughout
the history of the Paralympic Games and Movement.
The International Journal of Sport and Society 1(3):
81–93.

Wolken, Dan. 2013. Golfers' gambling concerns
NCAA. *USA Today* (May 7): 1–2C.

Wolverton, Brad. 2013. Education' Dept.'s guidance
on disabled athletes could lead to changes in college
sports. *The Chronicle of Higher Education*
(January 28): http://chronicle.com/blogs/players
/education-departments-guidance-on-disabled-
athletes-could-lead-to-changes-in-college-
sports/32579.

Wolverton, Brad. 2013. With God on our side.
Chronicle of Higher Education (November 24):
http://chronicle.com/article/With-God-on-Our-
Side/143231/.

Wolverton, Brad. 2014. At meeting of Knight
Commission, old ideas are new again. The Chronicle

of Higher Education (September 9): http://chronicle
.com/article/At-Meeting-of-Knight/148709/

Wolverton, Brad; Ben Hallman, Shane Shifflett and
Sandhya Kambhampati. 2015. The $10-billion sports
tab: How college students are funding the athletics
arms race. *Huffington Post* (November 15): http://
chronicle.com/interactives/ncaa-subsidies-main.

Worden, Minky. 2008. *China's great leap: The Beijing
games and Olympian human rights challenges.* New
York: Seven Stories Press.

Wright, Darlene, and Kevin Fitzpatrick. 2006. Social
capital and adolescent violent behavior correlates of
fighting and weapon use among secondary school
students. *Social Forces* 4: 1435–1453.

Wright, Erik Olin. 2011. Real utopias for a global
sociology. *International Sociological Association*
(July 18): http://www.isa-sociology.org/global-
dialogue/.

Wright, Jan, and Lisette Burrows. 2006. Re-conceiving
ability in physical education: A social analysis. *Sport,
Education and Society* 11(3): 275–291.

Yamane, David, Charles Mellies, and Teresa Blake.
2010. Playing for whom? Sport, religion, and the
double movement of secularization in America. In
Earl Smith, ed., *Sociology of sport and social theory
I* (pp. 81–94). Champaign, IL: Human Kinetics.

Yang, Chih-Hai, and Hsuan-Yu Lin. 2011. Is there
salary discrimination by nationality in the NBA?
Foreign talent or foreign market. *Journal of Sports
Economics* 13(1): 53–75.

Yep, Kathleen S. 2009. *Outside the paint: When
basketball ruled at the Chinese playground.* Temple
University Press.

Yep, Kathleen S. 2010. Playing rough and tough:
Chinese American women basketball players in the
1930s and 1940s. *Frontiers: A Journal of Women's
Studies* 31(1): 123–141.

Yep, Kathleen S. 2012. Peddling sport: Liberal
multiculturalism and the racial triangulation of
blackness, Chineseness and Native American-ness
in professional basketball. *Ethnic and Racial Studies*
35(6): 971–987.

Yochim, Emily Chivers. 2010. *Skate life: Re-imagining
white masculinity.* Ann Arbor, MI: University of
Michigan Press.

Yoo, Jin. 2001. Coping profile of Korean competitive
athletes. *International Journal of Sport Psychology,*
32(3): 290–303.

Yost, Mark. 2010. *Varsity green: A behind the scenes look at culture and corruption in college athletics.* Stanford, CA: Stanford University Press.

Yost, Mark. 2011. The price of football that even nonfans pay. *Wall Street Journal* (February 3): D6. Online: http://online.wsj.com/article/SB1000142405 2748703439504576116680460638092.html.

Youn, Anthony. 2012. What *Lin* means to *Asian Americans. USA Today* (February 24): 13A.

Young, Kevin. 2000. Sport and violence. In J. Coakley & E. Dunning, eds., *Handbook of sport studies* (pp. 382–407). London: Sage.

Young, Kevin. 2007a. Violence among athletes. In George Ritzer, ed., *Encyclopedia of sociology* (pp. 5199–5202). London/New York: Blackwell.

Young, Kevin. 2007b. Violence among fans. In George Ritzer, ed., *Encyclopedia of sociology* (pp. 5202–5206). London/New York: Blackwell.

Young, Kevin. 2012. *Sport, violence and society.* London and New York: Routledge.

Younghan, Cho, Charles Leary, and Stephen J. Jackson. 2012. Glocalization and sports in Asia. *Sociology of Sport Journal* 29(4): 421–432.

Yu, Junwei. 2011. Promoting Buddhism through modern sports: The case study of Fo Guang Shan in Taiwan. *Physical Culture and Sport. Studies and Research* 53: 28–38.

Yu, Junwei, and Alan Bairner. 2010. Schooling Taiwan's aboriginal baseball players for the nation. *Sport, Education and Society* 15(1): 63–82.

Yu, Junwei, and Alan Bairner. 2012. Confucianism, baseball and ethnic stereotyping in Taiwan. *International Review for the Sociology of Sport* 47(6): 690–704.

Zaremba, Alan Jay. 2009. *The madness of March: Bonding and betting with the boys in Las Vegas.* Lincoln, NE: University of Nebraska Press.

Zeitler, Ezra J. 2008. Geographies of indigenous-based team name and mascot use in American secondary schools. A dissertation presented to the Faculty of The Graduate College at the University of Nebraska In partial fulfillment of requirements for the degree of doctor of philosophy. Lincoln, NE. Online: http://digitalcommons.unl.edu/cgi/viewcontent .cgi?article=1006&context=geographythesis.

Zenic, Natasa, Marija Stipic, and Damir Sekulic. 2013. Religiousness as a factor of hesitation against doping behaviour in college-age athletes. *Journal of Religion and Health* 52(2): 386–396.

Zernicke, Ronald F., Kathryn A. Antle, Scott G. McLean, Riann M. Palmieri-Smith, James A. Ashton Miller & Edward M. Wojtys. 2009. Play at your own risk: Sport and the injury epidemic. *Journal of Intercollegiate Sports* 2(1): 42–63.

Zillgitt, Jeff. 2011. Aspiring power has doubters. *USA Today* (August 18): 1–2C.

Zimbalist, Andrew. 2010. Reflections on salary shares and salary caps. *Journal of Sports Economics* 11(1): 17–28.

Zimbalist, Andrew. 2013. Inequality in intercollegiate athletics: Origins, trends, and policies. *Journal of Intercollegiate Sport* 6(1): 5–24.

Zimbalist, Andrew, and Allen Sack, 2013. Thoughts on amateurism, the O'Bannon case and the viability of college sport. *The Drake Group:* https:// drakegroupblog.files.wordpress.com/2013/04/drake-statement-obannon1.doc.

Zimmerman, Matthew H. 2012. Interview with Pat Donahue, coordinator of digital media, Los Angeles Kings. *International Journal of Sport Communication* 5(4): 457–461.

Zirin, Dave. 2004. An interview with Adonal Foyle: Rebounder for reforms, master of the lefty lay-up. *CounterPunch* (July 16): http://www.counterpunch .org/2004/07/16/rebounder-for-reforms-master-of-the-lefty-lay-up/.

Zirin, Dave. 2005. *What's my name, fool? Sports and resistance in the United States.* Chicago, IL: Haymarket Books.

Zirin, Dave. 2008a. *A people's history of sports in the United States.* New York/London: The New Press.

Zirin, Dave. 2010a. *Bad sports: How owners are ruining the games we love.* New York: Scribner.

Zirin, Dave. 2010b. The beautiful game, a beautiful cause: Why I root for Argentina. *The Nation* (June 28): http:// www.thenation.com/article/why-i-root-argentina/.

Zirin, Dave. 2011a. Soccer clubs central to ending Egypt's "dictatorship of fear." *Sports Illustrated* (January 31): http://sportsillustrated.cnn.com/2011 /writers/dave_zirin/01/31/egypt.soccer/index.html (retrieved 5-29-13).

Zirin, Dave. 2011b. Understanding Vancouver's 'Hockey riot'. *The Nation* (June 16): http://www .thenation.com/article/understanding-vancouvers-hockey-riot/.

Zirin, Dave. 2011c. When sports met the world. *The New Yorker* (December 22): http://www.newyorker.com /news/news-desk/2011-when-sports-met-the-world.

Zirin, Dave. 2011e. Green Bay Packers sound off against Gov. Scott 'Hosni' Walker. *The Nation* (February 16): http://www.thenation.com/article/green-bay-packers-sound-against-gov-scott-hosni-walker/.

Zirin, Dave. 2012a. In Egypt: How a tragic 'soccer riot' may have revived a revolution. *The Nation* (February 7): http://www.thenation.com/article/how-tragic-soccer-riot-may-have-revived-egyptian-revolution/?nc=1.

Zirin, Dave. 2012b. Preserving the bounty: Gregg Williams, the Saints, and the audio the NFL wants you to hear. *The Nation* (April 6): http://www.thenation.com/article/preserving-bounty-gregg-williams-saints-and-audio-nfl-wants-you-hear/.

Zirin, Dave. 2012c. Jeremy Lin and ESPN's "accidental" racism. *The Nation* (February 19): http://www.thenation.com/article/jeremy-lin-and-espns-accidental-racism/.

Zirin, Dave. 2013a. The cesspool: Why youth sports tend to suck. *Edge of Sports* (May 9): http://www.edgeofsports.com/2013-05-09-839/index.html.

Zirin, Dave. 2013b. The ring and the rings: Vladimir Putin's mafia Olympics. *The Nation* (June 16): http://www.thenation.com/article/ring-and-rings-vladimir-putins-mafia-olympics/.

Zirin, Dave. 2013c. Redskins: The clock is now ticking on changing the name. *The Nation* (February 11): http://www.thenation.com/article/redskins-clock-now-ticking-changing-name/.

Zirin, Dave. 2013d. Enough: An open letter to Dan Snyder. *Grantland* (June 13): http://www.grantland.com/story/_/id/9376010/rename-washington-redskins.

Zirin, Dave. 2013e. *ESPN* journalists speak out on concussion documentary. *The Nation* (August 26): http://www.thenation.com/article/espn-journalists-speak-out-concussion-documentary/?nc=1.

Zirin, Dave. 2013g. Soccer and Egypt's "state of emergency." *The Nation* (January 29): http://www.thenation.com/article/soccer-and-egypts-current-state-emergency/?nc=1.

Zirin, Dave. 2013h. NHL takes 'historic step' for LGBT equality. *The Nation* (April 12): http://www.thenation.com/article/nhl-takes-historic-step-lgbt-equality/.

Zirin, Dave. 2013i. "It's a new world": The Super Bowl becomes a platform for LGBT equality. *The Nation* (January 25): http://www.thenation.com/article/its-new-world-super-bowl-becomes-platform-lgbt-equality/.

Zirin, Dave. 2013j. *Game over: How politics has turned the sports world upside down.* NY: The New Press.

Zirin, Dave. 2014a. The Super Bowl's military fables. *The Nation* (February 3): http://www.thenation.com/article/super-bowls-military-fables/?nc=1.

Zirin, Dave. 2015a. 3 Lessons from University of Missouri President Tim Wolfe's resignation. *The Nation* (November 9): http://www.thenation.com/article/3-lessons-from-university-of-missouri-president-tim-wolfes-resignation/?nc=1.

Zirin, Dave. 2015b. Serena Williams is today's Muhammad Ali. *The Nation* (July 14): http://www.thenation.com/article/serena-williams-is-todays-muhammad-ali/.

Zirin, Da. 2015c. A year since the killing of Michael Brown, a year of sports being shaped by struggle. *The Nation* (August 7): http://www.thenation.com/article/a-year-since-the-killing-of-michael-brown-a-year-of-sports-being-shaped-by-struggle/.

Zirin, Dave. 2015d. Hurricane Katrina and the revival of the political athlete. *The Nation* (August 17): http://www.thenation.com/article/hurricane-katrina-and-the-revival-of-the-political-athlete/

Zweig, David. 2012. What the NFL won't show you. *The Atlantic* (January 31): http://www.theatlantic.com/entertainment/archive/2012/01/what-the-nfl-wont-show-you/252240/.

NAME INDEX

Note: Page numbers followed by *n*, *f*, and *t* indicate notes, figures, and tables, respectively.

SUBJECT INDEX

Note: Page numbers followed by *n, f,* and *t* indicate notes, figures, and tables, respectively.

A

ABC, 378*f*
  sports programming, 389
ABC Sports, 381
ability, 290–334. *See also* disability
  differences, meaning of, 320
  meaning of, 307–308, 314–319
  sport and, 326–328
  variations in, 307
able-bodied
  definition of, 292, 331
  privileging of, 331
ableism: attitudes, actions, and
    policies based on the belief that
    people classified as physically
    or intellectually disabled are
    incapable of full participation in
    mainstream activities and inferior
    to people with "normal" abilities,
    17, 295
ableist ideology:interrelated ideas and
    beliefs that are widely used to
    identify people as physically or
    intellectually disabled, to justify
    treating them as inferior, and
    to organize social worlds and
    physical spaces without taking
    them into account, 17, 293
  dominant, central constructs of, 17
  and sports, 17
absolutist approach: when studying
    deviance, it is based on the
    assumption that social norms
    are based on essential principles
    that constitute an unchanging
    foundation for identifying good
    and evil and distinguishing right
    from wrong, 107–108, 107*f,* 131
abuse
  institutional corruption and, 116–117
  sexual, Penn State scandal, 472
academic cheating, 121–122

academic issues. *See* education
academic progress rate (APR), 454
academic support programs, for college
  athletes, 455
Accra, Ghana, panic in, as venue
  violence, 160
achieved status, in Protestant ethic, 488
ACL. *See* anterior cruciate ligament
  (ACL) injury(ies)
action sports
  children in, 89–90, 90*f*
  media content on, 379
ADA. *See* Americans with Disabilities
  Act (ADA)
Adidas, 346
administrative jobs
  gender inequities in, 195–198, 278
  racial inequities in, 250
adolescence, burnout during, 59
advertising. *See also* media
  and media coverage of sports, 393
  in newspaper sports pages, 387–388
aesthetic orientation: a perspective
    emphasizing the beauty and
    pleasure of movement and
    other factors related to the
    skills and interests of players in
    entertainment of mass audiences,
    349–350, 349*f*
Afghanistan, 421
  buzkashi in, 339*f*
African Americans. *See also* race and
  ethnicity
  arrest rates, 123
  athletics-as-destiny concept, 226
  boxers, social world of, 71–72
  career opportunities in sports,
    278–281
  college basketball players, social
    world of, 71
  in college sports, graduation rates,
    452

  as ethnic group, 217
  female, physical appearance, racial
    ideology and, 228–229
  "jumping genes" in, 224–225
  male, athletic achievements,
    sociological hypothesis for,
    226, 227*f*
  Muslim, and sports, 492
  as race, 217
  sport participation among, 230–233
  and sport participation by childhood,
    56
age
  and ability, 301–303
  meaning of, 295–303
  of professional athletes, 277
age discrimination, 294, 332
ageism: an evaluative perspective
    that favors one age groupusually
    younger people over others and
    justifies discrimination against
    particular age groups that are
    assumed to be incapable of full
    participation in mainstream
    activities, 293–295, 294*f,* 297,
    301, 332
  challenges to, 308, 312
agent(s), for athletes in individual
  sports, 364
agents of change, 522–527
  athletes as, 528–530, 529*f*
agents of change
  challenges to, 527–530
  creating new or alternative sports, 525
  effective, characteristics of, 530
  joining "opposition" groups, 525
  theories used by, 526–527
  working inside sports organizations,
    525
  working outside sports, 525–526
age relations, and youth sports, 258
age segregation, 294*f,* 299–301

Gonzaga University, sports as
recruiting and public relations tool
for, 499
goons, 148
governing bodies, politics in,
433–434
governments: formal organizations with
the power to make and enforce
rules in a particular territory or
among a collection of people, 408
cash awards to Olympic medal
winners, 412–413
and dominant political ideology, 416
and economic development,
417–418
and fairness, 411
and health and fitness, 412
and human rights, 411
involvement in sports, 419
and national identity, 413–416,
413*n,* 414*f*
and national unity, 413–416
and prestige and power, 412–413
and public order, 409–411
and social development, 417–418
sponsorship of sports events,
410–411
support for, sports and, 416–417
graduation success rate (GSR), 454
great sport myth (GSM), 11, 11*f,* 62,
65, 104, 115, 117, 124–125, 129,
418, 423*f,* 498, 506, 528
Greenpeace, 408
group dynamics
of high-performance athletes, 112
of special groups, 112
growth, as goal of change, 523, 525
GSM. *See* great sport myth (GSM)
gymnastics
athletic scholarships for, 285
women in, 175
gymnast(s), elite, disengagement from
sport, 60

H
handball
men's team, "best places to work"
for, 430
Olympic, women's, 175
women's team, "best places to work"
for, 430

handicapped: a term that means
being held back, weighed down,
and marked as inferior due to
perceived physical or intellectual
impairments, 303
handicaps, in athletic events, 303*f*
Hanes underwear, 75
harassment, in sports organizations,
115–117
Harlem Globetrotters, 233*f*
harm reduction approach, to injuries,
134
hazing: a private, interpersonal process
that reaffirms a hierarchical status
difference between incoming
and existing group members,
119–121, 120*f*
head trauma
and brain damage, 149–150
and chronic traumatic
encephalopathy, 149
deviant overconformity and, 111
Frontline program on, 375–376
in high school and college sports,
465–466
in NFL players, 66
rules and guidelines related to, 150
health, social class and, 265
health advocate(s), 134
health and fitness. *See also* pleasure
and participation sports
social class and, 263
sports and, 65–66
youth sports and, 94
health and fitness movement
government involvement in, 412
and pleasure and participation sports,
516*f,* 517
and women's sports, 186–187, 187*f*
health-care insurance, need for, sports
and, 66
health education, for athletes, 134
hearing-impaired athletes, 315, 322,
324
hegemonic masculinity, 182, 207–208
hegemony: a process of maintaining
leadership and control by gaining
the consent and approval of other
groups, including those who are
being led or controlled, 74, 262
helmet(s), 151

heroic orientation: a perspective
emphasizing the danger and
excitement of movement and
other factors that entertain a mass
audience, in entertainment of
mass audiences, 349*f,* 350
high school, student culture in,
444–447
high school athletes, 441–444
academic implications for, 443
filtering-out process and, 442
gender differences, 443
in-season control of, 442
selection-in process and, 442
and sexual activity, 443
social activity of, 444
social class and, 443
high school sports. *See also*
interscholastic sports
athletes' and parents' changing
orientations and expectations
regarding, 465
branding of, 346–347
commercialism and, 345
and cost containment, 463–464
crowd violence at, 157
educational relevance of, 466–467
effects on adult life, 444
and fighting off the field, 154
funding of, 458–459
gang violence at, 157
gender inequity in, 467–470, 468*t*
and ideology, 446–447
issues facing, 462–471
as learning experiences, 447,
466–467
and opportunities for students with
disabilities, 470–471
participation in, pre-and post-Title
IX comparisons, 185
participation inequity in, 186, 188–190
player safety in, 150
and popularity, 445–446, 445*f*
program inequality in, 463–464
and school spirit, 456–458
significance of, gender differences
in, 445, 445*f*
social consequences of, 446–447
spending on, 467
status dynamics of, 154
Title IX and, 185